ACCP Updates in Therapeutics®:

Pharmacotherapy Preparatory Review and Recertification Course

ACCP Updates in Therapeutics®:

Pharmacotherapy Preparatory Review and Recertification Course

2015 Edition

Volume I

accp

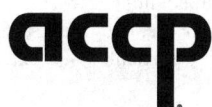

American College of Clinical Pharmacy
Lenexa, Kansas

Director of Professional Development: Nancy M. Perrin, M.A., CAE
Project Manager, Education: Zangi Miti, B.S.
Medical Editor: Carol Anne Peschke
Graphic Designer/Desktop Publisher: Steven M. Brooker

For order information or questions, contact:
American College of Clinical Pharmacy
13000 W. 87th St. Parkway
Lenexa, KS 66215-4530
Telephone: (913) 492-3311
Fax: (913) 492-0088
accp@accp.com
http://www.accp.com

Printed in the United States of America.

To properly cite this book:
Author(s). Chapter name. In: Burke J, Cauffield J, El-Ibiary S, et al. Updates in Therapeutics®: The Pharmacotherapy Preparatory Review and Recertification Course, 2015 ed. Lenexa, KS: American College of Clinical Pharmacy, **year:pages.**

Note: The authors and publisher of the Pharmacotherapy Preparatory Review and Recertification Course recognize that the development of this material offers many opportunities for error. Despite our very best efforts, some errors may persist into print. Drug dosage schedules are, we believe, accurate and in accordance with current standards. Readers are advised, however, to check other published sources to be certain that recommended dosages and contraindications are in agreement with those listed in this book. This is especially important in new, infrequently used, or highly toxic drugs.

Library of Congress Control Number: 2014958696
ISBN: 978-1-939862-12-9

Errata: The errata for the Pharmacotherapy Preparatory Review and Recertification Course, 2015 edition, can be found at www.accp.com/media/ppc15/errata.pdf.

Continuing Pharmacy Education:
The American College of Clinical Pharmacy is accredited by the Accreditation Council for Pharmacy Education as a provider of continuing pharmacy education. The Universal Activity Numbers are as follows: Pharmacotherapy Preparatory Review and Recertification Course for home study, 2015 Edition: Pediatrics, Geriatrics, and Gastrointestinal Disorders, Activity No. 217-0000-15-014-H01-P; 3.5 contact hours; Ambulatory Care and Critical Care, Activity No. 0217-0000-15-015-H01-P; 3.0 contact hours; Nephrology, Infectious Diseases, and HIV/Infectious Diseases, Activity No. 0217-0000-15-016-H01-P; 3.0 contact hours; Pharmacokinetics: A Refresher, Biostatistics: A Refresher, and Study Designs: Fundamentals of Interpretation, Activity No. 0217-0000-15-017-H04-P; 3.5 contact hours; Neurology and General Psychiatry, Activity No. 0217-0000-15-018-H01-P; 2.75 contact hours; Fluids, Electrolytes, and Nutrition, and Endocrine and Metabolic Disorders, Activity No. 0217-0000-15-019-H01-P; 3.0 contact hours; Cardiology I and Cardiology II, Activity No. 0217-0000-15-020-H01-P; 3.0 contact hours; Men's and Women's Health and Oncology Supportive Care, Activity No. 0217-0000-15-021-H01-P; 3.0 contact hours.

To earn continuing pharmacy education credit for the home study version of the 2015 Pharmacotherapy Preparatory Review and Recertification Course, you must successfully complete and submit the Web-based posttest associated with each activity within the course by October 31, 2016. Statements of continuing pharmacy education credit will be available at CPE monitor within 2-3 business days after the successfully completed Web-based posttest is submitted.

The American College of Clinical Pharmacy (ACCP) has compiled the materials in this course book for pharmacists to use in preparing for the Board of Pharmacy Specialties (BPS) Pharmacotherapy Specialty Certification Examination. There is no intent or assurance that all of the knowledge on the examination will be covered in the ACCP process. Although ACCP does use the BPS Content Outline in creating the material for this course, ACCP does not know the specific content of any particular BPS examination. BPS guidelines prohibit any overlap of individuals writing the examination and developing preparatory materials.

Board Certified Pharmacotherapy Specialist (BCPS) Recertification Credit
The Pharmacotherapy Preparatory Review and Recertification Course is part of a Board of Pharmacy Specialties (BPS)-approved professional development program for BCPS recertification credit. To be eligible to earn the 24.75 contact hours of pharmacotherapy recertification credit for the Pharmacotherapy Preparatory Review and Recertification Course, you must purchase and successfully submit the completed Web-based posttest by 11:59 p.m. (CDT) on September 1, 2015. Please note the course must be completed in its entirety. Partial recertification credit is not available.

PROGRAM GOALS AND TARGET AUDIENCE

Updates in Therapeutics®: The Pharmacotherapy Preparatory Review and Recertification Course is designed to help pharmacists who are preparing for the Board of Pharmacy Specialties certification examination in Pharmacotherapy as well as those seeking a general review and refresher on disease states and therapeutics. The program goals are as follows:

1. To present a high-quality, up-to-date overview of disease states and therapeutics;
2. To provide a framework to help attendees prepare for the specialty certification examination in pharmacotherapy; and
3. To offer participants an effective learning experience using a case-based approach with a strong focus on the thought processes needed to solve patient care problems in each therapeutic area.

FACULTY

John M. Burke, Pharm.D., FCCP, BCPS
Professor of Pharmacy Practice
Associate Dean for Post-Graduate Education
St. Louis College of Pharmacy
St. Louis, Missouri

Jacintha S. Cauffield, Pharm.D., BCPS
Associate Professor of Pharmacy Practice
The Lloyd L. Gregory School of Pharmacy
Palm Beach Atlantic University
West Palm Beach, Florida

Anna Legreid Dopp, Pharm.D.
Clinical Pharmacist
Drug Policy Program
University of Wisconsin Hospital and Clinics
Madison, Wisconsin

Shareen El-Ibiary, Pharm.D., BCPS
Associate Professor of Pharmacy Practice
Department of Pharmacy Practice
Midwestern University College of Pharmacy-Glendale
Glendale, Arizona

Shannon W. Finks, Pharm.D., FCCP, BCPS
Associate Professor
University of Tennessee College of Pharmacy
Clinical Pharmacy Specialist, Cardiology
Veterans Affairs Medical Center
Memphis, Tennessee

Linda Gore Martin, Pharm.D., MBA, BCPS
Dean
Professor, Social and Administrative Pharmacy
University of Wyoming School of Pharmacy
Laramie, Wyoming

Leslie A. Hamilton, Pharm.D., BCPS
University of Tennessee Health Science Center
College of Pharmacy
Knoxville, Tennessee

Dana Hammer, Ph.D., Pharm.D.
Senior Lecturer and Director of Teaching Certificate
Program in Pharmacy Education
Department of Pharmacy
University of Washington
Seattle, Washington

Ila M. Harris, Pharm.D., FCCP, BCPS
Associate Professor
University of Minnesota Medical School
Minneapolis, Minnesota

Brian A. Hemstreet, Pharm.D., FCCP, BCPS
Assistant Dean for Student Affairs
Associate Professor
Regis University School of Pharmacy
Rueckert-Hartman College for Health Professions
Denver, Colorado

Lisa C. Hutchison, Pharm.D., MPH, FCCP, BCPS
Professor
Department of Pharmacy Practice
University of Arkansas for Medical Sciences
College of Pharmacy
Little Rock, Arkansas

Brian K. Irons, Pharm.D., FCCP, BCPS, BCACP, BC-ADM
Associate Professor of Pharmacy Practice
Division Head – Ambulatory Care
Texas Tech University Health Sciences Center
Lubbock, Texas

LeAnn B. Norris, Pharm.D., BCPS, BCOP
Clinical Assistant Professor
Department of Clinical Pharmacy and Outcomes
Sciences
South Carolina College of Pharmacy
Columbia, South Carolina

Kirsten H. Ohler, Pharm.D., BCPS
Clinical Assistant Professor
University of Illinois Hospital and Health Sciences
System
Chicago, Illinois

Christopher A. Paciullo, Pharm.D., FCCM, BCPS
Clinical Specialist, Cardiothoracic Surgery/
Critical Care
Emory University Hospital
Atlanta, Georgia

Melody Ryan, Pharm.D., FCCP, BCPS
Associate Professor
University of Kentucky
Lexington, Kentucky

Curtis L. Smith, Pharm.D., BCPS
Professor
Ferris State University
Grand Ledge, Michigan

Kevin M. Sowinski, Pharm.D., FCCP
Professor of Pharmacy Practice
Purdue University College of Pharmacy
Adjunct Professor of Medicine
Indiana University School of Medicine
Indianapolis, Indiana

**Barbara S. Wiggins, Pharm.D., FCCP, FNLA,
FAHA, BCPS, CLS, AACC**
Clinical Pharmacy Specialist – Cardiology
Department of Pharmacy Services
Medical University of South Carolina
Adjunct Associate Professor
South Carolina College of Pharmacy
Charleston, South Carolina

FACULTY DISCLOSURES

Clinical Investigator: Lisa Hutchison (Boehringer Ingelheim)

Nothing to Disclose: John Burke, Jacintha Cauffield, Anna Legreid Dopp, Shareen El-Ibiary, Shannon Finks, Linda Gore Martin, Leslie Hamilton, Dana Hammer, Ila Harris, Brian Hemstreet, Brian Irons, LeAnn Norris, Kirsten Ohler, Christopher Paciullo, Melody Ryan, Curtis Smith, Kevin Sowinski, Barbara Wiggins

REVIEWER DISCLOSURES

The following reviewers have indicated conflicts of interest:

Consultancies: Mary Bridgeman (Merck Consumer Health, Inc.)
Received grand funding/research support: Mary Bridgeman (CareFusion Foundation), Douglas Fish (Merck & Co.)
Speakers Bureau: Kim Benner (FluMist)

ACKNOWLEDGMENTS

Teresa M. Bailey, Pharm.D., BCPS
Professor
College of Pharmacy
Ferris State University
Big Rapids, Michigan

Debra J. Barnette, Pharm.D., BCPS
Assistant Professor of Clinical Pharmacy
Pharmacy Practice and Administration
The Ohio State University College of Pharmacy
Columbus, Ohio

Lisa Anne Boothby, Pharm.D., BCPS
Clinical Research Pharmacist
Drug Information Coordinator
Pharmacy Administration
Columbus Regional Healthcare System
Columbus, Georgia

Linda R. Bressler, Pharm.D., BCOP
Clinical Associate Professor
Department of Pharmacy Practice
College of Pharmacy
Director of Regulatory Affairs
Cancer and Leukemia Group B
University of Illinois
Chicago, Illinois

John M. Burke, Pharm.D., FCCP, BCPS
Professor of Pharmacy Practice
Associate Dean for Post-Graduate Education
St. Louis College of Pharmacy
St. Louis, Missouri

Sheryl Chow, Pharm.D., FCCP, BCPS (AQ Cardiology)
Associate Professor of Pharmacy Practice and
 Administration
College of Pharmacy Western University of Health
 Sciences
Los Angeles, California

G. Robert DeYoung, Pharm.D., BCPS
PGY-1 Residency Program Director
Mercy Health Saint Mary's Campus
Clinical Pharmacist
Mercy Health Physician Partners
Grand Rapids, Michigan

Anna Legreid Dopp, Pharm.D.
Clinical Pharmacist
Drug Policy Program
University of Wisconsin Hospital and Clinics
Madison, Wisconsin

Jennifer M. Dugan, Pharm.D., BCPS
Primary Care Clinical Pharmacy Specialist
Kaiser Permanente Colorado
Evergreen, Colorado

Shareen El-Ibiary, Pharm.D., BCPS
Associate Professor of Pharmacy Practice
Department of Pharmacy Practice
Midwestern University College of Pharmacy-Glendale
Glendale, Arizona

Shannon W. Finks, Pharm.D., FCCP, BCPS
Associate Professor
University of Tennessee College of Pharmacy;
Clinical Pharmacy Specialist, Cardiology
Veterans Affairs Medical Center
Memphis, Tennessee

Edward F. Foote, Pharm.D., FCCP, BCPS
Professor
Wilkes University
Wilkes-Barre, Pennsylvania

Linda Gore Martin, Pharm.D., MBA, BCPS
Dean
Professor, Social and Administrative Pharmacy
University of Wyoming School of Pharmacy
Laramie, Wyoming

Leslie A. Hamilton, Pharm.D., BCPS
University of Tennessee Health Science Center
College of Pharmacy
Knoxville, Tennessee

Dana Hammer, Ph.D., Pharm.D.
Senior Lecturer and Director of Teaching Certificate
 Program in Pharmacy Education
Department of Pharmacy
University of Washington
Seattle, Washington

Ila M. Harris, Pharm.D., FCCP, BCPS
Associate Professor
Department of Family Medicine and Community Health
University of Minnesota
Bethesda Family Medicine
St. Paul, Minnesota

Brian A. Hemstreet, Pharm.D., FCCP, BCPS
Assistant Dean for Student Affairs
Associate Professor
Regis University School of Pharmacy
Rueckert-Hartman College for Health Professions
Denver, Colorado

Lisa C. Hutchison, Pharm.D., MPH, BCPS, FCCP
Professor
Department of Pharmacy Practice
University of Arkansas for Medical Sciences
College of Pharmacy
Little Rock, Arkansas

Trudy M.R. Hodgman, Pharm.D., FCCM, BCPS
Associate Professor of Pharmacy Practice
Clinical Coordinator/Critical Care Specialist
Northwest Community Hospital
Arlington Heights, Illinois

Brian K. Irons, Pharm.D., FCCP, BCPS, BCACP, BC-ADM
Associate Professor of Pharmacy Practice
Division Head – Ambulatory Care
Texas Tech University Health Sciences Center
Lubbock, Texas

William A. Kehoe, Pharm.D., MA, FCCP, BCPS
Professor, Department of Pharmacy Practice
Director of Student Academic Success
T.J. Long School of Pharmacy and Health Sciences
Stockton, California

Judith Kristeller, Pharm.D., BCPS
Associate Professor
Wilkes University
Wilkes-Barre, Pennsylvania

Kelly C. Lee, Pharm.D., M.A.S., BCPP
Associate Professor of Clinical Pharmacy
Associate Dean for Assessment and Accreditation
Skaggs School of Pharmacy and Pharmaceutical Sciences
University of California San Diego
La Jolla, California

LeAnn Norris, Pharm.D., BCPS, BCOP
Clinical Assistant Professor
Department of Clinical Pharmacy and Outcomes
 Sciences
South Carolina College of Pharmacy
Columbia, South Carolina

Kirsten H. Ohler, Pharm.D., BCPS
Pediatric Clinical Specialist
Florida Children's Hospital
Orlando, Florida

Norma J. Owens, Pharm.D., FCCP, BCPS
Professor and Chair
Pharmacy Department
University of Rhode Island
Providence, Rhode Island

Christopher A. Paciullo, Pharm.D., FCCM, BCPS
Clinical Specialist, Cardiothoracic Surgery/
 Critical Care
Emory University Hospital
Atlanta, Georgia

Robert Lee Page II, Pharm.D., FCCP, FAHA, BCPS
Associate Professor of Clinical Pharmacy and Physical
 Medicine
Schools of Pharmacy and Medicine
University of Colorado
Aurora, Colorado

Jo Ellen Rodgers, Pharm.D., BCPS
Clinical Assistant Professor
Division of Pharmacotherapy and Experimental
 Therapeutics
School of Pharmacy
University of North Carolina
Chapel Hill, North Carolina

Melody Ryan, Pharm.D., BCPS
Associate Professor
Department of Pharmacy Practice and Science
College of Pharmacy, University of Kentucky
Lexington, Kentucky

Gordan S. Sacks, Pharm.D., FCCP, BCNSP
Department Head
Professor, Pharmacy Practice
Auburn University Harrison School of Pharmacy
Auburn, Alabama

Lisa A. Sanchez, Pharm.D.
President
PE Applications
Highlands Ranch, Colorado

Curtis L. Smith, Pharm.D., BCPS
Professor
Ferris State University
Lansing, Michigan

Kevin M. Sowinski, Pharm.D., FCCP
Professor of Pharmacy Practice
Purdue University College of Pharmacy;
Adjunct Professor of Medicine
Indiana University School of Medicine
Indianapolis, Indiana

Anne P. Spencer, Pharm.D., FCCP, BCPS,
AQ-Cardiology
Associate Professor of Pharmacy and Clinical Sciences
College of Pharmacy
Medical University of South Carolina
Charleston, South Carolina

Ceressa T. Ward, Pharm.D., BCPS
Clinical Coordinator
Emory Crawford Long Hospital
Atlanta, Georgia

Barbara S. Wiggins, Pharm.D., FCCP, FNLA, FAHA, BCPS, CLS, AACC
Clinical Pharmacy Specialist – Cardiology
Department of Pharmacy Services
Medical University of South Carolina
Adjunct Associate Professor
South Carolina College of Pharmacy
Charleston, South Carolina

Eric T. Wittbrodt, Pharm.D., FCCP, BCPS
Principal Health Outcomes Liaison
Daiichi Sankyo, Inc.
Parsippany, New Jersey

REVIEWERS

The American College of Clinical Pharmacy and the authors would like to thank the following individuals for their reviews of the Updates of Therapeutics®: Pharmacotherapy Preparatory Review and Recertification Course.

Kevin E. Anger Pharm.D., BCPS
Clinical Pharmacy Specialist
Brigham and Women's Hospital
Boston, Massachusetts

Lindsay Arnold, Pharm.D., BCPS
Cardiology & Anticoagulation Clinical Specialist
Boston Medical Center
Boston, Massachusetts

**William L. Baker, Pharm.D., FCCP, BCPS
(AQ Cardiology)**
Assistant Professor of pharmacy Practice
University of Connecticut School of Pharmacy
Storrs, Connecticut

Kim W. Benner, Pharm.D., FASHP, FPPAG, BCPS
Professor of Pharmacy Practice
Samford University McWhorter School of Pharmacy
Birmingham, Alabama

Todd Brackins Pharm.D., BCPP
Assistant Professor of Pharmacy Practice
Compass Psychiatric Hospital
Searcy, Arkansas

Wayne E. Bradley, Pharm.D., MBA, BCPS
Predictive Therapeutica Consulting, LLC
Johns Creek, Georgia

Mary Elizabeth Briand, Pharm.D., BCPS, CGP, AE-C
Clinical Pharmacy Practitioner
Baptist Medical Center Jacksonville
Jacksonville, Florida

Mary M. Bridgeman, Pharm.D., BCPS, CGP
Clinical Associate Professor
Ernest Mario School of Pharmacy
Rutgers, The State University of New Jersey
Piscataway, New Jersey

Kamaria K. Brown, Pharm.D., BCPS
Clinical Care Team Leader
CMC Biddlepoint
Carolinas Healthcare System
Charlotte, North Carolina

Kathleen Bungay, Pharm.D., M.S.
Associate Professor, Department of Pharmacy Practice
Bouvé College of Health Sciences
Northeastern University
Boston, Massachusetts

Hope Campbell, Pharm.D., BCPS
Assistant Professor of Pharmacy Practice
Belmont University College of Pharmacy
Nashville, Tennessee

Lingtak-Neander Chan, Pharm.D., BCNSP
Associate Professor
University of Washington
Seattle, Washington

Lindsey Childs-Kean, Pharm.D., MPH, BCPS
Clinical Assistant Professor
University of Florida College of Pharmacy
Seminole, Florida

Jennifer N. Clements, Pharm.D., BCPS, BCACP, CDE
Chair and Associate Professor of Pharmacy Practice
Presbyterian College School of Pharmacy
Clinton, South Carolina

Kristen Cook, Pharm.D., BCPS
Assistant Professor Pharmacy Practice
University of Nebraska Medical Center College of
    Pharmacy
Omaha, Nebraska

Michael P. Dorsch, Pharm.D., MS, BCPS (AQ-CV)
Clinical Associate Professor
University of Michigan
Ann Arbor, Michigan

Elizabeth Farrington, Pharm.D., FCCP, FCCM, FPPAG, BCPS
Pharmacist III - Pediatrics
New Hanover Regional Medical Center
Wilmington, North Carolina

Douglas N. Fish, Pharm.D., FCCP, FCCM, BCPS (AQ-ID)
Professor and Chair, Department of Clinical Pharmacy
University of Colorado Skaggs School of Pharmacy and
  Pharmaceutical Sciences
Aurora, Colorado

Derek Griffing, Pharm.D., MPH
Research Associate
The Brookings Institution, Engelberg Center for Health
  Care Reform
Washington, D.C

Olga Hilas, Pharm.D., MPH, BCPS, CGP
Associate Clinical Professor
Clinical Pharmacy Practice
St. John's University College of Pharmacy and Health
  Sciences
Queens, New York

Samantha Karr, Pharm.D., FCCP, BCPS, BCACP, BC-ADM
Associate Professor
Midwestern University College of Pharmacy-Glendale
Glendale, Arizona

Tyree H. Kiser, Pharm.D., FCCP, FCCM, BCPS
Associate Professor
University of Colorado Skaggs School of Pharmacy and
  Pharmaceutical Sciences
Aurora, Colorado

M. Shawn McFarland, Pharm.D., BCPS, BCACP, BC-ADM
Associate Service Chief of Pharmacy
Clinical & Educational Programs
VA Tennessee Valley Healthcare System
Nashville, Tennessee

Jean L. Mesaros, Pharm.D., BCPS
Assistant Consulting Professor
Duke University School of Medicine
Physician Assistant Program
Durham, North Carolina

Nicole L. Metzger, Pharm.D., BCPS
Clinical Associate Professor
Mercer University College of Pharmacy
Atlanta, Georgia

Molly G. Minze, Pharm.D., BCACP
Assistant Professor of Pharmacy Practice
Texas Tech University Health Sciences Center School of
  Pharmacy
Abilene, Texas

Jessica Njoku Pharm.D., BCPS
Director of Pharmacy/Infectious Diseases/Antimicrobial
  Stewardship
Baylor University Medical Center
Dallas, Texas

Carrie S. Oliphant, Pharm.D., BCPS (AQ Cardiology)
Clinical Pharmacy Specialist
Methodist University Hospital;
Associate Professor
University of Tennessee College of Pharmacy
Memphis, Tennessee

Erin C. Raney, Pharm.D., BCPS, BC-ADM
Professor of Pharmacy Practice
Midwestern University College of Pharmacy-Glendale
Glendale, Arizona

Shannon Reidt, Pharm.D., MPH, BCPS
Assistant Professor
University of Minnesota College of Pharmacy
Minneapolis, Minnesota

Brea O. Rowan, Pharm.D., BCPS
Clinical Pharmacy Specialist
Princeton Baptist Medical Center
Birmingham, Alabama

Cynthia A. Sanoski, Pharm.D., B.S., FCCP, BCPS
Chair and Associate Professor
Thomas Jefferson University, Jefferson School of
  Pharmacy
Philadelphia, Pennsylvania

Anne P. Spencer, Pharm.D., FCCP, BCPS, (AQ-Cardiology)
Associate Professor of Pharmacy and Clinical Sciences
Medical University of South Carolina College of
  Pharmacy
Charleston, South Carolina

Maureen Sullivan Pharm.D. BCPS
Associate Professor and Chair of Pharmacy Practice
Touro College of Pharmacy
New York, New York

Cheryl L. Szabo, Pharm.D., BCPS
Assistant Professor
Wayne State University;
Clinical Pharmacist Specialist
Detroit Medical Center
Detroit, Michigan

Kimberly Tallian, Pharm.D., FCCP, FASHP, BCPP
Pharmacy Clinical Manager
Scripps Memorial Hospital;
Associate Clinical Professor
University of California, San Diego
Skaggs School of Pharmacy & Pharmaceutical Sciences
La Jolla, California

Kristina E. Ward, Pharm.D., BCPS
Clinical Associate Professor and Director
Drug Information Services
University of Rhode Island College of Pharmacy
Kingston, Rhode Island

Sheila M. Wilhelm, Pharm.D., FCCP, BCPS
Associate Professor of Pharmacy Practice
Wayne State University Eugene Applebaum College of
  Pharmacy;
Clinical Pharmacy Specialist of Internal Medicine
Harper University Hospital
Detroit, Michigan

Elizabeth Wilpula, Pharm.D., BCPS
Clinical Pharmacy Specialist, Nephrology & Transplant
Harper University Hospital
Detroit, Michigan

Brenda Winger, Pharm.D., BCPS, BCOP
Pharmacy Manager
Intermountain Homecare and Hospice Pharmacy
Salt Lake City, Utah

Susan R. Winkler, Pharm.D., FCCP, BCPS
Professor and Chair
Department of Pharmacy Practice
Midwestern University Chicago College of Pharmacy
Downers Grove, Illinois

Abigail M. Yancey, Pharm.D., BCPS
Associate Professor of Pharmacy Practice
St. Louis College of Pharmacy
St. Louis, Missouri

Daisy Yang, Pharm.D., BCOP
Clinical Pharmacy Specialist
The University of Texas MD Anderson Cancer Center
Houston, Texas

TABLE OF CONTENTS

ACCP Updates in Therapeutics®:

Pharmacotherapy Preparatory Review and Recertification Course

Pediatrics

Kirsten H. Ohler, Pharm.D., BCPS

University of Illinois Hospital & Health Sciences System
Chicago, Illinois

Pediatrics

Kirsten H. Ohler, Pharm.D., BCPS

University of Illinois Hospital & Health Sciences System
Chicago, Illinois

Learning Objectives

1. Describe the most common pathogens associated with neonatal and pediatric sepsis and meningitis.
2. Describe current therapeutic options for the management of neonatal and pediatric sepsis and meningitis.
3. Identify the drugs available for preventing and treating respiratory syncytial virus.
4. Describe the most common causative organisms of otitis media and potential treatment options.
5. Identify the recommended pediatric immunization schedule and barriers to routine immunization.
6. Discuss the differences in anticonvulsant pharmacokinetics and adverse effects between children and adults.
7. Describe the current drug therapy for treating patients with attention-deficit/hyperactivity disorder.

Self-Assessment Questions

Answers and explanations to these questions can be found at the end of this chapter.

1. A 15-year-old boy with a history of exercise-induced asthma presents with fever, tachypnea, headache, and myalgia. Which is most likely to be isolated from this patient?
   A. Respiratory syncytial virus (RSV).
   B. *Streptococcus pneumoniae.*
   C. Group B *Streptococcus.*
   D. *Pseudomonas aeruginosa.*

2. Which is the best assessment of the risk of severe RSV infection and subsequent need for prophylaxis in a 3-month-old girl born at 30 weeks' gestation?
   A. This patient should receive prophylaxis if she is 6 months or younger at the beginning of RSV season.
   B. This patient is at risk only if she has chronic lung disease (i.e., necessitating more than 21% oxygen for at least the first 28 days of life).
   C. All neonates born during RSV season should receive prophylaxis.

   D. This patient should receive prophylaxis only if she has additional risk factors such as day care attendance or school-aged siblings.

3. Which is the most accurate statement about prophylaxis of bacterial meningitis?
   A. Close contacts of patients with pneumococcal meningitis should receive prophylaxis.
   B. Close contacts of patients with *Haemophilus influenzae* meningitis require prophylaxis only if their immunizations are not up-to-date.
   C. Rifampin is a first-line agent for prophylaxis against meningococcal meningitis.
   D. Prophylaxis against bacterial meningitis is no longer recommended regardless of the causative organism.

4. A 6-month-old baby who was born at 24 weeks' gestation is brought to the clinic in October for a routine checkup and immunizations. Which is the best recommendation to make for this patient's immunization schedule?
   A. Only two of the five immunizations due should be given at the same time; schedule another appointment for the next week to administer the rest.
   B. Oral polio vaccine should be used to reduce the number of injections required to complete the schedule.
   C. Vaccines should be based on his corrected gestational age rather than on his chronologic age because he was born prematurely.
   D. Influenza vaccine should be administered with all other scheduled vaccinations.

5. A physician asks for your recommendation for treating a 5-year-old child with his first case of acute otitis media (AOM). Which statement is the best advice?
   A. A blood culture should be obtained to identify the causative organism.
   B. Antibiotics may not be warranted at this time.
   C. Initiate azithromycin to treat atypical organisms (e.g., mycoplasma).
   D. Administer intramuscular ceftriaxone.

6. A 16-year-old girl with asthma, a history of ventricular septal defect, and attention-deficit/hyperactivity disorder (ADHD) was initially treated with methylphenidate immediate release, but her ADHD symptoms persisted at home and at school. Her therapy was then changed to methylphenidate OROS (Concerta). The dose was maximized during the next several weeks; however, her symptoms were still not well controlled throughout the day. She and her family report adherence to the treatment regimen. Which is the best recommendation to make for treating her ADHD?

    A. Switch to clonidine.
    B. Switch to extended-release mixed amphetamine salts (i.e., Adderall XR).
    C. Switch to methylphenidate transdermal system (i.e., Daytrana).
    D. Switch to atomoxetine.

7. A 7-year-old child with absence seizures is having breakthrough episodes on ethosuximide. Which is the most appropriate alternative therapy?

    A. Valproic acid.
    B. Phenytoin.
    C. Phenobarbital.
    D. Gabapentin.

8. In a retrospective study of the risk of loss of appetite in adolescents taking a specific stimulant agent for ADHD management, 7 of 200 patients exposed to the stimulant showed appetite loss, compared with 1 of 198 control subjects (unexposed). Which choice best reflects the correct odds ratio of developing loss of appetite for the case subjects compared with the control subjects?

    A. 3.
    B. 6.
    C. 7.
    D. 8.

9. An investigator wants to establish a causal relationship between the use of ceftriaxone in premature neonates and the incidence of kernicterus. Which study design is best to use?

    A. Case series.
    B. Randomized controlled.
    C. Retrospective cohort.
    D. Crossover.

10. An 8-month-old, former 36-week gestational-age infant with hypoplastic left heart disease is admitted during RSV season for stage II (of III) repair of his heart defect. Which statement is most accurate about the use of palivizumab for RSV prophylaxis in this patient?

    A. He is not at significant risk of severe RSV infection; therefore, palivizumab is not indicated.
    B. Palivizumab is indicated to reduce nosocomial transmission of RSV in high-risk patients.
    C. Palivizumab is not indicated because he has undergone surgical repair of his heart defect.
    D. A dose of palivizumab should be administered postoperatively and continued throughout the RSV season.

I. SEPSIS AND MENINGITIS

A. Clinical Presentation
   1. Signs and symptoms
      a. Neonates: Temperature instability, feeding intolerance, lethargy, grunting, flaring, retractions, apnea, bulging fontanelle, and seizures
      b. Children: Fever, loss of appetite, emesis, myalgias, arthralgias, cutaneous manifestations (e.g., petechiae, purpura, rash), nuchal rigidity, back pain, Kernig sign, Brudzinski sign, headache, photophobia, altered mental status, and seizures
   2. Early versus late neonatal sepsis
      a. Onset
         i. Early: Within 72 hours of birth
         ii. Late: After the first 3 days of life
      b. Risk factors
         i. Early: Very low birth weight, prolonged rupture of amniotic membranes, prolonged labor, maternal endometritis, or chorioamnionitis
         ii. Late:
            (a) Unrelated to obstetric risk factors
            (b) Usually related to iatrogenic factors (e.g., endotracheal tubes, central venous catheters)
      c. Incidence
         i. Early
            (a) 0.7–3.7 of 1000 live births (8 of 1000 very-low-birth-weight infants)
            (b) Meningitis occurs in less than 10% of cases.
         ii. Late
            (a) 0.5–1.8 of 1000 live births
            (b) Meningitis occurs in 60% of cases.
   3. Cerebrospinal fluid findings

Table 1. Cerebrospinal Fluid Findings

Laboratory Value	Normal Child	Normal Newborn	Bacterial Meningitis	Viral Meningitis
WBC (cells/mL)	0–6	0–30	>1000	100–500
Neutrophils (%)	0	2–3	>50	<40
Glucose (mg/dL)	40–80	32–121	<30	>30
Protein (mg/dL)	20–30	19–149	>100	50–100
RBC (cells/mL)	0–2	0–2	0–10	0–2

RBC = red blood cell count; WBC = white blood cell count.

Adapted with permission from the American Academy of Pediatrics. Wubbel L, McCracken GH. Management of bacterial meningitis: 1998. Pediatr Rev 1998;19:78-84.

Patient Case

1. A baby born at 36 weeks' gestation develops respiratory distress, hypotension, and mottling at 5 hours of life. The baby is transported to the neonatal intensive care unit, where he has a witnessed seizure, and cultures are drawn. Maternal vaginal cultures are positive for group B *Streptococcus,* and three doses of penicillin were given to the mother before delivery. Which is the best empiric antibiotic regimen?

    A. Vancomycin.

    B. Ampicillin plus gentamicin.

    C. Ampicillin plus ceftriaxone.

    D. Ceftazidime plus gentamicin.

    B.   Common Pathogens

Table 2. Common Pathogens

Age	Organism
0–1 month	Group B *Streptococcus* *Escherichia coli* *Listeria monocytogenes* Viral (e.g., herpes simplex virus) Coagulase-negative staphylococcus (nosocomial) Gram-negative bacteria (e.g., *Pseudomonas* spp., *Enterobacter* spp.; nosocomial)
1–3 months	Neonatal pathogens (see above) *Haemophilus influenzae* type B *Neisseria meningitidis* *Streptococcus pneumoniae*
3 months–12 years	*H. influenzae* type B[a] *N. meningitidis* *S. pneumoniae*
>12 years	*N. meningitidis* *S. pneumoniae*

[a]*H. influenzae* is no longer a common pathogen in areas where the vaccine is routinely used.

    C.   Potential Antibiotic Regimens

Table 3. Potential Antibiotic Regimens

Age	Regimen
0–1 month	Ampicillin + gentamicin OR ampicillin + cefotaxime
1–3 months	Ampicillin + cefotaxime/ceftriaxone
3 months–12 years	Ceftriaxone ± vancomycin[a]
>12 years	Ceftriaxone ± vancomycin[a]

[a]Addition of vancomycin should be based on the regional incidence of resistant *Streptococcus pneumoniae.*

Patient Cases

2. Culture results for the patient in question 1 reveal gram-negative rods in the cerebrospinal fluid. Which recommendation regarding antibiotic prophylaxis is best?

   A. The patient's 5-month-old stepsister is at high risk because she is not fully immunized; the patient should therefore receive rifampin.

   B. The patient should receive rifampin to eliminate nasal carriage of the pathogen.

   C. Antibiotic prophylaxis is not indicated in this case.

   D. All close contacts should receive rifampin for prophylaxis.

3. A 6-year-old boy presents to the emergency department with a temperature of 104°F, altered mental status, and petechiae. There is no history of trauma. A toxicology screen is negative. A complete blood cell count reveals 32×10^3 cells/mm³ white blood cells/mcL with 20% bands. Culture results are pending. The patient has no known drug allergies. Which antibiotic regimen provides the best empiric coverage?

   A. Ampicillin plus gentamicin.

   B. Cefuroxime.

   C. Ceftriaxone plus vancomycin.

   D. Rifampin.

    D. Sequelae of Meningitis
   1. Hearing loss
   2. Mental retardation and learning deficits
   3. Visual impairment
   4. Seizures
   5. Hydrocephalus

    E. Chemoprophylaxis of Bacterial Meningitis
   1. Purpose: Prevent the spread of *H. influenzae* and *Neisseria meningitidis*
   2. High-risk groups
      a. Household contacts
      b. Nursery or day care center contacts
      c. Direct contact with index patient's secretions
   3. Regimen

Table 4. Regimens for Chemoprophylaxis[a]

Drug	*Neisseria meningitidis*	*Haemophilus influenzae*
Rifampin	<1 month old: 5 mg/kg/dose PO every 12 hours × 2 days ≥1 month old: 10 mg/kg/dose PO every 12 hours × 2 days Adults: 600 mg PO every 12 hours × 2 days	20 mg/kg/dose (maximum 600 mg) PO daily × 4 days
Ceftriaxone	<15 years old: 125 mg IM × 1 dose ≥15 years old: 250 mg IM × 1 dose	Not indicated

[a]Ciprofloxacin and azithromycin are possible alternatives but not routinely recommended.
IM = intramuscularly; PO = orally.

II. RESPIRATORY SYNCYTIAL VIRUS INFECTION

A. Clinical Presentation
1. Seasonal occurrence: Typically November through April, depending on geographic location
2. Signs and symptoms
   a. Neonates and infants: Lower respiratory tract symptoms (e.g., bronchiolitis and pneumonia), wheezing, lethargy, irritability, poor feeding, and apnea
   b. Older children: Upper respiratory tract symptoms

B. Risk Factors for Severe Disease
1. Premature birth
2. Chronic lung disease or bronchopulmonary dysplasia
3. Cyanotic or complicated congenital heart disease
4. Immunodeficiency
5. Airway abnormalities or neuromuscular conditions compromising the handling of respiratory secretions
6. Other
   a. Lower socioeconomic status
   b. Passive smoking
   c. Day care attendance
   d. Siblings younger than 5 years

Patient Case

4. You are screening babies during the current respiratory syncytial virus (RSV) season for risk factors associated with the development of severe RSV infection. Which is the best recommendation about the use of palivizumab for RSV prophylaxis?

   A. Palivizumab should be prescribed for an 18-month-old, former 26-week premature infant with a history of chronic lung disease who has not received oxygen or medications during the past 8 months.

   B. Palivizumab should be prescribed for a 5-month-old, former 28-week premature infant with a history of chronic lung disease who was discharged from the hospital without oxygen or medications.

   C. Palivizumab should be prescribed for a 41-day-old baby, born at 31 weeks' gestation, without a history of chronic lung disease who will attend day care.

   D. Palivizumab should be prescribed for a 10-month-old baby, born at 37 weeks' gestation, with a surgically repaired congenital heart defect.

C. Prophylaxis
1. Nonpharmacologic: Avoid crowds during RSV season and conscientiously use good handwashing practice.
2. Palivizumab (Synagis)
   a. Dosing: 15 mg/kg/dose intramuscularly, given monthly during RSV season   Nov. – March
   b. Effects on outcomes
      i. A 55% reduction in hospitalizations for RSV
      ii. Safe in patients with cyanotic congenital heart disease. There is a 58% decrease in palivizumab serum concentration after cardiopulmonary bypass; therefore, a postoperative dose of palivizumab is recommended as soon as the patient is medically stable.

      iii.   No reduction in overall mortality

      iv.   Does not interfere with the response to vaccines

      v.   Not recommended for the prevention of nosocomial transmission of RSV

   c. American Academy of Pediatrics (AAP) recommendations for use were updated in 2014 (Table 5) and contain several significant changes from their 2009 policy statement.

      i.   Routine prophylaxis is no longer recommended for neonates born at 29 weeks' gestation or later; previously all neonates born at less than 32 weeks' gestation were recommended to receive routine prophylaxis.

      ii.   Risk factors for RSV infection such as day care attendance or siblings younger than 5 years of age are no longer considered when determining the need for prophylaxis.

      iii.   Prophylaxis is not recommended in the second year of life based on a history of prematurity alone; previously neonates born at less than 28 weeks' gestation could be considered for prophylaxis during their second RSV season.

      iv.   Prophylaxis should be discontinued if an RSV hospitalization occurs; previously palivizumab was continued to complete 5 monthly doses regardless of hospitalization.

Table 5. AAP Guidelines for Palivizumab Use

Gestational Age (weeks)	Age at Start of RSV Season (months)	Other Required Criteria	Maximal Doses
<29 + 0 days	<12		5
<32 + 0 days	<12	Chronic lung disease requiring more than 21% oxygen for at least the first 28 days of life	5
<32 + 0 days	<24	Consider prophylaxis for a second RSV season if chronic lung disease requiring medical therapy within the 6 months preceding the start of RSV season	5
Any	<12	Hemodynamically significant acyanotic[a] congenital heart disease receiving medication for congestive heart failure AND will require cardiac surgery	5
Any	<12	Moderate to severe pulmonary hypertension	5
Any	<12	Congenital abnormalities of airway or neuromuscular disease	5
Any	<24	Profound immunocompromise	5

[a]Infants with **cyanotic** heart defects may be considered for prophylaxis after consultation with a pediatric cardiologist.

AAP = American Academy of Pediatrics.

Patient Case

5. An 18-month-old baby with a history of premature birth and chronic lung disease is admitted to the pediatric intensive care unit with fever, respiratory distress requiring intubation, and a 3-day history of cold-like symptoms. A nasal swab is positive for RSV. Which is the best intervention?

   A. Palivizumab.

   B. Corticosteroids.

   C. Cefuroxime.

   D. Intravenous fluids and supportive care.

D. Treatment
   1. Supportive care
      a. Hydration
      b. Supplemental oxygen
      c. Mechanical ventilation as needed
   2. Ribavirin
      a. Active against RSV replication
      b. Not shown to reduce mortality in immunocompetent patients
      c. Not shown to reduce ventilator days, stay in the intensive care unit or hospital, or hospital cost
      d. The AAP states that ribavirin "may be considered" in a select group of high-risk patients (e.g., those with complicated congenital heart disease, chronic lung disease or bronchopulmonary dysplasia, immunocompromise).
   3. β_2-Agonists, racemic epinephrine
      a. Not shown to improve outcome measures
      b. Some practitioners may give a trial of these therapies, but this is not considered the standard of care.
   4. Corticosteroids
      a. Not shown to improve outcome measures
      b. Use is not recommended.
   5. Hypertonic saline _Nebulized_
      a. Should not be administered in the emergency department
      b. May be considered for hospitalized patients; however, the evidence supporting use is weak.
   6. Antibiotics: Not indicated unless secondary bacterial infection develops

III. OTITIS MEDIA

A. Clinical Presentation
   1. Definitions
      a. Acute otitis media (AOM): Presence of middle ear effusion and evidence of middle ear inflammation
         i. Middle ear effusion may be indicated by bulging tympanic membrane, decreased or no mobility of the tympanic membrane, purulent fluid in the middle ear.
         ii. Inflammation of the middle ear may be indicated by erythema of the tympanic membrane or otalgia.
      b. Otitis media with effusion (OME): Fluid in the middle ear without evidence of local or systemic illness

    c.   Recurrent AOM: Three or more episodes of acute otitis within 6 months or four episodes within 1 year

2. Risk factors

    a.   Day care attendance

    b.   Family history of AOM

    c.   Positioning during feeding (e.g., supine position during bottle-feeding allows reflux into eustachian tubes)

    d.   Lower socioeconomic status

    e.   Smokers in the household

    f.   Craniofacial abnormalities or cleft palate

B. Common Pathogens

  1. Viral

  2. *S. pneumoniae*

  3. Nontypeable *H. influenzae*

  4. *Moraxella catarrhalis*

C. Treatment

  1. General principles

    a.   Clinical resolution will occur in a significant number of cases without antibiotic therapy.

    b.   Immediate antibiotic therapy is warranted for AOM with bulging tympanic membrane, perforation, or otorrhea.

    c.   Delayed antibiotic prescribing (i.e., treatment only if otalgia persists for more than 48–72 hours or temperature greater than 39°C in past 48 hours) is an acceptable strategy in children older than 2 years with AOM without severe systemic symptoms.

        i.   Analgesics are more beneficial than antibiotics for relieving otalgia within the first 24 hours and are recommended regardless of antibiotic use.

        ii.   Antibiotics also may be deferred in otherwise healthy children between 6 months and 2 years of age if their symptoms are mild and otitis media is unilateral (as opposed to bilateral).

        iii.   Caregiver must be reliable to recognize worsening of condition and gain immediate access to medical care, if needed.

        iv.   Not recommended for infants younger than 6 months

    d.   Persistence of middle ear fluid is likely after treatment for AOM and does not warrant repeated treatment.

    e.   Antibiotics are not generally warranted for OME because of the high rate of spontaneous resolution.

        i.   Antibiotics are recommended only if bilateral effusions persist for more than 3 months.

        ii.   Corticosteroids, antihistamines, and decongestants are not recommended.

  2. Suggested treatment algorithm

Confirmed AOM

Otorrhea or severe symptoms?

NO

Age 6 mo–2 yr?

NO

YES

YES

Bilateral
or
unilateral
AOM?

Unilateral

Bilateral

Delayed antibiotic prescribing
- Not recommended if child is <6 months
- Antibiotics prescribed only if child worsens or does not improve within 48–72 hours

— *OR* —

Antibiotic therapy
- If child is < 6 months old or if reliable follow-up cannot be ensured

Antibiotic therapy
- First-line agents
  - Amoxicillin 80–90 mg/kg/day
  - Amoxicillin/clavulanate – Consider if amoxicillin taken within past 30 days
- Alternatives (if penicillin allergic)
  - Cefdinir
  - Cefuroxime
  - Cefpodoxime
  - Ceftriaxone

Reevaluate at 48–72 hours
Failure of initial treatment strategy?

NO

YES

- Continue current treatment strategy

- Antibiotic duration
  - Optimal duration is unknown
  - <2 yr or severe symptoms: 10 days
  - 2–5 yr with mild–moderate symptoms: 7 days
  - >6 yr with mild–moderate symptoms: 5–7 days

- Start antibiotic if prescribing was delayed

- Consider changing antibiotic regimen
  - Amoxicillin/clavulanate 90 mg/kg/day
  - Ceftriaxone x 3 days
  - Clindamycin ± 3rd-generation cephalosporin

- Consider tympanocentesis

- Consider tympanostomy tubes
  - Most beneficial for children with persistent OME and significant hearing loss (e.g., >25-dB hearing loss bilaterally >12 weeks)

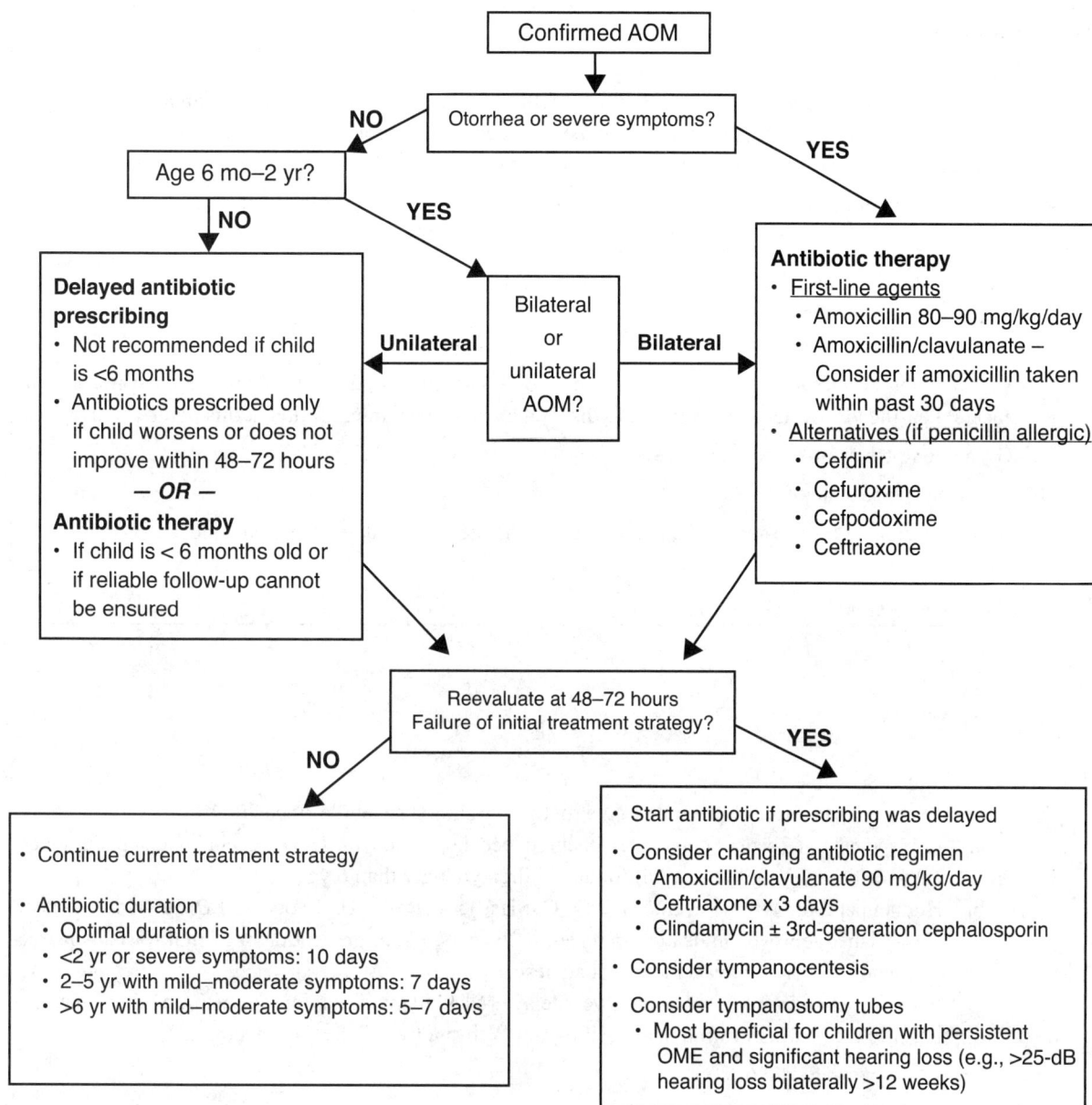

Figure 1. AOM Suggested Treatment Algorithm

D. Prevention Strategies
   1. Antibiotic prophylaxis
      a. Reduces occurrence by about one episode per year
      b. The risk of promoting bacterial resistance may outweigh the slight benefit.
      c. AAP recommends against routine use for children with recurrent AOM.
   2. Immunization – Pneumococcal and influenza vaccines should be administered according to the AAP and Advisory Committee on Immunization Practices (ACIP) recommendations.

Patient Cases

6. A 5-month-old infant who was born at term and is otherwise healthy was treated for her first case of otitis media with amoxicillin 45 mg/kg/day for 7 days. On follow-up examination, her pediatrician noticed fullness in the middle ear and a cloudy tympanic membrane with decreased mobility. She is now afebrile and eating well. Which is the best recommendation for her treatment?

    A. No antibiotics at this time.

    B. High-dose (90 mg/kg/day) amoxicillin for 7 days.

    C. Decongestant and antihistamine daily until resolution.

    D. Azithromycin.

7. A 4-year-old boy receives a diagnosis of his fourth case of otitis media within 12 months. He has not shown evidence of hearing loss or delay in language skills. Which is the best intervention at this point?

    A. Giving long-term antibiotic prophylaxis.

    B. Inserting tympanostomy tubes.

    C. Administering high-dose amoxicillin and ensuring that he is up to date on his pneumococcal and influenza vaccines.

    D. No antibiotic therapy warranted.

IV. IMMUNIZATIONS

    A. Recommended Schedule

        1. Few major changes have been made to the routine childhood schedule since 2009.

            a. Replacement of 7-valent conjugated pneumococcal vaccine with 13-valent conjugated pneumococcal vaccine (PCV13, Prevnar 13) for all children younger than 6 years

            b. Human papillomavirus vaccine (HPV4, Gardasil) received a U.S. Food and Drug Administration (FDA) label-approved indication in males 9–26 years old for prevention of genital warts. Now recommended for routine vaccination of adolescent males

            c. For children and adolescents who have a delayed start to immunizations, a catch-up schedule exists.

            d. Refer to the National Immunization Program Web site (www.cdc.gov/vaccines).

Patient Case

8. A 1-year-old boy with a history of Kawasaki disease treated 4 months ago with intravenous immunoglobulin (IVIG) is being seen by his pediatrician for a well-child checkup. He is due for the measles, mumps, and rubella (MMR) and varicella vaccines. He has no known drug allergies, but he has many food allergies, including peanuts, eggs, and shellfish. His mother has several concerns about administering these vaccines. Which concern is the best reason to defer administering vaccines in this patient?

    A. Association between MMR vaccine administration and the development of autism.

    B. Allergic reaction after MMR administration in a patient with an egg allergy.

    C. Many concurrent vaccines can overload the patient's immune system.

    D. Decreased vaccine efficacy because of previous IVIG administration.

2. Combination vaccines
   a. Main advantage: Reduction in the number of injections required to complete recommended schedule
   b. The FDA mandates that the safety and efficacy of combination products not be less than those of the individual components.
   c. Products
      i. The DTaP-Hib (*H. influenzae* type B) combination
         (a) The Hib antibody response is markedly lower after the combination product is administered than when the Hib vaccine is administered separately for primary immunization.
         (b) Product (TriHIBit) withdrawn from U.S. market
      ii. The DTaP-IPV (inactivated poliovirus) combination
         (a) Studies indicate that this combination has no consistent effect on antibody responses.
         (b) Indicated only for the fifth dose of DTaP and fourth dose of IPV in the routine series
         (c) Kinrix
      iii. The DTaP-HepB (hepatitis B) combination: Product is available outside the United States and provides good safety and antibody concentrations.
      iv. The DTaP-HepB-Hib combination: The Hib antibody levels are lower than after separate administration.
      v. The DTaP-HepB-IPV combination
         (a) At least as immunogenic as individual components when administered at 2, 4, and 6 months
         (b) Not indicated for infants younger than 6 weeks or children older than 7 years
         (c) Pediarix
      vi. The HepB-Hib combination
         (a) Not indicated for infants younger than 6 weeks because of possible decreased immune response
         (b) Comvax
      vii. The Hib-DTaP-IPV combination
         (a) Approved for use in children 6 weeks through 4 years of age
         (b) Pentacel
      viii. The HepA-HepB combination
         (a) Approved for use in adults 18 years and older
         (b) Twinrix
      ix. The MMR vaccine and varicella combination
         (a) Research from the Centers for Disease Control and Prevention and manufacturer indicated a higher incidence of febrile seizures in children 12–23 months of age who received the combination product compared with those who received the separate MMR and varicella vaccines.
         (b) Since June 2009, ACIP has expressed a preference for separate MMR and varicella vaccines as the first dose given to children 12–47 months of age. The combination product may be used for the second dose at any age and for the first dose in children 48 months or older.
         (c) ProQuad
      x. Adding HepB to combination products may result in an extra dose being provided (e.g., monovalent HepB given at birth and then combination products at 2, 4, and 6 months); however, ACIP states that this is a safe practice.
3. Interchangeability of products
   a. ACIP recommends that the same product be used throughout the primary series; however, if the previous product's identity is not known or is no longer available, any product may be used.
   b. For DTaP: The current standard of care is to use the same product for at least the first three doses of the five-dose series; however, if the product used previously is not known or is unavailable, any product may be used.

    c. For Tdap: BOOSTRIX or ADACEL may be used for the booster dose, regardless of the manufacturer of the DTaP product administered during the primary immunization series.

    d. For HepB: It is acceptable to use ENGERIX-B and RECOMBIVAX HB interchangeably.

    e. For polio: Oral polio vaccine and inactivated poliovirus vaccine provide equivalent protection against paralytic poliomyelitis; however, because the only cases of polio in the United States since 1979 have been vaccine associated (i.e., from the live virus in oral polio vaccine), oral polio vaccine is no longer recommended.

    f. For Hib: These products may be used interchangeably; however, if the regimen is completed using PedvaxHIB exclusively, only three doses are required; regimens using HibTITER or ActHIB require four doses.

    g. For HPV: The products differ in the HPV types against which they provide protection. HPV4 (Gardasil) protects against types 6, 11, 16, and 18. HPV2 (Cervarix) protects against types 16 and 18. HPV types 6 and 11 are associated with genital warts; types 16 and 18 are associated with gynecologic, anal, and penile cancers.

B. Barriers to Routine Immunization

  1. Contraindications

    a. Anaphylactic reaction to vaccine or any of its components

      i. Inactivated poliovirus vaccine, MMR, and varicella contain neomycin.

      ii. Influenza vaccine: Live attenuated influenza vaccine (LAIV) should be avoided in patients with severe egg allergy; inactivated influenza vaccine may be administered with close monitoring.

      iii. Severe egg allergy is not considered a contraindication to MMR, which is grown in chick embryo tissue.

    b. Acute moderate to severe febrile illness

    c. Immunodeficiency: Oral polio vaccine, MMR, varicella

    d. Pregnancy: MMR, varicella

    e. Recent administration of immune globulin: MMR, varicella

      i. Delay administration of vaccine product.

      ii. Interval between immune globulin dose and administration of vaccine depends on indication for and dose of immune globulin.

    f. Encephalopathy within 7 days after administration of a previous dose of DTaP

    g. History of intussusception: rotavirus vaccine

  2. Misconceptions about contraindications (i.e., these are NOT contraindications)

    a. Mild acute illness

    b. Current antimicrobial therapy

    c. Reaction to DTaP involving only soreness, redness, or swelling at the site

    d. Pregnancy of the mother of the vaccine recipient

    e. Breastfeeding

    f. Allergies to antibiotics other than neomycin or streptomycin

    g. Family history of an adverse effect after vaccine administration

  3. Other factors associated with underimmunization

    a. Low socioeconomic status

    b. Late start of vaccination series

    c. Missed opportunities

      i. Provider unaware that vaccination is due

      ii. Failure to provide simultaneous vaccines

      iii. Inappropriate contraindications (see previous discussion)

    d. Concern about potential adverse reactions
        i. Autism: The association with MMR vaccine has not been proved.
       ii. Guillain-Barré syndrome: The association with meningococcal conjugate vaccine has not been proved.
           (a) 15 reported cases in adolescents after receiving meningococcal vaccine
           (b) ACIP continues to recommend the routine use of meningococcal vaccine.
      iii. Intussusception: An association with rotavirus vaccine led to the market withdrawal of RotaShield; two currently available products:
           (a) Live, oral human-bovine reassortant rotavirus vaccine (RotaTeq, licensed in 2006)
           (b) Live, attenuated human rotavirus vaccine (Rotarix, licensed in 2008)
           (c) Neither product has been associated with intussusception.

Patient Case

9. The following patients are seeing their pediatrician today and are due for immunizations according to the routine schedule. For which patient would it be best to recommend deferring immunizations until later?

    A. A 12-month-old boy who recently completed a cycle of chemotherapy for acute lymphocytic leukemia.

    B. A 6-month-old girl receiving amoxicillin for otitis media.

    C. A 12-month-old HIV-positive boy whose most recent CD4 count was greater than 1000.

    D. A 12-year-old girl completing a prednisone "burst" (1 mg/kg/day for 5 days) for asthma exacerbation.

C. Considerations in Special Populations
  1. Preterm infants
    a. Immunize according to chronologic age.
    b. Do not lower vaccine doses.
    c. If birth weight is less than 2 kg, delay HepB vaccine because of reduced immune response until the patient is 30 days old or at hospital discharge if it occurs before 30 days of age (unless the mother is positive for HepB surface antigen).
  2. Children who are immunocompromised
    a. Should not receive live vaccines
    b. Inactivated vaccines and immune globulins are appropriate.
    c. Household contacts should not receive oral polio vaccine; however, MMR, influenza, varicella, and rotavirus vaccines are recommended.
  3. Patients receiving corticosteroids
    a. Live vaccines may be administered to patients receiving the following:
        i. Topical corticosteroids
       ii. Physiologic maintenance doses
      iii. Low or moderate doses (less than 2 mg/kg/day of prednisone equivalent)
    b. Live vaccines may be given immediately after discontinuation of high doses (2 mg/kg/day or more of prednisone equivalent) of systemic steroids given for less than 14 days.
    c. Live vaccines should be delayed at least 1 month after discontinuing high doses (2 mg/kg/day or more of prednisone equivalent) of systemic steroids given for more than 14 days.
  4. Patients with HIV infection
    a. MMR should be administered unless patient is severely immunocompromised.
    b. Varicella should be considered for asymptomatic or mildly symptomatic patients.
    c. Inactivated vaccines should be administered routinely.

Vaccine	Birth	1 mo	2 mos	4 mos	6 mos	9 mos	12 mos	15 mos	18 mos	19–23 mos	2–3 yrs	4–6 yrs	7–10 yrs	11–12 yrs	13–15 yrs	16–18 yrs
Hepatitis B[1] (HepB)	1st dose	←— 2nd dose —→			←————————— 3rd dose —————————→											
Rotavirus[2] (RV) RV1 (2-dose series); RV5 (3-dose series)			1st dose	2nd dose	See footnote 2											
Diphtheria, tetanus, & acellular pertussis[3] (DTaP: <7 yrs)			1st dose	2nd dose	3rd dose		←——— 4th dose ———→					5th dose				
Tetanus, diphtheria, & acellular pertussis[4] (Tdap: ≥7 yrs)														(Tdap)		
Haemophilus influenzae type b[5] (Hib)			1st dose	2nd dose	See footnote 5		←— 3rd or 4th dose, See footnote 5 —→									
Pneumococcal conjugate[6] (PCV13)			1st dose	2nd dose	3rd dose		←— 4th dose —→									
Pneumococcal polysaccharide[6] (PPSV23)																
Inactivated poliovirus[7] (IPV: <18 yrs)			1st dose	2nd dose	←————————— 3rd dose —————————→							4th dose				
Influenza[8] (IIV; LAIV) 2 doses for some: See footnote 8					Annual vaccination (IIV only) 1 or 2 doses						Annual vaccination (LAIV or IIV) 1 or 2 doses		Annual vaccination (LAIV or IIV) 1 dose only			
Measles, mumps, rubella[9] (MMR)					See footnote 9		←— 1st dose —→					2nd dose				
Varicella[10] (VAR)							←— 1st dose —→					2nd dose				
Hepatitis A[11] (HepA)							←—— 2-dose series, See footnote 11 ——→									
Human papillomavirus[12] (HPV2: females only; HPV4: males and females)							See footnote 13							(3-dose series)		
Meningococcal[13] (Hib-MenCY ≥ 6 weeks; MenACWY-D ≥9 mos; MenACWY-CRM ≥ 2 mos)														1st dose		Booster

Legend:
- Range of recommended ages for all children
- Range of recommended ages for catch-up immunization
- Range of recommended ages during which catch-up is encouraged and for certain high-risk groups
- Range of recommended ages for certain high-risk groups
- Not routinely recommended

This schedule includes recommendations in effect as of January 1, 2015. Any dose not administered at the recommended age should be administered at a subsequent visit, when indicated and feasible. The use of a combination vaccine generally is preferred over separate injections of its equivalent component vaccines. Vaccination providers should consult the relevant Advisory Committee on Immunization Practices (ACIP) statement for detailed recommendations, available online at http://www.cdc.gov/vaccines/hcp/acip-recs/index.html. Clinically significant adverse events that follow vaccination should be reported to the Vaccine Adverse Event Reporting System (VAERS) online (http://www.vaers.hhs.gov) or by telephone (800-822-7967). Suspected cases of vaccine-preventable diseases should be reported to the state or local health department. Additional information, including precautions and contraindications for vaccination, is available from CDC online (http://www.cdc.gov/vaccines/recs/vac-admin/contraindications.htm) or by telephone (800-CDC-INFO [800-232-4636]).

This schedule is approved by the Advisory Committee on Immunization Practices (http://www.cdc.gov/vaccines/acip), the American Academy of Pediatrics (http://www.aap.org), the American Academy of Family Physicians (http://www.aafp.org), and the American College of Obstetricians and Gynecologists (http://www.acog.org).

NOTE: The above recommendations must be read along with the footnotes of this schedule.

Figure 2. Recommended immunization schedule for persons aged 0-18 years — 2015

For those who fall behind or start late, see the catch-up schedule at http://www.cdc.gov/vaccines/schedules/hcp/imz/catchup.html

Footnotes — Recommended immunization schedule for persons aged 0 through 18 years—United States, 2015

For further guidance on the use of the vaccines mentioned below, see: http://www.cdc.gov/vaccines/hcp/acip-recs/index.html.
For vaccine recommendations for persons 19 years of age and older, see the Adult Immunization Schedule.

Additional information

- For contraindications and precautions to use of a vaccine and for additional information regarding that vaccine, vaccination providers should consult the relevant ACIP statement available online at http://www.cdc.gov/vaccines/hcp/acip-recs/index.html.
- For purposes of calculating intervals between doses, 4 weeks = 28 days. Intervals of 4 months or greater are determined by calendar months.
- Vaccine doses administered 4 days or less before the minimum interval are considered valid. Doses of any vaccine administered ≥5 days earlier than the minimum interval or minimum age should not be counted as valid doses and should be repeated as age-appropriate. The repeat dose should be spaced after the invalid dose by the recommended minimum interval. For further details, see MMWR, General Recommendations on Immunization and Reports / Vol. 60 / No. 2; Table 1. Recommended and minimum ages and intervals between vaccine doses available online at http://www.cdc.gov/mmwr/pdf/rr/rr6002.pdf.
- Information on travel vaccine requirements and recommendations is available at http://wwwnc.cdc.gov/travel/destinations/list.
- For vaccination of persons with primary and secondary immunodeficiencies, see Table 13, "Vaccination of persons with primary and secondary immuno-deficiencies," in General Recommendations on Immunization (ACIP), available at http://www.cdc.gov/mmwr/pdf/rr/rr6002.pdf.; and American Academy of Pediatrics. "Immunization in Special Clinical Circumstances," in Pickering LK, Baker CJ, Kimberlin DW, Long SS eds. Red Book: 2012 report of the Committee on Infectious Diseases. 29th ed. Elk Grove Village, IL: American Academy of Pediatrics.

1. Hepatitis B (HepB) vaccine. (Minimum age: birth)
Routine vaccination:
At birth:
- Administer monovalent HepB vaccine to all newborns before hospital discharge.
- For infants born to hepatitis B surface antigen (HBsAg)-positive mothers, administer HepB vaccine and 0.5 mL of hepatitis B immune globulin (HBIG) within 12 hours of birth. These infants should be tested for HBsAg and anti-body to HBsAg (anti-HBs) 1 to 2 months after completion of the HepB series at age 9 through 18 months (preferably at the next well-child visit).
- If mother's HBsAg status is unknown, within 12 hours of birth adminis-ter HepB vaccine regardless of birth weight. For infants weighing less than 2,000 grams, administer HBIG in addition to HepB vaccine within 12 hours of birth. Determine mother's HBsAg status as soon as possible and, if mother is HBsAg-positive, also administer HBIG for infants weighing 2,000 grams or more as soon as possible, but no later than age 7 days.

Doses following the birth dose:
- The second dose should be administered at age 1 or 2 months. Monovalent HepB vaccine should be used for doses administered before age 6 weeks.
- Infants who did not receive a birth dose should receive 3 doses of a HepB-containing vaccine on a schedule of 0, 1 to 2 months, and 6 months starting as soon as feasible. See Figure 2.
- Administer the second dose 1 to 2 months after the first dose (minimum interval of 4 weeks), administer the third dose at least 8 weeks after the second dose AND at least 16 weeks after the first dose. The final (third or fourth) dose in the HepB vaccine series should be administered no earlier than age 24 weeks.
- Administration of a total of 4 doses of HepB vaccine is permitted when a combination vaccine containing HepB is administered after the birth dose.

Catch-up vaccination:
- Unvaccinated persons should complete a 3-dose series.
- A 2-dose series (doses separated by at least 4 months) of adult formulation Recombivax HB is licensed for use in children aged 11 through 15 years.
- For other catch-up guidance, see Figure 2.

2. Rotavirus (RV) vaccines.
(Minimum age: 6 weeks for both
RV1 [Rotarix] and RV5 [RotaTeq])
Routine vaccination:
Administer a series of RV vaccine to all infants as follows:
1. If Rotarix is used, administer a 2-dose series at 2 and 4 months of age.
2. If RotaTeq is used, administer a 3-dose series at ages 2, 4, and 6 months.
3. If any dose in the series was RotaTeq or vaccine product is unknown for any dose in the series, a total of 3 doses of RV vaccine should be administered.

Catch-up vaccination:
- The maximum age for the first dose in the series is 14 weeks, 6 days; vaccina-tion should not be initiated for infants aged 15 weeks, 0 days or older.
- The maximum age for the final dose in the series is 8 months, 0 days.
- For other catch-up guidance, see Figure 2.

3. Diphtheria and tetanus toxoids and acellular
pertussis (DTaP) vaccine. (Minimum age: 6 weeks.
Exception: DTaP-IPV [Kinrix]: 4 years)
Routine vaccination:
- Administer a 5-dose series of DTaP vaccine at ages 2, 4, 6, 15 through 18 months, and 4 through 6 years. The fourth dose may be administered as early as age 12 months, provided at least 6 months have elapsed since the third dose. However, the fourth dose of DTaP need not be repeated if it was administered at least 4 months after the third dose of DTaP.

Catch-up vaccination:
- The fifth dose of DTaP vaccine is not necessary if the fourth dose was admin-istered at age 4 years or older.
- For other catch-up guidance, see Figure 2.

4. Tetanus and diphtheria toxoids and acellular pertussis (Tdap) vaccine. (Minimum age: 10 years for both Boostrix and Adacel)
Routine vaccination:
- Administer 1 dose of Tdap vaccine to all adolescents aged 11 through 12 years.
- Tdap may be administered regardless of the interval since the last tetanus and diphtheria toxoid-containing vaccine.
- Administer 1 dose of Tdap vaccine to pregnant adolescents during each preg-nancy (preferred during 27 through 36 weeks' gestation) regardless of time since prior Td or Tdap vaccination.

Catch-up vaccination:
- Persons aged 7 years and older who are not fully immunized with DTaP vaccine should receive Tdap vaccine as 1 dose (preferably the first) in the catch-up series; if additional doses are needed, use Td vaccine. For children 7 through 10 years who receive a dose of Tdap as part of the catch-up series, an adolescent Tdap vaccine dose at age 11 through 12 years should NOT be administered. Td should be administered instead 10 years after the Tdap dose.
- Persons aged 11 through 18 years who have not received Tdap vaccine should receive a dose followed by tetanus and diphtheria toxoid (Td) booster doses every 10 years thereafter.
- Inadvertent doses of DTaP vaccine:
  -- If administered inadvertently to a child aged 7 through 10 years may count as part of the catch-up series. This dose may count as the adolescent Tdap dose, or the child can later receive a Tdap booster dose at age 11 through 12 years.
  -- If administered inadvertently to an adolescent aged 11 through 18 years, the dose should be counted as the adolescent Tdap booster.
- For other catch-up guidance, see Figure 2.

5. *Haemophilus influenzae* type b (Hib) conjugate vaccine.
(Minimum age: 6 weeks for PRP-T [ACTHIB, DTaP-IPV/
Hib (Pentacel) and Hib-MenCY (MenHibrix)], PRP-OMP
[PedvaxHIB or COMVAX], 12 months for PRP-T [Hiberix])
Routine vaccination:
- Administer a 2- or 3-dose Hib vaccine primary series and a booster dose (dose 3 or 4 depending on vaccine used in primary series) at age 12 through 15 months to complete a full Hib vaccine series.
- The primary series with ActHIB, MenHibrix, or Pentacel consists of 3 doses and should be administered at 2, 4, and 6 months of age. The primary series with PedvaxHIB or COMVAX consists of 2 doses and should be administered at 2 and 4 months of age; a dose at age 6 months is not indicated.
- One booster dose (dose 3 or 4 depending on vaccine used in primary series) of any Hib vaccine should be administered at age 12 through 15 months. An exception is Hiberix. Hiberix should only be used for the booster (final) dose in children aged 12 months through 4 years who have received at least 1 prior dose of Hib-containing vaccine.
- For recommendations on the use of MenHibrix in patients at increased risk for meningococcal disease, please refer to the meningococcal vaccine footnotes and also to MMWR February 28, 2014 / 63(RR01);1-13, available at http://www.cdc.gov/mmwr/PDF/rr/rr6301.pdf.

Catch-up vaccination:
- If dose 1 was administered at ages 12 through 14 months, administer a second (final) dose at least 8 weeks after dose 1, regardless of Hib vaccine used in the primary series.
- If both doses were PRP-OMP (PedvaxHIB or COMVAX), and were admin-istered before the first birthday, the third (and final) dose should be adminis-tered at age 12 through 59 months and at least 8 weeks after the second dose.
- If the first dose was administered at age 7 through 11 months, administer the second dose at least 4 weeks later and a third (and final) dose at age 12 through 15 months or 8 weeks after second dose, whichever is later.

- If first dose is administered before the first birthday and second dose administered at younger than 15 months, a third (and final) dose should be given 8 weeks later.
- For unvaccinated children aged 15 months or older, administer only 1 dose.
- For other catch-up guidance, see Figure 2. For catch-up guidance related to MenHibrix, please see the meningococcal vaccine footnotes and also MMWR February 28, 2014 / 63(RR01);1-13, available at http://www.cdc.gov/mmwr/PDF/rr/rr6301.pdf.

Vaccination of persons with high-risk conditions:

- Children aged 12 through 59 months who are at increased risk for Hib disease, including chemotherapy recipients and those with anatomic or functional asplenia (including sickle cell disease), human immunodeficiency virus (HIV) infection, immunoglobulin deficiency, or early component complement deficiency, who have received either no doses or only 1 dose of Hib vaccine before 12 months of age, should receive 2 additional doses of Hib vaccine 8 weeks apart; children who received 2 or more doses of Hib vaccine before 12 months of age should receive 1 additional dose.
- For patients younger than 5 years of age undergoing chemotherapy or radiation treatment who received a Hib vaccine dose(s) within 14 days of starting therapy or during therapy, repeat the dose(s) at least 3 months following therapy completion.
- Recipients of hematopoietic stem cell transplant (HSCT) should be revaccinated with a 3-dose regimen of Hib vaccine starting 6 to 12 months after successful transplant, regardless of vaccination history; doses should be administered at least 4 weeks apart.
- A single dose of any Hib-containing vaccine should be administered to unimmunized* children and adolescents 15 months of age and older undergoing an elective splenectomy; if possible, vaccine should be administered at least 14 days before procedure.
- Hib vaccine is not routinely recommended for patients 5 years or older. However, 1 dose of Hib vaccine should be administered to unimmunized* persons aged 5 years or older who have anatomic or functional asplenia (including sickle cell disease) and unvaccinated persons 5 through 18 years of age with human immunodeficiency virus (HIV) infection.

  Patients who have not received a primary series and booster dose or at least 1 dose of Hib vaccine after 14 months of age are considered unimmunized.

6. Pneumococcal vaccines. (Minimum age: 6 weeks for PCV13, 2 years for PPSV23)
Routine vaccination with PCV13:
- Administer a 4-dose series of PCV13 vaccine at ages 2, 4, and 6 months and at age 12 through 15 months.
- For children aged 14 through 59 months who have received an age-appropriate series of 7-valent PCV (PCV7), administer a single supplemental dose of 13-valent PCV (PCV13).

Catch-up vaccination with PCV13:
- Administer 1 dose of PCV13 to all healthy children aged 24 through 59 months who are not completely vaccinated for their age.
- For other catch-up guidance, see Figure 2.

Vaccination of persons with high-risk conditions with PCV13 and PPSV23:
- All recommended PCV13 doses should be administered prior to PPSV23 vaccination if possible.
- For children 2 through 5 years of age with any of the following conditions: chronic heart disease (particularly cyanotic congenital heart disease and cardiac failure); chronic lung disease (including asthma if treated with high-dose oral corticosteroid therapy); diabetes mellitus; cerebrospinal fluid leak; cochlear implant; sickle cell disease and other hemoglobinopathies; anatomic or functional asplenia; HIV infection; chronic renal failure; nephrotic syndrome; diseases associated with treatment with immunosuppressive drugs or radiation therapy, including malignant neoplasms, leukemias, lymphomas, and Hodgkin's disease; solid organ transplantation; or congenital immunodeficiency:
  1. Administer 1 dose of PCV13 if any incomplete schedule of 3 doses of PCV (PCV7 and/or PCV13) were received previously.
  2. Administer 2 doses of PCV13 at least 8 weeks apart if unvaccinated or any incomplete schedule of fewer than 3 doses of PCV (PCV7 and/or PCV13) were received previously.
  3. Administer 1 supplemental dose of PCV13 if 4 doses of PCV7 or other age-appropriate complete PCV7 series was received previously.
  4. The minimum interval between doses of PCV (PCV7 or PCV13) is 8 weeks.
  5. For children with no history of PPSV23 vaccination, administer PPSV23 at least 8 weeks after the most recent dose of PCV13.
- For children aged 6 through 18 years who have cerebrospinal fluid leak; cochlear implant; sickle cell disease and other hemoglobinopathies; anatomic or functional asplenia; congenital or acquired immunodeficiencies; HIV infection; chronic renal failure; nephrotic syndrome; diseases associated with treatment with immunosuppressive drugs or radiation therapy, including malignant neoplasms, leukemias, lymphomas, and Hodgkin's disease; generalized malignancy; solid organ transplantation; or multiple myeloma:

  1. If neither PCV13 nor PPSV23 has been received previously, administer 1 dose of PCV13 now and 1 dose of PPSV23 at least 8 weeks later.
  2. If PCV13 has been received previously but PPSV23 has not, administer 1 dose of PPSV23 at least 8 weeks after the most recent dose of PCV13.
  3. If PPSV23 has been received but PCV13 has not, administer 1 dose of PCV13 at least 8 weeks after the most recent dose of PPSV23.
- For children aged 6 through 18 years with chronic heart disease (particularly cyanotic congenital heart disease and cardiac failure), chronic lung disease (including asthma if treated with high-dose oral corticosteroid therapy), diabetes mellitus, alcoholism, or chronic liver disease, who have not received PPSV23, administer 1 dose of PPSV23. If PCV13 has been received previously, then PPSV23 should be administered at least 8 weeks after any prior PCV13 dose.
- A single revaccination with PPSV23 should be administered 5 years after the first dose to children with sickle cell disease or other hemoglobinopathies; anatomic or functional asplenia; congenital or acquired immunodeficiencies; HIV infection; chronic renal failure; nephrotic syndrome; diseases associated with treatment with immunosuppressive drugs or radiation therapy, including malignant neoplasms, leukemias, lymphomas, and Hodgkin's disease; generalized malignancy; solid organ transplantation; or multiple myeloma.

7. Inactivated poliovirus vaccine (IPV). (Minimum age: 6 weeks)
Routine vaccination:
- Administer a 4-dose series of IPV at ages 2, 4, 6 through 18 months, and 4 through 6 years. The final dose in the series should be administered on or after the fourth birthday and at least 6 months after the previous dose.

Catch-up vaccination:
- In the first 6 months of life, minimum age and minimum intervals are only recommended if the person is at risk of imminent exposure to circulating poliovirus (i.e., travel to a polio-endemic region or during an outbreak).
- If 4 or more doses are administered before age 4 years, an additional dose should be administered at age 4 through 6 years and at least 6 months after the previous dose.
- A fourth dose is not necessary if the third dose was administered at age 4 years or older and at least 6 months after the previous dose.
- If both OPV and IPV were administered as part of a series, a total of 4 doses should be administered.
- Regardless of the child's current age. IPV is not routinely recommended for U.S. residents aged 18 years or older.
- For other catch-up guidance, see Figure 2.

8. Influenza vaccines. (Minimum age: 6 months for inactivated influenza vaccine [IIV], 2 years for live, attenuated influenza vaccine [LAIV])
Routine vaccination:
- Administer influenza vaccine annually to all children beginning at age 6 months. For most healthy, nonpregnant persons aged 2 through 49 years, either LAIV or IIV may be used. However, LAIV should NOT be administered to some persons, including 1) persons who have experienced severe allergic reactions to LAIV, any of its components, or to a previous dose of any other influenza vaccine; 2) children 2 through 17 years receiving aspirin or aspirin-containing products; 3) persons who are allergic to eggs; 4) pregnant women; 5) immunosuppressed persons; 6) children 2 through 4 years of age with asthma or who had wheezing in the past 12 months; or 7) persons who have taken influenza antiviral medications in the previous 48 hours. For all other contraindications and precautions to use of LAIV, see MMWR August 15, 2014 / 63(32);691-697 [40 pages] available at http://www.cdc.gov/mmwr/pdf/wk/mm6332.pdf.

For children aged 6 months through 8 years:
- For the 2014-15 season, administer 2 doses (separated by at least 4 weeks) to children who are receiving influenza vaccine for the first time. Some children in this age group who have been vaccinated previously will also need 2 doses. For additional guidance, follow dosing guidelines in the 2014-15 ACIP influenza vaccine recommendations, MMWR August 15, 2014 / 63(32);691-697 [40 pages] available at http://www.cdc.gov/mmwr/pdf/wk/mm6332.pdf.
- For the 2015–16 season, follow dosing guidelines in the 2015 ACIP influenza vaccine recommendations.

For persons aged 9 years and older:
- Administer 1 dose.

9. Measles, mumps, and rubella (MMR) vaccine. (Minimum age: 12 months for routine vaccination)
Routine vaccination:
- Administer a 2-dose series of MMR vaccine at ages 12 through 15 months and 4 through 6 years. The second dose may be administered before age 4 years, provided at least 4 weeks have elapsed since the first dose.
- Administer 1 dose of MMR vaccine to infants aged 6 through 11 months before departure from the United States for international travel. These children should be revaccinated with 2 doses of MMR vaccine, the first at age 12 through 15 months (12 months if the child remains in an area where disease risk is high), and the second dose at least 4 weeks later.

- Administer 2 doses of MMR vaccine to children aged 12 months and older before departure from the United States for international travel. The first dose should be administered on or after age 12 months and the second dose at least 4 weeks later.

Catch-up vaccination:
- Ensure that all school-aged children and adolescents have had 2 doses of MMR vaccine; the minimum interval between the 2 doses is 4 weeks.

10. **Varicella (VAR) vaccine. (Minimum age: 12 months)**
   Routine vaccination:
   - Administer a 2-dose series of VAR vaccine at ages 12 through 15 months and 4 through 6 years. The second dose may be administered before age 4 years, provided at least 3 months have elapsed since the first dose. If the second dose was administered at least 4 weeks after the first dose, it can be accepted as valid.

   Catch-up vaccination:
   - Ensure that all persons aged 7 through 18 years without evidence of immunity (see MMWR 2007 / 56 [No. RR-4], available at http://www.cdc.gov/mmwr/pdf/rr/rr5604.pdf) have 2 doses of varicella vaccine. For children aged 7 through 12 years, the recommended minimum interval between doses is 3 months (if the second dose was administered at least 4 weeks after the first dose, it can be accepted as valid); for persons aged 13 years and older, the minimum interval between doses is 4 weeks.

11. **Hepatitis A (HepA) vaccine.**
   (Minimum age: 12 months)
   Routine vaccination:
   - Initiate the 2-dose HepA vaccine series at 12 through 23 months; separate the 2 doses by 6 to 18 months.
   - Children who have received 1 dose of HepA vaccine before age 24 months should receive a second dose 6 to 18 months after the first dose.
   - For any person aged 2 years and older who has not already received the HepA vaccine series, 2 doses of HepA vaccine separated by 6 to 18 months may be administered if immunity against hepatitis A virus infection is desired.

   Catch-up vaccination:
   - The minimum interval between the two doses is 6 months.

   Special populations:
   - Administer 2 doses of HepA vaccine at least 6 months apart to previously unvaccinated persons who live in areas where vaccination programs target older children, or who are at increased risk for infection. This includes persons traveling to or working in countries that have high or intermediate endemicity of infection; men having sex with men; users of injection and non-injection illicit drugs; persons who work with HAV-infected primates or with HAV in a research laboratory; persons with clotting-factor disorders; persons with chronic liver disease; and persons who anticipate close personal contact (e.g., household or regular babysitting) with an international adoptee during the first 60 days after arrival in the United States from a country with high or intermediate endemicity. The first dose should be administered as soon as the adoption is planned, ideally 2 or more weeks before the arrival of the adoptee.

12. **Human papillomavirus (HPV) vaccines.**
   (Minimum age: 9 years for HPV2 [Cervarix]
   and HPV4 [Gardasil])
   Routine vaccination:
   - Administer a 3-dose series of HPV vaccine on a schedule of 0, 1-2, and 6 months to all adolescents aged 11 through 12 years. Either HPV4 or HPV2 may be used for females, and only HPV4 may be used for males.
   - The vaccine series may be started at age 9 years.
   - Administer the second dose 1 to 2 months after the first dose (minimum interval of 4 weeks); administer the third dose 24 weeks after the first dose and 16 weeks after the second dose (minimum interval of 12 weeks).

   Catch-up vaccination:
   - Administer the vaccine series to females (either HPV2 or HPV4) and males (HPV4) at age 13 through 18 years if not previously vaccinated.
   - Use recommended routine dosing intervals (see Routine vaccination above) for vaccine series catch-up.

13. **Meningococcal conjugate vaccines.**
   (Minimum age: 6 weeks for Hib-MenCY
   [MenHibrix], 9 months for MenACWY-D [Menactra],
   2 months for MenACWY-CRM [Menveo])
   Routine vaccination:
   - Administer a single dose of Menactra or Menveo vaccine at age 11 through 12 years, with a booster dose at age 16 years.

- Adolescents aged 11 through 18 years with human immunodeficiency virus (HIV) infection should receive a 2-dose primary series of Menactra or Menveo with at least 8 weeks between doses.
- For children aged 2 months through 18 years with high-risk conditions, see below.

Catch-up vaccination:
- Administer Menactra or Menveo vaccine at age 13 through 18 years if not previously vaccinated.
- If the first dose is administered at age 13 through 15 years, a booster dose should be administered at age 16 through 18 years with a minimum interval of at least 8 weeks between doses.
- If the first dose is administered at age 16 years or older, a booster dose is not needed.
- For other catch-up guidance, see Figure 2.

Vaccination of persons with high-risk conditions and other persons at increased risk of disease:
- Children with anatomic or functional asplenia (including sickle cell disease):
   1. Menveo
      o Children who initiate vaccination at 8 weeks through 6 months: Administer doses at 2, 4, 6, and 12 months of age.
      o Unvaccinated children 7 through 23 months: Administer 2 doses, with the second dose at least 12 weeks after the first dose AND after the first birthday.
      o Children 24 months and older who have not received a complete series: Administer 2 primary doses at least 8 weeks apart.
   2. MenHibrix
      o Children 6 weeks through 18 months: Administer doses at 2, 4, 6, and 12 through 15 months of age.
      o If the first dose of MenHibrix is given at or after 12 months of age, a total of 2 doses should be given at least 8 weeks apart to ensure protection against serogroups C and Y meningococcal disease.
   3. Menactra
      o Children 24 months and older who have not received a complete series: Administer 2 primary doses at least 8 weeks apart. If Menactra is administered to a child with asplenia (including sickle cell disease), do not administer Menactra until 2 years of age and at least 4 weeks after the completion of all PCV13 doses.
- Children with persistent complement component deficiency:
   1. Menveo
      o Children who initiate vaccination at 8 weeks through 6 months: Administer doses at 2, 4, 6, and 12 months of age.
      o Unvaccinated children 7 through 23 months: Administer 2 doses, with the second dose at least 12 weeks after the first dose AND after the first birthday.
      o Children 24 months and older who have not received a complete series: Administer 2 primary doses at least 8 weeks apart.
   2. MenHibrix
      o Children 6 weeks through 18 months: Administer doses at 2, 4, 6, and 12 through 15 months of age.
      o If the first dose of MenHibrix is given at or after 12 months of age, a total of 2 doses should be given at least 8 weeks apart to ensure protection against serogroups C and Y meningococcal disease.
   3. Menactra
      o Children 9 through 23 months: Administer 2 primary doses at least 12 weeks apart.
      o Children 24 months and older who have not received a complete series: Administer 2 primary doses at least 8 weeks apart.
- For children who travel to or reside in countries in which meningococcal disease is hyperendemic or epidemic, including countries in the African meningitis belt or the Hajj, administer an age-appropriate formulation and series of Menactra or Menveo for protection against serogroups A and W meningococcal disease. Prior receipt of MenHibrix is not sufficient for children traveling to the meningitis belt or the Hajj because it does not contain serogroups A or W.
- For children at risk during a community outbreak attributable to a vaccine serogroup, administer or complete an age- and formulation-appropriate series of MenHibrix, Menactra, or Menveo.
- For booster doses among persons with high-risk conditions, refer to MMWR 2013 / 62(RR02);1-22, available at http://www.cdc.gov/mmwr/preview/mmwr html/rr6202a1.htm.

For other catch-up recommendations for these persons, and complete information on use of meningococcal vaccines, including guidance related to vaccination of persons at increased risk of infection, see MMWR March 22, 2013 / 62(RR02);1-22, available at http://www.cdc.gov/mmwr/pdf/rr/rr6202.pdf.

V. PEDIATRIC SEIZURE DISORDERS

A. Treatment Options Based on Seizure Type

Table 6. Treatment Options Based on Seizure Type

Seizure Type	Drugs of Choice	Alternatives
Focal (formerly "partial")	VPA, CBZ, PHT	PB, gabapentin, lamotrigine, tiagabine, topiramate, oxcarbazepine, zonisamide, levetiracetam, lacosamide
Generalized		
Tonic-clonic	VPA, CBZ, PHT	Lamotrigine, topiramate, zonisamide, levetiracetam
Myoclonic	VPA	Topiramate, zonisamide, levetiracetam
Absence	Ethosuximide, VPA	Lamotrigine, zonisamide, levetiracetam
Lennox-Gastaut	VPA, topiramate, lamotrigine	Rufinamide, clobazam, felbamate, zonisamide
Infantile spasms	ACTH	Vigabatrin, lamotrigine, tiagabine, topiramate, VPA, zonisamide

ACTH = adrenocorticotropic hormone; CBZ = carbamazepine; PB = phenobarbital; PHT = phenytoin; VPA = valproic acid.

B. Comparison of Available Antiepileptic Drugs

Table 7. Comparison of Available Antiepileptic Drugs

Drug	Adverse Effects	Pharmacokinetic Considerations	Other Comments
Carbamazepine	Rash Hyponatremia ↓ Bone density Teratogenic	Autoinduction ↓ Effectiveness of OCs	Significant drug interactions
Clobazam	Somnolence	Dose adjustment required in hepatic impairment Dose adjustment required in CYP2C19 poor metabolizers	
Felbamate	Anorexia, nausea, weight loss Insomnia, somnolence Aplastic anemia Hepatic failure	Clearance ~50:50 renal/hepatic	Significant drug interactions Aplastic anemia: Adults > children Requires signed informed consent
Gabapentin	Somnolence Weight gain	↑ Clearance in children <6 years Dose adjustment required in renal insufficiency Nonlinear pharmacokinetics	Minimal drug interactions Minimal cognitive effects May worsen Lennox-Gastaut
Lacosamide	Prolonged PR interval Dizziness Headache Diplopia	Dose adjustment required in severe renal insufficiency	Use with caution if severe cardiac disease or conduction problems No clinically significant drug interactions
Lamotrigine	Rash Stevens-Johnson syndrome	Autoinduction	Rash: Children > adults Minimal cognitive effects

Table 7. Comparison of Available Antiepileptic Drugs *(continued)*

Drug	Adverse Effects	Pharmacokinetic Considerations	Other Comments
Levetiracetam	Headache Somnolence	Linear pharmacokinetics Renal excretion Clearance 40% ↑ in children No effect on CYP system	Minimal drug interactions
Oxcarbazepine	Hyponatremia (>CBZ) Rash (<CBZ)	Linear pharmacokinetics Clearance 40% ↑ in children <6 years Induces CYP3A4 Inhibits CYP2C19	Hyponatremia more common in adults than in children Minimal cognitive effects
Phenobarbital	Cognitive dysfunction Sedation Rash ↓ Bone density	Linear pharmacokinetics ↓ Effectiveness of OCs	Significant drug interactions
Phenytoin	Rash Gingival hyperplasia Hirsutism ↓ Bone density Teratogenic	Nonlinear pharmacokinetics ↓ Effectiveness of OCs	Significant drug interactions
Rufinamide	Somnolence Rash QT interval shortening	↑ Level with concurrent VPA	Somnolence: Minimized with slow dose titration Rash: All reported cases are in children
Tiagabine	Dizziness Nonconvulsive status epilepticus (case reports)	Clearance 50% ↑ in children	Minimal cognitive effects
Topiramate	Cognitive dysfunction Weight loss Glaucoma Oligohidrosis	↑ Clearance in children Dose adjustment required in renal insufficiency	Weight loss more common in obese patients Children at higher risk of oligohidrosis than adults
Valproic acid	Weight gain Menstrual irregularities Polycystic ovarian syndrome Hyperandrogenism Hepatotoxicity Teratogenic Thrombocytopenia	CYP induction > in children	Significant drug interactions Most cases of hepatotoxicity in children <2 years
Vigabatrin	Vision loss Weight gain		Available only through restricted distribution program
Zonisamide	Weight loss Rash Oligohidrosis Somnolence Agitation Hallucinations	Linear pharmacokinetics Primarily renal excretion No effect on CYP system	Better tolerated by children than by adults

CBZ = carbamazepine; CYP = cytochrome P450; OC = oral contraceptive; PHT = phenytoin; VPA = valproic acid.

Patient Case

10. A 14-year-old moderately obese girl comes to the clinic with an erythematous pruritic rash. She was initiated on oxcarbazepine about 3 weeks ago for the management of partial seizures. Her medical history is significant only for seizures. She recently became sexually active with a male and admits inconsistent contraceptive use. Which intervention is best for her?

    A. Change to carbamazepine.

    B. Change to levetiracetam.

    C. Change to valproic acid.

    D. No change in therapy is necessary.

VI. ATTENTION-DEFICIT/HYPERACTIVITY DISORDER

A. Clinical Presentation
   1. *Diagnostic and Statistical Manual for Mental Disorders* (*DSM-V*) criteria
      a. Either (i) or (ii):
         i. Six or more of the following symptoms of inattention have been present for at least 6 months to a point that is disruptive and inappropriate:
         Inattention
            (a) Often does not give close attention to detail/makes careless mistakes
            (b) Often has trouble keeping attention on tasks/activities
            (c) Often does not seem to listen
            (d) Often does not follow instructions
            (e) Often has trouble organizing activities
            (f) Often avoids or dislikes things that require long periods of mental effort
            (g) Often loses things needed for tasks or activities
            (h) Often is easily distracted
            (i) Often is forgetful
         ii. Six or more of the following symptoms of hyperactivity-impulsivity have been present for at least 6 months to a point that is disruptive and inappropriate:
         Hyperactivity
            (a) Often fidgets or squirms
            (b) Often is unable to remain seated when it is expected
            (c) Often runs or climbs when and where it is not appropriate
            (d) Often has difficulty with quiet play or activities
            (e) Often is "on the go"
            (f) Often talks excessively
         Impulsivity
            (g) Often blurts out answers
            (h) Often has difficulty waiting one's turn
            (i) Often interrupts
      b. Some symptoms were present before 7 years of age.
      c. Some impairment from the symptoms is present in two or more settings.
      d. Clear evidence of significant impairment exists in social, school, or work functioning.
      e. No other mental disorder better describes the symptoms.
   2. Comorbid disease states: 44%–87% of children with ADHD have at least one other disorder:
      a. Oppositional defiant disorder

   i. Most common comorbid disorder in adolescents

   ii. Presence of ADHD increases the odds of oppositional defiant disorder almost 11-fold.

  b. Anxiety disorder: May exist in about 25% of children with ADHD

  c. Tics

   i. 21%–90% of children with Tourette syndrome may also have ADHD.

   ii. May not be exacerbated by stimulant agents, as once thought

---

Patient Case

11. A 9-year-old boy has a new diagnosis of ADHD. At school, he is disruptive, talks when the teacher is talking, and runs around the classroom. His parents report extreme difficulty in getting him to do his homework after school. Which is best for his initial drug therapy?

 A. Methylphenidate (OROS) (Concerta) given once daily.

 B. Methylphenidate immediate release (Ritalin) given twice daily, with doses administered 4 hours apart.

 C. Guanfacine given at bedtime.

 D. D-Methylphenidate (Focalin) given twice daily, with doses administered 4 hours apart.

 B. Classification: Based on *DSM-V* Criteria (see previous section)

  1. ADHD, Combined Type: Criteria (i) and (ii) both are met.

  2. ADHD, Predominantly Inattentive Type: Criterion (i) is met, but (ii) is not met.

  3. ADHD, Predominantly Hyperactive-Impulsive Type: Criterion (ii) is met, but (i) is not met.

 C. Treatment Options: Combination of pharmacotherapy and behavioral therapy is more beneficial than either intervention alone.

  1. Factors affecting choice of pharmacologic agent

   a. Desired length of coverage time for symptoms

    i. Consider time of day when symptoms occur.

    ii. Consider time of day when child's activities occur (e.g., when is homework done, at what time are teenagers driving, when is child's bedtime).

   b. Child's ability to swallow pills or capsules

   c. Concomitant disease states (e.g., tic disorders)

   d. Adverse effect profile

   e. Concerns about abuse or diversion potential

    i. Children with ADHD are more likely to have a concurrent substance use disorder than those without ADHD.

    ii. Treatment with stimulant medication may reduce the risk of developing a substance use disorder.

    iii. Children treated with stimulants at a younger age are less likely to misuse or abuse substances than those in whom treatment is delayed.

   f. Expense

  2. Available pharmacologic agents

   a. Stimulant medications: Some children with ADHD respond better to one stimulant type than another; therefore, both methylphenidate- and amphetamine-containing products should be tried before stimulant treatment is deemed a failure.

    i. Methylphenidate-containing products

     (a) Ramp effect: behavioral effects are proportional to the rate of methylphenidate absorption into the central nervous system.

       (b) See Table 8 for a comparison of available products.

       (c) Adverse effects and precautions

           (1) Headache, stomachache, loss of appetite, and insomnia

           (2) Use with caution in patients with glaucoma, tics, psychosis, and concomitant monoamine oxidase inhibitor use.

           (3) Insomnia, anorexia, and tics occur more often with transdermal patch, also mild skin reactions.

    ii. Amphetamine-containing products

       (a) See Table 8 for a comparison of available products.

       (b) Adverse effects and precautions

           (1) Loss of appetite, insomnia, abdominal pain, and nervousness

           (2) May exacerbate preexisting hypertension and tic disorders

           (3) Labeling change warns of potential association with sudden cardiac death (SCD); therefore, not recommended for patients with known structural heart defects.

    iii. Potential association with SCD

       (a) No established evidence of causative relationship between stimulants and SCD

       (b) The frequency of SCD is no higher in children taking stimulants than in the general pediatric population.

       (c) The AAP recommends targeted cardiac history and careful physical examination before initiating stimulant therapy.

           (1) Routine electrocardiography is not recommended unless history and physical examination suggest cardiac disease.

           (2) For otherwise healthy children, stimulant therapy should not be withheld because of the inability to obtain an electrocardiogram or assessment by a pediatric cardiologist.

b. Nonstimulant medications

    i. Norepinephrine reuptake inhibitors (see Table 9)

       (a) Adverse effects: Dyspepsia, decreased appetite, weight loss, and fatigue

       (b) Labeling change warns of potential for severe liver injury, although routine monitoring of hepatic function is not required.

       (c) Black box warning about increased risk of suicidal ideation in children and adolescents

       (d) Does not exacerbate tics

    ii. α-Adrenergic receptor agonists: See Table 9 for a comparison of available products.

    iii. Antidepressants: Non-FDA label approved for the treatment of ADHD

       (a) Noradrenergic antidepressant (e.g., bupropion [Wellbutrin])

           (1) May use immediate- or extended-release product given in two or three doses

           (2) Contraindicated for children with active seizure disorder

       (b) Tricyclic antidepressants (e.g., imipramine, nortriptyline)

           (1) Baseline electrocardiogram is recommended before therapy initiation and after each dose increase.

           (2) Desipramine should be used with extreme caution because of reports of sudden death.

Table 8. Stimulant Agents for the Treatment of ADHD

Methylphenidate-Containing Products				
Medication	**Doses per Day**	**Onset of Effect**	**Duration of Effect (hours)**	**Other Comments**
Methylphenidate immediate release (Ritalin)	2 or 3	20–60 minutes	3–5	50:50 racemic mixture of L-threo and D-threo isomers
Dexmethylphenidate (Focalin)	2 or 3	20–60 minutes	3–5	Only D-threo isomer, thought to be pharmacologically active enantiomer D-Threo isomer has not been shown to hinder effectiveness or increase adverse effects Recommended doses are half those of methylphenidate immediate release Offers no proven pharmacoeconomic benefit over methylphenidate immediate-release products
Methylphenidate sustained release (Ritalin SR)	1 or 2	1–3 hours	2–6	
Methylphenidate extended release (Ritalin LA)	1	20–60 minutes	6–8	Contains 50% immediate-release and 50% extended-release beads Capsule may be opened and sprinkled on applesauce Efficacy may wane in after-school or late-afternoon hours, necessitating addition of methylphenidate immediate release for later-day coverage
Methylphenidate modified release (Metadate CD)	1	20–60 minutes	6–8	Capsule contains 30% immediate-release and 70% extended-release beads (slowly released about 4 hours after ingestion) Capsule may be opened and sprinkled on applesauce Efficacy may wane in after-school or late-afternoon hours, necessitating addition of methylphenidate immediate release for later-day coverage
Methylphenidate extended release (Methylin ER)	1	20–60 minutes	8	
Dexmethylphenidate extended release (Focalin XR)	1	20–60 minutes	8–12	Bimodal drug release results in peak serum concentrations at 1½ and 6½ hours after dose administration Shorter duration of action than methylphenidate OROS, so afternoon symptom control is not as good
Methylphenidate OROS (Concerta)	1	20–60 minutes	12	Outer capsule contains ~22% of the drug, allowing immediate release; tablet core contains remainder of drug, which is released over 10 hours, minimizing peak to trough fluctuations Swallow whole; do NOT chew, crush, or divide

Table 8. Stimulant Agents for the Treatment of ADHD *(continued)*

Methylphenidate-Containing Products				
Medication	**Doses per Day**	**Onset of Effect**	**Duration of Effect (hours)**	**Other Comments**
Methylphenidate transdermal system (Daytrana)	1	60 minutes	11–12	Apply to hip 2 hours before effect is needed Recommended to remove 9 hours after application, may be worn up to 16 hours Duration of effect is ~3 hours after patch removal May be worn while swimming or exercising
Amphetamine-Containing Products				
Medication	**Doses per Day**	**Onset of Effect**	**Duration of Effect (hours)**	**Other Comments**
Mixed amphetamine salts immediate release (Adderall)	1 or 2	20–60 minutes	6	
Mixed amphetamine salts extended release (Adderall XR)	1	20–60 minutes	10	Contains 50% immediate-release and 50% extended-release beads (released 4 hours after ingestion) May be sprinkled on applesauce
Lisdexamfetamine dimesylate (Vyvanse)	1	60 minutes	10–12	Prodrug with D-amphetamine covalently bound to L-lysine Designed for less abuse potential than amphetamine No clinical evidence of superiority over other amphetamine products

Table 9. Nonstimulant Agents for the Treatment of ADHD

Norepinephrine Reuptake Inhibitor				
Medication	**Doses per Day**	**Onset of Effect (weeks)**	**Duration of Effect (hours)**	**Other Comments**
Atomoxetine (Strattera)	1 or 2	1–2	10–12	May be considered first-line therapy for children with active substance abuse problem, comorbid anxiety, or tics Metabolized through cytochrome P450 2D6
α-Adrenergic Receptor Agonists				
Clonidine extended release (Kapvay)	1 or 2	1–2	10–12	May be more effective for hyperactivity than for inattention symptoms Lessens severity of tics, especially when used in combination with methylphenidate Primary adverse effect is sedation
Guanfacine extended release (Intuniv)	1	1–2	10–12	Improves comorbid tic disorder Less sedating than clonidine Abrupt discontinuation may cause rebound hypertension

Patient Case

12. The patient in question 11 has been doing well in school since methylphenidate (OROS) (Concerta) was initiated 6 months ago. His late-afternoon symptoms are well controlled; however, he has had insomnia since drug therapy initiation. Which is the best modification to his treatment regimen?

    A. Administer the Concerta dose later in the day.

    B. Change to methylphenidate modified release (Metadate CD) once a day.

    C. Change to methylphenidate transdermal patch (Daytrana).

    D. Change to atomoxetine at bedtime.

REFERENCES

Sepsis and Meningitis

1. American Academy of Pediatrics (AAP). Meningococcal infections. In: Pickering LK, ed. 2012 Red Book: Report of the Committee on Infectious Diseases, 29th ed. Elk Grove Village, IL: American Academy of Pediatrics, 2012:500-9.

2. Brierly J, Carcillo JA, Choong K, et al. Clinical practice parameters for hemodynamic support of pediatric and neonatal septic shock: 2007 update from the American College of Critical Care Medicine. Crit Care Med 2009;37:666-88.

3. Dellinger RP, Levy MM, Rhodes A, et al. Surviving sepsis campaign: international guidelines for management of severe sepsis and septic shock: 2012. Crit Care Med 2013;41:580-637.

4. Polin RA; Committee on Fetus and Newborn. Sepsis management of neonates with suspected or proven early onset bacterial sepsis. Pediatrics 2012;129:1006-15.

5. Wubbel L, McCracken GH. Management of bacterial meningitis: 1998. Pediatr Rev 1998;19:78-84.

Respiratory Syncytial Virus Infection

1. American Academy of Pediatrics Committee on Infectious Diseases and Bronchiolitis Guidelines Committee. Policy statement: updated guidance for palivizumab prophylaxis among infants and young children at increased risk of hospitalization for respiratory syncytial virus infection. Pediatrics 2014;134:415-20.

2. American Academy of Pediatrics Committee on Infectious Diseases and Bronchiolitis Guidelines Committee. Technical report: updated guidance for palivizumab prophylaxis among infants and young children at increased risk of hospitalization for respiratory syncytial virus infection. Pediatrics 2014;134:e620-e638.

3. American Academy of Pediatrics (AAP). Respiratory syncytial virus. In: Pickering LK, ed. 2012 Red Book: Report of the Committee on Infectious Diseases, 29th ed. Elk Grove Village, IL: American Academy of Pediatrics, 2012:609-18.

4. Mendonca EA, Phelan KJ, Zorc JJ, et al. Clinical practice guideline: the diagnosis, management, and prevention of bronchiolitis. Pediatrics 2014;134: e1474-e1502.

5. Patel H, Platt RW, Pekeles GS, et al. A randomized, controlled trial of the effectiveness of nebulized therapy with epinephrine compared with albuterol and saline in infants hospitalized for acute viral bronchiolitis. J Pediatr 2002;141:818-24.

Otitis Media

1. American Academy of Pediatrics (AAP). Principles of appropriate use for upper respiratory tract infections. In: Pickering LK, ed. 2012 Red Book: Report of the Committee on Infectious Diseases, 29th ed. Elk Grove Village, IL: American Academy of Pediatrics, 2012:802-5.

2. Lieberthal AS, Carrol AE, Chonmaitree T, et al. Clinical practice guideline: diagnosis and management of acute otitis media. Pediatrics 2013;131:e964-e999.

3. Rettig E, Tunkel DE. Contemporary concepts in management of acute otitis media in children. Otolaryngol Clin N Am 2014;47:651-72.

Immunizations

1. American Academy of Pediatrics (AAP). Active and passive immunization. In: Pickering LK, ed. 2012 Red Book: Report of the Committee on Infectious Diseases, 29th ed. Elk Grove Village, IL: American Academy of Pediatrics, 2012:1-109.

2. Feldman S. Interchangeability of vaccines. Pediatr Infect Dis J 2001;20:S23-9.

3. Santoli JM, Szilagyi PG, Rodewald LE. Barriers to immunization and missed opportunities. Pediatr Ann 1998;27:366-74.

Pediatric Seizure Disorders

1. Anderson GD. Children versus adults: pharmacokinetic and adverse-effect differences. Epilepsia 2002;43(suppl 3):53-9.

2. Asconape JJ. Some common issues in the use of antiepileptic drugs. Semin Neurol 2002;22:27-39.

3. Sarco DP, Bourgeois BFD. The safety and tolerability of newer antiepileptic drugs in children and adolescents. CNS Drugs 2010;24:399-430.

4. Sheth R, Gidel B. Optimizing epilepsy management in teenagers. J Child Neurol 2006;21:273-9.

Attention-Deficit/Hyperactivity Disorder

1. American Academy of Pediatrics (AAP). Subcommittee on attention-deficit/hyperactivity disorder. ADHD: clinical practice guideline for the diagnosis, evaluation, and treatment of attention-deficit/hyperactivity disorder in children and adolescents. Pediatrics 2011;128:1007-22.

2. American Psychiatric Association. Diagnostic and Statistical Manual of Mental Disorders, 5th ed. Arlington, VA: American Psychiatric Association, 2013.

3. Cortese S, Holtmann M, Banaschewski T, et al. Practitioner review: current best practice in the management of adverse events during treatment with ADHD medications in children and adolescents. J Child Psychol Psychiatry 2013;54:227-46.

4. Harstad E, Levy S, and Committee on Substance Abuse. Attention-deficit/hyperactivity disorder and substance abuse. Pediatrics 2014;134:e293-301.

5. Kaplan G, Newcorn JH. Pharmacotherapy for child and adolescent attention-deficit hyperactivity disorder. Pediatr Clin North Am 2011;58:99-120.

ANSWERS AND EXPLANATIONS TO PATIENT CASES

1. Answer: B

Group B *Streptococcus, Escherichia coli, Klebsiella* spp., and *Listeria* are the most likely pathogens of neonatal sepsis or meningitis. Ampicillin plus gentamicin administered in meningitic doses would provide reasonable empiric coverage. Although coagulase-negative *Staphylococcus* is the most likely cause of nosocomial neonatal sepsis, this patient's early presentation makes a hospital-acquired pathogen extremely unlikely. Therefore, vancomycin is unnecessary. Ampicillin plus ceftriaxone would provide adequate empiric antimicrobial coverage for the most likely pathogens. However, ceftriaxone use can result in biliary sludging, leading to reduced elimination of bilirubin and a potential risk of kernicterus in neonates. Ceftazidime plus gentamicin lacks coverage for *Listeria* and group B *Streptococcus,* which is still necessary empirically even though the mother received penicillin before delivery. In addition, empiric double-coverage of gram-negative organisms is not necessary for early neonatal sepsis.

2. Answer: C

Given this patient's age and culture results, the most likely infecting organism is *E. coli* or *Klebsiella* spp. (gram-negative rods), for which antimicrobial prophylaxis is not indicated. The most common pathogens causing meningitis in neonates do not warrant antimicrobial prophylaxis. If this patient had been older and infected with *N. meningitidis* or *H. influenzae,* antibiotic prophylaxis with rifampin would have been indicated for all close contacts, regardless of age or immunization status. Rifampin prophylaxis to eliminate nasal carriage is also indicated for people who receive index diagnoses of *N. meningitidis* and treatment with an antibiotic other than ceftriaxone.

3. Answer: C

The most likely causative organisms of sepsis or meningitis in this age group are *S. pneumoniae* and *N. meningitidis.* Therefore, a regimen of ceftriaxone plus vancomycin would provide appropriate empiric coverage. Depending on the regional incidence of resistant *S. pneumoniae,* empiric vancomycin may not be necessary. Ampicillin plus gentamicin would not provide adequate coverage. Cefuroxime does not provide

reliable penetration into the cerebrospinal fluid, so it would not be appropriate empiric coverage because this patient's presentation suggests he has meningitis. Rifampin would be the drug of choice for the prophylaxis of close contacts if this patient receives a diagnosis of meningococcal meningitis; however, it is inadequate for treatment.

4. Answer: B

Palivizumab is the drug of choice for prophylaxis against RSV infection in high-risk patient populations, including those born before 29 weeks' gestation, regardless of risk factors, who are 12 months or younger during RSV season. Patients born between 29 weeks' gestation and 32 weeks' gestation are no longer considered high risk based solely on their gestational age. To be considered as candidates for palivizumab prophylaxis, these infants must have a disease state (e.g., chronic lung disease, hemodynamically significant heart disease, airway anomalies, neuromuscular disease, or profound immunodeficiency) that puts them at risk for severe RSV infection. Other potential risk factors (e.g., siblings younger than 5 years or day care attenders) are no longer considered when determining the appropriateness of palivizumab prophylaxis. Patients with complex heart defects requiring surgical repair are at high risk of developing severe RSV infections; however, after the repair is complete, palivizumab is no longer warranted. Patients with a history of chronic lung disease who are 24 months or younger and who are receiving, or have received in the past 6 months, oxygen or medical management for chronic lung disease are also at risk of severe RSV infection.

5. Answer: D

There is no specific treatment of RSV infection. Intravenous fluids, oxygen, and mechanical ventilation, if needed, are indicated. Palivizumab is the drug of choice for RSV prophylaxis, but it has no role in treatment. Corticosteroids have not been shown to be of benefit and are therefore not indicated. Secondary bacterial infection with *H. influenzae* or *M. catarrhalis* may occur; however, empiric antibiotic therapy is not indicated.

6. Answer: A

Persistence of middle ear fluid after an episode of AOM is common. If these findings are not associated with signs and symptoms of infection, a diagnosis of OME is made. The AAP practice guideline for the management of OME recommends watchful waiting. A watch-and-wait approach would not be appropriate for this patient if she were given a diagnosis of AOM rather than OME because she is younger than 6 months. Spontaneous resolution of OME occurs within 3 months in 75%–90% of cases after AOM without residual morbidities. Children at high risk of speech and learning problems (e.g., craniofacial anomalies, Down syndrome, severe visual impairment) may require earlier, more aggressive intervention (e.g., tympanostomy tubes). Decongestants and antihistamines do not promote resolution or improve symptoms. Antibiotics are not effective in treating OME. However, high-dose amoxicillin (80–100 mg/kg/day) is considered first-line therapy for AOM, so if this patient's treatment with the initial course of lower-dose amoxicillin fails (which is not a recommended regimen) or if she develops new signs of infection, then high-dose amoxicillin will be an appropriate treatment choice. Up to 74% of streptococcal strains have been reported to be resistant to azithromycin, which also has poor activity against *H. influenzae,* so this would not be the best antibiotic option if an infection developed.

7. Answer: C

Four cases of otitis media in 12 months is considered recurrent otitis media, for which the watch-and-wait approach is not recommended. Previously, this patient would have been a candidate for antibiotic prophylaxis; however, this practice has fallen out of favor because of the significant risk of antimicrobial resistance compared with the minor reduction in the occurrence of otitis media. Tympanostomy tubes are typically reserved for patients in whom aggressive antibiotic therapy fails and may be effective only in otitis with bulging tympanic membrane. In addition, the greatest benefit of tympanostomy tubes may be in patients with persistent OMEs resulting in significant hearing loss. As long as this patient continues to respond to high-dose amoxicillin, this will be considered a first-line regimen. In addition, the pneumococcal and influenza vaccines should be administered according to the recommended schedule because these organisms are common causes of AOM.

8. Answer: D

Vaccines are often deferred for inappropriate reasons, leading to missed opportunities for immunization. Previous administration of IVIG can decrease the efficacy of live vaccines such as MMR and varicella, but it does not affect the efficacy of inactivated products. The suggested interval between an IVIG dose and the administration of live vaccines depends on the immune globulin product and indication. Concerns about an association between MMR vaccine and the development of autism and immunizations overwhelming the immune system have been disproved by scientific evaluation. The MMR vaccine is grown in chick embryo tissue; however, an egg allergy is not a contraindication to its administration.

9. Answer: A

Immunocompromised patients should not receive live vaccines; therefore, the MMR and varicella vaccines should be deferred in these patients. Mild cold-like symptoms, or administration of antibiotics for mild illnesses such as otitis media, are not a contraindication to vaccination, and deferring immunizations for such reasons is considered a missed opportunity. Patients with HIV, especially those with asymptomatic disease, should be considered candidates for all age-appropriate vaccines, including those containing live virus and the pneumococcal vaccine. Corticosteroid administration is an indication for deferral of live vaccines only if the patient is receiving high doses (more than 2 mg/kg/day of prednisone equivalent) for more than 14 days.

10. Answer: B

Rash associated with antiepileptic drugs is a common adverse effect and generally resolves within a few days after discontinuation. There is no reliable method to determine whether the rash will remain benign or progress to a more severe skin reaction, so discontinuation of the offending drug is warranted. Carbamazepine has a higher incidence of rash than oxcarbazepine, and cross-reactivity has been noted. Valproic acid is a good choice for managing partial seizures and has a low incidence of rash. However, the principal adverse effects of valproic acid include weight gain and menstrual irregularities, both of which would be undesirable in this overweight teenage girl. In addition, valproic acid is a known teratogen (pregnancy category D) that should be avoided if other options are available in females of reproductive age who are unreliable in their use of contraception. Levetiracetam (pregnancy category C) has a low incidence of rash and minimal drug interactions.

11. Answer: A

Stimulants, especially methylphenidate, are generally considered first-line therapy for treating ADHD. Because this patient shows symptoms at school and at home, the short duration of action (about 6–8 hours) of a twice-daily methylphenidate immediate-release regimen will probably not provide adequate symptom relief. Likewise, D-methylphenidate has a short duration of action. In addition, D-methylphenidate is no more effective and has no fewer adverse effects than methylphenidate immediate release. Therefore, D-methylphenidate is generally not considered cost-beneficial. Extended-release guanfacine was recently FDA label approved for the treatment of ADHD, but it should be reserved for patients with ADHD and tic disorders or those who have not responded to stimulant agents. Methylphenidate (OROS) with its longer duration of action (10–12 hours) would provide the best coverage. Therapy with this drug may be initiated without previous titration using methylphenidate immediate release.

12. Answer: C

Changing to a methylphenidate transdermal patch allows flexibility in the duration of drug effect. Wearing the patch for 9 hours results in about 12 hours of therapeutic effect; however, the patch may be removed sooner, thus reducing the duration of effect and allowing serum concentrations to decrease before bedtime. Response rates to atomoxetine are lower than to methylphenidate (OROS) in children with ADHD. In addition, the onset of therapeutic effect for atomoxetine is delayed (typically 2–4 weeks). Atomoxetine does not have the adverse effect of insomnia. Rather, fatigue and drowsiness are more common, the tolerability of which is improved with the initiation of atomoxetine at low doses with a gradual titration. The dose may also be administered in the evening to improve tolerability. Because this patient responded well to stimulant therapy with methylphenidate and there are disadvantages to atomoxetine (i.e., lower response rates and delayed onset), it would be best to manage the adverse effect of insomnia by altering the stimulant regimen. Administering methylphenidate OROS later in the day would probably worsen the insomnia. A better recommendation would be to administer methylphenidate OROS earlier in the morning, which would allow more time in the late afternoon and evening for the serum concentration to decrease before bedtime. Changing to a shorter-acting methylphenidate product (e.g., methylphenidate CD or LA) might improve the insomnia, but because of its shorter duration of action, it might compromise late-afternoon symptom control.

ANSWERS AND EXPLANATIONS TO SELF-ASSESSMENT QUESTIONS

1. Answer: B
The pathogens most likely to cause pediatric sepsis or meningitis are *S. pneumoniae, N. meningitidis,* and *H. influenzae. P. aeruginosa* is more commonly associated with nosocomial sepsis. Adolescents who develop an RSV infection typically present with mild upper respiratory tract symptoms, whereas this patient's presentation suggests meningitis.

2. Answer: B
Before the 2014 publication of the AAP's updated guidelines, infants who were born before 31 weeks', 6 days' gestation who were 6 months or younger at the beginning of RSV season were considered at high risk of severe infection; therefore, routine palivizumab prophylaxis was recommended based solely on their prematurity. The 2014 guidelines changed the prematurity-based criteria for routine palivizumab prophylaxis to include only infants born before 29 weeks' gestation who are younger than 12 months at the beginning of RSV season. According to the new guidelines, infants born between 29 weeks' and 32 weeks' gestation must have chronic lung disease, hemodynamically significant congenital heart disease, airway anomalies, neuromuscular disease, or profound immunocompromise to be considered candidates for palivizumab prophylaxis. Risk factors such as day care attendance and school-aged siblings are no longer considered when determining whether prophylaxis is warranted. Routine prophylaxis for otherwise healthy, full-term neonates is not recommended because evidence of benefit is lacking.

3. Answer: C
Prophylaxis with rifampin is recommended for close contacts of patients with *N. meningitidis* or *H. influenzae,* regardless of their immunization status. Postexposure prophylaxis against pneumococcal meningitis is not recommended.

4. Answer: D
All scheduled immunizations should be given during the same visit. Delaying some vaccines until a later date is considered a missed opportunity. Oral polio vaccine is no longer recommended as part of the routine schedule because of the risk of vaccine-associated poliomyelitis, which accounts for most newly diagnosed cases in the United States since 1979. Premature neonates should be vaccinated according to chronologic age, and doses should not be reduced. As of 2008, influenza vaccine is recommended for all children 6 months to 18 years of age during influenza season.

5. Answer: B
Otitis media is most commonly caused by *S. pneumoniae, H. influenzae, M. catarrhalis,* and viruses. Blood culture results do not predict causative organisms of otitis media. If the patient is older than 2 years and does not have severe symptoms (i.e., moderate to severe otalgia or temperature of 39°C or greater), delaying the decision to prescribe antibiotics is an acceptable strategy. If otalgia or fever persists for more than 48–72 hours, then antibiotic therapy is acceptable, but if these symptoms resolve spontaneously within this time, antibiotics are not necessary. If antibiotics are warranted and the patient does not have an allergy, high-dose amoxicillin is the treatment of choice rather than azithromycin. Broad-spectrum antibiotics such as ceftriaxone should be reserved for resistant cases.

6. Answer: D
In general, patients who do not respond to one stimulant agent should be treated with a different stimulant before they are considered not to have responded to this class of drug therapy. However, switching from a methylphenidate-containing stimulant to extended-release mixed amphetamine salts (a different stimulant) should be avoided in this patient because amphetamine-containing products have been associated with SCD in children with structural heart defects. The methylphenidate transdermal system has a duration of action and efficacy similar to those of methylphenidate OROS; therefore, it is unlikely to benefit this patient because her therapy with methylphenidate immediate release and methylphenidate OROS has already failed. If adherence or difficulty swallowing pills were a suspected cause of treatment failure in this patient, a patch might be a reasonable alternative. Clonidine may be added as an adjunctive therapy for patients whose treatment with a single stimulant agent fails; however, it should not be used as the sole agent for treating ADHD. Atomoxetine, a nonstimulant, would be a

reasonable alternative to the stimulant class of agents in this patient because some patients respond better to one class of agent than another.

7. Answer: A

Valproic acid is considered a first-line therapy for treating absence seizures. If the patient is having breakthrough seizures on ethosuximide—also a first-line therapy—and the dose has been maximized, it is reasonable to switch to valproic acid. Phenytoin, phenobarbital, and gabapentin have not been shown effective in treating absence seizures.

8. Answer: C

	Adverse Event (loss of appetite)	
	Yes	No
Exposure (stimulant)		
Yes	7 (*a*)	193 (*b*)
No	1 (*c*)	197 (*d*)

Odds ratio = (*a*/*c*)/(*b*/*d*)
= (7/1)/(193/197)
= 7.15

9. Answer: C

A case series does not reliably establish a causal relationship but rather suggests a potential hypothesis to be further studied. Given the current knowledge about the potential risk of kernicterus related to ceftriaxone use, obtaining investigational review board approval for a randomized controlled or a crossover trial design would be difficult, given ethical considerations, although this study design is the gold standard for establishing a causal relationship. Therefore, a retrospective cohort would be best to investigate a causal relationship in this instance.

10. Answer: D

Patients with congenital heart defects, particularly those with hemodynamically significant lesions, are at high risk of severe RSV infection regardless of their gestational age. These patients are considered to be at high risk if they are younger than 12 months at the beginning of RSV season and have not undergone definitive surgical repair of their heart defect. It is not recommended that palivizumab be initiated as routine prophylaxis in hospitalized patients because it does not reduce the incidence of nosocomial-acquired RSV infection. However, patients currently receiving a course of palivizumab (one dose per month for 5 months) at the time of hospital admission should have that intervention continued. In addition, cardiopulmonary bypass reduces palivizumab serum concentrations; therefore, patients undergoing congenital heart defect repair during RSV season should receive a postoperative dose of palivizumab as soon as they are medically stable, regardless of when their next scheduled dose is due.

Geriatrics

Lisa C. Hutchison, Pharm.D., MPH, BCPS, FCCP

University of Arkansas for Medical Sciences
College of Pharmacy
Little Rock, Arkansas

Geriatrics

Lisa C. Hutchison, Pharm.D., MPH, BCPS, FCCP

University of Arkansas for Medical Sciences
College of Pharmacy
Little Rock, Arkansas

Learning Objectives

1. Summarize common age-related pharmacokinetic and pharmacodynamic changes in older adults.
2. Evaluate the pharmacotherapeutic regimens of older adults to support optimal risk and benefit of medications.
3. Assess inappropriate medication prescribing in older adults using accepted tools.
4. Recommend appropriate pharmacotherapy for patients with dementia.
5. Evaluate the risks and benefits of antipsychotic use in older adults with dementia.
6. Recommend appropriate interventions for patients with behavioral and psychological symptoms related to dementia (BPSD).
7. Differentiate between the types of urinary incontinence and recommend appropriate treatments.
8. Recommend an appropriate benign prostatic hypertrophy (BPH) treatment based on the American Urological Association Symptom Index (AUASI).
9. Recommend appropriate analgesic therapy for older adults with osteoarthritis.
10. Discuss the risks and benefits of medication classes used to treat rheumatoid arthritis and associated comorbidities.

Self-Assessment Questions

Answers and explanations to these questions can be found at the end of this chapter.

Questions 1 and 2 pertain to the following case:
A.R. is an 85-year-old man who presents to the primary care clinic after the death of his spouse 1 month ago. His medical history is significant for hypertension, hyperlipidemia, BPH, and major depressive disorder. His current medications include lisinopril 10 mg daily, atorvastatin 20 mg daily, tamsulosin 0.4 mg daily, diazepam 5 mg at bedtime as needed for sleep, and escitalopram 10 mg daily. His daughter reports that he has been more lethargic and unsteady walking during the past 3 days. The patient reports trouble sleeping and taking diazepam every night this past week. His blood pressure (BP) is 135/72 mm Hg, and his heart rate (HR) is 76 beats/minute. Urinalysis was negative, thyroid-stimulating hormone (TSH) was within the reference range, and Geriatric Depression Scale (GDS) score was 6/15.

1. Which medication is contributing most to this patient's lethargy and confusion?
   - A. Diazepam.
   - B. Lisinopril.
   - C. Atorvastatin.
   - D. Escitalopram.

2. Which age-related change in pharmacokinetics is most likely to underlie this patient's medication-related problem?
   - A. Delayed oral absorption.
   - B. Decreased renal excretion.
   - C. Slowed metabolism in the liver.
   - D. Decreased volume of distribution.

Questions 3–5 pertain to the following case:
P.J., a 76-year-old woman, was recently admitted to a long-term care facility for rehabilitation after multiple falls at home. Her medical history is significant for hypertension, hypothyroidism, Alzheimer disease (AD), hyperlipidemia, and osteoarthritis. She currently takes metoprolol succinate 50 mg daily, levothyroxine 75 mcg daily, atorvastatin 10 mg daily, and donepezil 10 mg daily. Her BP is 126/80 mm Hg and heart rate is 66 beats/minute. Basic metabolic panel results were all within reference ranges; 25-hydroxy vitamin D level was 20 ng/mL, TSH 1.89 mU/L, total cholesterol 180 mg/dL, low-density lipoprotein cholesterol 140 mg/dL, high-density lipoprotein cholesterol 35 mg/dL, and triglycerides 176 mg/dL. Her Mini–Mental State Examination (MMSE) score was 16/30, and her GDS score was 2/15.

3. Which recommendation would be most appropriate to reduce the risk of falls in this patient?
   - A. Begin memantine titration.
   - B. Initiate vitamin D 1000 units daily.
   - C. Decrease metoprolol succinate to 25 mg daily.
   - D. Initiate calcium carbonate 500 mg twice daily.

4. Which is the best intervention for reducing the incidence of ischemic stroke in this patient?
   - A. Initiate aspirin 81 mg daily.
   - B. Increase atorvastatin to 20 mg daily.

C. Initiate hydrochlorothiazide 25 mg daily.

D. Increase metoprolol succinate to 100 mg daily.

5. Which would be most appropriate for complaints of osteoarthritic knee pain?

A. Ibuprofen 200 mg four times daily.

B. Acetaminophen 650 mg three times daily.

C. Tramadol 50 mg three times daily as needed for pain.

D. Hydrocodone/acetaminophen 5/325 mg every 4 hours as needed for pain.

Questions 6–8 pertain to the following case:
T.W. is an 80-year-old woman who presents to your clinic accompanied by her daughter, who no longer feels comfortable leaving her mother alone because of her mother's "increasing forgetfulness." T.W.'s medical history is significant for type 2 diabetes mellitus, hypertension, coronary artery disease, congestive heart failure, and osteoarthritis. She is taking the following medications: acetaminophen 650 mg every 6 hours as needed for pain, lisinopril 20 mg daily, furosemide 20 mg daily, potassium chloride 20 mEq daily, carvedilol 12.5 mg twice daily, and glipizide 5 mg daily. Her MMSE score was 18/30. Blood work drawn last week revealed a normal basic metabolic panel, with the exception of a serum glucose reading of 65 mg/dL. Her hemoglobin A1C result was 5.6%. A urinalysis was negative. No nutritional deficiencies were noted. The patient's BP is 130/80 mm Hg, and her HR is 60 beats/minute. She receives a diagnosis of AD.

6. Which initial intervention would be most appropriate to help with this patient's cognitive function?

A. Donepezil 10 mg daily.

B. Galantamine ER 24 mg daily.

C. Memantine 10 mg twice daily.

D. Rivastigmine patch 4.6 mg daily.

7. Which intervention would be most appropriate to prevent an adverse drug reaction?

A. Discontinue glipizide.

B. Discontinue lisinopril.

C. Reduce carvedilol to 6.25 mg twice daily.

D. Reduce potassium chloride to 10 mEq daily.

8. One year later, the patient returns to clinic. She has moved in with her daughter. Lately she is wandering around the house continuously. She frequently changes clothes and asks repetitive questions. Her current medication regimen includes donepezil 10 mg daily, which she has been taking for the past 6 months. Which would be most appropriate for this patient's new behavioral symptoms?

A. Initiate olanzapine 5 mg daily.

B. Initiate risperidone 0.5 mg twice daily.

C. Change donepezil dosage to 23 mg daily.

D. Change acetaminophen to 650 mg every 6 hours around the clock.

9. A.S. is an 80-year-old woman who had a total right knee replacement 3 days ago after conservative strategies for osteoarthritis failed. Her medical history is significant for hypothyroidism, osteoarthritis, and hyperlipidemia. Her current medications include simvastatin 20 mg daily, risedronate 35 mg weekly, levothyroxine 75 mcg daily, and oxycodone/acetaminophen 5/325 mg 1 tablet every 4 hours as needed for moderate pain. She is in the hospital preparing for discharge. As the pharmacist is counseling the patient on her discharge medication, the patient reports experiencing a new onset of "losing her water" the day before and again overnight. Which intervention would be most appropriate for this patient?

A. Urinalysis.

B. Pelvic floor exercises.

C. Tolterodine 2 mg daily.

D. Duloxetine 20 mg daily.

Questions 10 and 11 pertain to the following case:
J.P., a 69-year-old man with hypertension and BPH, is admitted after being involved in a motorcycle collision. He sustained serious injuries, resulting in a left leg above-the-knee amputation, and has undergone several surgeries and rehabilitation in the past 2 weeks. His current medications include tamsulosin 0.4 mg daily, atenolol 25 mg daily, amlodipine 10 mg daily, senna/docusate 8.6/50 mg twice daily, oxycodone controlled release 10 mg every 12 hours, and hydromorphone 4 mg every 3 hours as needed for breakthrough pain (uses 1–2 daily). His current BP is 155/88 mm Hg, HR

is 84 beats/minute, and postvoid residual (PVR) volume is 400 mL after voiding 110 mL. His chronic medical conditions are unremarkable except for hypertension, BPH, and gastroesophageal reflux disease (GERD).

10. Which intervention would be most appropriate for this patient?

    A. Increase tamsulosin to 0.8 mg.

    B. Increase atenolol to 50 mg daily.

    C. Change tamsulosin to terazosin 5 mg daily.

    D. Reduce hydromorphone to 2 mg every 3 hours as needed for breakthrough pain.

11. One year later, J.P. complains of osteoarthritis of his right knee. His current medications are amlodipine 10 mg daily, acetaminophen 1000 mg three times daily, omeprazole 40 mg daily, and aspirin 81 mg daily. Which agent would be best to initiate for this patient's knee pain?

    A. Celecoxib 200 mg daily

    B. Naproxen 500 mg twice daily

    C. Diclofenac 1% gel apply 4 g to knee every 6 hours.

    D. Methylprednisolone 40 mg injected into affected joint.

Questions 12 and 13 pertain to the following case:
D.C., a 72-year-old woman whose medical history is significant for rheumatoid arthritis, type 2 diabetes mellitus, GERD, and hypothyroidism, presents to the clinic with inflammation of the joints of the hands and stiffness lasting 1–2 hours in the morning. She is a smoker, weighs 82 kg, and is 66 inches tall. Her current medications include pantoprazole 40 mg daily, metformin 850 mg twice daily, levothyroxine 100 mcg daily, folic acid 1 mg daily, methotrexate 12.5 mg weekly, naproxen 500 mg twice daily, calcium 600 mg twice daily, and vitamin D 1000 units twice daily. Her blood work reveals a negative rheumatoid factor but positive anti–cyclic citrullinated peptides. The physician determines that this is a flare of moderate disease.

12. Which would be the most appropriate intervention for this patient's rheumatoid arthritis?

    A. Change naproxen to prednisone 20 mg daily.

    B. Change methotrexate to 25 mg intramuscularly.

    C. Switch methotrexate to leflunomide 20 mg daily.

    D. Add sulfasalazine 500 mg twice daily and hydroxychloroquine 400 mg daily.

13. Three months later she has responded to therapy. A bone mineral density T-score of –2.0 is reported from her latest scan. Her vitamin D level is 40 ng/mL. Which recommendation would be most appropriate to help reduce the risk of major osteoporotic fractures in this patient?

    A. Raloxifene 60 mg daily.

    B. Risedronate 35 mg weekly.

    C. Teriparatide 20 mcg subcutaneously daily.

    D. Increase to calcium 600 mg and vitamin D 2000 mg twice daily.

I. **OPTIMIZING PHARMACOTHERAPY IN OLDER ADULTS**

    A. Aging

        1. Aging definition: A normal process whereby the human body declines after peak growth and development. Generally aging results as the body responds to environmental stressors according to the person's health and lifestyle factors together with genetic makeup. If environmental stressors are severe enough or individual factors have too small of a reserve capacity, aging causes frailty, disability, and increased vulnerability to disease and death.

        2. At present, 13.3% (2010 U.S. Census) of Americans are 65 years or older. This figure is projected to rise to 20% by 2050. Older adults are about 13% of the population, but they are responsible for:

            a. 34% of medication costs

            b. 36% of hospital stays

            c. 40% of medication-related hospitalizations

            d. 50% of medication-related deaths

        3. At least $30 billion/year is spent on medication-related morbidity.

        4. There is large heterogeneity in older people: Diversity is increasing, and incomes have a wide range; some people live independently into their 90s and beyond, whereas others become frail and dependent at a younger age. Measurement of aging with years of life is insensitive to the differences between older people.

            a. If one survives to age 65, it is likely that he or she will live an additional 13–20 years.

            b. If one survives to age 85, it is likely that he or she will live an additional 6–7 years.

    B. Pharmacokinetic Changes Associated with Aging

        1. Common physiologic changes occur in most older adults, but they are highly variable because of differences in genetics, lifestyle, and environment.

Table 1. Common Physiologic Changes with Age That May Change Drug Pharmacokinetics

Organ System	Physiologic Change with Aging	Effect on Pharmacokinetics
Gastrointestinal	↑ Or no change in stomach pH ↓ GI blood flow Slowed gastric emptying Slowed GI transit	↓ Absorption of some drugs and nutrients requiring acid environment Absorption rate may be prolonged
Skin	Thinning of dermis Loss of subcutaneous fat	↓ Or no change to drug reservoir formation with transdermal formulation
Body composition	↓ Total body water ↓ Lean body mass ↑ Body fat ↓ Or unchanged serum albumin ↑ α_1-Acid glycoprotein	↑ Volume of distribution and accumulation of lipid-soluble drugs ↓ Volume of distribution of water-soluble drugs ↑ Free fraction of highly protein-bound drugs
Liver	↓ Liver mass ↓ Blood flow to the liver ↓ Or no change in CYP enzymes	↓ First-pass extraction and metabolism ↑ Half-life and ↓ clearance of drugs with a high first-pass extraction and metabolism ↓ Or no change in phase I metabolism No change in phase II drug metabolism
Renal	↓ Glomerular filtration rate ↓ Renal blood flow ↓ Tubular secretion ↓ Renal mass	↓ Renal elimination of many medications ↑ Half-life of renally eliminated drugs and metabolites

CYP = cytochrome P450; GI = gastrointestinal.

2. Absorption
    a. Iron, vitamin B_{12}, antifungals, and calcium are decreased with hypochlorhydria or achlorhydria.
    b. Slower gastric emptying can increase risk of ulceration from aspirin, nonsteroidal anti-inflammatory drugs (NSAIDs), or potassium chloride tablets.
    c. Most drugs are absorbed by passive diffusion without significant age-related changes.
    d. Transdermal formulations usually require a subcutaneous fat layer to form a drug reservoir for absorption. Use with caution in patients who are thin or cachetic.
3. Distribution
    a. Lipid-soluble benzodiazepines such as diazepam have an increased half-life in older people.
    b. Highly albumin-bound drugs such as phenytoin may have a larger fraction of free (active) drug.
    c. P-glycoprotein, an efflux transporter for several organs including the brain, decreases with aging, which may lead to higher brain concentrations of medications. One example is opioid analgesics.
4. Metabolism
    a. Morphine and propranolol clearance are substantially reduced because of a reduction in first-pass metabolism.
    b. Changes in metabolism through phase I (oxidative) and cytochrome P450 (CYP) enzymes are variable and confounded by age, sex, concomitant drugs, and genetics.
    c. Lorazepam, oxazepam, and temazepam are dependent on phase II metabolism and are less affected by age-related changes in metabolism.
5. Elimination
    a. Drugs eliminated through glomerular filtration must be dosed according to individual estimated renal function.
    b. The Cockcroft-Gault equation is a validated method to estimate creatinine clearance (CrCl) for drug dosing in older adults.
    c. The National Kidney Foundation recommends using the Chronic Kidney Disease Epidemiology Collaboration (CKD-EPI) Creatinine Equation (2009) to estimate glomerular filtration rate. However, this recommendation has not been validated in older adults.

Table 2. Differences in Renal Estimation with Common Formulas

Patient: 85-year-old person with an SCr of 1 mg/dL	Cockcroft-Gault Creatinine Clearance (mL/minute)	MDRD Estimated Glomerular Filtration Rate (mL/minute)	CKD-EPI Creatinine Clearance Equation
64-inch-tall white woman weighing 60 kg	39	56	51 (stage 3)
64-inch-tall African American woman weighing 60 kg	39	68	60 (stage 2)
70-inch-tall white man weighing 75 kg	57	75	68 (stage 2)
70-inch-tall African American man weighing 75 kg	57	91	79 (stage 2)
Cockcroft-Gault: CrCl = [(140 − age) × weight in kg]/[(72 × SCr)] × 0.85 if female [use actual weight if it is less than ideal body weight]			
MDRD: estimated GFR = 186 × $SCr^{1.154}$ × $Age^{-0.203}$ × 1.21 if black × 0.742 if female			
CKD-EPI Creatinine Equation 2009[a]: CKD-EPI equation expressed as a single equation: GFR = 141 × [min(SCr/κ, 1)$^{\alpha}$ × max(SCr/κ, 1)$^{-1.209}$ × $Age^{-0.993}$] × 1.018 [if female] × 1.159 [if African American]			

[a]SCr is standardized serum creatinine in milligrams per deciliter; κ is 0.7 for women and 0.9 for men, α is −0.329 for women and −0.411 for men, min indicates the minimum of SCr/κ or 1, and max indicates the maximum of SCr/κ or 1.

CKD-EPI = Chronic Kidney Disease Epidemiology Collaboration; MDRD = Modified Diet Renal Disease.

d. Some clinicians round the serum creatinine concentration (SCr) up to 1 mg/dL because older adults have lower muscle mass, which produces less creatinine, and extremely low SCr would overestimate renal function with these formulas. This rounding is not supported by evidence and remains controversial. Also, clinicians may use adjusted weight for obese patients with formulas used for younger adults.

C. Pharmacodynamic Changes Common with Aging
  1. Increased sensitivity
    a. Benzodiazepines
    b. Opioids
    c. Antipsychotics, metoclopramide: extrapyramidal effects and tardive dyskinesia
    d. Tricyclic antidepressants, α-blockers, antihypertensives: orthostatic hypotension
    e. Warfarin
    f. NSAIDs: gastrointestinal (GI) bleeding
    g. Anticholinergic agents
  2. Decreased sensitivity
    a. β-blockers
    b. β-agonists
  3. Impaired homeostasis
    a. Diuretics, angiotensin-converting enzyme inhibitors: sodium and electrolytes
    b. Diuretics: hydration status

Patient Cases

1. N.H. is an 85-year-old woman who resides at home with her daughter. She weighs 65 kg. Her medical history is significant for type 2 diabetes mellitus and hypertension, and 1 year ago she sustained a right hip fracture after a fall. Her regularly scheduled medications include glyburide 10 mg daily, lisinopril 10 mg daily, metformin 500 mg twice daily, aspirin 81 mg daily, and a multivitamin daily. Her as-needed medications include melatonin 6 mg at bedtime as needed for sleep, meclizine 25 mg ½ tablet three times daily as needed for dizziness, and docusate 100 mg twice daily. Her laboratory results reveal fasting plasma glucose 90 mg/dL, sodium 138 mEq/L, potassium 4.5 mEq/L, chloride 102 mEq/L, CO_2 25 mEq/L, blood urea nitrogen (BUN) 30 mg/dL, SCr 1.8 mg/dL, and thyroid-stimulating hormone (TSH) 4.0 mU/L. Considering potential for altered pharmacokinetics, which medications are the most likely potential problems for N.H.?

  A. Aspirin and melatonin.
  B. Lisinopril and meclizine.
  C. Lisinopril and metformin.
  D. Glyburide and metformin.

2. Considering potential for increased pharmacodynamic sensitivity, which medications are the most likely potential problems for N.H.?

  A. Aspirin and melatonin.
  B. Lisinopril and meclizine.
  C. Lisinopril and metformin.
  D. Glyburide and metformin.

D. Optimal Pharmacotherapy in Older People
   1. An optimal pharmacotherapeutic regimen is one in which the benefit of the therapy outweighs risk for adverse effects.
   2. To reduce risk, doses of many medications must be adjusted in older people because of age-associated changes in drug pharmacokinetics and pharmacodynamics.
   3. Alternate medications may be more appropriate because of these changes.
   4. Therapeutic window becomes smaller even with dose and drug adjustments.

E. Drug-Related Assessment for Risk in Older Adults
   1. Overuse of medications
      a. Unnecessary drugs: Use of more medications than clinically indicated and unneeded therapeutic duplication
      b. Common unnecessary drugs: GI agents, central nervous system agents, vitamins, minerals
      c. May be caused by
         i. Prescribing cascade: When drug is prescribed for treatment of another drug's side effects
         ii. Multiple prescribers
         iii. Care transitions
   2. Underuse of medications
      a. Omitted but necessary or indicated drug therapy or inadequate dosing
      b. Commonly underused drugs: anticoagulants, statins, antihypertensives
      c. Medications considered appropriate according to guidelines may be omitted because prescriber or patient is overly wary of adverse drug effects.
   3. Nonadherence
      a. Unintentional nonadherence caused by complex drug regimen
      b. Dementia or other cognitive impairment increases risk.
      c. Cost of medications is another barrier.
      d. Intentional nonadherence because of patient health beliefs or concerns
   4. Withdrawal syndromes
      a. Abrupt discontinuation of medication may cause rebound symptoms or delirium.
      b. Common culprits: antihypertensives, antidepressants, anxiolytics, pain medications
   5. Inappropriate medications
      a. Explicit tools frequently used to identify for quality measure. Best known is the Beers List of Drugs to Avoid in the Elderly, updated in 2012.
         i. Evidence-based list of drugs likely to cause problems
         ii. Adopted by many federal agencies and Part D plans
         iii. Arranged as drugs and drug classes to always avoid, drugs to avoid in certain diseases or conditions, and drugs to be used with caution
         iv. Examples: anticholinergics, long half-life benzodiazepines, sedative-hypnotics, older anti-psychotics, certain opiates or pain medications, hypoglycemics, NSAIDs and GI drugs
      b. Implicit tools are patient-centered, take more time to apply. Best studied is the Medication Appropriateness Index.
         i. 10 questions to ask about each medication regarding indication, effect, dosing, directions, interactions, duration, and cost
         ii. Indication, effectiveness, and correct dosage have most weight.
   6. Choosing Wisely Campaign
      a. Two sets of five things to question in older adults
      b. Seven of the 10 items are drug related.
         i. Antipsychotics in patients with dementia should be avoided.
         ii. Target hemoglobin A1C in diabetes management 7.5% or higher

   iii. Avoid benzodiazepines and sedative-hypnotics for insomnia, agitation, or delirium.

   iv. Do not start antimicrobials to treat bacteriuria without symptoms.

   v. Assess benefit and risk of cholinesterase inhibitors.

   vi. Appetite stimulants not helpful for anorexia or cachexia

   vii. Drug regimen review is necessary with every new prescription.

F. Function with Aging

 1. Quality of life, place of residence, social and physical function may become more important than duration of life.

 2. Instrumental activities of daily living (IADLs)

  a. Examples: housekeeping, using phone, managing medications, shopping, cooking, managing money

  b. Need to do these to live independently

 3. Activities of daily living (ADLs)

  a. Examples: feeding, dressing, bathing, toileting, transferring

  b. Nursing home or home caregivers required if ADLs cannot be performed

 4. Cognitive screening: Mini–Mental State Examination (MMSE), Montreal Cognitive Assessment (MoCA), St. Louis University Mental Status (SLUMS) Examination

 5. Mood: Geriatric Depression Scale

 6. Gait and balance: Timed Up and Go, Berg Balance Scale

 7. Drugs can alter cognition, mood, and mobility.

G. Geriatric Syndromes

 1. Geriatric syndromes follow a concentric model, with multiple risk factors and numerous etiologies contributing to a clinical presentation rather than the linear model with one etiology following a defined pathogenesis.

 2. Falls

  a. Possible etiologies: psychoactive medications, polypharmacy, orthostatic hypotension, hyponatremia, myocardial infarction, urinary tract infection

  b. Examples of contributing risk factors: vitamin D deficiency, poor balance, poor vision, environment

 3. Delirium

  a. Possible etiologies: psychoactive medications, polypharmacy, hyponatremia, myocardial infarction, urinary tract infection

  b. Example of contributing risk factors: dementia, stroke, vitamin B_{12} deficiency, poor hearing, lack of sleep

 4. Hazards of hospitalization

  a. Usual aging involves a decline in numerous organ systems, which are further compromised when an older patient is admitted to the hospital and expected to remain in bed.

   i. Immobilization leads to deconditioning. Regaining what was lost takes longer in older adults.

   ii. Immobilization and inability to obtain water lead to decreased plasma volume, which can lead to syncope, falls, and fractures.

   iii. Sensory deprivation from isolation and lack of glasses or hearing aids can lead to delirium, which may be treated with restraints or antipsychotics.

   iv. Immobilization and "tethers" (e.g., intravenous lines, oxygen lines, catheters) necessitate nursing assistance to bathroom. Unavoidable delay may lead to incontinence, catheters, infections, and pressure sores.

   v. Prescribed diets or nothing-by-mouth status lead to dehydration, malnutrition, insertion of feeding tubes, and aspiration pneumonia.

b. Preventable adverse drug events are frequent contributors to increased morbidity and mortality in older hospitalized adults.

c. Functional decline typically follows a hospitalization and is referred to as a cascade to dependency.

d. One study showed subjects that had a loss of ADLs at discharge had a higher mortality rate (40% at 12 months), with only 30% returning to baseline function.

e. Early mobility, adequate nutrition, reduced polypharmacy, and early discharge planning may reduce functional disability and length of stay.

Patient Cases

3. N.H. is admitted to the hospital with a broken arm after a fall. While in the hospital she was on bedrest most of the time, lost 2 kg (current weight 63 kg), and had trouble sleeping. She is to be discharged to a rehabilitation facility for 2–3 weeks of therapy. Her medications at discharge are glipizide 5 mg daily, lisinopril 10 mg daily, aspirin 81 mg daily, multivitamin daily, mirtazapine 15 mg at bedtime, calcium 500 mg twice daily, and tramadol 25 mg every 8 hours as needed for pain. When recommending medication changes for this patient, which functional assessment is most important to evaluate?

   A. IADLs

   B. Depression

   C. Pressure sores

   D. Gait and balance

4. To maintain and improve function in N.H., which intervention is best to implement?

   A. Add simvastatin 10 mg daily.

   B. Increase lisinopril to 20 mg daily.

   C. Add vitamin D 1000 units twice daily.

   D. Change tramadol to naproxen 500 mg twice daily as needed for pain.

II. DEMENTIA

A. Epidemiology
   1. Affects 4–5 million in the United States
   2. Of people 65 years and older, 6% have dementia, increasing to 30–50% of those 85 years and older.

B. Dementia Definition: Cognitive decline in complex attention, executive function, learning and memory, language, perceptual–motor or social cognition AND interferes with work or social functions
   1. Delirium should be ruled out first.
      a. Delirium: A disturbance in attention and awareness developing over hours to days with fluctuation over the course of the day
      b. It is a geriatric syndrome, with age, underlying dementia, functional impairment, medical comorbidities as risk factors.
      c. Etiologies include medications such as sedative hypnotics, antidepressants, anticholinergics, opioids, anticonvulsants, and antiparkinson drugs.
   2. Mild cognitive impairment (MCI) is a term used for people with some deficits in cognition that do not meet criteria for dementia.
   3. Alzheimer disease (AD) is most common type of dementia.

4. Theories of pathogenesis include cholinergic, β-amyloid plaques, tau protein (neurofibrillary tangles), genetics (apolipoprotein E4), and inflammation (cytokines, prion).

5. Multiple other types of dementia exist; few are reversible.

Table 3. Comparisons of Memory Impairment and Dementias with AD

Disease	Differences from AD	Treatment Notes
Common Irreversible Causes		
MCI	No interference with work or social functions 1 in 5 progress to AD	Eliminate or control risk factors for dementia May use CIs, which reduced risk for progression by 40% in 1 study
Vascular dementia	Includes focal neurological signs and symptoms Radiologic evidence of stroke Onset within 3–6 months of stroke Abrupt deterioration followed by stepwise progression	Control of cardiac and vascular risk factors
Lewy body dementia	Fluctuating cognition with pronounced variation in attention and alertness Recurrent visual hallucinations Motor features of PD	Avoid typical antipsychotics, which may worsen motor symptoms
Dementia of advanced PD	PD onset predates cognitive impairment Usually at latter stages of PD	May use CIs or memantine
Frontotemporal dementia	Affects personality, behavior, self-care, and language Onset in ages 45–65 with a 2- to 10-year course	CIs may worsen behavior and cause agitation
Reversible Causes		
Vitamin B_{12} deficiency	Progressive memory loss Vitamin B_{12} serum concentration <300 pg/mL May be anemic also, but folic acid may disguise the anemia	Replace vitamin B_{12} per standard protocols
Hypothyroidism	Deficient or inadequate replacement of thyroxine	Levothyroxine replacement per standard protocols
Depression	Trouble concentrating and memory Apathy and "I don't care" responses	Treatment of depression per standard protocols
NPH	Triad of progressive memory loss, incontinence, and gait abnormality Symptoms improve after lumbar puncture	Surgical placement of ventricular shunt

AD = Alzheimer disease; CI = cholinesterase inhibitor; MCI = mild cognitive impairment; NPH = normal pressure hydrocephalus; PD = Parkinson disease.

C. Assessment Tools
1. Folstein MMSE
    a. 30-point scale; higher is better function.
    b. Untreated AD: Score usually decreases 3–4 points a year.
    c. Heavily relies on verbal and language skills so less accurate if education is poor
2. SLUMS Examination
    a. 30-point scale; higher number is better function.
    b. Includes adjustment of scores for lower educational status
3. MoCA
    a. 30-point scale; higher number is better function.
    b. Less reliant on verbal or language skills
4. Mini-Cog Assessment
    a. 5-point scale; higher number is better function.
    b. Easiest to administer; takes 3 minutes
5. Research instruments
    a. AD Assessment Scale–Cognitive: (ADAS-Cog): 70-point scale
    b. AD Cooperative Study Activities of Daily Living Inventory: (ADCS-ADL): 54-point scale
    c. Clinician Interview–Based Impression of Change: (CIBIC-Plus): 1–7 points, with 4 points indicating no change
    d. Functional Assessment Staging Test: 7 major stages
    e. Severe Impairment Battery: 100-point scale

D. New Diagnostic Guidelines
1. Recognizes three phases
    a. Preclinical, asymptomatic phase
    b. Symptomatic, predementia phase (MCI)
    c. Dementia phase
2. Diagnosis may be identified for research purposes by:
    a. Biomarkers of increased tau or decreased β-amyloid levels in cerebrospinal fluid
    b. Reduced glucose uptake in brain on positron emission tomography scanning using florbetapir F18 or flutemetamol F18
    c. Atrophy of specific brain areas on magnetic resonance imaging
3. Preclinical and predementia phases are targets for investigational studies to halt progression
4. For clinicians, usually diagnosis given without these biomarkers or imaging

E. Clinical Presentation and Classification

Table 4. Stages of Alzheimer Disease

	MMSE (out of 30)	**Examples of Cognitive Loss**	**Examples of Functional Loss**
Mild	20–24	Some short-term memory loss; word-finding problems	Loss of IADLs such as laundry, housekeeping, and managing medications; may get lost in familiar places
Moderate	10–19	Disorientation to time and place, inability to engage in activities and conversation	Needs assistance with ADLs such as bathing, dressing, and toileting
Severe	<10	Loss of speech and ambulation, incontinence of bowel and bladder	Dependency in basic ADLs such as feeding oneself; often needs around-the-clock care

ADLs = activities of daily living; IADLs = instrumental activities of daily living; MMSE = Mini–Mental State Examination

F. Management
   1. Goals are to maintain function and cognition.
      a. Functional management and safety issues
      b. Legal considerations
   2. Nonpharmacologic therapy
      a. Education, especially with caregiver
      b. Physical exercise and mental exercise
      c. Management of comorbid conditions
      d. Avoid alcohol and medications that worsen mentation.
   3. Medical food: caprylidene triglyceride
      a. Mechanism is to provide ketone bodies for brain to use as energy source when glucose metabolism is impaired.
      b. Not routinely used because study measures became nonsignificant

---

Patient Case

5. M.B. is an 84-year-old widow living at home alone. She is able to perform ADLs and most IADLs with some assistance from her daughter. Her medications are hydrochlorothiazide 12.5 mg daily for hypertension, tolterodine LA 4 mg daily for incontinence, escitalopram 20 mg daily for depression, acetaminophen 650 mg as needed for arthritis, and calcium/vitamin D for prevention of osteoporosis. Her physician administers the MMSE, and M.B.'s score is 23. On physical examination no cogwheel rigidity or tremor is noted. What medication change is indicated at this time?

A. Add donepezil 5 mg daily.

B. Discontinue tolterodine and reassess M.B.

C. Add vitamin B_{12} 1000-mg injection monthly.

D. Switch hydrochlorothiazide to lisinopril 5 mg daily.

---

4. Pharmacologic therapy

Table 5. Comparison of Drugs for the Treatment of AD

Drug	Starting Dose	Maintenance Dose	Dosage Forms	Pharmacologic Properties	Comments
Cholinesterase Inhibitors					
Donepezil	5 mg daily	10 mg daily May increase to 23 mg/day	Tablets Orally disintegrating tablets	Acetylcholinesterase inhibitor; metabolized in part by CYP2D6 and CYP3A4 Protein binding 96%	Labeled for mild to moderate and moderate to severe AD
Rivastigmine	1.5 mg twice daily 4.6-mg patch daily	3–6 mg twice daily 9.5-mg patch daily; may increase to 13.3-mg patch daily	Capsules Oral solution Transdermal patch	Acetyl- and butyryl-cholinesterase inhibitor Nausea, vomiting, and diarrhea seem more intense than with other CIs	Labeled for mild to moderate and moderate to severe AD as well as mild to moderate dementia with Parkinson disease Skin reactions with patch
Galantamine	4 mg twice daily	8–12 mg twice daily 8–24 mg ER once daily	Tablets Oral solution ER capsules	Selective competitive, reversible acetylcho-linesterase inhibitor and nicotine receptor modulator Metabolized in part by CYP2D6 and CYP3A4	Preferable to administer with food Renal dosing adjustment necessary
Glutamatergic Therapy					
Memantine	5 mg once daily 7 mg ER once daily	10 mg twice daily 28 mg ER once daily	Tablets Oral solution ER capsules	*N*-methyl-D-aspartate receptor antagonist that blocks glutamate transmission	Labeled for moderate to severe AD; may be used in combination with acetylcholinesterase inhibitors.

AD = Alzheimer disease; CI, cholinesterase inhibitor; ER = extended release.

  a. Adverse effects of cholinesterase inhibitors (CIs)
     i. GI: nausea, vomiting, diarrhea, elevated risk of GI bleeding
     ii. Central nervous system: headache, insomnia, dizziness
     iii. Cardiac: bradycardia, orthostatic hypotension, syncope (Beers List notes CIs as inappropriate drugs in patients with syncope)
     iv. Genitourinary: incontinence
  b. Adverse effects of memantine: agitation, urinary incontinence, insomnia, diarrhea, dizziness, confusion, headache
5. Consensus treatment guidelines in United States, 2001 (partially outdated)
  a. Initiate CI in patients with mild to moderate AD.
  b. No evidence one agent is superior to others
  c. Titrate to recommended maintenance dose as tolerated.
  d. May increase to maximum dose if tolerated and maintenance dose no longer effective

    e. In moderate to severe disease may use CI, or memantine, or both CI and memantine

    f. Study in 2012 found no benefit with combination therapy.

    g. Study in 2011 found no benefit of memantine in mild AD.

6. Controversy over clinically significance responses

Table 6. Evidence for Response to Drugs for AD

Drug	Test	Testing Range	Response Difference Compared with Placebo	
			Mean	Range
Cholinesterase inhibitor	AD Assessment Scale–Cognitive	0–70	–2.7	–2.73 to –2.01
Memantine	Severe Impairment Battery	0–100	2.97	1.68 to 4.26

7. Duration of therapy

    a. Generally need 3–6 months to evaluate for objective benefit with tools

    b. Longest study was for 52 weeks, but many are maintained for years.

    c. Choosing Wisely campaign recommends evaluating at 12 weeks and considering discontinuation if goals of therapy not obtained.

    d. Generally discontinue at advanced stages of disease. Recommend tapering if on high dose.

    e. May see some rebound agitation

8. Herbals and dietary supplements

    a. Vitamin E was not shown effective in large prospective trials.

    b. Gingko biloba was not shown effective in prevention.

    c. Curcumin (turmeric) observational studies support effect.

Patient Cases

6. An 87-year-old man with AD is receiving rivastigmine 6 mg twice daily. His family notes improvement in his functional ability but reports that he is experiencing nausea and vomiting that appear to be related to rivastigmine. Which recommendation is best for this patient at this time?

    A. Advise the patient to take rivastigmine with an antacid.

    B. Change rivastigmine to the patch that delivers 9.5 mg daily.

    C. Discontinue rivastigmine and initiate memantine 5 mg twice daily.

    D. Add prochlorperazine 25 mg by rectal suppository with each rivastigmine dose.

7. A 75-year-old woman with AD who lives at home with her husband has been treated with donepezil 10 mg daily for about 3 years. When she began therapy, her MMSE was 21/30; her present MMSE is 17/30. The patient cannot perform most IADLs but can perform most ADLs with cueing. About 2 months ago, her donepezil was increased to 23 mg, but she could not tolerate it, and it was reduced back to 10 mg daily. Her husband asks about changing her drug treatment to help maintain her function. Which is the next best course of action?

    A. Retry donepezil 23 mg daily.

    B. Initiate memantine 5 mg daily.

    C. Add vitamin E 400 units twice daily.

    D. Switch donepezil to rivastigmine 9.5-mg patch daily.

III. BEHAVIORAL AND PSYCHOLOGICAL SYMPTOMS OF DEMENTIA (BPSD)

A. Epidemiology
   1. As disease progresses from mild to moderate, BPSD occur. They tend to wane as disease progresses to severe.
   2. Up to 90% of patients with dementia have BPSD at some point in disease progression.
   3. Associated with high rate of disability, functional decline, poor health outcomes, physical injury, nursing home placement, and emergency services

Table 7. Symptoms Seen During Disease Progression

MMSE Score	Stage	Symptoms
25 20	Mild	Memory loss Apathy Poor drawing Mood swings[a] Mild executive function Mild personality changes[a]
15 10	Moderate	Unable to learn Aphasia, apraxia Wandering, agitation[a] Aggression, psychosis[a] Confusion, insomnia[a] Need ADL assistance
5 0	Severe	Gait changes[a] Incontinence Loss of ADLs Bed bound

[a]Noncognitive symptoms.
ADLs = activities of daily living; MMSE = Mini–Mental State Examination.

B. Assessment Tools: Higher scores indicate more severe symptoms.
   1. Neuropsychiatric Inventory
   2. Behavioral Pathology in Alzheimer's Disease (BEHAVE-AD)
   3. Cohen-Mansfield Agitation Inventory
   4. Scales rarely used in nursing home or clinical practice, but it is important to identify the target behavior, how often it is occurring, and how severe it is in order to assess the response to treatment.
   5. Assess for medical reason that may precipitate and treat, if found
      a. Pain is frequent issue that patient cannot communicate.
      b. Treat with scheduled acetaminophen.

C. Nonpharmacologic Treatment: cornerstone of therapy
   1. Theory is that behavior is communication of unmet need.
   2. Eliminate antecedents and triggers.
   3. Person-centered interventions: Consider long-standing habits, values, and beliefs of patient; use distraction, music, aromatherapy.
   4. Symptoms likely to respond: wandering, hoarding, hiding objects, repetitive questioning, withdrawal, social inappropriateness, apathy

D. Pharmacologic Treatment: None of these are U.S. Food and Drug Administration (FDA) labeled indications.
1. Agency for Healthcare Research and Quality has published a summary on the use of atypical antipsychotic agents for off-label indications.
   a. Atypical antipsychotics improve behavioral symptoms of dementia, but effect sizes are small, and adverse effects are significant.
   b. It lists the risk of death at 1 for every 100 patients treated.

Table 8. Drug Treatment for BPSD

Symptom	Presentation	Treatment Options After Nonpharmacologic Efforts Ineffective
Anxiety	Part of this is caused by the fact that they cannot remember things	Buspirone or SSRI/SNRI or gabapentin Limit benzodiazepines
Apathy	One of earliest symptoms	Cholinesterase inhibitors
	Nonpharmacologic, tailored to patient's activities	Methylphenidate, modafinil effective in small, short-term studies
Depression	Up to 80% of patients with AD have depression	SSRI or mirtazapine
Insomnia	Sleep/wake cycle is disrupted	Melatonin
Wandering	Walk so much they begin to lose weight	No drug will stop wandering
Paranoia Hallucinations Sundowning	They may think because they cannot find something, you stole it Frequently accuse spouse of infidelity If psychosis and delusions do not bother anyone, do not use drugs	Risperidone, olanzapine, or quetiapine. Use very low doses. ADEs may offset any benefit.
Aggression, resistance to care	Most difficult and best response is to nonpharmacologic treatment	Prazosin is in investigation for agitation

ADE = adverse drug effect; BPSD = behavioral and psychological symptoms of dementia; SNRI = serotonin-norepinephrine reuptake inhibitor; SSRI = selective serotonin reuptake inhibitor

Patient Cases

8. You are evaluating the medication profile of an 87-year-old woman who resides in a secure advanced dementia unit. Her medical history includes dementia (likely AD), Parkinson disease, and osteoarthritis. She needs assistance with all ADLs including total assistance with bathing and dressing and help with feeding. She ambulates with the assistance of a four-wheeled walker. Her medication regimen includes donepezil 10 mg daily, memantine 10 mg twice daily, carbidopa/levodopa 25/100 mg four times daily, oxybutynin extended release 5 mg daily, and a multivitamin supplement daily. The patient's most recent MMSE score is 5/30. When reviewing the nursing notes, you note several references to the patient's continuously crying out, "Help me, help me." She is medically evaluated, and reversible causes of her hypervocalization are ruled out. Which additional assessment tool is most necessary for appropriate assessment of this patient?

A. Geriatric Depression Scale.

B. Functional Assessment Staging Test.

C. Neuropsychiatric Inventory.

D. MoCA.

9. Which is the best approach to treating her behavioral symptoms?

    A. Begin music therapy with songs patient enjoyed when younger.

    B. Turn the television on to comedy shows.

    C. Add quetiapine 25 mg at 4 p.m. daily.

    D. Add citalopram 10 mg daily.

IV. URINARY INCONTINENCE

  A. Epidemiology
1. Prevalence in community-dwelling elderly women is 38%.
2. Less common in elderly men: 17%.
3. Up to 75% of nursing home residents have urinary incontinence (UI).
4. Transient incontinence can occur due to DRIP:
   D = Drugs, Delirium
   R = Retention, Restricted Mobility
   I = Impaction, Infection, Inflammation
   P = Polyuria, Prostatitis

  B. Physiology
1. During filling, β_3-adrenergic stimulation relaxes detrusor to increase capacity.
2. α-Adrenergic stimulation tightens the internal bladder sphincter.
3. Acetylcholine (M_3) mediates involuntary and volitional bladder contractions.
4. Normal bladder emptying occurs with a decrease in urethral resistance and contraction of the bladder muscle.
5. Aging effects include decreased bladder elasticity and capacity, more frequent voiding, decline in bladder outlet and urethral resistance in women with loss of estrogen, and decrease in flow rate in men with prostatic enlargement.

C. Types of UI

Table 9. Common Types of UI and Drug-Induced Causes

Type of Incontinence	Description	Drug-Induced Causes
Urge or overactive bladder	Loss of a moderate amount of urine with an increased need to void Detrusor instability can be caused by central nervous system damage from a stroke	Cholinergic agents that stimulate the bladder such as bethanechol and cholinesterase inhibitors
Stress incontinence	Loss of small amounts of urine with increased abdominal pressure (e.g., sneezing, coughing) Stress UI is more common in postmenopausal women	α-Blockers such as prazosin decrease urethral sphincter tone
Overflow incontinence	Loss of urine because of excessive bladder volume caused by outlet obstruction or an acontractile detrusor PVR is often high (>300 mL), indicating incomplete emptying	Anticholinergic agents, calcium channel blockers, and opioids decrease detrusor muscle contractions
Functional incontinence	Inability to reach the toilet because of mobility constraints	Sedating drugs that cause confusion Diuretics increase voiding
Mixed incontinence	UI that has more than one cause, usually stress and overactive bladder	

PVR = postvoid residual; UI = urinary incontinence.

D. Nonpharmacologic Interventions
   1. Pelvic floor exercises (Kegel exercises) are first line for stress, urge, or mixed UI.
   2. Exercise and weight loss for patients with BMI >30
   3. Bladder training to increase time between voiding in urge incontinence
   4. Biofeedback to teach pelvic floor exercises
   5. Scheduled and timed voiding may be helpful for patients with dementia.
   6. Stress incontinence usually responds to surgical repair.
   7. Pessaries, collagen, or other bulking agent injections also help stress incontinence.
   8. Prostatectomy in men or self-catheterization for severe overflow incontinence

E.   Drug Treatment

Table 10. Recommended Drug Treatment by Type of Incontinence

Type of Incontinence	Drug Treatment	Comments
Urge or overactive bladder	**Antimuscarinic and anticholinergic agents** Oxybutynin, tolterodine, fesoterodine, trospium, solifenacin, darifenacin	Magnitude of clinical efficacy is modest Differences in adverse reactions exist, but clinical differences in efficacy between these agents have not been shown Longer-acting formulations may be better tolerated
	β₃-Agonist Mirabegron	Recently approved in 2012; appears well tolerated but has not been compared with antimuscarinics
	Botulinum toxin A intravesical injections	Prevents stimulation of detrusor muscle May cause voiding difficulty
Stress	**α-Adrenergic agonists** Pseudoephedrine, phenylephrine	Efficacy evidence is limited
	Topical estrogens Conjugated estrogen vaginal cream or estradiol vaginal insert or ring	Use if other symptoms of estrogen deficiency Vaginal estrogens may improve severity of stress incontinence
	Serotonin/norepinephrine reuptake inhibitor Duloxetine	Not FDA labeled for stress UI; may reduce the severity of incontinence Not significantly different from placebo for symptoms Adverse effects may limit its usefulness
Overflow	**α-Adrenergic antagonists** Alfuzosin, tamsulosin, silodosin, doxazosin, terazosin, prazosin	Adverse effects vary depending on selectivity to receptors in the bladder or prostate (alfuzosin, silodosin, and tamsulosin are more specific)
	5-α-reductase inhibitors Finasteride, dutasteride	To slow progression
	Cholinomimetics Bethanechol	Stimulates the detrusor muscle but also systemic cholinomimetic effects
	Phosphodiesterase-5 inhibitors Tadalafil	5 mg once daily approved for BPH
Functional	No drug treatments	Consider interventions to remove any potential cause, barriers or obstacles; provide schedules or prompted toileting; assistance may be required to transfer on and off commode
Mixed	Focus on symptoms that dominate	Consider treatments for individual components (i.e., stress and urge)

BPH = benign prostatic hypertrophy; FDA = U.S. Food and Drug Administration; UI = urinary incontinence.

Table 11. Comparison of Adverse Effects from Urinary Antimuscarinic Agents[a]

Drug	Dry Mouth (%)	Constipation (%)	Dizziness (%)
Oxybutynin	88	32	38
Oxybutynin ER/XL	68	9	11
Oxybutynin TDS	10	5	4
Oxybutynin gel	8	1	3
Tolterodine IR, ER	50, 39	10, 10	4, 3
Fesoterodine	99	14	2
Trospium	33	11	?
Solifenacin	34	19	1
Darifenacin	59	28	0

[a]Treatment of Overactive Bladder in Women. Agency for Healthcare Research and Quality publication no. 09-E017. August 2009. Mirabegron is not available for comparison.

ER/XL = extended release; IR = immediate release; TDS = transdermal delivery system.

Patient Case

10. A 75-year-old woman reports urinary urgency, frequency, and loss of urine when she cannot make it to the bathroom in time. She also wears a pad at night that she changes two or three times because of incontinence. Her medical history is significant for mild cognitive impairment (MMSE = 25), osteoarthritis, and hypothyroidism. A urinalysis is negative. Physical examination is normal, and her postvoid residual (PVR) is normal (less than 100 mL). Which therapy would be best to initiate in this patient at this time?

   A. Pelvic floor exercises.

   B. Bethanechol.

   C. Darifenacin.

   D. Tolterodine.

V. BENIGN PROSTATIC HYPERTROPHY

   A. Epidemiology
   1. Benign prostatic hypertrophy (BPH) usually develops after age 40.
   2. By age 60, half of all men have BPH; by age 85, 90% have BPH.

   B. Pathophysiology and Clinical Presentation
   1. Type II 5-α-reductase facilitates conversion of testosterone to dihydrotestosterone (DHT), resulting in prostate growth.
   2. Lower urinary tract symptoms (LUTS) are seen in 25% of men.
       a. Voiding (obstructive) symptoms: decreased force, hesitancy, dribbling
       b. Storage (irritative) symptoms: urinary urgency, frequency, nocturia, dysuria
   3. The American Urological Association Symptom Index (AUASI) can help determine severity and appropriate treatment. The index consists of seven questions evaluating the severity of LUTS on a 0–5 scale. Higher numbers indicate more severe symptoms.

C. Evaluation
 1. Medical history, digital rectal examination, BUN, serum creatinine, and urinalysis
 2. If suspect prostate cancer, plan treatment with 5-α reductase inhibitor, prostate-specific antigen (PSA)
 3. If suspect significant urinary retention, need to assess PVR. If PVR is greater than 50 mL, patients have an elevated risk of infection.
 4. Assess for medications that may exacerbate BPH symptoms.
    a. α-Adrenergic agonists (decongestants) can stimulate smooth muscle contraction in the prostate and urethra, obstructing urinary flow through the urethra.
    b. Anticholinergic drugs (urinary and GI antispasmodics, antihistamines, tricyclic antidepressants, phenothiazines) can reduce the ability of the bladder detrusor muscle to contract and empty the bladder.
    c. Diuretics can increase urinary frequency and volume.
    d. Testosterone replacement can stimulate prostate growth.
 5. If AUASI score is 0–7 (mild), then watchful waiting.
 6. Patients with high AUASI scores of 20 and up (severe disease) should be assessed for prostatectomy.
 7. Patients with moderate disease (scores 8–19) are candidates for medical treatment.

D. Drug Treatment
 1. α-Adrenergic blockers: Relieve LUTS in men with moderate or severe AUASI scores by reducing smooth muscle contractions in the urethra and surrounding tissues
    a. Nonspecific α-adrenergic blockers such as doxazosin and terazosin also lower BP significantly.
    b. Newer agents are uroselective antagonists of α_1-adrenergic receptors (tamsulosin, silodosin) and selective antagonists of postsynaptic α_1-adrenergic receptors (alfuzosin) in the prostate and bladder. They may have less associated hypotension.
    c. All α-blockers can cause hypotension.
    d. Compared with placebo, the α-blockers lower the AUASI by 4 to 6 points in patients with LUTS and BPH.
    e. All α-blockers are metabolized through the CYP3A4 pathway and have drug interactions with strong CYP3A4 inhibitors and inducers.
    f. Intraoperative floppy iris syndrome is a concern with α-blockers, especially tamsulosin. Men with LUTS being offered α-blockers should be asked about planned cataract surgery. Men with planned cataract surgery should avoid the initiation of α-blockers until their cataract surgery is completed.
 2. α-Reductase inhibitors
    a. These agents prevent the conversion of testosterone to DHT, modify the disease course, and may reduce the risk of urinary retention and surgical interventions.
       i. Finasteride competitively inhibits type II 5-α-reductase and lowers prostatic DHT by 80%–90%.
       ii. Dutasteride is a nonselective inhibitor of both type I and II 5-α-reductase. Prostatic DHT production is quickly suppressed with this agent.
       iii. Despite these pharmacologic differences, no differences between these two agents were observed in trials; both reduce prostate size.
    b. α-Reductase inhibitors do not immediately reduce LUTS and should be reserved for use in men with large prostate volume (more than 40 g). At least 6 months of therapy is usually needed to achieve clinical benefit. Prostate size may be reduced by about 25% during this interval.
    c. PSA concentrations are used to monitor for prostate cancer. Because these agents lower PSA concentrations, a baseline PSA test is recommended before initiating treatment with α-reductase inhibitors.
    d. Long-term therapy with an α-reductase inhibitor can increase the risk of high-grade tumors of the prostate in healthy men without a history of prostate cancer.

3. Phosphodiesterase type-5 inhibitors
   a. Tadalafil 5 mg once daily is approved for use in BPH.
   b. Mechanism is thought to be caused by phosphodiesterase-induced smooth muscle relaxation in the bladder, urethra, and prostate.
   c. Studied as monotherapy; the FDA does not recommend in combination with α-blockers because the combination has not been adequately studied for the treatment of BPH, and there is a risk of lowering BP. May be used in practice to treat both BPH and erectile dysfunction with a 4-hour separation of doses.
4. Combination therapy
   a. May be needed in men with LUTS, a larger prostate size, and an elevated PSA
   b. Finasteride and doxazosin most studied; dutasteride is FDA label approved for use with tamsulosin in symptomatic men having an enlarged prostate.
   c. Two large clinical trials [Medical Therapy of Prostatic Symptoms (MTOPS) and the Combination of Avodart and Tamsulosin studies (CombAT)] evaluated monotherapy versus combination therapy and concluded that in men with LUTS and an enlarged prostate, further benefit can be achieved by using the two drugs in combination.
5. Supplements
   a. Saw palmetto plant extract (*Serenoa repens*)
   b. Conflicting evidence about the efficacy of saw palmetto in relieving LUTS; two recent trials suggested no benefit over placebo.
   c. Use of this agent with 5-α-reductase inhibitors may reduce the efficacy of the reductase inhibitors.
6. Surgery is preferred in men with severe symptoms and in those with moderate symptoms who have not adequately responded to medical options.
7. Anticholinergic agents can be appropriate and effective treatment alternatives in men without an elevated PVR when LUTS are predominantly storage (irritative) symptoms.

Table 12. Comparison of Drugs for the Treatment of Benign Prostatic Hypertrophy

Medication	Dose Range	Adverse Effects	Comments
Terazosin Doxazosin	1–10 mg daily 1–8 mg daily	Orthostatic hypotension	Initiate at low dose; can titrate up every 2–7 days Start at bedtime
Alfuzosin ER	10 mg daily	Orthostatic hypotension	No need to titrate Take after a meal
Tamsulosin modified release	0.4–0.8 mg daily	May cause less orthostasis Causes ejaculatory dysfunction	Start at bedtime
Silodosin	8 mg daily 4 mg daily if CrCl 30–50 mL/minute	Causes ejaculatory dysfunction; appears less sedating	Contraindicated if CrCl < 30 mL/minute Take with food
Finasteride Dutasteride Dutasteride/tamsulosin	5 mg daily 0.5 mg daily 0.5/0.4 mg daily	Decreased libido Pregnancy category X	Onset of action is usually 6 months Monitor PSA
Tadalafil	5 mg daily	Orthostatic hypotension	Avoid use with α-blockers No data in combination or with long-term use

CrCl = creatinine clearance; ER extended release; PSA = prostate-specific antigen.

Patient Case

11. An 85-year-old man with LUTS visits his physician, who determines his AUASI score is 15. His BP is 118/70 mm Hg sitting. A digital rectal examination confirms the diagnosis of BPH, and the physician schedules a further workup including a prostate ultrasound, which shows a prostate volume of 31 g. Which therapy is best at this time?

  A. Terazosin.

  B. Finasteride plus saw palmetto.

  C. Tamsulosin.

  D. Finasteride plus tamsulosin.

VI. OSTEOARTHRITIS

  A. Epidemiology
  1. Osteoarthritis (OA) is the most prevalent form of arthritis, affecting more than 46 million Americans.
  2. Highly associated with aging
  3. Women are afflicted more often than men.
  4. Large weight-bearing joints (e.g., hip and knee) are commonly affected.

  B. Etiology and Pathophysiology
  1. Risk factors include age, female sex, obesity, genetics, sports activities, occupation, previous injury, acromegaly
  2. Loss of cartilage occurs in the joint as the balance of chondrocyte function shifts from formation to destruction. Secondary inflammation and production of cytokines play a role.
  3. Subchondral bone and the synovium are damaged, and the joint space narrows.
  4. Single injuries or repeated micro-injuries may initiate or accelerate process.
  5. Symptoms of pain result from activation of nociceptive nerve endings in the damaged joint.
  6. Therapy goals: To relieve pain and swelling, maintain or improve joint function, prevent loss of function, and maintain or improve quality of life

  C. Nonpharmacologic Treatment
  1. Patient education: lifestyle, expectations, when to seek care
  2. Weight loss decreases the biomechanical load on large weight-bearing joints; even a small amount of weight loss helps decrease pain and disability.
  3. Exercise
  4. Physical and occupational therapy
  5. Surgery

  D. Drug Therapy
  1. Acetaminophen is first line, with as-needed doses followed by scheduled dosing to maximum of 4 g daily in divided doses.
     a. 1000 mg every 6 hours for three times daily or 650 mg every 6 hours
     b. Ensure that patient knows to watch for "hidden" acetaminophen in other products.
     c. Monitor for hepatotoxicity in patients with elevated risk of liver disease (previous liver problems, heavy alcohol consumption) with periodic liver function tests.

---

2. NSAIDs are used if acetaminophen response inadequate in select patients.
   a. Avoid chronic use or, if necessary, use a COX-2 selective NSAID, or add a proton pump inhibitor to reduce the risk of GI bleeding.
   b. If one NSAID is not effective, switch to others.
   c. Monitor for adverse effects: rash, abdominal pain, GI bleeding, renal impairment, hypertension, heart failure, and drug-drug interactions.
   d. For patients taking aspirin (for cardiac disease), a proton pump inhibitor may be recommended for gastric protection. Patients should be educated to take aspirin at least 30 minutes before their first daily dose of NSAID in the morning to avoid any interactions or reductions in aspirin efficacy. Naproxen appears to be safest with respect to cardiac risk.
   e. Monitor in chronic users: complete blood cell count, BUN, serum creatinine, and aspartate amino-transferase at least annually

3. Topical agents: Helpful for knees or smaller joints near surface of skin. Limited efficacy for widespread joint pain.
   a. Capsaicin difficult to administer: Wear gloves, avoid contact with eyes, and do not skip doses. Local irritation occurs in 40%.
   b. Diclofenac 1% gel (or patch is FDA labeled for minor trauma): Four short-term trials showed a 50% reduction in pain in 40% of subjects (number needed to treat = 5); longer-term trials had number needed to treat = 10. Comparative trials with oral administration showed no difference in proportion who received pain relief.

4. Intra-articular glucocorticoid injections
   a. Methylprednisolone or triamcinolone 10- to 40-mg injection depending on size of joint; may be repeated every 3 months
   b. Primary adverse effects are risk for septic arthritis, synovitis.

5. Intra-articular hyaluronans may be used if glucocorticoid injections are ineffective.
   a. Meta-analysis indicates effects last up to 30 weeks.
   b. Frequency of injection undetermined: annual or more often?

6. Alternative dietary supplements: Glucosamine sulfate, 400–500 mg taken three times daily, with or without chondroitin, may be considered for chronic therapy to prevent joint degradation and relieve pain.
   a. Evidence to support treatment is contradictory. Sulfate vs. HCl salt
   b. The adverse effect profile of glucosamine is similar to that of placebo and includes GI complaints

7. Opioids
   a. Patients with persistent, moderate to severe pain from OA who do not respond to more conservative strategies are candidates for treatment with opioids. The American Geriatrics Society recommends treatment with opioids for OA when older patients do not respond to initial acetaminophen therapy rather than chronic use of NSAIDs.
   b. Hydrocodone/acetaminophen combination now Schedule II.
   c. Tramadol alone or in combination with acetaminophen is an alternative when NSAIDs are ineffective or contraindicated.
   d. Stronger opioids can be more effective but can incur more significant adverse effects.
   e. Monitor and anticipate opioid adverse effects and treat accordingly.

Patient Case

12. An 85-year-old man presents with pain from hip OA. He has hypertension, coronary artery disease, and BPH. For his OA, he has been taking acetaminophen 650 mg three times daily. He reports that acetaminophen helps but that the pain persists and limits his ability to walk. Which is the best next step for this patient?

    A. Change acetaminophen to celecoxib.

    B. Add hydrocodone.

    C. Change acetaminophen to ibuprofen.

    D. Add glucosamine.

VII. RHEUMATOID ARTHRITIS

A. Epidemiology
   1. A systemic disease characterized by a bilateral inflammatory arthritis that usually affects the small joints of the hands, wrists, and feet
   2. The prevalence is estimated to be between 1% and 2%, with women predominating until after age 60, when it becomes equal.
   3. Rheumatoid arthritis (RA) can occur at any age but has an increasing prevalence up to age 70.
   4. RA is an autoimmune disease with a strong genetic predisposition.

B. Pathophysiology and Clinical Presentation
   1. Chronic inflammation of the synovium leads to proliferation and development of a pannus.
   2. The pannus invades joint cartilage and eventually causes erosion of the bone and joint destruction.
   3. The cause of the initial inflammatory activation is unknown, but once activated, the immune system produces antibodies and cytokines that accelerate cartilage and joint destruction.
   4. Patients present with joint pain and stiffness, fatigue, and other inflammatory symptoms. Symptoms also include warmth, redness, and swelling of the joints, usually with symmetrical distribution.
   5. Laboratory tests often reveal a positive rheumatoid factor (RF), elevated sedimentation rate, C-reactive protein, anti–cyclic citrullinated peptide antibodies, and normochromic normocytic anemia.
   6. RA can also affect other organs, causing pulmonary fibrosis, vasculitis, and dry eyes.

C. Treatment
   1. The treatment goal is to control the inflammatory process so that disease remission occurs. This should lead to relief of pain, maintenance of function, and improved quality of life. Treatment response can be measured by:
      a. Reduction in the number of affected joints and in joint tenderness and swelling
      b. Improvement in pain
      c. Decreased amount of morning stiffness
      d. Reduction in serologic markers such as RF
      e. Improvement in quality-of-life scales
   2. Nonpharmacologic treatment: concurrent with pharmacologic treatment
      a. Rest during periods of disease exacerbation
      b. Occupational and physical therapy to support mobility and maintain function
      c. Maintenance of a normal weight (avoid overweight and obesity) to reduce biomechanical stress on joints
      d. Assistive devices if needed
      e. Surgery for tendons or joints

---

3. Disease-modifying antirheumatic drugs (DMARDs)
   a. Start DMARD within 3 months of diagnosis.
   b. Step-down approach: Start with DMARD (1 or more depending on disease severity) along with anti-inflammatory drug (NSAID, steroid). As pain is controlled, reduce anti-inflammatory agent. As joint damage is controlled, reduce DMARD.
   c. Nonbiologic DMARDs are first line.
      i. Methotrexate has most long-term data and better outcomes.
      ii. Hydroxychloroquine has slow onset of action.
      iii. Sulfasalazine is drug of choice in pregnancy but has slow onset too.
      iv. Leflunomide
      v. Some patients with poor prognostic indicators such as functional limitation, extra-articular disease, positive RF, anti–cyclic citrullinated peptide antibodies, or bony erosions on radiography may be candidates for combination DMARD therapy.
   d. Biologic DMARDs are used in combination for severe disease or as alternatives if nonbiologic DMARDs are ineffective or contraindicated. Etanercept, infliximab, abatacept, or rituximab are most often used.
4. NSAIDs, glucocorticosteroids, or both can be used to provide immediate treatment of pain and inflammation.
   a. NSAIDs do not affect disease progression in RA; their anti-inflammatory effect occurs within 1–2 weeks of daily dosing, whereas the analgesic effect begins within several hours of administration.
   b. Glucocorticosteroids (dosed at 10 mg daily or less) are not recommended for long-term use because of their many adverse effects and long-term complications. They are often used as bridge therapy to provide anti-inflammatory effects while waiting for the DMARDs to take effect.

Table 13. Selected DMARDs for Rheumatoid Arthritis

Drug	Customary Dose	Comments
Nonbiologic DMARDs		
Methotrexate	7.5–15 mg every week	Probably first-line DMARD; monitor for myelosuppression, liver dysfunction, and pulmonary fibrosis; a teratogen
Leflunomide (Arava)	10–20 mg/day	Similar to methotrexate; an initial loading dose may give therapeutic response within the first month
Hydroxychloroquine (Plaquenil)	200–300 mg twice daily	Must routinely monitor for ocular toxicity; however, this agent has a better adverse effect profile overall
Sulfasalazine	500–1000 mg twice daily	GI adverse effects often limit the use of this agent
Biologic DMARDs		
Etanercept (Enbrel)	50 mg SC weekly	Binds to TNF, inactivating this cytokine; generally well tolerated; usually used in those whose methotrexate therapy fails; monitor for infection; check baseline PPD
Infliximab (Remicade)	3 mg/kg IV at 0, 2, and 6 weeks, then every 8 weeks thereafter	A mouse/human chimeric antibody to TNF; used in combination with methotrexate to prevent formation of antibodies to this protein; monitor for infection; check baseline PPD
Adalimumab (Humira)	40 mg SC every 2 weeks	Human antibody to TNF; less antigenic than other TNF antibodies; monitor for infection; check baseline PPD

Table 13. Selected DMARDs for Rheumatoid Arthritis *(continued)*

Drug	Customary Dose	Comments
Biologic DMARDs		
Anakinra (Kineret)	100 mg SC daily	IL-1 receptor antagonist; avoid combination therapy with TNF agents because of elevated risk of infection
Rituximab (Rituxan)	Two infusions of 1000 mg given 2 weeks apart	Chimeric antibody to CD20 protein on B lymphocytes; corticosteroid infusions help reduce infusion reactions; used in combination with methotrexate to improve response
Abatacept (Orencia)	Weight-based dose every 2 weeks for 2 doses and then monthly (i.e., 750 mg for those weighing 60–100 kg)	Inhibits interactions between antigens and T cells; may be useful in those who do not respond to TNF inhibitors; monitor for infusion reactions
Golimumab (Simponi)	50 mg SC every month	Monoclonal antibody against TNF Intended for use in combination with methotrexate Monitor for infections
Certolizumab pegol (Cimzia)	400 mg SC at 0, 2, and 4 weeks, then 200 mg every other week	Monoclonal antibody against TNF; may have best response when used in combination with methotrexate Monitor for infections
Tocilizumab (Actemra)	4 mg/kg IV infusion every 4 weeks; can increase to 8 mg/kg on the basis of clinical response	Anti–human IL-6 receptor monoclonal antibody; indicated for patients who have not responded to TNF inhibitors Monitor for infections
Tofacitinib (Xeljanz)	5 mg twice daily	Oral Janus kinase inhibitor; intended as second-line therapy Can be used as monotherapy or in combination with methotrexate

DMARD = disease-modifying antirheumatic drug; GI = gastrointestinal; IL = interleukin; IV = intravenous(ly); NSAID = nonsteroidal anti-inflammatory drug; PPD = purified protein derivative; SC = subcutaneously; SSRI = selective serotonin reuptake inhibitor; TNF = tumor necrosis factor.

D. Comorbid Conditions
1. Patients with RA are more likely to develop other chronic diseases either from the effects of RA or from medications used to treat RA.
2. Cardiovascular disease (myocarditis and heart failure) causes 40% of all deaths in patients with RA. Low-dose aspirin, omega-3 fatty acids, statins, or combination therapy should be considered.
   a. Follow standard guidelines to lower cardiovascular risk factors.
   b. European guidelines recommend multiplying risk score by 1.5 for patients with RA who have disease of 10 years or more, are positive for RF or anti–cyclic citrullinated peptide, or have severe extra-articular disease manifestations (two of the three should be present).
3. Infection risk is elevated, particularly pulmonary infections and sepsis. A history of tuberculosis or hepatitis B calls for extra vigilance. Tuberculosis screening is required for patients who are considered for therapy with biologic DMARDs.
4. Malignancy is more common, particularly GI cancers and lymphoproliferative disorders. Also, melanoma and lung cancer rates were elevated in one cohort study.
5. Osteoporosis is more common in patients with RA. Calcium and vitamin D are recommended. In addition, bisphosphonates should be considered for prevention if prednisone 5 mg or more daily is prescribed.

Patient Case

13. A 65-year-old woman received a diagnosis of RA 1 year ago. At the time of her diagnosis, her RF titer was 1:64; she presented with joint inflammation in both hands and about 45 minutes of morning stiffness. She began therapy with oral methotrexate and currently receives 15 mg weekly, folic acid 2 mg daily, ibuprofen 800 mg three times daily, and omeprazole 20 mg daily. At today's clinic visit, the patient reports the recurrence of her symptoms. Radiographic evaluation of her hand joints shows progression of joint space narrowing and bone erosion. Which is the next best step for this patient?

    A. Administer etanercept.

    B. Change to leflunomide.

    C. Add prednisone bridge therapy.

    D. Switch to hydroxychloroquine.

Acknowledgment: The contributions of the previous authors, Drs. Norma Owens, Jennifer Dugan, and Dominick Trombetta, are acknowledged.

REFERENCES

Principles to Promote Optimal Medication Use in Older People

1. American Geriatrics Society (AGS). Updated Beers Criteria for potentially inappropriate medication use in older adults. American Geriatrics Society 2012 Beers Criteria Update Expert Panel. J Am Geriatr Soc 2012;60:616-31.

2. AGS Expert Panel on the Care of Older Adults with Multimorbidity. Patient-centered care for older adults with multiple chronic conditions: a stepwise approach from the American Geriatrics Society. J Am Geriatr Soc 2012;60:1957-68.

3. AGS. Ten things physicians and patients should question. Released February 21, 2013 (1–5) and February 27, 2014 (6–10). Available at www.choosingwisely.org/doctor-patient-lists/american-geriatrics-society/. Accessed November 25, 2014.

4. Dowling TC, Wang ES, Ferrucci L, Sorkin JD. Glomerular filtration rate equations overestimate creatinine clearance in older individuals enrolled in the Baltimore Longitudinal Study on aging: impact on renal drug dosing. Pharmacotherapy 2013;33:912-21.

5. Elliott DP. Pharmacokinetics and pharmacodynamics in the elderly. In: Schumock G, Brundage D, Chapman M, et al., eds. Pharmacotherapy Self-Assessment Program, 5th ed. Lenexa, KS: American College of Clinical Pharmacy, 2004:115-30.

6. Hajjar ER, Gray SL, Slattum PW, et al. Chapter e8. Geriatrics. In: DiPiro JT, Talbert RL, Yee GC, et al., eds. Pharmacotherapy: A Pathophysiologic Approach, 9th ed. Available at: http://accesspharmacy.mhmedical.com/content.aspx?bookid=689&sectionid=48811433. Accessed November 25, 2014.

7. Handler SM, Wright RM, Ruby CM, et al. Epidemiology of medication-related adverse events in nursing homes. Am J Geriatr Pharmacother 2006;4:264-72.

8. Higashi T, Shekelle PG, Solomon DH, et al. The quality of pharmacologic care for vulnerable older patients. Ann Intern Med 2004;140:714-20.

9. Hutchison LC, O'Brien CE. Changes in pharmacokinetics and pharmacodynamics in the elderly patient. J Pharm Pract 2007;20(1):4-12.

10. Inouye SK, Studenski S, Tinetti ME, Kuchel GA. Geriatric syndromes: clinical, research and policy implications of a core geriatric concept. J Am Geriatr Soc 2007;55:780-91.

11. Labella AM, Merel SE, Phelan EA. Ten ways to improve the care of elderly patients in the hospital. J Hosp Med 2011;6:351-7.

12. Moore TJ, Cohen MR, Furberg CD. Serious adverse drug events reported to the Food and Drug Administration, 1998–2005. Arch Intern Med 2007;167:1752-9.

13. National Kidney Foundation. Glomerular Filtration Rate. Available at www.kidney.org/professionals/kls/pdf/12-10-4004_KBB_FAQs_AboutGFR-1.pdf. Accessed November 25, 2014.

14. Onder G, van der Cammen TJM, Petrovic M, et al. Strategies to reduce the risk of iatrogenesis in complex older adults. Age Ageing 2013;42:284-91.

15. Schwartz JB. The current state of knowledge on age, sex, and their interactions on clinical pharmacology. Clin Pharmacol Ther 2007;82:87-96.

Dementia

1. American Geriatrics Society (AGS). A Guide to Dementia Diagnosis and Treatment. 2010. Available at http://dementia.americangeriatrics.org. Accessed November 25, 2014.

2. Birks J. Cholinesterase inhibitors for Alzheimer's disease. Cochrane Database Syst Rev 2006;1:CD005593.

3. Dubois B, Feldman HH, Jacova C, et al. Research criteria for the diagnosis of Alzheimer's disease: revising the NINCDS-ADRDA criteria. Lancet Neurol 2007;6:734-46.

4. Gill SS, Anderson GM, Fischer HD, et al. Syncope and its consequences in patients with dementia receiving cholinesterase inhibitors. Arch Intern Med 2009;169:867-73.

5. Grimmer T, Kurz A. Effects of cholinesterase inhibitors on behavioural disturbances in Alzheimer's disease: a systematic review. Drugs Aging 2006;23:957-67.

6. Hilas O, Ezzo DC. Dementias and related neuropsychiatric issues. In: Richardson M, Chant C, Cheng JWM, et al., eds. Pharmacotherapy Self-Assessment Program, 7th ed. Neurology and psychiatry. Lenexa, KS: American College of Clinical Pharmacy, 2012:91-110.

7. Howard R, Lindesay J, Ritchie C, et al. Donepezil and memantine for moderate-to-severe Alzheimer's disease. N Engl J Med 2012;366:893-903.

8. Linnebur SA. Geriatric assessment, chapter 4 In: Hutchison LC, Sleeper RB, eds. Fundamentals of Geriatric Pharmacotherapy. Bethesda, MD: American Society of Health-System Pharmacists, 2010:71-90.

9. Inouye SK, Westendorp RG, Saczynski JS. Delirium in elderly people. Lancet 2014;383(9920):911-22.

10. National Institute on Aging. Alzheimer's diagnostic guidelines. Available at www.nia.nih.gov/research/dn/alzheimers-diagnostic-guidelines. Accessed November 25, 2014.

11. Qaseam A, Snow V, Cross JT, et al. Current pharmacologic treatment of dementia: a clinical practice guideline from the American College of Physicians and the American Academy of Family Physicians. Ann Intern Med 2008;148:370-8.

12. Rubin CD. The primary care of Alzheimer disease. Am J Med Sci 2006;332(6):314-33.

13. Slattum PW, Peron EP, Hill AM. Chapter 38: Alzheimer's Disease. In: DiPiro JT, Talbert RL, Yee GC, et al., eds. Pharmacotherapy: A Pathophysiologic Approach, 9th ed. Available at: http://accesspharmacy.mhmedical.com/content.aspx?bookid=689&sectionid=45310488.

Behavioral Symptoms of Dementia

1. Agency for Heath Care Research and Quality. Off-label use of atypical antipsychotics: an update. Aug 1, 2012. Available at: http://effectivehealthcare.ahrq.gov/ehc/products/150/1193/off_lab_ant_psy_clin_fin_to_post.pdf. Accessed November 25, 2014.

2. Ballard C, Hanney ML, Theodoulou M, et al. The dementia antipsychotic withdrawal trial (DART-AD): long-term follow-up of a randomized placebo-controlled trial. Lancet Neurol 2009;8:151-7.

3. Ballard CG, Waite J, Birks J. Atypical antipsychotics for aggression and psychosis in Alzheimer's disease. Cochrane Database Syst Rev 2006;1:CD003476.

4. Banerjee S, Hellier J, Romeo R, et al. Study of the use of antidepressant for depression in dementia: the HTA-SADD trial—a multicentre, randomized, double-blind, placebo-controlled trial of the clinical effectiveness and cost effectiveness of sertraline and mirtazapine. Health Technol Assess 2013;17:1-166.

5. Howard RJ, Juszczak E, Ballard CG, et al. Donepezil for the treatment of agitation in Alzheimer's disease. N Engl J Med 2007;357:1382-92.

6. Maher AR, Maglione M, Bagley S, et al. Efficacy and comparative effectiveness of atypical antipsychotic medications for off-label uses in adults. JAMA 2011;306:1359-69.

7. Sadowsky CH, Galvin JE. Guidelines for the management of cognitive and behavioral problems in dementia. JABFM 2012;25:350-66.

8. Schneider LS, Dagerman KS, Insel P. Risk of death with atypical antipsychotic drug treatment for dementia. Meta-analysis of randomized placebo-controlled trials. JAMA 2005;294:1934-43.

9. Schneider LS, Tariot PN, Dagerman KS, et al. Effectiveness of atypical antipsychotic drugs in patients with Alzheimer's disease. N Engl J Med 2006;355:1525-38.

10. Sink KM, Holden KF, Yaffe K. Pharmacological treatment of neuropsychiatric symptoms of dementia. A review of the evidence. JAMA 2005;293:596-8.

11. Sutor B, Rummans TA, Smith GE. Assessment and management of behavioral disturbances in nursing home patients with dementia. Mayo Clin Proc 2001;76:540-50.

12. Wang PS, Schneeweiss S, Avorn J, et al. Risk of death in elderly users of conventional vs. atypical antipsychotic medications. N Engl J Med 2005;353:2335-41.

13. Yury CA, Fisher JE. Meta-analysis of the effectiveness of atypical antipsychotics for the treatment of behavioural problems in persons with dementia. Psychother Psychosom 2007;76:213-8.

Urinary Incontinence and Benign Prostatic Hypertrophy

1. American Urological Association. Clinical Guidelines. Management of Benign Prostatic Hyperplasia. 2010. Available at www.auanet.org/content/guidelines-and-quality-care/clinical-guidelines.cfm?sub=bph. Accessed November 25, 2014.

2. Chughtai B, Levin R, De E. Choice of antimuscarinic agents for overactive bladder in the older patient: focus on darifenacin. Clin Interv Aging 2008;3:503-9.

3. Edwards JL. Diagnosis and management of benign prostatic hyperplasia. Am Fam Physician 2008;77:1403-10.

4. Filson CP, Hollingsworth JM, Clemens JQ, Wei JT. The efficacy and safety of combined therapy with α-blockers and anticholinergics for men with benign prostatic hyperplasia: a meta-analysis. J Urol 2013;190:2153-65.

5. Gormley EA, Lightner DJ, Burglio KL, et al. Diagnosis and treatment of overactive bladder (non-neurogenic) in adults: AUA/SUFU Guideline. American Urological Association, May 2012, updated 2014. Available at www.auanet.org/common/pdf/education/clinical-guidance/Overactive-Bladder.pdf. Accessed November 25, 2014.

6. Huang A. Nonsurgical treatments for urinary incontinence in women. Summary of primary findings and conclusions. JAMA 2013;173:1463-4.

7. Kaplan SA, Roehrborn CG, McConnell JD, et al. Long-term treatment with finasteride results in a clinically significant reduction in total prostate volume compared to placebo over the full range of baseline prostate sizes in men enrolled in the MTOPS trial. J Urol 2008;180:1030-3.

8. Porst H, Oelke M, Goldfischer ER, et al. Efficacy and safety of tadalafil 5 mg once daily for lower urinary tract symptoms suggestive of benign prostatic hyperplasia: subgroup analyses of pooled data from 4 multinational, randomized, placebo-controlled clinical studies. Urology 2013; 82:667-73.

9. Rees J, Bultitude M, Challacombe B. The management of lower urinary tract symptoms in men. BMJ 2014;348:g3861 doi:10.1136/bmj.g3861.

10. Roehrborn CG, Siami P, Barkin J, et al. The effects of dutasteride, tamsulosin and combination therapy on lower urinary tract symptoms in men with benign prostatic hyperplasia and prostatic enlargement: 2-year results from the CombAT study. J Urol 2008;179:616-21.

11. Rogers R. Urinary stress incontinence in women. N Engl J Med 2008;358:1029-36.

12. Yamaguchi O, Nishizawa O, Takeda M, et al. Clinical guidelines for overactive bladder. Int J Urol 2009;16:126-42.

13. Sherman JJ. Health issues in older men. In: Dunsworth T, Richardson M, Chant C, et al., eds. Pharmacotherapy Self-Assessment Program, 6th ed. Women's and Men's Health. Lenexa, KS: American College of Clinical Pharmacy, 2008:163-80.

Osteoarthritis and Rheumatoid Arthritis

1. Bruce SP. Rheumatoid arthritis. In: Richardson M, Chant C, Cheng JWM, et al., eds. Pharmacotherapy Self-Assessment Program, 6th ed. Chronic Illness II. Lenexa, KS: American College of Clinical Pharmacy, 2009:73-90.

2. Clegg DO, Reda DJ, Harris CL, et al. Glucosamine, chondroitin sulfate, and the two in combination for painful knee osteoarthritis. N Engl J Med 2006;354:795-808.

3. Eriksson J, Neovius M, Bratt J, et al. Biological vs conventional combination treatment and work loss in early rheumatoid arthritis. A randomized trial. JAMA Intern Med 2013;173:1407-14.

4. Fosbol E, Folke F, Jacobsen S, et al. Cause-specific cardiovascular risk associated with nonsteroidal antiinflammatory drugs among healthy individuals. Circ Cardiovasc Qual Outcomes 2010;3:395-405.

5. Hochberg, MC, Altman RD, April KT, et al. American College of Rheumatology 2012 recommendations for the use of nonpharmacologic and pharmacologic therapies in osteoarthritis of the hand, hip, and knee. Arthritis Care Res 2012;64:465-74.

6. McAlindon TE, LaValley MP, Gulin JP, et al. Glucosamine and chondroitin for treatment of osteoarthritis: a systematic quality assessment and meta-analysis. JAMA 2000;283:1469-75.

7. O'Dell JR, Curtis JR, Mikuls TR, et al. Validation of the methotrexate-first strategy in patients with early, poor-prognosis rheumatoid arthritis: results from a two-year randomized, double-blind trial. Arthritis Rheum 2013;65:1985.

8. AGS. Pharmacological management of persistent pain in older persons. J Am Geriatr Soc 2009;57:1331-46.

9. Peters MJL, Symmons DPM, McCarey D, et al. EULAR evidence-based recommendations for cardiovascular risk management in patients with rheumatoid arthritis and other forms of inflammatory arthritis. Ann Rheum Dis 2010;69:325-31.

10. Singh JA, Furst DE, Bharat A, et al. 2012 update of the 2008 American College of Rheumatology recommendations for the use of disease-modifying antirheumatic drugs and biologic agents in the treatment of rheumatoid arthritis. Arthritis Care Res 2012;64:625-39.

11. U.S. Food and Drug Administration (FDA). Acetaminophen information. Available at www.fda.gov/Drugs/DrugSafety/InformationbyDrugClass/ucm165107.htm. Accessed February 13, 2012.

ANSWERS AND EXPLANATIONS TO PATIENT CASES

1. Answer: D
Renal elimination is usually the most significantly changed pharmacokinetic value in older people. In this patient, her advanced age and diseases will add to her loss of renal function. Using the Cockcroft-Gault equation, this patient's estimated CrCl is 24 mL/minute. Creatinine clearance = $[(140 - 85)65/(72 \times 1.8)] \times 0.85$. At this level of function, glyburide elimination would be prolonged, and metformin use is contraindicated.

2. Answer: B
Common pharmacodynamic changes associated with aging include impaired homeostasis for electrolytes with angiotensin-converting enzyme inhibitors such as lisinopril and increased sensitivity to anticholinergic side effects from drugs such as meclizine.

3. Answer: D
This patient experienced a geriatric syndrome (a fall) and hazards of hospitalization (decline in organ systems and function) seen with many elderly patients. At this time, she has several risk factors for another fall, including a history of falls, diseases such as diabetes and hypertension, dizziness, and use of several drugs. An assessment of gait and balance would help determine the severity of her risk.

4. Answer: C
Efforts to maintain bone and muscle strength are more important for this patient than primary prevention of cardiovascular disease with simvastatin or lisinopril. Most older people do not consume a diet rich in vitamin D, have less sun exposure, and are more likely to be deficient in vitamin D, which is a risk factor for falls and reduced muscle strength. Furthermore, naproxen is not a good alternative for N.H. because of her poor renal function.

5. Answer: B
This patient has a positive screen for mild dementia. However, when evaluating her cognitive loss, it is important to limit the use of any drug that could contribute to confusion. Anticholinergics such as tolterodine can cause confusion, so it would be best to discontinue this agent and reassess cognition before beginning treatment for AD. Also, before beginning vitamin B_{12}

injections, the patient should first have laboratory evidence of deficiency. There is no reason to anticipate that hydrochlorothiazide would cause her cognitive decline, so a switch to lisinopril is not indicated at this time.

6. Answer: B
Rivastigmine is a potent inhibitor of acetyl and butyryl cholinesterase, leading to significant cholinergic adverse effects such as nausea, vomiting, and diarrhea. However, use of the transdermal delivery system generates even plasma concentrations and lessens the incidence of cholinergic adverse effects. Because the maintenance dose has been achieved with rivastigmine 12 mg, this man can switch to the patch that delivers 9.5 mg/day.

7. Answer: B
Over 3 years, this patient has declined only 4 points on her MMSE, which suggests a treatment response to donepezil. Furthermore, the patient is still able to live at home with her husband, and she has maintained some function in her basic ADLs. However, she has failed a higher donepezil dose, and there is no evidence that retrying it later is useful. Switching from one cholinesterase inhibitor to another has not been shown effective. Because she has benefited from donepezil use, she should not abruptly discontinue it. Some, but not all, clinical trials with memantine show an additional treatment response when memantine is added to donepezil therapy. When the benefits, risks, and costs have been openly discussed and family preferences are to consent to therapy, a time-based trial is reasonable. Memantine should be initiated at 5 mg daily. Donepezil can be evaluated for tapering after memantine titration is achieved. Vitamin E has shown no effect in large prospective trials of AD and should not be initiated.

8. Answer: C
Patients in the late stages of dementia (as evidenced by an MMSE of 5/30) would be unable to cooperate for administration of the Geriatric Depression Scale. The Functional Assessment Staging Test may help identify prognosis but would not benefit her in the management of her BPSD. The MoCA might validate the findings of the MMSE but would not help in management of BPSD. The Neuropsychiatric Inventory would provide

an objective baseline of BPSD so that interventions implemented could be assessed for effectiveness with a reevaluation.

9. Answer: A
Adding quetiapine would probably result in sedation and increase her risk of mortality. Although the behavior might decrease during periods of sedation, a chemical restraint is inappropriate for behavior not likely to harm the patient or others, and the behavior often returns when the patient adjusts to or develops a tolerance for the sedative properties. Citalopram does not have much evidence of effectiveness in the literature for symptoms besides depression. Television shows often confuse patients with severe AD because they cannot follow the activities or the plot and become frustrated. A behavioral approach with music therapy is the best method to try in this patient.

10. Answer: C
This patient shows symptoms of urge incontinence. There is some evidence that darifenacin, a selective muscarinic blocker, does not worsen cognition, and it would be preferred to tolterodine in this patient with MCI. Bethanechol is an option for overflow incontinence and could worsen her urge symptoms. Pelvic floor exercises are best used in stress incontinence.

11. Answer: C
Pharmacologic therapy targeted at reducing urethral sphincter pressure has proved effective in reducing BPH symptoms. Tamsulosin is an α-adrenergic blocker with more specific activity for the genitourinary system. Given that the patient already has low normal blood pressure, tamsulosin would be preferred to terazosin. Orthostatic hypotension can still occur with all α-adrenergic blockers, so patients should be monitored when therapy is initiated. Finasteride, an α-reductase inhibitor, and combination therapy with these agents are recommended when there is evidence of large prostate size. Saw palmetto is not recommended in combination with 5-α-reductase inhibitors because it may reduce the efficacy of the reductase inhibitors.

12. Answer: B
The American Geriatrics Society recommends treatment with opioids for OA when older patients do not respond to initial therapy with acetaminophen. The NSAIDs and COX-2 inhibitors are seldom considered when a thorough assessment of the patient shows that the risk of treatment (GI bleeding and renal disease) does not outweigh the potential benefit. Glucosamine can be added to this patient's medication regimen; however, even if effective, it will not provide immediate pain relief.

13. Answer: A
This woman has indicators of a poor prognosis with rheumatoid arthritis (positive RF, many symptoms) and has not responded to methotrexate therapy. Although the next treatment step is not entirely clear, her best choices are between double or triple combination DMARD therapy and a biologic agent. Leflunomide or hydroxychloroquine would not be recommended as monotherapy for someone who has not responded to methotrexate. Etanercept has a response in 60%–75% of patients whose therapy with methotrexate has failed. Glucocorticosteroids are used as adjunctive therapy for the first several months of treatment with a disease-modifying agent and would not be adequate treatment at this time.

ANSWERS AND EXPLANATIONS TO SELF-ASSESSMENT QUESTIONS

1. Answer: A

Diazepam is a long-acting benzodiazepine that can accumulate in older patients, resulting in excessive lethargy, sedation, and unsteady gait, and the patient admits taking it every night over the past week. A worsening of the patient's depression is evident with the recent bereavement; however, that would not explain the unsteady gait. Lisinopril is not likely to cause this problem with his blood pressure at target.

2. Answer: C

In older patients, the volume of distribution of lipid-soluble drugs such as diazepam is increased, not decreased. In addition, changes in metabolism through phase I (oxidation) are diminished. Diazepam tends to accumulate with reduced capacity for elimination, resulting in excessive sedation and an increased risk of falls in older patients.

3. Answer: B

The patient is not experiencing any symptoms of hypotension; therefore, no changes in her metoprolol therapy are warranted. Insufficient information is provided to determine the need to add memantine at this time. Adding vitamin D to this resident's regimen, given her deficient serum levels, may help reduce falls. Adding calcium carbonate may be helpful but will not reduce fall risk.

4. Answer: A

The U.S. Preventive Services Task Force recommends aspirin use in women 55–79 years of age to prevent ischemic strokes in women with a low risk of GI bleeding. This patient has no history of GI bleeding and would probably benefit from low-dose aspirin. Increasing the dose of metoprolol or adding hydrochlorothiazide might increase the risk of falls without providing additional risk reduction at her current BP. Similarly, increasing her atorvastatin dose might marginally improve her low-density lipoprotein cholesterol but would not significantly change her risk of ischemic stroke. Furthermore, given this patient's age over 75, the newest guidelines for prevention of cardiovascular disease do not recommend titration above moderate intensity statin therapy.

5. Answer: B

An initial trial of acetaminophen at doses less than 3 g/day is a reasonable option for frail patients with OA pain. Ibuprofen and tramadol would be alternatives when more conservative medications have failed a trial of 1–2 weeks. As-needed hydrocodone/acetaminophen should be used cautiously in older patients who have significant osteoarthritic pain and are unable to tolerate other drugs.

6. Answer: D

All cholinesterase inhibitors have similar efficacy. The rivastigmine transdermal patch is better tolerated than the oral dosage formulation. Donepezil tends to be better tolerated than the other oral cholinesterase inhibitors. Doses of cholinesterase medications should be titrated slowly to prevent GI upset. The initial dose of donepezil is 5 mg daily at bedtime, and for galantamine ER, the dose is 8 mg once daily. The rivastigmine patch 4.6 mg is the appropriate initial starting dose. Memantine has not shown any beneficial effect in maintaining cognitive function as measured by MMSE scores.

7. Answer: A

This patient's current fasting blood glucose of 65 mg/dL and A1C value of 5.6% should prompt the pharmacist to request glipizide discontinuation. The recommendation for A1C goal for older patients with several comorbid conditions is to keep it above 7.5%. The goals of therapy are to prevent hypoglycemia in older patients at greatest risk of this adverse drug reaction. There is no rationale for reducing the dose of carvedilol, and given a normal basic metabolic panel and her blood pressure, reducing potassium chloride or discontinuing lisinopril is not indicated at this time.

8. Answer: D

There is no evidence at this time that would support increasing the dose of donepezil to 23 mg to manage behavioral symptoms of dementia. The off-label use of atypical antipsychotic medications in patients with behavioral symptoms of dementia should be reserved for patients who pose a danger to themselves or others or experience hallucinations or delusions that are stressful to them. Adding acetaminophen to treat possible pain that could be causing T.W.'s behavior should be tried before more aggressive strategies.

9. Answer: A

Any new symptom of UI in an older adult should be thoroughly evaluated to determine whether there is a reversible cause. Infection, or the "I" in the mnemonic DRIP, may be the cause of the new symptoms in this patient. Urinalysis would be the most appropriate intervention to treat this reversible cause of incontinence. Tolterodine is used in urge incontinence that does not respond to an adequate pelvic floor muscle trial. Duloxetine has been used off-label for stress incontinence. Pelvic floor muscle exercises or Kegel exercises should be first-line therapy for stress, urge, or mixed incontinence in women.

10. Answer: C

In this patient with comorbid conditions of hypertension and BPH, the choice of α-blockers is based on the adverse effect profiles. This patient has an elevated PVR volume, so changing tamsulosin to terazosin might achieve a reduction in both BP and urinary retention. Increasing the atenolol dose would address just the increased BP, with no effect on the current problem of acute urinary retention. The patient is receiving moderate doses of controlled-release opioid, so reducing the hydromorphone dose for breakthrough pain is unlikely to help reduce the obstruction that may be worsened by the narcotics.

11. Answer: C

This patient is currently receiving 3 g of acetaminophen daily without adequate response, so a change in treatment is indicated. Diclofenac gel may provide adequate relief without systemic side effects. He has a history of GERD and is on aspirin, so naproxen is not preferred. Evidence indicates that initially GI bleeding is reduced with celecoxib, but this is not maintained with chronic use. Methylprednisolone injection is more aggressive treatment and may be considered if topical diclofenac is ineffective.

12. Answer: D

In patients with recurring rheumatoid arthritis symptoms, moderate disease activity, and presence of a poor prognostic factor (anti–cyclic citrullinated peptides), adding sulfasalazine and hydroxychloroquine

to methotrexate follows guidelines from the 2012 American College of Rheumatology recommendations update for the treatment of rheumatoid arthritis. Specifically, they recommend either double or triple combination DMARD therapy for patients with an inadequate response to methotrexate. Prednisone may be used as bridge therapy, but continued therapy may not be supported by a risk-benefit analysis. Changing the administration of methotrexate from the oral route to the intramuscular route would not confer any significant advantage in this case. Similarly, changing methotrexate to monotherapy with leflunomide would not provide any significant benefits.

13. Answer: B

Patients with a low bone mass and a T-score of –2.5 or less at the femoral neck, total hip, or lumbar spine, with a 10-year probability of having a major osteoporosis-related fracture of 20% or greater on the basis of the World Health Organization Fracture Risk Assessment Tool would benefit from an osteoporosis medication. This patient's risk fits that category, and she is already on adequate calcium and vitamin D. Adding a bisphosphonate is the most appropriate intervention at this time. Adding raloxifene or teriparatide is inappropriate for the treatment of this patient right now but might be appropriate care in a different scenario.

Gastrointestinal Disorders

Brian A. Hemstreet, Pharm.D., FCCP, BCPS

Regis University School of Pharmacy
Rueckert-Hartman College for Health Professions
Denver, Colorado

Gastrointestinal Disorders

Brian A. Hemstreet, Pharm.D., FCCP, BCPS

Regis University School of Pharmacy
Rueckert-Hartman College for Health Professions
Denver, Colorado

Learning Objectives

1. Review and apply national guideline treatment strategies to the following gastrointestinal (GI) disorders: gastroesophageal reflux disease (GERD), peptic ulcer disease (PUD), ulcerative colitis (UC), Crohn disease (CD), viral hepatitis, chronic liver disease, constipation, diarrhea, irritable bowel syndrome (IBS), nausea, vomiting, pancreatitis, and upper GI bleeding, including prevention of stress-related mucosal disease (SRMD).

2. Recommend appropriate pharmacologic and non-pharmacologic interventions for the management of GERD.

3. Differentiate between clinical signs, symptoms, risk factors, and treatment of PUD associated with both *Helicobacter pylori* and nonsteroidal anti-inflammatory drugs.

4. Discuss the role of pharmacologic intervention in the treatment of nonvariceal upper GI bleeding and the prevention of SRMD.

5. Review the clinical differences in signs, symptoms, and treatment of CD and UC.

6. Identify the common manifestations of chronic liver disease and their treatment.

7. Review the treatment and prevention of both acute and chronic viral hepatitis.

8. Recognize pertinent information for educating patients and prescribers about the appropriate use of pharmacologic agents for various GI disorders.

9. Recommend appropriate pharmacologic and non-pharmacologic interventions for diarrhea and constipation.

10. Review recommendations for the treatment and prevention of nausea and vomiting.

11. Discuss the clinical and treatment differences between acute and chronic pancreatitis.

12. Discuss the role of pharmacologic intervention in the treatment of IBS.

13. Discuss commonly encountered statistical tests and concepts, using GI disorders as examples.

Self-Assessment Questions

Answers and explanations to these questions can be found at the end of the chapter.

1. A 58-year-old African American man presents with a 2-month history of burning epigastric pain and intermittent difficulty swallowing. The pain is unrelieved by positional changes or by eating, and he has tried over-the-counter (OTC) antacids with minimal relief. He takes amlodipine 5 mg/day for hypertension and ibuprofen for occasional back pain. Which is best for this patient?

    A. Initiate famotidine 20 mg/day.

    B. Refer for possible endoscopic evaluation.

    C. Initiate omeprazole 20 mg twice daily.

    D. Change amlodipine to hydrochlorothiazide.

2. A 50-year-old woman is seen today in the clinic for severe pain related to the swelling of three of her metacarpophalangeal joints on each hand and swelling of her right wrist. She is unable to write or perform her usual household activities. Radiograms of these joints reveal bony decalcifications and erosions. A serum rheumatoid factor is obtained, which is elevated. Her medical history includes type 2 diabetes mellitus, hypertension, and dyslipidemia. Her medications include metformin 1000 mg twice daily, glyburide 10 mg/day, metoprolol 100 mg twice daily, aspirin 81 mg/day, and rosuvastatin 5 mg/day. The primary care provider would like to initiate systemic anti-inflammatory therapy for this patient's rheumatoid arthritis with high-dose nonsteroidal anti-inflammatory drug (NSAID) therapy; however, the primary care provider is worried about potential gastrointestinal (GI) toxicity. Which regimen is best for treating this patient's pain while minimizing the risk of GI toxicity?

    A. Celecoxib 400 mg twice daily.

    B. Indomethacin 75 mg/day plus ranitidine 150 mg/day.

    C. Naproxen 500 mg twice daily plus omeprazole 20 mg/day.

    D. Piroxicam 20 mg/day plus misoprostol 600 mcg three times/day.

3. A 68-year-old Hispanic man is assessed in the emergency department for a 36-hour history of black, tarry stools; dizziness; confusion; and vomiting a substance resembling coffee grounds. He has a medical history of osteoarthritis, hypertension, myocardial infarction (MI) in 1996 and 1998, and seasonal allergies. He has been taking naproxen 500 mg twice daily for 4 years, metoprolol 100 mg twice daily, aspirin 325 mg/day, and loratadine 10 mg/day. Nasogastric (NG) aspiration is positive for blood, and subsequent endoscopy reveals a 3-cm antral ulcer with a visible vessel. The vessel is obliterated using an epinephrine solution, and a rapid urease test is negative for *Helicobacter pylori*. Which recommendation is best for this patient?

A. Intravenous ranitidine 50 mg/hour for 5 days.

B. Sucralfate 1 g four times/day by NG tube.

C. Oral lansoprazole 15 mg/day by NG tube.

D. Pantoprazole 80 mg intravenous bolus, followed by an 8-mg/hour infusion.

4. A 38-year-old white woman presents with an 8-week history of new-onset cramping abdominal pain together with two to four bloody stools per day. She has a medical history of urinary tract infection and reports an allergy to "sulfa"-containing medications (shortness of breath). Colonoscopy reveals diffuse superficial colonic inflammation consistent with ulcerative colitis (UC). The inflammation is continuous and extends to the hepatic flexure. Which drug therapy is best?

A. Sulfasalazine 4 g/day.

B. Hydrocortisone enema 100 mg every night.

C. 6-mercaptopurine (6-MP) 75 mg/day.

D. Mesalamine (Delzicol) 1.6 g orally three times/day.

5. A 45-year-old African American man with a history of alcoholic cirrhosis (Child-Pugh class B) was seen in the clinic today for a follow-up. He was recently referred for screening endoscopy, which revealed several large esophageal varices. He has no history of bleeding; 1 month ago, propranolol 10 mg orally three times/day was initiated. At that time, his vital signs included temperature 98.7°F, heart rate (HR) 85 beats/minute, respiratory rate (RR) 15 breaths/minute, and blood pressure (BP) 130/80 mm Hg. At his evaluation today, he seems to be tolerating the propranolol dose and has no new concerns. His vital signs now include temperature 98.6°F, HR 79 beats/minute, RR 14 breaths/minute, and BP 128/78 mm Hg. Which is the best course of action?

A. Continue current therapy, with a close follow-up in 4 weeks.

B. Increase propranolol to 20 mg orally three times/day.

C. Add isosorbide dinitrate 10 mg orally three times/day.

D. Change propranolol to atenolol 25 mg orally once daily.

6. A new stool antigen test to detect *H. pylori* was tested in 1000 patients with suspected peptic ulcer disease (PUD), and 865 had a positive result. All patients had also undergone a concomitant endoscopy with biopsy and culture as the gold standard comparative test, and 900 had a positive result. Of these 900 patients with confirmed disease, only 850 also had a positive result with the new stool antigen test. From these results, which best represents the sensitivity and specificity of the new stool antigen test?

A. Sensitivity 82%, specificity 86%.

B. Sensitivity 85%, specificity 97%.

C. Sensitivity 94%, specificity 85%.

D. Sensitivity 96%, specificity 90%.

7. A 50-year-old Asian woman is seeking advice about a recent possible exposure to hepatitis A virus (HAV). She saw on the local news report that a chef at a local restaurant where she had eaten about 3 weeks earlier had active HAV. Having heard that HAV could be transmitted through food, she would like to know her options. She has not previously received the HAV vaccine. Which is the best recommendation for this patient?

A. Initiate HAV vaccine.

B. Administer HAV immune globulin.

C. Continue to observe the patient for symptoms.

D. Initiate HAV vaccine and immune globulin.

8. A 48-year-old woman is admitted to the general medicine floor with abdominal pain, severe nausea and vomiting, and abdominal distension secondary to alcoholic hepatitis. She has a history of alcohol abuse for 20 years and takes no current medications. Her serum creatinine (SCr) is 0.5 mg/dL, aspartate aminotransferase (AST) 250 IU/L, alanine aminotransferase (ALT) 60 IU/L, total bilirubin 10.3 mg/dL, prothrombin time 19 seconds (control 12 seconds), and albumin 2.1 g/L. An abdominal paracentesis shows no evidence of spontaneous bacterial peritonitis. She reports no known drug allergies. What treatment is best for this patient's alcoholic hepatitis?

   A. Naproxen 220 mg orally twice daily.

   B. Octreotide 50 mcg/hour intravenously.

   C. Prednisolone 40 mg/day.

   D. Midodrine 7.5 mg three times daily.

9. A 50-year-old, 80-kg man with a history of intravenous drug abuse and chronic hepatitis C virus (HCV) (genotype 2) was initiated on pegylated interferon (PEG-IFN) 180 mcg subcutaneously and ribavirin 400 mg orally twice daily 2 weeks ago. He returns to the clinic today with fatigue, scleral icterus, and pallor. There is no clinical evidence of bleeding. Laboratory values reveal the following: hematocrit 31% (baseline 39%), total bilirubin 3.2 mg/dL (indirect 2.7 mg/dL, direct 0.5 mg/dL), AST 150 IU/mL (baseline 300 IU/mL), ALT 180 IU/mL (baseline 400 IU/mL), SCr 0.7 mg/dL, HCV RNA 1×10^6 IU/mL (baseline 2.3×10^6 copies/mL), white blood cell count (WBC) 7.8×10^3 cells/mm^3, and platelet count 160,000/mm^3. Which is the most likely cause of this patient's current symptoms?

   A. Worsening of his liver disease secondary to inadequate treatment.

   B. An adverse effect secondary to treatment with PEG-IFN.

   C. Systemic manifestations of chronic HCV disease.

   D. An adverse effect secondary to treatment with ribavirin.

10. A 35-year-old man with a history of Crohn disease (CD) is in the clinic today with a chief concern of mucopurulent drainage from an erythematous region on his abdomen. Examination reveals a moderate-size enterocutaneous fistula in the left upper abdominal area. He takes mesalamine (Pentasa) 250 mg 4 capsules three times/day and azathioprine 150 mg/day. His physician wants to prescribe infliximab. Which recommendation is best when initiating infliximab therapy?

    A. Rule out tuberculosis by purified protein derivative or QuantiFERON-TB test.

    B. Administer a test dose before the initial infusion.

    C. Admit to the hospital for the administration of all doses.

    D. Obtain an echocardiogram to assess cardiac function.

11. A 41-year-old woman with a history of bipolar disorder and recurrent urinary tract infections is admitted to the general medicine service with severe nausea, vomiting, fever, and back pain. On examination, she has fever, dry mucous membranes, and right-sided costovertebral tenderness. A urinalysis, which reveals many bacteria, is positive for leukocyte esterase. Her SCr is 1.3 mg/dL and blood urea nitrogen (BUN) is 29 mg/dL, and she is 65 inches tall and weighs 70 kg. She takes risperidone 6 mg twice daily and sertraline 150 mg/day. She reports an allergy to trimethoprim/sulfamethoxazole that causes a rash. Which drug would be best for treating this patient's nausea?

    A. Prochlorperazine 10-mg tablet orally twice daily.

    B. Metoclopramide orally disintegrating tablets (ODTs) 5 mg three times/day.

    C. Ondansetron 4 mg intravenously three or four times/day.

    D. Diphenhydramine 50 mg intravenously three or four times/day.

12. A 75-year-old man with a history of hypertension, type 2 diabetes mellitus, and chronic low back pain is admitted to the hospital for abdominal pain lasting 2 days. He denies fever, chills, or sick contacts. His last bowel movement was 3–4 days ago. On examination, he is afebrile and has moderate left upper and lower quadrant tenderness. An abdominal radiograph reveals large amounts of stool in the colon with no signs of obstruction. He currently takes lisinopril 20 mg/day, verapamil 240 mg once daily, acetaminophen 500 mg four times/day, oxycodone sustained release 20 mg twice daily, and oxycodone/acetaminophen 5/325 mg as needed for pain. His SCr is 1.8 mg/dL (baseline 1.7 mg/dL); he is 58 inches tall and weighs 68 kg. Which therapy would be best to manage this patient's constipation?

    A. Sodium phosphate oral solution.

    B. Bisacodyl suppository.

    C. Methylcellulose tablets.

    D. Methylnaltrexone injection.

13. A 65-year-old man with a history of hypothyroidism, heart failure, and MI is admitted to the intensive care unit with severe community-acquired pneumonia. Six hours after admission, he develops acute respiratory failure, hypotension, and acute kidney injury from presumed sepsis; he is placed on mechanical ventilation. An NG tube is placed. He currently takes ramipril 10 mg/day, metoprolol 100 mg twice daily, levothyroxine 125 mcg/day, and aspirin 81 mg/day. His WBC is 25×10^3 cells/mm³, platelet count 170,000/mm³, SCr 3.8 mg/dL (baseline 1.1 mg/dL), potassium 4.9 mEq/L, BUN 65 mg/dL, international normalized ratio (INR) 1.1, AST 30 IU/mL, and ALT 45 IU/mL. He is 68 inches tall and weighs 79 kg. Which approach is most appropriate for preventing stress-related mucosal disease (SRMD) in this patient?

    A. Sucralfate 1 g four times/day by NG tube.

    B. Magnesium hydroxide 30 mL four times/day by NG tube.

    C. Cimetidine 8-mg/hour intravenous infusion.

    D. Pantoprazole 40 mg intravenously once daily.

14. A newly available NSAID was designed to reduce the incidence of adverse GI events compared with traditional NSAIDs. A large retrospective cohort study compares the incidence of ulceration and bleeding associated with the use of this new NSAID with that of ibuprofen and naproxen. The results indicate that the new agent is associated with no statistically or clinically significant reduction in ulceration or bleeding with long-term use compared with ibuprofen and naproxen. The investigators of the study argue that the lack of difference in safety is because the drug is being promoted as safer; therefore, most patients receiving it are at a much higher baseline risk of NSAID-induced ulceration and bleeding. If this phenomenon did indeed affect the study results, which potential source of bias would probably be present?

    A. Recall bias.

    B. Misclassification bias.

    C. Interviewer bias.

    D. Channeling bias.

15. A new enzyme immunoassay for HCV RNA has a reported sensitivity of 95% and a specificity of 92%. If the prevalence of HCV in a cohort of 500 patients is 40%, which best represents the positive predictive value of this new test?

    A. 75%.

    B. 89%.

    C. 92%.

    D. 96%.

I. **GASTROESOPHAGEAL REFLUX DISEASE (GERD)**

A. Definition
   1. "GERD is defined by consensus and as such is a disease comprising symptoms, end-organ effects and complications related to the reflux of gastric contents into the esophagus, oral cavity, and/or the lung" Strength of guideline evidence is rated by the GRADE system (Level of Evidence and Strength).

Table 1. Level of Evidence and Strength

Level of Evidence	Definition
High	Further research was unlikely to change the authors' confidence in the estimate of the effect
Moderate	Further research would probably affect confidence in the estimate of effect
Low	Further research would be expected to have an important impact on the confidence in the estimate of the effect and would be likely to change the estimate
Strength of Evidence	
Strong	The desirable effects of an intervention clearly outweigh the undesirable effects
Conditional	There is uncertainty about the trade-offs

   2. Definition subdivides GERD into the following categories:
      a. Symptoms without erosions on endoscopy (nonerosive reflux disease)
      b. Symptoms with erosions on endoscopy (erosive reflux disease)
   3. Symptoms
      a. Typical symptoms: heartburn (pyrosis), regurgitation, acidic taste in the mouth
      b. Extraesophageal or atypical symptoms: Chronic cough, asthma-like symptoms, recurrent sore throat, laryngitis or hoarseness, dental enamel loss, and noncardiac chest pain; sinusitis, pneumonia, bronchitis, and otitis media are less common atypical symptoms.
      c. Alarm symptoms: dysphagia, odynophagia, bleeding, weight loss, choking, chest pain, and epigastric mass. These symptoms warrant immediate referral for more invasive testing.
      d. Aggravating factors: recumbency (gravity), elevated intra-abdominal pressure, reduced gastric motility, decreased lower esophageal sphincter (LES) tone, and direct mucosal irritation
      e. Long-term complications: esophageal erosion, strictures or obstruction, Barrett esophagus, and reduction in patient's quality of life

B. Diagnosis
   1. Symptoms
      a. A presumptive diagnosis of GERD can be established in the setting of typical symptoms of heartburn and regurgitation. Empiric therapy with a proton pump inhibitor (PPI) is recommended if patient has typical symptoms of heartburn or regurgitation. (Strong recommendation/Moderate level of evidence)
      b. Screening for *H. pylori* is *not* recommended. (Strong/Low)
      c. Patients with noncardiac chest pain that is suspected of having been caused by GERD should have a diagnostic evaluation before institution of therapy. (Strong/Low)
   2. Endoscopy: Upper endoscopy is not necessary in the presence of typical GERD symptoms. Endoscopy is recommended in the presence of alarm symptoms and in the screening of patients at high risk of complications. Repeat endoscopy is not indicated in patients without Barrett esophagus in the absence of new symptoms. (Strong/Moderate)

3. Manometry: Recommended for preoperative evaluation but has no role in the diagnosis of GERD (Strong/Low)

4. Ambulatory pH testing

    a. Ambulatory esophageal reflux monitoring is indicated before considering endoscopic or surgical therapy in patients with nonerosive reflux disease as part of the evaluation of patients who are refractory to PPI therapy and in situations when the diagnosis of GERD is in question. (Strong/Low)

    b. Ambulatory reflux monitoring is the only test that can assess reflux symptom association. (Strong/Low)

    c. Ambulatory reflux monitoring is not necessary in the presence of short- or long-segment Barrett esophagus to establish a diagnosis of GERD. (Strong/Moderate)

C. Treatment Strategies for GERD

1. Nonpharmacologic interventions and lifestyle modifications are unlikely to control symptoms in most patients. The American Gastroenterological Association (AGA) guidelines cite insufficient evidence to advocate lifestyle modifications for all patients; rather, they advocate use in targeted populations. Thus, the following lifestyle modifications should be implemented only in the patient populations specified.

    a. Dietary modifications in patients whose symptoms are associated with certain foods or drinks. Routine global elimination of food triggers *not* recommended according to the 2013 guidelines. (Conditional/Low)

        i. Avoid aggravating foods and beverages; some may reduce LES pressure (alcohol, caffeine, chocolate, citrus juices, garlic, onions, peppermint or spearmint) or cause direct irritation (spicy foods, tomato juice, coffee).

        ii. Reduce fat intake (high-fat meals slow gastric emptying) and portion size.

        iii. Avoid eating 2–3 hours before bedtime.

        iv. Remain upright after meals.

    b. Weight loss if overweight or recent weight gain (Conditional/Mod)

    c. Reduce or discontinue nicotine use in patients who use tobacco products (affects LES).

    d. Elevate head of bed and avoid meals 2–3 hours before bedtime if nocturnal symptoms. (Conditional/Low)

    e. Avoid tight-fitting clothing (decreases intra-abdominal pressure).

    f. Avoid medications that may reduce LES pressure, delay gastric emptying, or cause direct irritation: α-adrenergic antagonists, anticholinergics, benzodiazepines, calcium channel blockers, estrogen, nitrates, opiates, tricyclic antidepressants, theophylline, NSAIDs, and aspirin.

2. Pharmacologic therapies

    a. Initial treatment depends on the severity, frequency, and duration of symptoms.

        i. "Step-down" treatment: Starting with maximal therapy, such as therapeutic doses of PPIs, is always appropriate as a first-line strategy in patients with documented esophageal erosion. Advantages: Rapid symptom relief, avoidance of overinvestigation. Disadvantages: Potential overtreatment, higher drug cost, increased potential for adverse effects

        ii. "Step-up" treatment: Start with lower-dose over-the-counter (OTC) products. Advantages: Avoids overtreatment, has lower initial drug cost. Disadvantages: Potential undertreatment (partial symptom relief; may take longer for symptom control; may lead to overinvestigation)

    b. The AGA treatment guideline recommendation summary follows.

Table 2. AGA Treatment Guideline Recommendation

Area	Recommendation (Level/Strength)
Treatment	• Erosive esophagitis should be treated with an 8-week course of PPIs; no major differences in products (Strong/High)
	• Use maintenance PPIs if return of symptoms or complications (Strong/Moderate)
	• Bedtime histamine-2 receptor antagonists can be used if a.m. PPI and nighttime symptoms, but tachyphylaxis develops (Conditional/Low)
	• Further testing needed before use of metoclopramide or baclofen (Conditional/Mod)
Dosing	• Traditional PPIs should be given 30–60 minutes before meals (Strong/Moderate)
	• Newer PPIs offer dosing flexibility in relation to meals (Conditional/Moderate)
	• Initiate PPIs once daily before a.m. meal (Strong/Moderate)
	• Twice-daily PPIs if partial response to once-daily PPIs or nighttime symptoms (Strong/Low)
	• Twice daily if partial response to once daily or can switch to another PPI (Conditional/Low)

PPI = proton pump inhibitor.

    c. Pharmacologic agents
      i. Antacids
        (a) Calcium-, aluminum-, and magnesium-based products are available OTC in a wide variety of formulations (capsules, tablets, chewable tablets, and suspensions).
        (b) Neutralizing acid and raising intragastric pH results in decreased activation of pepsinogen and increased LES pressure; rapid onset of action but short duration, necessitating frequent dosing
        (c) Some products (Gaviscon) contain the antirefluxant alginic acid, which forms a viscous layer on top of gastric contents to act as a barrier to reflux (variable added efficacy).
        (d) Used as first-line therapy for intermittent (less than twice weekly) symptoms or as breakthrough therapy for those on PPI/histamine-2 receptor antagonist (H2RA) therapy; not appropriate for healing established esophageal erosions
        (e) Adverse reactions: Constipation (aluminum), diarrhea (magnesium), accumulation of aluminum and magnesium in renal disease with repeated dosing
        (f) Drug interactions: Chelation (fluoroquinolones, tetracyclines); reduced absorption because of increases in pH (ketoconazole, itraconazole, iron, atazanavir, delavirdine, indinavir, nelfinavir) or increases in absorption, leading to potential toxicity (raltegravir, saquinavir)
      ii. Histamine-2 receptor antagonists
        (a) Reversibly inhibit histamine-2 receptors on the parietal cell
        (b) All agents available as prescription and OTC products; a variety of formulations available; generics exist for all prescription products

Table 3. Histamine-2 Receptor Antagonists

Agent	Oral OTC Formulations	Oral Prescription Formulations
Ranitidine (Zantac)	75-mg tablet (Zantac 75) 150-mg tablet (Zantac 150)	150-mg tablets/EFFERdose tablets/granules 300-mg tablet 15 mg/mL of syrup
Cimetidine (Tagamet)	200-mg tablet (Tagamet-HB)	300-, 400-, 800-mg tablets 300 mg/5 mL of solution
Nizatidine (Axid)	75-mg tablet (Axid AR)	150-mg/300-mg capsules 15 mg/mL of solution
Famotidine (Pepcid) Pepcid Complete	10-mg tablets, gelatin capsules, chewable tablets (Pepcid AC) 20-mg tablets 10 mg + 800 mg of calcium carbonate + 165 mg of magnesium hydroxide chewable tablets	20-mg/40-mg tablets 20-mg/40-mg rapidly disintegrating tablet 40-mg/5-mL suspension

OTC = over the counter.

   (c) OTC H2RA products may be used for on-demand therapy for intermittent mild–moderate GERD symptoms; preventive dosing before meals or exercise is also possible for all agents. Higher prescription doses are often necessary for more severe symptoms or for maintenance dosing. Prolonged use is associated with the development of tolerance and reduced efficacy (tachyphylaxis).

   (d) Therapy with H2RAs is less efficacious than therapy with PPIs in healing erosive esophagitis.

   (e) Adverse effects: Most are well tolerated. Central nervous system (CNS) effects such as headache, dizziness, fatigue, somnolence, and confusion are the most common. Older adults and patients with reduced renal function are more at risk. Prolonged cimetidine use is associated with rare development of gynecomastia.

   (f) Drug interactions: May affect the absorption of drugs dependent on lower gastric pH (e.g., ketoconazole, itraconazole, iron, atazanavir, delavirdine, indinavir, nelfinavir) or increases in absorption leading to potential toxicity (raltegravir, saquinavir). Cimetidine also inhibits cytochrome P450 (CYP) enzymes 1A2, 2C9, 2D6, and 3A4. Warfarin, theophylline, and other agents metabolized by these enzymes may be affected. Cimetidine may also compete with medications and creatinine for tubular secretion in the kidney.

  iii. Proton pump inhibitors

   (a) Irreversibly inhibit the final step in gastric acid secretion; greater degree of acid suppression achieved and typically longer duration of action than H2RAs

   (b) Most effective agents for short- and long-term management of GERD and for management of erosive disease

   (c) Most costly agents: Omeprazole and lansoprazole now available as generic prescription-strength products and OTC. The OTC products are considered safe and effective for intermittent short-term (2 weeks) use in patients with typical heartburn symptoms. Long-term use of OTC products should be discussed with prescriber to prevent loss of follow-up or to assess for potential undertreatment.

   (d) Most effective when taken orally before meals; for divided dosing, give evening dose before evening meal instead of at bedtime.

Table 4. Proton Pump Inhibitors

Product	Dosage Forms
Esomeprazole (Nexium)	Delayed-release capsule (20 mg/40 mg) IV solution (20- and 40-mg vials) Delayed-release oral suspension (2.5-, 10-, 20-, 40-mg packets)
Omeprazole (Prilosec) Prilosec OTC Zegerid OTC	Delayed-release capsule (10 mg/20 mg/40 mg); delayed-release 20-mg tablet (magnesium salt) Immediate-release powder for oral suspension (20- and 40-mg packets); sodium bicarbonate buffer = 460 mg of Na⁺/dose (2 20-mg packets are not equivalent to 1 40-mg packet) Zegerid OTC 20-mg immediate-release capsules with sodium bicarbonate (1100 mg/capsule)
Lansoprazole (Prevacid) Lansoprazole (Prevacid 24HR)	Prevacid 24HR 15-mg delayed-release capsule Delayed-release capsule (15 mg/30 mg) Delayed-release oral suspension (15 mg/30 mg) Delayed-release orally disintegrating tablet (15 mg/30 mg)
Rabeprazole (AcipHex)	Delayed-release enteric-coated tablet (20 mg)
Pantoprazole (Protonix)	Delayed-release tablet (20 mg/40 mg) IV solution (40 mg/vial) Pantoprazole granules 40 mg/packet
Dexlansoprazole (Dexilant)	Delayed-release capsule (30 mg/60 mg)
Esomeprazole strontium	Delayed-release capsule (20 mg/40 mg base)
Product	**Alternative Administration Technique**
Omeprazole (Prilosec) Esomeprazole (Nexium) Zegerid	Open capsules; mix with applesauce or juice Simplified omeprazole suspension; contents dissolved in bicarbonate (NG/OG) Open esomeprazole capsules and mix with 60 mL of water by NG tube, or dissolve oral suspension in 15 mL of water and administer by NG tube; IV bolus, or continuous infusion Zegerid mix packet with 20 mL water in syringe (NG)
Lansoprazole (Prevacid)	Open capsules; mix with applesauce, ENSURE, cottage cheese, pudding, yogurt, or strained pears, or 60 mL of tomato, orange, or apple juice Open capsules + 40 mL of apple juice (NG/OG) Simplified lansoprazole suspension; contents dissolved in bicarbonate (NG/OG) *DO NOT* use oral suspension for NG/OG; mix packet with 30 mL of water and swallow Orally disintegrating tablet by oral syringe: Use 4 mL for 15 mg or 10 mL for 30 mg Orally disintegrating tablet by NG tube (>8 French): Same preparation as for oral syringe
Rabeprazole (AcipHex)	*DO NOT CRUSH*
Pantoprazole (Protonix)	*DO NOT CRUSH* IV (bolus or continuous infusion) Pantoprazole suspension (compounded with bicarbonate)
Dexlansoprazole (Dexilant)	Open capsules and sprinkle on applesauce

IV = intravenous; NG = nasogastric; OG = orogastric.

(e) Adverse reactions
  (1) Overall, well tolerated; possible adverse effects include headache, dizziness, nausea, diarrhea, and constipation. Long-term use is not associated with significant increases in endocrine neoplasia or symptomatic vitamin B_{12} deficiency. As an option, the 2013 AGA guidelines list the switching of PPIs in patients experiencing adverse effects. (Conditional/Low)
  (2) Summary of major adverse effects of PPIs and prevention and management strategies

Table 5. Summary of Major Adverse Effects of PPIs and Prevention and Management Strategies

Adverse Effect	Prevention and Management
Risk of fracture (hip, wrist, spine)	• Concern about fractures should not affect decision to use PPIs, except in patients with other known risk factors for hip fracture (Conditional/Moderate) • Patients with osteoporosis can remain on PPIs • Limit dose and duration • Ensure adequate calcium and vitamin D • BMD screening if at risk of low bone mass • Weight-bearing exercise
Hypomagnesemia	• Reevaluate need • Limit dose and duration • Consider baseline testing (presence of diuretics, digoxin) • Supplementation
Clostridium difficile–associated diarrhea	• Reevaluate need • Limit dose and duration • Evaluate for *C. difficile* if patient receiving PPI has diarrhea that is not improving • Have patients report diarrhea
Community-acquired pneumonia	• Short-term use may increase risk; long-term risk is not elevated (Conditional/Moderate) • Assess for vaccine status

BMD = bone mineral density; PPI = proton pump inhibitor.

(f) Drug interactions
  (1) Inhibition of CYP450: Omeprazole inhibits the metabolism of substrates such as diazepam through CYP2C19 inhibition.
    (A) Recent data suggest a reduced effectiveness of clopidogrel through CYP2C19-mediated inhibition of conversion to active metabolite by omeprazole. Recommendations according to the U.S. Food and Drug Administration (FDA) are to avoid omeprazole and to use pantoprazole as an alternative. The 2013 AGA guidelines consider the PPI/clopidogrel interaction NOT clinically significant. (Strong/High)
    (B) Interaction with high-dose intravenous methotrexate. The labeling for both intravenous methotrexate and the PPIs has been updated to include this interaction, which places patients at higher risk of methotrexate toxicity. Proposed mechanisms include reduced methotrexate excretion by PPI inhibition of BCRP or reduced renal excretion by inhibition of renal H+/K+-ATPase. Patients receiving high-dose intravenous methotrexate should avoid PPI use, with a switch to ranitidine if needed. There is some thought that holding the PPI dose for 2 days before and after methotrexate administration may prevent the interaction.

(2) Drugs with pH-dependent absorption (e.g., ketoconazole, itraconazole, protease inhibitors)

    iv. Promotility agents

        (a) The 2013 guidelines state that therapy for GERD other than acid suppression, including prokinetic therapy or baclofen, should not be used in patients with GERD without diagnostic evaluation. (Conditional/Mod)

        (b) Work through cholinergic mechanisms to facilitate increased gastric emptying.

        (c) Metoclopramide: Dopamine antagonist; must be dosed several times a day; associated with many adverse effects such as dizziness, fatigue, somnolence, drowsiness, extrapyramidal symptoms (EPS), and hyperprolactinemia. New 5- and 10-mg ODT formulations (metoclopramide [Metozolv ODT]) are now available. Indications for GERD and diabetic gastroparesis

        (d) Bethanechol: Cholinergic agonist; poorly tolerated because of adverse effects such as diarrhea, blurred vision, and abdominal cramping; may also increase gastric acid production

        (e) Cisapride: Available only on a restricted basis for patients whose other therapies have failed; cisapride was withdrawn from the market initially because of cardiac arrhythmia (torsades de pointes) when used in combination with drugs inhibiting CYP3A4.

    v. Surgical therapy

        (a) Surgical therapy is a treatment option for long-term therapy in patients with GERD. (Strong/High)

        (b) Surgical therapy is generally not recommended in patients who do not respond to PPI therapy. (Strong/High)

        (c) Surgical therapy is as effective as medical therapy for carefully selected patients with chronic GERD when performed by an experienced surgeon. (Strong/High)

        (d) Obese patients contemplating surgical therapy for GERD should be considered for bariatric surgery. Gastric bypass would be the preferred operation in these patients. (Conditional/Moderate)

Patient Case

1. A 55-year-old man with an 8-month history of GERD symptoms 4 or 5 days/week has been receiving lansoprazole 15 mg daily by mouth, with the use of magnesium hydroxide for breakthrough symptoms. His symptoms are still present 3–4 days/week and are disruptive to his daily life. He has implemented lifestyle modifications and has been adherent to the lansoprazole. His medical history is significant for hypothyroidism. He takes levothyroxine 100 mcg once daily. An endoscopy perfumed last week revealed no ulcers or erosions. Which treatment approach is best for this patient?

    A. Add metoclopramide 10 mg 4 times/day.

    B. Increase lansoprazole to 15 mg twice daily

    C. Switch to omeprazole 20 mg daily.

    D. Add sucralfate 1000 mg 4 times/day.

II. PEPTIC ULCER DISEASE

A. Classification of peptic ulcer disease (PUD)
   1. Duodenal ulcer
      a. Common causes: *H. pylori* infection (95%), NSAIDs, low-dose aspirin
      b. Uncommon causes: Zollinger-Ellison syndrome, hypercalcemia, granulomatous diseases, neoplasia, infections (cytomegalovirus, herpes simplex, tuberculosis), ectopic pancreatic tissue
      c. Clinical signs and symptoms: Epigastric pain, possibly worse at night; often, pain occurs 1–3 hours after a meal and may be relieved by eating. Pain may also be episodic. Associated symptoms may include heartburn, belching, a bloated feeling, nausea, and anorexia.
   2. Gastric ulcer
      a. Common causes: NSAIDs, *H. pylori* infection
      b. Uncommon causes: Crohn disease (CD), infections (cytomegalovirus, herpes simplex)
      c. Clinical signs and symptoms: Epigastric pain, which is often made worse by eating; associated symptoms may include heartburn, belching, a bloated feeling, nausea, and anorexia.
   3. Complications of PUD
      a. Bleeding
      b. Gastric outlet obstruction
      c. Perforation
   4. Patients at risk of NSAID-induced GI toxicity

Table 6. Risk Factors for NSAID-Induced GI Complications

Category	Risk Factors
High risk	1. History of complicated ulcer 2. Several (>2) risk factors 3. Concomitant use of corticosteroids, anticoagulants, or antiplatelet drugs
Moderate risk (1 or 2 risk factors)	1. Age >65 years 2. High-dose NSAID therapy 3. History of uncomplicated ulcer 4. Concurrent use of aspirin (including low dose), corticosteroids, or anticoagulants
Low risk	No risk factors

GI = gastrointestinal; NSAID = nonsteroidal anti-inflammatory drug.

   a. Some NSAIDs such as ibuprofen, diclofenac, and nabumetone are intrinsically less toxic to the GI tract than naproxen, which is considered moderate risk. Other agents such as piroxicam, indomethacin, and ketorolac are considered high-risk drugs.
   b. Duration of NSAID use (higher risk in first 3 months). Presence of chronic debilitating disorders such as rheumatoid arthritis or cardiovascular (CV) disease may also contribute to the increased GI toxicity of NSAIDs, but these are not generally considered independent risk factors.
   c. *H. pylori* infection is thought to confer additive risk of GI toxicity in NSAID users.
   5. Diagnosis
      a. Symptom presentation
      b. Testing for *H. pylori* infection: Practitioners must be willing to treat if testing is positive because *H. pylori* is a known carcinogen.
         i. Testing is indicated for patients with active ulcer disease, history of PUD, or gastric mucosa–associated lymphoid tissue lymphoma.
         ii. The test-and-treat strategy for identifying *H. pylori*–positive patients is also acceptable for patients with unevaluated dyspepsia who have no alarm symptoms and are younger than 55 years

    c. Diagnostic tests for *H. pylori* infection

        i. Invasive (endoscopic)

            (a) Histology: 90%–95% sensitive, 98%–99% specific, subject to sampling error

            (b) Rapid urease tests (*Campylobacter*-like organism [CLO] test, Hp-fast, and PyloriTek): Detect the presence of ammonia (NH_3) in a sample generated by *H. pylori* urease activity; 80%–95% sensitive, 95%–100% specific. False negatives may result from a partly treated infection, GI bleeding, achlorhydria, or use of PPIs, H2RAs, or bismuth. Patients should discontinue antisecretory agents for at least 1 week before test is performed.

            (c) Culture: Costly, time-consuming, and technically difficult, although 100% specific

        ii. Noninvasive

            (a) Serologic tests (QuickVue *H. pylori* gII, FlexSure HP): Detect immunoglobulin G (IgG) to *H. pylori* in the serum by enzyme-linked immunosorbent assay (ELISA); 85% sensitive, 79% specific. Cannot distinguish between active infection and past exposure. Because antibodies persist for long periods after eradication, cannot use to test for eradication after treatment. Newly available tests will detect the presence of CagA or VacA antibodies.

            (b) Urea breath test (BreathTek UBT, PYtest): Detects the exhalation of radiolabeled CO_2 after the ingestion of ^{13}C- or ^{14}C-radiolabeled urea. *H. pylori* hydrolysis of the radiolabeled urea results in CO_2 production; 97% sensitive, 95% specific. Used to make a diagnosis and to test for eradication. Recent use of antibiotics or PPIs may result in false negatives in up to 40% of patients. Patients should discontinue antisecretory agents or antibiotics at least 2 weeks before UBT testing or wait 4 weeks after treatment has ended before having the UBT performed.

            (c) Stool antigen tests (Premier Platinum HpSA, ImmunoCard STAT! HpSA): Polyclonal or monoclonal antibody tests that detect the presence of *H. pylori* in the stool; 88%–92% sensitive, 87% specific. Can be used to make a diagnosis and confirm eradication. Recent use of bismuth, antibiotics, or PPIs may also result in false negatives. Patients should discontinue antisecretory agents or antibiotics at least 2 weeks before stool antigen testing or wait 4 weeks after treatment has ended before having the stool antigen test performed.

B. Treatment of *H. pylori*–Associated Ulcers

    1. General recommendations, based on the American College of Gastroenterology (ACG) guidelines, are to include an antisecretory agent (preferably a PPI) plus at least two antibiotics (clarithromycin and amoxicillin or metronidazole) in the eradication regimen.

    2. Therapy duration is 7–14 days, depending on the regimen chosen. The ACG guidelines state that 14 days is preferred. Most regimens last for 10 days.

    3. Follow-up testing for eradication should be performed in patients with a history of ulcer complication, gastric mucosa–associated lymphoid tissue lymphoma, early gastric cancer, or recurrence of symptoms.

    4. UBTs or stool antigen tests are preferred for confirming eradication (should wait at least 4 weeks after treatment for both).

    5. Quadruple-based therapy with bismuth subsalicylate, metronidazole, tetracycline, and a PPI is considered a first-line treatment and can also be used for 14 days if triple-based therapy fails or if the patient has an intolerance of or allergy to components of the triple-drug therapy. Pylera, a quadruple-based therapy formulated with tetracycline, bismuth, and metronidazole in 1 capsule, contains the bismuth subcitrate salt rather than the subsalicylate salt.

    6. Sequential therapy involved administration of a PPI and amoxicillin given first for the first 5 days, followed by a PPI, clarithromycin, and tinidazole for an additional 5 days. This therapy requires further validation before widespread use will be accepted.

    7. A bismuth-based quadruple therapy for 14 days or a levofloxacin-based triple therapy for 10 days can be used in patients who have not responded to initial regimens as salvage therapy.

Table 7. *H. pylori* Treatment Regimens

Regimen[a,b]	Duration (days)	Efficacy (%)[c]
Lansoprazole 30 mg BID + amoxicillin 1000 mg BID + clarithromycin 500 mg BID	10–14	81–86
Esomeprazole 40 mg once daily + amoxicillin 1000 mg BID + clarithromycin 500 mg BID	10–14	70–85
Omeprazole 20 mg BID + amoxicillin 1000 mg BID + clarithromycin 500 mg BID	10–14	70–85
Rabeprazole 20 mg PO BID + amoxicillin 1000 mg BID + clarithromycin 500 mg BID	7	70–85
Bismuth subsalicylate 525 mg QID + metronidazole 500 mg TID + tetracycline 500 mg QID + PPI BID	14	75–90
Bismuth subcitrate 420 mg + tetracycline 375 mg + metronidazole 375 mg 3 capsules QID + PPI BID[d]	10	85–92
Sequential therapy: PPI + amoxicillin 1 g BID for 5 days; then PPI, clarithromycin 500 mg BID + tinidazole 500 mg BID for 5 days	10 (5 each treatment)	>90

[a]Pantoprazole 40 mg BID or dexlansoprazole does not have an FDA-approved indication for *H. pylori* eradication; however, it could be substituted in any of the 10- to 14-day regimens.

[b]Metronidazole 500 mg BID can be substituted for amoxicillin or clarithromycin in patients with penicillin or macrolide allergy for the triple-drug regimens. Treat for 14 days in this instance.

[c]Rates are based on intention to treat.

[d]Triple-capsule formulation.

BID = twice daily; PO = orally; PPI = proton pump inhibitor; QID = 4 times/day; TID = 3 times/day.

C. Primary Prevention of NSAID-Induced Ulcers
1. Implement risk factor modification.
2. Test and treat for *H. pylori* if patient is beginning long-term NSAID therapy.
3. Determine level of GI-related risk (low, medium, high) using Table 6.
4. Because of the association of increased risk of CV events with NSAID use, patient's CV risk should be determined as well. The ACG guidelines define those at *high CV risk* as patients who require low-dose aspirin for prevention of cardiac events. Naproxen is the only NSAID that has been touted as not appearing to increase the risk of CV events; therefore, its use is preferred in patients with CV risk factors per the ACG guidelines. However, in February 2014 an FDA panel voted against label changes that would indicate a lower cardiovascular thrombotic risk (http://www.fda.gov/AdvisoryCommittees/Calendar/ucm380871.htm).

Table 8. Preventive Strategies Based on Risk of NSAID-Related GI Complications and CV Risk

If low CV risk and: Low GI risk[a] → NSAID (lowest dose of least ulcerogenic agent) Moderate GI risk[b] → NSAID + PPI or misoprostol High GI risk[c] → COX-2 inhibitor + PPI or misoprostol
If high CV risk (requirement for low-dose aspirin) and: Low GI risk[a] → Naproxen + PPI or misoprostol Moderate GI risk[b] → Naproxen + PPI or misoprostol High GI risk[c] → Avoid NSAIDs or COX-2 inhibitors

[a]No risk factors.

[b]One or two risk factors present.

[c]Positive history of ulcer complication or several (more than 2) risk factors or use of steroids and anticoagulants.

COX-2 = cyclooxygenase-2; CV = cardiovascular; GI = gastrointestinal; NSAID = nonsteroidal anti-inflammatory drug; PPI = proton pump inhibitor.

5. Misoprostol (Cytotec) should be given at full doses (800 mcg/day in divided doses); however, this therapy is poorly tolerated because of excessive nausea, vomiting, diarrhea, and abdominal cramping.

6. Concomitant use of antiplatelet agents and NSAIDs
   a. Need for antiplatelet therapy should first be evaluated.
   b. If antiplatelet therapy is deemed necessary, assess for the presence of GI risk factors (see Table 6). These guidelines also cite dyspepsia or GERD symptoms as risk factors.
   c. Test and treat for *H. pylori* in patients with a history of a nonbleeding ulcer and in those with a history of an ulcer-related complication. Eradicating *H. pylori* before beginning long-term antiplatelet therapy is optimal.
   d. PPIs are the preferred gastroprotective agents for both treatment and prevention of aspirin- and NSAID-associated GI injury.
   e. Gastroprotective therapy should be prescribed for patients with GI risk factors who require the use of any NSAID (including OTC and cyclooxygenase-2 [COX-2] inhibitors) in conjunction with cardiac-dose aspirin.
   f. Gastroprotective therapy should be prescribed for patients with GI risk factors who require preventive doses of aspirin. Aspirin doses greater than 81 mg/day should not be used in patients with GI risk factors during the long-term phase of aspirin therapy.
   g. PPIs should be prescribed for patients receiving concomitant aspirin and anticoagulant therapy (unfractionated heparin, low-molecular-weight heparin, warfarin, dabigatran, rivaroxaban, apixaban, and fondaparinux).
   h. A target international normalized ratio (INR) of 2–2.5 should be used in patients for whom warfarin is added to concomitant aspirin and clopidogrel therapy. The combination of both aspirin and clopidogrel with warfarin should be used only when benefit outweighs risk.
   i. Clopidogrel is not recommended as a substitute for patients with recurrent ulcer bleeding. Aspirin plus a PPI is superior to clopidogrel.
   j. The health care provider (HCP) who decides to discontinue aspirin therapy in patients with short-term bleeding episodes should weigh the risks of subsequent GI or cardiac events.
   k. For patients receiving dual antiplatelet therapy (aspirin plus clopidogrel) who require elective endoscopy (particularly colonoscopy and polypectomy), consider deferring if patient is at high risk of cardiac events. Elective endoscopy should be deferred for 1 year after the placement of drug-eluting stents.

D. Treatment and Secondary Prevention of NSAID-Induced Ulcers
1. Risk factor modification
2. Discontinue or lower NSAID dose, if possible. Ulcers will heal with appropriate treatment, but healing may take longer with continued NSAID use.
3. Test for *H. pylori* and treat, if present.
4. Drug therapy
   a. PPIs: Drugs of choice for healing and secondary prevention of NSAID-induced ulcers. Combination product Vimovo contains esomeprazole with naproxen in the same tablet (375 mg/20 mg or 500 mg/20 mg).
   b. Misoprostol: Appears to be as effective as PPIs for healing and secondary prevention however, it necessitates several doses per day and is poorly tolerated because of the high incidence of diarrhea and abdominal pain.
   c. Cyclooxygenase inhibitors: Celecoxib was shown to have rates of ulcer recurrence and bleeding comparable to those of a diclofenac plus omeprazole combination; use of celecoxib may be limited by its recent association with CV effects. Use of celecoxib is uncertain in combination with low-dose aspirin for secondary prevention of GI events.
   d. Combination of a COX-2 inhibitor and a PPI is not well studied but may be considered in high-risk patients such as older adults, especially if they are receiving aspirin plus steroids or warfarin or have a history of a recent complicated GI event and require continued NSAID or aspirin use.
   e. The H2RAs: Inferior to misoprostol and PPIs in healing and preventing recurrence
   f. Clopidogrel is not recommended as a substitute in patients with recurrent ulcer bleeding. Aspirin plus a PPI is superior to clopidogrel.
3. CV safety of COX-2 inhibitors and NSAIDs
   a. The main theory underlying the development of excess thrombotic events with COX-2 inhibitor use is that when COX-2–mediated prostacyclin production is reduced, the prothrombic prostaglandin thromboxane A continues to be produced by COX-1, leading to the development of a prothrombic state. The degree of development of these events does not appear to be equal across the class of COX-2 inhibitors.
   b. Guidelines for appropriate use and safety of NSAIDs, aspirin, and COX-2 inhibitors have been published by both the AHA and a multidisciplinary clinical group.
   c. Celecoxib was not associated with increases in CV events until the Adenoma Prevention with Celecoxib trial for cancer prevention was terminated in December 2004. Daily doses of 400 and 800 mg of celecoxib conferred a 2.5- and 3.4-fold higher risk of fatal and nonfatal MI, which suggests a dose-related response for this toxicity.
   d. A stepped approach is recommended for patients with CV disease or risk factors for ischemic heart disease who require analgesic treatment of musculoskeletal symptoms based on recommendations from the AHA.
      i. Consider using acetaminophen, aspirin, tramadol, or short-term narcotics first.
      ii. Nonacetylated salicylates can be considered next.
      iii. Non–COX-2-selective NSAIDs can be used next, followed by NSAIDs with some COX-2 activity. Use the lowest dose possible to control symptoms.
      iv. The COX-2 inhibitors should be reserved as last line. In patients at increased risk of thromboembolic events, coadministration with aspirin and a PPI may be considered.
      v. Routinely monitor BP, renal function, and signs of edema or GI bleeding.

e. Methods to reduce CV risk such as tobacco cessation, BP reductions, lipid control, and glucose control are recommended for NSAID users but have not been proved to reduce NSAID-associated CV risk. In patients for whom the risk of GI bleeding outweighs the CV risk, lower-risk NSAIDs such as ibuprofen, etodolac, diclofenac, or celecoxib should be used. In patients for whom the CV risk outweighs the risk of GI bleeding, COX-2 inhibitors should be avoided. Limit the dose and therapy duration if possible.

f. An FDA article also reviews the effects of ibuprofen on the attenuation of aspirin's antiplatelet effects. The AHA recommends that ibuprofen be taken at least 30 minutes after or 8 hours before the ingestion of immediate-release low-dose aspirin to prevent this interaction.

g. In February 2014 an FDA panel voted against label changes that would indicate a lower cardiovascular thrombotic risk with naproxen compared with other NSAIDs. (http://www.fda.gov/AdvisoryCommittees/Calendar/ucm380871.htm). This was despite a 2013 meta-analysis that demonstrated that naproxen had lower CV risk compared with high-dose diclofenac and ibuprofen (Lancet 2013;382:769–79).

Patient Cases

2. A 68-year-old woman referred to a gastroenterologist has intermittent upper abdominal pain with anemia and heme-positive stools. She has a history of type 2 diabetes mellitus with peripheral neuropathy and hypertension. She reports no known drug allergies and takes metformin 1000 mg twice daily, aspirin 325 mg/day, lisinopril 20 mg once daily, and gabapentin 1000 mg three times/day. In addition, she reports using OTC ketoprofen daily for the past 2 months secondary to uncontrolled pain. Her colonoscopy is negative, but her endoscopy reveals a 1-cm gastric ulcer with an intact clot. A rapid urease test (CLO) performed on the ulcer biopsy specimen is negative. Which treatment is best for this patient's ulcer?

   A. Ranitidine 150 mg twice daily for 4 weeks.

   B. Lansoprazole 30 mg twice daily plus amoxicillin 1000 mg twice daily plus clarithromycin 500 mg twice daily for 10 days.

   C. Lansoprazole 30 mg/day for 8 weeks.

   D. Misoprostol 200 mcg two times/day for 8 weeks.

3. A 42-year-old man is in the clinic with the chief concern of sharp epigastric pain for the past 6 weeks. He states that the pain is often worse with eating and that it is present at least 5 days/week. He states that although he initially tried OTC antacids with some relief, the pain returns about 3 hours after each dose. He does not currently take any other medications. He reports an allergy to sulfa-containing medications (rash). His practitioner is concerned about a potential peptic ulcer and tests him for *H. pylori* using a UBT, the result of which is positive. Which treatment for *H. pylori* is best?

   A. Amoxicillin 1 g twice daily plus clarithromycin 500 mg twice daily plus omeprazole 20 mg twice daily for 5 days.

   B. Cephalexin 1 g twice daily plus clarithromycin 500 mg twice daily plus omeprazole 20 mg twice daily for 10 days.

   C. Bismuth subsalicylate 525 mg four times/day plus tetracycline 500 mg four times/day plus metronidazole 500 mg three times/day plus omeprazole 20 mg twice daily for 14 days.

   D. Levofloxacin 500 mg once daily plus metronidazole 500 mg twice daily plus omeprazole 20 mg twice daily for 21 days.

III. UPPER GI BLEEDING

A. Background: Prevalence is 170 cases/100,000 adults; associated annual costs are about $750 million, and mortality is 6%–10%.

B. Causes of Upper GI Bleeding
1. Peptic ulcer disease (40%–70%)
   a. NSAIDs and low-dose aspirin use
   b. *H. pylori*
2. Esophagitis
3. Erosive disease
4. Esophageal varices
5. Mallory-Weiss tear
6. Neoplasm
7. Stress ulcers (critically ill patients)

C. Clinical Symptoms and Presentation
1. Hematemesis or "coffee-ground" emesis
2. Hematochezia
3. Nausea, vomiting
4. Melena
5. Shock (tachycardia, clammy skin)
6. Hypotension
7. Associated organ dysfunction (renal, hepatic, cardiac, cerebral hypoperfusion)

Table 9. Clinical Predictors of Death Associated with Nonvariceal Upper GI Bleeding

Advanced age (>75 years at highest risk)	Red blood on rectal examination
Shock or hypotension	Elevated serum urea
>1 comorbid condition	Serum creatinine >150 µmol/L (1.7 mg/dL)
Continued bleeding or rebleeding	Elevated aminotransferases
Blood in gastric aspirate	Sepsis
Hematemesis	Onset of bleeding during hospitalization for other causes

Table 10. Predictors of Persistent or Recurrent Upper GI Bleeding

Age >65 years	Initial hemoglobin <10 g/dL or hematocrit <30%
Shock (systolic blood pressure <100 mm Hg)	Coagulopathy
Comorbid illness	Endoscopic findings:
Erratic mental status	Active bleeding on endoscopy
Ongoing bleeding	Presence of high-risk stigmata
Red blood on rectal examination	Adherent clot
Melena	Ulcer size ≥2 cm
Blood in gastric aspirate	Gastric or duodenal ulcer
Hematemesis	Location of ulcer on superior or posterior wall

D. Management of Ulcer-Related GI Bleeding
   1. Volume resuscitation and hemodynamic stabilization
      a. Placement of one or two large-bore intravenous catheters
      b. Replacement with crystalloid such as 0.9% normal saline is preferred; colloids such as blood can be given after initial resuscitation in patients with hemoglobin of less than 7 g/dL to maintain a hemoglobin concentration of 8–10 g/dL.
   2. Risk stratification
      a. Clinical signs and symptoms
      b. Use of clinical scoring scales such as Blatchford or Rockall scores to determine the risk of early rebleeding and the need for urgent versus nonemergency intervention. Patients with low risk of rebleeding may be discharged after endoscopy.
      c. Placing an NG tube for aspiration can be considered but is not required.
      d. Endoscopy (within 24 hours if possible or within 12 hours with high-risk clinical features)
      e. Assessment of comorbid illnesses (liver disease, coagulopathies, cardiac status)
   3. Endoscopic therapy
      a. Endoscopic therapy associated with reductions in rebleeding, need for surgery, and mortality. Perform within 12–24 hours of presentation.
      b. Observation of low-risk stigmata (a clean-based ulcer or a nonprotuberant pigmented dot in an ulcer bed) is not an indication for hemostatic therapy.
      c. Clots visible in an ulcer bed should be irrigated, with treatment of underlying lesions.
      d. The presence of high-risk stigmata warrants immediate hemostatic therapy.
   4. Endoscopic strategies
      a. The combination of injection and coaptive therapy is the most efficacious approach.
      b. The use of either technique plus pharmacotherapy is superior to monotherapy.
      c. Sclerotherapy: No single solution for injection is superior to another.
         i. Epinephrine with or without ethanolamine is inferior by itself. Combine with another endoscopic therapy.
         ii. Cyanoacrylate
         iii. Thrombin
         iv. Sodium tetradecyl sulfate
         v. Polidocanol
      d. Thermal coaptive therapy: No single method is superior to another.
         i. Heater probe thermocoagulation
         ii. Multipolar electrocoagulation
         iii. Laser coagulation (not often used because of cost)
         iv. Argon plasma coagulation
      e. Placement of hemostatic clips
   5. Pharmacotherapeutic management of nonvariceal upper GI bleeding
      a. Treatment guidelines apply to bleeding NSAID-induced ulcers as well.
      b. Remove medications that are contributing to bleeding (e.g., NSAIDs).
      c. Pre-endoscopic erythromycin, 250 mg intravenously, can be considered to improve diagnostic yield, but this has not been shown to improve outcomes (conditional recommendation).
      d. PPI therapy
         i. Use of a pre-endoscopic dose (80-mg intravenous bolus, followed by an 8-mg/hour intravenous infusion) of PPI may be considered. This does not result in reduced mortality, surgery, or rate of rebleeding, but it may reduce the lesion size, the possibility of finding a high-risk lesion, and the need for endoscopic therapy. PPIs may be given if endoscopy will be delayed or cannot be performed.

       ii.   Bolus 80 mg plus a continuous infusion of 8 mg/hour for 72 hours after endoscopic therapy for patients with active bleeding or nonbleeding visible vessel or with adherent clot. Intravenous pantoprazole or esomeprazole can be used; most data are with intravenous omeprazole (used in Europe).

       iii. Associated with decreases in rebleeding, mortality, and need for surgery in patients with active bleeding who have undergone successful endoscopic intervention.

       iv. Oral once-daily PPI therapy can be used for patients with a flat spot or clean-based ulcer.

   e.   Use of H2RAs or somatostatin-octreotide is *not* recommended.

   f.   Test for *H. pylori* and treat if results are positive. If negative, retest. No need for a PPI after eradication

   g.   Assess the need for continued secondary prevention with PPI therapy. If needed, a single daily oral dose of a PPI is recommended.

   h.   Assess the need for NSAID or aspirin use. If NSAID therapy is needed, then use of a COX-2 inhibitor plus a PPI is recommended, barring any significant CV risk. Otherwise, a PPI should be used.

   i.   If use of low-dose aspirin is required, reinitiate when CV risk is thought to outweigh GI risk. Use a PPI and reinitiate within 1–3 days, if not within 1 week. Clopidogrel has a higher rate of rebleeding than aspirin.

   j.   Long-term PPI therapy is recommended for ulcers not associated with NSAIDs or *H. pylori*.

  E. Prophylaxis of Stress-Related Mucosal Disease (SRMD) in Critically Ill Patients

    1. Stress-related injury: Superficial diffuse upper GI ulceration

    2. Stress ulcer: Deeper mucosal ulceration; may lead to bleeding and hemodynamic compromise

    3. Contributing factors to SRMD development

      a. Hypoperfusion of the GI tract

      b. Altered susceptibility to gastric acid

      c. Loss of defense mechanisms: Mucous/bicarbonate layer, prostaglandins, cellular renewal

      d. Alterations in gastric motility; may affect absorption of drugs

    4. Pharmacologic prevention

      a. Not routinely recommended in non–intensive care unit settings

      b. Recommended in patients in an intensive care unit setting with the risk factors listed in Table 11.

Table 11. Risk Factors for Initiation of Prophylaxis for SRMD

Mechanical ventilation >48 hours[a]	Two or more of the following:
Coagulopathy (platelet count <50,000/mm³, INR >1.5)[a]	Sepsis syndrome
Thermal injury (>35% BSA)	ICU stay >1 week
Severe head or spinal cord injury	Occult bleeding
GI bleeding or ulceration within past year	High-dose corticosteroids
Multiple trauma (injury severity score >16)	(250 mg of hydrocortisone equivalent)
Perioperative transplant period	Hepatic failure
Low intragastric pH	Acute renal insufficiency
Major surgery (lasting >4 hours)	Hypotension
Acute lung injury	Anticoagulation

[a]Independent risk factors for SRMD.

BSA = body surface area; GI = gastrointestinal; ICU = intensive care unit; INR = international normalized ratio; SRMD = stress-related mucosal disease.

5. Preventive treatment options
   a. Antacids: Effectively raise pH and prevent bleeding; require several oral doses per day or administration by NG tube; possibility of diarrhea, constipation, and electrolyte abnormalities
   b. Sucralfate
      i. Works by providing a direct mucosal barrier; also modulates pepsin, mucus activity, bicarbonate secretion, and tissue growth repair
      ii. Use has fallen out of favor. Requires many oral doses or administration by NG tube. May lead to aluminum accumulation and constipation. No effect on platelet count and is associated with lower rates of pneumonia development. Possibility of binding to other drugs in GI tract
      iii. General efficacy regarding bleeding considered similar to that of H2RAs
   c. Histamine-2 receptor antagonists
      i. Reduce gastric acid secretion by inhibition of histamine stimulation of the parietal cell; may be associated with the development of tolerance or tachyphylaxis with continued use
      ii. Considered efficacious in the prevention of clinically significant bleeding; oral, intravenous intermittent dosing, and continuous infusion are all possible options; high-dose intravenous (ranitidine, cimetidine, or famotidine) use can be considered first-line therapy. Cimetidine is the only H2RA that is FDA approved for SRMD prevention.
      iii. Associated with CNS adverse effects and the rare development of thrombocytopenia; require adjustment for renal dysfunction
   d. Proton pump inhibitors
      i. The American Society of Health-System Pharmacists guidelines include minimal recommendations for PPI use because of the lack of data at that time; however, PPIs are commonly used for SRMD prevention.
      ii. PPIs are similar to H2RAs in safety and efficacy.
      iii. Oral or intravenous routes may be used. Alternative formulations exist for patients with difficulty swallowing or with feeding tubes (see section on GERD).
      iv. Oral PPIs are also as efficacious as intravenous PPI therapy for maintaining equivalent pH
      v. Intravenous PPI therapy is generally considered equivalent to high-dose intravenous H2RA therapy.
      vi. Recent associations with *C. difficile* infections in hospitalized patients

IV. INFLAMMATORY BOWEL DISEASE

A. Background
   1. Inflammatory bowel disease (IBD) includes both UC and CD. In some instances, UC may be indistinguishable from CD. This is referred to as indeterminate or intermediate colitis.
   2. Pathophysiology: Continuing inflammation of the GI mucosa; exact cause is unknown, but it is thought that the inflammation is secondary to an antigen-driven response
   3. Contributing factors
      a. Defects in the intestinal epithelial barrier and immune system
      b. Genetic: Definite genetic association; first-degree relatives of affected patients have a 4–20 times higher risk of developing IBD
      c. Environmental
         i. NSAIDs: Worsen IBD, probably secondary to alteration of epithelial barrier
         ii. Smoking: Worsens CD; however, is associated with improvement in UC symptoms

        iii. Luminal bacteria: Endogenous intestinal bacteria thought to be highly involved in stimulating the intestinal inflammatory response observed in IBD

        iv. Dietary: Dietary antigens may also contribute to ongoing inflammation.

    d. Various proinflammatory cytokines, including interleukin-1, interleukin-6, and tumor necrosis factor (TNF), release and contribute to the ongoing inflammatory process.

B. Clinical Features

    1. Presenting symptoms common to both diseases include fever, abdominal pain, diarrhea (may be bloody, watery, or mucopurulent), rectal bleeding, and weight loss. Symptoms may vary depending on disease location.

Table 12. Clinical Features of Inflammatory Bowel Disease

Clinical Findings	Ulcerative Colitis	Crohn Disease
Bowel involvement	Confined to rectum and colon Terminal ileal involvement (backwash ileitis) occurs in a minority of patients	May be anywhere from mouth to anus (66% of cases located in ileum)
Perianal involvement	Unlikely	Yes
Depth of ulceration	Superficial	May extend to submucosa or deeper
Continuous inflammation	Very common	Rarely, a patchy, "cobblestone" appearance
Histology	Nontransmural, crypt abscesses	Transmural lesions Granulomas
Fistula, perforation, or strictures	No	Yes
Development of toxic megacolon	Yes	No
Malabsorption or malnutrition	Rare	Yes, often vitamin deficiencies; possible growth retardation in children
Risk factor for colorectal cancer	Yes	Uncommon
Pseudopolyps	Common	Fairly uncommon

    2. Systemic manifestations

        a. Both UC and CD may present with concurrent systemic manifestations.

        b. Hepatobiliary: primary sclerosing cholangitis, cholangiocarcinoma, hepatitis or cirrhosis, cholelithiasis, steatosis

        c. Rheumatologic arthritis, sacroiliitis, ankylosing spondylitis

        d. Dermatologic: erythema nodosum, aphthous ulcers, pyoderma gangrenosum

        e. Ocular: iritis or uveitis, episcleritis

    3. Gauging clinical severity

        a. Ulcerative colitis (based on Truelove and Witt criteria)

Table 13. Clinical Severity of Ulcerative Colitis

Mild	Moderate	Severe	Fulminant
<4 stools/day (±blood) No fever, anemia, or tachycardia Normal ESR	>4 stools/day (±blood) Minimal signs of systemic toxicity	>6 stools/day with blood Temp >99.5°F HR >90 beats/minute ESR >30 mm/hour Hb <75% of normal Abdominal tenderness Bowel wall edema	>10 stools/day with continuous blood Temp >99.5°F HR >90 beats/minute ESR >30 mm/hour Transfusions required Abdominal pain Dilated colon

ESR = erythrocyte sedimentation rate; Hb = hemoglobin; HR = heart rate; Temp = temperature.

    b. Crohn disease
       i. Mild–moderate: Tolerates oral administration; absence of fever, dehydration, and abdominal tenderness; less than 10% weight loss
      ii. Moderate–severe: Failed treatment of mild–moderate; these symptoms usually present; possibly anemia, nausea and vomiting, considerable weight loss
     iii. Severe–fulminant: No response to outpatient steroids; high temperature, abdominal pain, persistent vomiting; possible obstruction, abscess, cachexia, rebound tenderness
  4. General management considerations
    a. Rule out possible infectious causes of bloody diarrhea in patients with acute symptoms.
    b. Most patients will receive a colonoscopy to confirm the diagnosis and extent of disease.
    c. Surgery is a viable option when complications (abscess, fistula, perforation) occur or when fulminant disease is unresponsive to medical treatment.
    d. Distribution and severity of disease will dictate the initial choice of therapeutic agents.
    e. Most patients will require maintenance therapy because of the high incidence of relapse after induction therapy; the relapse rate is 35%–80% at 2 years for CD and 50%–70% at 1 year for UC.

C. Medical Management of IBD
  1. Adjunctive therapies: Use with caution in active disease because reduction in motility may precipitate toxic megacolon.
  2. Loperamide (Imodium): May be useful for proctitis or diarrhea; 2 mg after each loose stool (16 mg/day maximum)
  3. Antispasmodics
    a. Dicyclomine (Bentyl), 10–40 mg orally four times/day
    b. Propantheline (Pro-Banthine), 7.5–15 mg orally three times/day
    c. Hyoscyamine (Levsin), 0.125–0.25 mg orally/slow release every 4 hours as needed
  4. Cholestyramine (Questran): Possibly for bile salt–induced diarrhea after ileal resection

D. Medications Used to Treat IBD
  1. Treatment is selected on the basis of disease location and severity.
  2. Aminosalicylates
    a. Used for both induction and maintenance of remission
    b. Sulfasalazine: Prototype agent (Azulfidine, Azulfidine-EN)
       i. The drug is cleaved by colonic bacteria to the active portion (5-aminosalicylate) and the inactive carrier molecule sulfapyridine.

    ii. Efficacy is best in colonic disease because of the colonic activation of the drug. Toxicity may be dose related and related to the sulfapyridine portion.

    iii. Dose-related adverse effects: GI disturbance, headache, arthralgia, folate malabsorption

    iv. Idiosyncratic adverse effects: rash, fever, pneumonitis, hepatotoxicity, bone marrow suppression, hemolytic anemia, pancreatitis, decreased sperm production in men

    v. Avoid in patients with a sulfa allergy.

    vi. Doses are 4–6 g/day for induction and 2–4 g/day for maintenance; available as immediate-release and enteric-coated products. Doses should be titrated beginning at 500–1000 mg once or twice daily to avoid adverse effects.

  c. 5-Aminosalicylates (non–sulfa containing)

    i. In general, better tolerated than sulfasalazine; considered first line in mild–moderate UC and CD

    ii. Product selection depends on location of disease.

    iii. Olsalazine is associated with secretory diarrhea in up to 25% of patients.

    iv. Rare instances of nephrotoxicity with use of 5-aminosalicylates

Table 14. Aminosalicylate Formulations

Drug	Trade Name	Formulation	Strength	Daily Dosage Range (g)	Site of Action
Mesalamine	Rowasa[a]	Enema	4 g/60 mL	4	Rectum Terminal colon
	Delzicol Asacol HD	Delayed-release capsule Delayed-release resin	400 mg 800 mg	1.6–4.8	Distal ileum Colon
	Canasa	Suppository	1000 mg	1	Rectum
	Pentasa	Microgranular-coated tablet	250 mg 500 mg	2–4	Small bowel Colon
	Lialda	MMX delayed-release tablet	1.2 g	2.4–4.8 (once daily)	Colon
	Apriso	INTELLICOR delayed- and extended-release capsule	0.375 g	0.375–1.5 (once daily)	Colon
Olsalazine	Dipentum	Dimer of mesalamine (capsule)	250 mg	1–3	Colon
Balsalazide	Colazal Giazo	Capsule Tablet	750 mg 1100 mg	2–6.75	Colon

[a]Generic mesalamine enema now available.

3. Corticosteroids

  a. Work quickly to suppress inflammation during acute flares

  b. No role in maintenance therapy; however, more than 50% of patients with severe disease may become steroid-dependent

  c. Budesonide is about 15 times more potent than prednisone; because of its high first-pass metabolism, allow a 2-week overlap when changing from prednisone to budesonide to prevent adrenal insufficiency. Formulated to release in the terminal ileum and treats only terminal ileal and ascending colonic disease

  d. Adverse effects (systemic therapy) are adrenal suppression, glucose intolerance, hypertension, sodium/water retention, osteoporosis, cataracts, and impaired wound healing.

Table 15. Corticosteroid Preparations

Route	Agents	Dose	Comments
Oral	Prednisone Prednisolone	20–60 mg/day	Taper ASAP
	Budesonide capsule (Entocort EC)	9 mg/day PO, then 6 mg/day Can be continued for up to 3 months	Minimal absorption; indicated for mild–moderate active CD involving terminal ileum or ascending colon
	Budesonide tablet (Uceris)	9 mg/day in the a.m. for 8 weeks	Minimal absorption; indicated for mild–moderate active UC
IV	Hydrocortisone Methylprednisolone	100 mg every 8 hours 15–48 mg/day	7- to 10-day course; change to PO when gut is functional
Topical (rectal)	Cortenema (100 mg/60 mL)	100 mg HS	Hydrocortisone-based products
	Cortifoam (90 mg/applicator)	90 mg/day BID	Used for patients with distal disease
	Anucort-HC 25 mg Proctocort 30 mg	25–50 PR BID	Suppositories; use for proctitis

ASAP = as soon as possible; BID = twice daily; CD = Crohn disease; HS = at bedtime; IV = intravenous; PO = by mouth; PR = rectally; UC = ulcerative colitis.

4. Immunomodulators
   a. 6-MP (or Purinethol), azathioprine (Imuran, Azasan; prodrug of 6-MP), or methotrexate
   b. Doses: Azathioprine 2–2.5 mg/kg/day orally, 6-MP 1–1.5 mg/kg/day orally, methotrexate 15–25 mg/week intramuscularly (CD only)
   c. Indicated only for maintenance because of its long onset of action (3–15 months)
   d. Use may result in a steroid-sparing effect.
   e. Azathioprine and 6-MP are metabolized by the enzyme thiopurine methyltransferase (TPMT); reduced expression of TPMT may result in slower metabolism and increased toxicity. TPMT activity or *TPMT* genotype or phenotype should be determined before initiating therapy.
   f. Adverse reactions
      i. Azathioprine and 6-MP: Pancreatitis (3%–15%), bone marrow suppression, nausea, diarrhea, rash, possible hepatotoxicity. Risk of hepatosplenic T-cell lymphoma, especially in younger male patients. Risk is great if combined with a TNFα antagonist.
      ii. Methotrexate: Bone marrow suppression, nausea, diarrhea, rash, pulmonary toxicity, hepatotoxicity
5. Infliximab (Remicade)
   a. Chimeric monoclonal antibody versus TNF
   b. Indicated for both CD and UC
      i. Moderate–severe active disease
      ii. Fistulizing CD
      iii. Maintenance of moderate–severe disease
   c. Available as intravenous infusion only; very expensive
   d. Studies of patients whose conventional therapy failed; response is about 40%–80%
   e. Dosing: Moderate–severe active disease or fistulizing disease: 5 mg/kg as single dose, followed by 5 mg/kg at 2 and 6 weeks, then every 8 weeks as maintenance. Patients losing response with time may be treated with a 10-mg/kg dose.

f. Adverse reactions

　　i. Infusion related: Hypotension, fever, chills, urticaria, pruritus; infuse over at least 2 hours (may pretreat with acetaminophen or antihistamine)

　　ii. Delayed hypersensitivity: May be associated with fever, rash, myalgia, headache, or sore throat 3–10 days after administration

　　iii. Infection: Use is associated with the reactivation of latent infections (bacterial, including disseminated tuberculosis, fungal, and sepsis); do not give to patients with active infections. Tuberculosis should be ruled out in patients before any biologic agents are initiated.

　　iv. Heart failure exacerbations: Contraindicated in New York Heart Association class III/IV heart failure; do not exceed 5-mg/kg dose in other patients with chronic heart failure.

　　v. Antibody induction: Up to 50% of patients may develop antinuclear antibodies; 19% may develop anti–double-stranded DNA antibodies.

　　vi. Bone marrow suppression (pancytopenia)

　　vii. Black box warning. Applies to all tumor necrosis factor alpha (TNFα) antagonists: Unusual cancers have been reported in children and teenage patients taking TNF blockers. Hepatosplenic T-cell lymphoma has occurred mostly in teenaged or young adult males with CD or UC who were taking infliximab and azathioprine or 6-MP.

　　viii. Hepatitis (reactivation of hepatitis B virus [HBV], autoimmune hepatitis); discontinue use if liver function tests rise to more than 5 times the upper limit of normal (ULN)

　　ix. Vasculitis with CNS involvement

6. Adalimumab (Humira)

　a. Fully humanized antibody to TNFα; therefore, theoretically, no development of antibodies

　b. Indicated for both induction and maintenance therapy for moderate–severe active CD and UC in patients unresponsive to conventional therapy; also indicated for patients who no longer respond to infliximab

　c. Dosing: Induction, 160 mg subcutaneously on day 1 (given as four separate 40-mg injections) or two 40-mg/day injections for 2 consecutive days, followed by 80 mg subcutaneously 2 weeks later (day 15). Then, can decrease dose to 40 mg subcutaneously every 2 weeks starting on day 29 of therapy

　d. Efficacy

　　i. Complete remission rates at week 4 ranges from 21% to 54%

　　ii. Efficacy rates for maintenance therapy range from 56% to 79% at week 4 to 36% to 46% at week 56.

　　iii. The adverse effect profile of adalimumab is similar to that of infliximab, except for the development of antibodies to adalimumab.

7. Certolizumab (Cimzia)

　a. Humanized monoclonal antibody fragment linked to polyethylene glycol (PEG), with murine-complimentary determining regions

　b. Indicated for maintenance therapy for moderate–severe active CD in patients unresponsive to conventional therapy

　c. Dosing: Induction, 400 mg subcutaneously, then 400 mg subcutaneously at weeks 2 and 4; maintenance dose is 400 mg subcutaneously every 4 weeks

　d. Efficacy

　　i. Patients with a C-reactive protein concentration greater than 10 mg/L have the best response. Up to 37% response at 6 weeks versus 26% for placebo.

　　ii. Up to 62% of patients with an initial response and a C-reactive protein concentration greater than 10 mg/L may be maintained in remission at 26 weeks.

　　iii. Certolizumab adverse effect profile is similar to that of other TNFα antagonists.

8. Golimumab (Simponi)
   a. Human IgG1κ monoclonal antibody
   b. Indicated for moderate to severe UC in patients intolerant of previous therapies or requiring continuous steroid therapy
   c. Dosing: 200 mg subcutaneously at week 0, then 100 mg at week 2, then 100 mg every 4 weeks
   d. Similar efficacy and toxicity profile compared with other TNFα antagonists.
9. Natalizumab (Tysabri)
   a. Humanized monoclonal antibody that antagonizes integrin heterodimers and inhibits α4 integrin-mediated leukocyte adhesion
   b. Indicated for inducing and maintaining clinical response and remission in adult patients with moderate–severe active CD who have had an inadequate response to, or are unable to tolerate, conventional therapies and inhibitors of TNFα
   c. Dosing
      i. All patients must be enrolled in the TOUCH program before the drug is dispensed because of its association with progressive multifocal leukoencephalopathy.
      ii. Induction and maintenance doses are both 300 mg intravenously every 4 weeks. If no effect after 12 weeks or inability to discontinue steroids within 6 months of beginning therapy, treatment should be discontinued
   d. Efficacy
      i. The ENACT 1 and 2 trials showed similar results for natalizumab and placebo at 10 weeks (56% vs. 49%; p=0.05). However, those who initially responded had rates of sustained response (61% vs. 28%; p=0.001) at week 36.
      ii. Discontinue if no response is observed by week 12 of treatment.
      iii. May also improve quality of life in patients who initially respond after 48 weeks of treatment.
   e. Safety
      i. Natalizumab is associated with the development of progressive multifocal leukoencephalopathy. Monitor for mental status changes while on treatment. Consider magnetic resonance imaging and lumbar puncture if mental status changes or weakness is observed.
      ii. Potential for hepatotoxicity; monitor for jaundice or other signs of liver disease
      iii. Increased risk of infection
      iv. Infusion-related reactions: Observe patient for 1 hour after infusion.
      v. The drug should not be used in combination with inhibitors of TNFα or immunosuppressants.
10. Vedolizumab (Entyvio)
   a. Humanized monoclonal antibody that targets α4β7-integrin–mediated leukocyte adhesion
   b. Indicated use as induction and maintenance therapy for patients with UC and CD for whom other therapies, including TNF-α antagonists, have failed
   c. Induction and maintenance doses are both 300 mg intravenously given at 0, 2, and 6 weeks, then given every 4 weeks. Discontinue if no evidence of improvement at 14 weeks.
   d. The GEMINI I study demonstrated efficacy in induction and maintenance for moderate–severe UC with a clinical response rate of 47% vs. 25% versus placebo at 6 weeks (p<0.001). The GEMINI II Study of induction and maintenance of moderate to severe CD demonstrated rates of remission of 14.5% vs. 6.8% for placebo at 6 weeks (p=0.02).
   e. Safety profile is similar to that of natalizumab, with the exception of a lower risk of progressive multifocal leukoencephalopathy because vedolizumab's mechanism is more specific for leukocyte honing in the gut. There is not a required prescribing program for this agent.
11. Medical management of UC: Treatment is selected according to disease location and severity
   a. Guideline definitions of UC distribution
      i. Distal disease: Distal to splenic flexure (may use oral/systemic or topical [rectal] therapy)
      ii. Extensive disease: Proximal to splenic flexure (requires systemic/oral therapy)

b. Mild–moderate distal disease

    i. First-line therapy: Topical (enema/suppository) aminosalicylates are preferred and are superior to oral aminosalicylates and topical corticosteroids (grade A evidence). Oral budesonide (Uceris) can be considered an alternative first-line therapy.

    ii. Patients refractory to oral aminosalicylates or topical corticosteroids may respond to mesalamine enemas or suppositories.

    iii. Oral mesalamine plus topical mesalamine can be considered, and this combination may be more effective than either agent alone (grade A evidence).

    iv. Patients refractory to the above agents may require 40–60 mg of oral prednisone or infliximab given as 5 mg/kg intravenously at weeks 0, 2, and 6.

    v. Maintenance

        (a) Mesalamine suppositories (1 g rectally every day or 1 g three times/week) are effective for maintaining remission in patients with proctitis.

        (b) Mesalamine enemas (2–4 g/day) are effective for maintaining remission in patients with distal disease extending to the splenic flexure and may also be given three times/week.

        (c) Oral treatment with sulfasalazine (2–4 g/day), mesalamine (1.5–4.8 g/day), or balsalazide (6.75 g/day) is also effective.

        (d) Combining oral and topical mesalamine is more effective than using either regimen alone.

        (e) Topical steroids have no role in maintenance therapy.

        (f) Nicotine replacement (15–25 mg/day transdermally) may improve symptoms as an adjunctive therapy. Effects seem to be most beneficial in ex-smokers.

        (g) Azathioprine, 6-MP, infliximab, or adalimumab may be necessary if patients do not respond to aminosalicylate therapy.

c. Mild–moderate active extensive disease

    i. First-line therapy: Oral sulfasalazine (4–6 g/day) or an alternative aminosalicylate at a dose equivalent to mesalamine 4.8 g/day or oral budesonide (Uceris) can be considered an alternative first-line therapy.

    ii. Patients refractory to the combination of oral and topical aminosalicylate agents may require oral corticosteroids (40–60 mg of prednisone).

    iii. Azathioprine or 6-MP may be used for patients who are unresponsive to oral steroids but not acutely ill enough to require intravenous treatment with infliximab or adalimumab.

    iv. Infliximab, adalimumab, golimumab, or certolizumab may be used for moderate active disease in patients who are steroid-refractory or steroid-dependent or are intolerant of, or unresponsive to, azathioprine or 6-MP.

    v. Maintenance

        (a) Aminosalicylates are the preferred agents for maintenance of remission.

        (b) Patients should not be treated with long-term steroids for maintenance therapy.

        (c) Azathioprine or 6-MP is an effective steroid-sparing agent for maintenance of remission; can be used in combination with aminosalicylates

        (d) Infliximab may be given for maintenance of moderate disease at a dose of 5 mg/kg every 8 weeks if patients are initially responsive. Adalimumab may also be used at a dose of 40 mg subcutaneously every 2 weeks. Certolizumab can be used at a dose of 100 mg subcutaneously every 4 weeks.

d. Severe disease

    i. Patients with severe symptoms refractory to oral/topical aminosalicylates or corticosteroids should be treated with a 7- to 10-day course of intravenous corticosteroids (hydrocortisone 300 mg or methylprednisolone equivalent 60 mg/day).

        ii.   Alternatively, infliximab, adalimumab, or certolizumab should be used for severe disease as a next step in therapy.

        iii.   Antibiotics, particularly metronidazole, have mixed results in the treatment of active UC. In the absence of infection, their use provides little clinical benefit. Antibiotics may be used in severe colonic disease or for patients with pouchitis.

        iv.   Patients refractory to 3–5 days of intravenous corticosteroids are candidates for intravenous cyclosporine (4 mg/kg/day; target concentration of 350–500 ng/mL), followed by oral therapy at 8 mg/kg/day with a target concentration of 200–350 ng/mL if initial response to intravenous cyclosporine is obtained. Adding azathioprine or 6-MP to oral cyclosporine has shown better long-term success in maintaining remission, and this should be implemented.

        v.   Patients refractory to the above are candidates for colectomy.

        vi.   Patients with toxic megacolon should undergo bowel decompression, treatment with broad-spectrum antibiotics, and possibly colectomy.

    e.   Management of pouchitis

        i.   Patients with ileoanal anastomosis who develop symptoms of pouchitis may be treated with metronidazole (250 mg or 20 mg/kg three times/day), ciprofloxacin 500 mg twice daily, or the combination of both antibiotics.

        ii.   Use of oral probiotics (VSL #3) may be beneficial in preventing recurrent pouchitis.

12. Medical management of CD

    a.   Treatment is selected according to disease location and severity.

    b.   Mild–moderate active disease: First line for ileal, ileocolonic, or colonic disease

        i.   Oral aminosalicylate (mesalamine 3.2–4 g/day or sulfasalazine 6 g/day). Commonly used but considered minimally effective

        ii.   Budesonide 9 mg/day is preferred for terminal ileal or ascending colonic disease.

        iii.   Metronidazole 10–20 mg/kg/day may be used in patients not responding to oral aminosalicylates, but it is generally more effective in patients with perianal or colonic disease.

        iv.   Ciprofloxacin 1 g/day is considered as effective as mesalamine (generally, second line) but is usually more effective in perianal or colonic disease and is typically used in combination with metronidazole.

    c.   Moderate–severe disease

        i.   Corticosteroids (prednisone 40–60 mg/day or budesonide 9 mg/day if terminal ileal involvement) until resolution of symptoms and resumption of weight gain

        ii.   Anti-TNFα agents in combination with thiopurines are the preferred therapies for induction of remission for moderate to severe CD. Thiopurine monotherapy or methotrexate is not recommended to induce remission in moderate to severe active CD according to the 2013 guideline update.

           (a) Infliximab 5 mg/kg is an alternative first-line treatment (improvement in up to 80% of patients). Infliximab may be combined with azathioprine in patients whose therapy with aminosalicylates and corticosteroids has failed and who are naive to biologic agents. This combination is superior to each drug given alone; however, there is a risk of hepatosplenic T-cell lymphoma.

           (b) Certolizumab 400 mg subcutaneously and then 400 mg subcutaneously at weeks 2 and 4, or adalimumab 160 mg subcutaneously initially followed by 80 mg subcutaneously 2 weeks later, may also be considered for use as an alternative therapy for moderate to severe disease, particularly in patients with C-reactive protein values greater than 10 mg/L.

           (c) Adalimumab may used as initial therapy or for patients who no longer respond to infliximab therapy because they developed antibodies to infliximab.

       iii. Natalizumab or vedolizumab 300 mg intravenously every 4 weeks may be considered for patients who did not respond to any other conventional medical therapy.

       iv. Methotrexate maintenance therapy (15–25 mg/week intramuscularly or subcutaneously) is effective in patients whose active disease has responded to intramuscular methotrexate and who have steroid-dependent or steroid-refractory disease.

  d. Severe–fulminant disease

       i. Severe symptoms despite oral corticosteroids or infliximab therapy

       ii. Assess need for surgical intervention (mass, obstruction, and abscess).

       iii. Administer intravenous corticosteroids (40–60 mg of prednisone equivalent).

       iv. Parenteral nutrition may be needed after 5–7 days.

       v. Possibly use intravenous cyclosporine if steroids fail.

  e. Maintenance therapy

       i. No role for long-term corticosteroid use, but budesonide may be used for up to 3 months in patients with mild–moderate disease having ileal involvement

       ii. Azathioprine/6-MP or infliximab, or the combination, can be used after induction with corticosteroids.

       iii. Azathioprine/6-MP or mesalamine (more than 3 g/day) may also be used after surgical resection to prevent recurrence.

       iv. Infliximab 5 mg/kg at 0, 2, and 6 weeks and then every 8 weeks or adalimumab 40 mg subcutaneously every other week (starting on day 29 of therapy)

       v. Natalizumab or vedolizumab 300 mg intravenously every 4 weeks may be considered for patients who did not respond to any other conventional medical therapy.

       vi. Methotrexate intramuscularly 25 mg for up to 16 weeks, followed by 15 mg/week intramuscularly, is effective for patients with chronic active disease.

  f. Perianal disease

       i. Simple perianal fistulas

         (a) Antibiotics: Metronidazole or ciprofloxacin

         (b) Azathioprine/6-MP

         (c) Infliximab, adalimumab, certolizumab

       ii. Complex perianal fistulas

         (a) Infliximab, adalimumab, or certolizumab

         (b) Antibiotics: Metronidazole or ciprofloxacin (mainly as adjunctive therapy in this case)

         (c) Azathioprine/6-MP or methotrexate

         (d) Cyclosporine or tacrolimus

Patient Cases

4. A 35-year-old man presents with newly diagnosed mild–moderately active UC affecting his descending colon and rectum (left-sided disease). He takes loratadine 10 mg/day for seasonal allergies. He has no known drug allergies. Which drug regimen is best?

  A. Balsalazide 750 mg twice daily.

  B. Methotrexate 25 mg intramuscularly once weekly.

  C. Infliximab 5 mg/kg intravenously.

  D. Mesalamine enema 1000 mg rectally once daily.

Patient Cases *(continued)*

5. A 25-year-old woman presents to the clinic with a 12-week history of cramping abdominal pain, fever, fatigue, and 3–4 bloody stools a day. A colonoscopy reveals patchy inflammation in the colon and terminal ileum consistent with moderately active Crohn disease. She has an allergy to penicillin (rash). Vital signs include temperature 98°F, HR 100 beats/minute, RR 18 breaths/minute, and BP 118/68 mm Hg. She is 65 inches tall and weighs 120 lb. Which therapeutic choice is best?

   A. Mesalamine (Pentasa) 1000 mg 4 times/day.

   B. Infliximab 275 mg intravenously and azathioprine 110 mg daily.

   C. Budesonide (Entocort) 9 mg orally once daily.

   D. Adalimumab 40 mg subcutaneously every 2 weeks.

V. COMPLICATIONS OF LIVER DISEASE

Scoring Systems for Severity of Liver Disease

Table 16. Child-Pugh Classification of the Severity of Cirrhosis

Variable	Score		
	1 Point	**2 Points**	**3 Points**
Encephalopathy	Absent	Mild–moderate	Severe to coma
Ascites	Absent	Slight	Moderate
Bilirubin (mg/dL)	<2	2–3	>3
Albumin (g/L)	>3.5	2.8–3.5	<2.8
Prothrombin time (seconds above normal)	1–4	4–6	>6

[a]Class A = total score of 5 or 6; class B = total score of 7–9; class C = total score of 10 or more.

Table 17. Model for End-Stage Liver Disease (MELD)

Version	Calculation	Comments
Original	$9.57 \times \ln(\text{creatinine}) + 3.78 \times \ln(\text{total bilirubin}) + 11.2 \times \ln(\text{INR}) + 6.43$	• Score ranges from 6 to 40 • Higher number indicates more severe disease • Used to predict mortality and prioritize patients for liver transplantation
MELD-Na	$\text{MELD} - \text{Na} - [0.025 \times \text{MELD} \times (140 - \text{Na})] + 140$	• Incorporates sodium • May better discriminate risk of death
UNOS modification	Original MELD equation with limits set on laboratory values that are entered	• Lower end of laboratory values for SCr, bilirubin, and INR are set at 1 with a maximum of 4 • If 2 or more dialysis treatments within the prior week or within 24 hours of CVVHD within the prior week, SCr concentration automatically set to 4.0 mg/dL

MELD Score Calculators available at www.mayoclinic.org/meld/mayomodel5.html.

CVVHD = continuous venovenous hemodialysis; INR = international normalized ratio; Na = sodium, SCr = serum creatinine; UNOS = United Network for Organ Sharing.

A. Ascites
   1. Definition: Free fluid in the abdominal cavity secondary to increased resistance within the liver (forces lymphatic drainage into the abdominal cavity) and reduced osmotic pressure within the bloodstream (hypoalbuminemia); develops at a 5-year cumulative rate of 30% in compensated liver disease
   2. Clinical features: Protuberant abdomen, shifting dullness, fluid wave, bulging flanks, abdominal pain
   3. Diagnosis
      a. Clinical features
      b. Abdominal ultrasonography
      c. Paracentesis. Can use serum-ascites albumin gradient, calculated by subtracting the ascites albumin concentration from the serum albumin concentration; a value greater than 1.1 indicates ascites secondary to portal hypertension
   4. Treatment
      a. Alcohol cessation if alcohol induced
      b. Attainment of negative sodium balance
         i. Dietary sodium restriction (less than 2000 mg/day), fluid restriction to less than 1.5 L/day if serum sodium is less than 120–125 mmol/L
         ii. Goal is excretion greater than 78 mmol/day of sodium. A random spot urine sodium concentration greater than the potassium concentration (ratio greater than 1) correlates with a 24-hour sodium excretion of greater than 78 mmol/day with 90% accuracy.
         iii. Diuretics
            (a) A combination of furosemide and spironolactone is preferable as initial therapy in most patients. When used in combination, a ratio of 40 mg of furosemide to every 100 mg of spironolactone is an appropriate starting regimen. Amiloride 10–40 mg/day may be substituted for spironolactone in patients who develop tender gynecomastia.
            (b) If tense ascites is present, may use large-volume paracentesis. Administer albumin at a dose of 6–8 g/L of ascitic fluid removed (if more than 5 L is removed at one time).
            (c) If refractory ascites is present, may consider midodrine 7.5 mg three times daily as add-on therapy to diuretics.
         iv. No upper limit of weight loss if massive edema is present, 0.5 kg/day in patients without edema
         v. Monitor for electrolyte imbalances, renal impairment, and gynecomastia (spironolactone).
      c. Discontinue drugs associated with sodium/water retention such as NSAIDs. Angiotensin-converting enzyme inhibitors and angiotensin receptor blockers should be avoided also to prevent renal failure.

B. Hepatic Encephalopathy
   1. Definition: Hepatic encephalopathy is a brain dysfunction caused by liver insufficiency or portosystemic shunting; it manifests as a wide spectrum of neurological or psychiatric abnormalities ranging from subclinical alterations to coma.
      a. Thought to be secondary to the accumulation of nitrogenous substances (mainly NH_3) arising from the gut; overall, NH_3 serum concentrations do not correlate well with mental status
      b. Other theories are related to the activation of GABA (γ-aminobutyric acid receptors) by endogenous benzodiazepine-like substances, possible zinc deficiency, or altered cerebral metabolism.
   2. Clinical features and criteria
      a. May result in acute encephalopathy with altered mental status and progress to coma if untreated; asterixis ("hand flap") is a classic physical finding.
      b. May be precipitated by various factors including constipation, GI bleeding, infection, hypokalemia, dehydration, hypotension, and CNS-active drugs (benzodiazepines and narcotics)
      c. The West Haven Criteria and the Glasgow Coma Scale can be used to classify and grade.

Table 18. Common Criteria and Clinical Symptoms for Hepatic Encephalopathy

West Haven Criteria	ISHEN[a]	Clinical Description
Unimpaired		No current or history of encephalopathy
Minimal	Covert	Psychometric or neuropsychological alterations of tests exploring psychomotor speed and executive functions or neurophysiological alterations without clinical evidence of mental change
Grade I		Trivial lack of awareness Euphoria or anxiety Shortened attention span Impairment of addition or subtraction Altered sleep rhythm
Grade II	Overt	Lethargy or apathy Disorientation for time Obvious personality change Inappropriate behavior Dyspraxia Asterixis
Grade III		Somnolence to semistupor Responsive to stimuli Confused Gross disorientation Bizarre behavior
Grade IV		Coma

[a]International Society for Hepatic Encephalopathy and Nitrogen Metabolism.

3. Classifications
   a. Subtypes according to underlying disease
      i. Type A: Due to acute liver failure
      ii. Type B: Due to portosystemic bypass or shunting
      iii. Type C: Due to cirrhosis
   b. Duration
      i. Episodic
      ii. Recurrent (occurs within a time frame of 6 months or less)
      iii. Persistent: Denotes a pattern of behavioral alteration that is always present and interspersed with relapses of overt hepatic encephalopathy (HE)
   c. Presence or absence of precipitating factors
      i. Precipitated
      ii. Nonprecipitated
4. Treatment
   a. Assess need for airway support and remove possible precipitating factors.
   b. Main treatments targeted at reducing the nitrogen load in the gut
   c. Treatment recommendations are based on type C

Table 19. Treatment of Hepatic Encephalopathy due to Cirrhosis (Type C)

Type	Recommendations
Episodic overt HE type C	Treat episodic overt HE and then use secondary prophylaxis
	Primary prophylaxis is not indicated unless cirrhosis and high risk for HE
	Lactulose is first-line treatment for overt HE
	Rifaximin can be used as add-on therapy with lactulose to prevent recurrence after the second episode of overt HE
	Oral BCAA or IV LOLA can be used as alternative or additional therapy in patients unresponsive to traditional therapies
	Neomycin or metronidazole can be used as alternative treatment

BCAA = branched chain amino acids; HE = hepatic encephalopathy; IV = intravenous; LOLA = L-ornithine L-aspartate.

    d. Lactulose
       i. Nonabsorbable disaccharide: Metabolized by colonic bacteria to acetic and lactic acid; NH_3 present in the GI lumen is reduced to ammonium ion (NH_4^+) through the reduction in pH ("ammonia trapping") and is therefore unable to diffuse back into the bloodstream. Lactulose may also alter bacterial metabolism, resulting in increased uptake of NH_3.
       ii. Dose: 45 mL orally every 1–2 hours until the patient has a loose bowel movement, then titrate to two or three loose bowel movements a day (typically, a 15- to 45-mL dose two or three times daily); may also administer as an enema (300 mL plus 700 mL of water retained for 1 hour). Powder formulation (KRISTALOSE) is available in 10- and 20-g packets that may be dissolved in 4 oz water (10 g = 15 mL traditional lactulose). This formulation is more palatable than the traditional syrup.
       iii. May be continued over the long term to prevent recurrent encephalopathy
       iv. Flatulence, diarrhea, and abdominal cramping are common adverse effects.
    e. Antibiotics
       i. Targeted at reducing the number of intraluminal urease-producing bacteria that may be associated with excess NH_3 production
       ii. Neomycin (3–6 g/day in three or four divided doses × 1–2 weeks, then 1–2 g/day maintenance) or metronidazole (250 mg orally twice daily) may be used; neomycin is considered as effective as lactulose.
       iii. From 1% to 3% of neomycin is absorbed, so use caution with long-term use in patients with renal insufficiency; long-term metronidazole use may result in peripheral neuropathy.
       iv. Rifaximin is as effective as lactulose and other nonabsorbable antibiotics and may be better tolerated. Approved dose for reduction in overt encephalopathy in patients 18 years and older is 550 mg twice daily. Drug cost may be greater, but this may be offset by fewer hospitalizations and shorter lengths of stay. Previous studies in the short-term setting have used 400 mg three times/day.
    f. Other possible treatments
       i. A recent trial demonstrated that PEG 3350 4 liters given orally or via nasogastric tube over 4 hours resulted in faster improvement in encephalopathy compared with lactulose (Rahimi RS, Singal AG, Cuthbert JA, et al. JAMA 2014;174(11):1727-33)
       ii. Benzodiazepine antagonists such as flumazenil may be used in cases of suspected benzodiazepine overdose.
       iii. Zinc supplementation should used in patients with documented zinc deficiency.

iv. Branched chain amino acids and IV L-ornithine L-aspartate are alternative or additional therapies in patients unresponsive to traditional therapies

v. Nutritional interventions include 35–40 kcal/kg/day based on IBW and 1.2–1.5 g/kg/day protein intake

C. Gastroesophageal Varices

1. Background

a. Resistance to blood flow within the liver secondary to cirrhosis results in the development of portal hypertension. Collateral blood vessels (e.g., esophageal varices) are formed because of this increased resistance to blood flow.

b. Variceal hemorrhage may occur in around 25%–35% of patients with cirrhosis and varices; mortality rates are as high as 30%–50% per bleed; recurrence rates are as high as 70% within the first 6 months after an initial bleed.

2. Management of acute variceal bleeding

a. Fluid resuscitation and hemodynamic stabilization. Maintain hemoglobin concentration of about 8 g/dL. Administration of fresh frozen plasma or platelet may be considered for patients with considerable coagulopathy.

b. Endoscopy to assess the extent of disease with potential intervention

i. Sclerotherapy: Effective in discontinuing bleeding in 80%–90% of patients; may be associated with complications such as perforation, ulceration, stricture, and bacteremia; possible sclerosing agents include ethanolamine and sodium tetradecyl sulfate

ii. Endoscopic variceal band ligation may be used as an alternative to sclerotherapy; fewer complications

c. Medical management of acute variceal bleeding

i. Should be instituted after fluid resuscitation (before endoscopy, if possible)

ii. Most therapies are targeted at reducing splanchnic blood flow and portal pressure; combination of endoscopic and vasoactive therapies most effective

iii. Vasopressin: 0.2–0.4 unit/minute plus nitroglycerin 40–400 mcg/minute for 3–5 days

(a) Vasopressin use results in splanchnic vasoconstriction; used less often secondary to the need for both drugs and coronary vasoconstriction/hypertension with vasopressin (nitroglycerin attenuates these effects to some extent)

(b) More adverse effects than octreotide, so overall, less preferable

iv. Octreotide or somatostatin

(a) Works possibly by preventing postprandial hyperemia, by reducing portal pressure (by reduced splanchnic blood flow) through inhibitory effects on vasoactive peptides such as glucagon, or by a local vasoconstrictor effect

(b) Preferred agent in combination with endoscopic interventions because of more favorable adverse effect profiles; main adverse effects include hyperglycemia and abdominal cramping

(c) Dosing

(1) Octreotide: 50-mcg intravenous bolus, then 50 mcg/hour intravenously for 3–5 days

(2) Somatostatin: 250-mcg intravenous bolus, then 250–500 mcg/hour intravenously for 3–5 days

v. Nondrug measures to control bleeding

(a) Typically used for medically unresponsive bleeding

(b) Minnesota or Blakemore tube: Balloon compression applied directly to bleeding varices

(c) Transjugular intrahepatic portosystemic shunt: Results in shunting of blood from the portal circulation; however, may be associated with complications such as bleeding and infection

(d) Surgery

vi. Antibiotic therapy

(a) Use of oral or intravenous prophylactic antibiotics in patients with cirrhosis with variceal bleeding reduces short-term mortality; these agents should be prescribed.

(b) Typical regimens include a fluoroquinolone (norfloxacin or ciprofloxacin) orally for 7 days. Intravenous therapy (ciprofloxacin) can be used if the oral route of administration is not an option. Ceftriaxone 1 g/day intravenously may be used if high rates of fluoroquinolone resistance are present.

d. Prevention of variceal bleeding

i. Primary prophylaxis

(a) A screening esophagogastroduodenoscopy is recommended to evaluate for esophageal and gastric varices when the diagnosis of cirrhosis is made.

(b) Pharmacologic therapy is not recommended to prevent the development of varices in patients with cirrhosis who have not yet developed varices.

(c) Patients who have small varices and no history of bleeding but meet the criteria for increased risk of bleeding (Child-Pugh class B or C, red wale marks on varices) should receive preventive drug therapy with nonselective β-blockers.

(d) Nonselective β-blockers can be considered; however, the long-term benefit is unclear in patients who have small varices and no history of bleeding but who do *not* meet the criteria for increased risk of bleeding.

(e) Nonselective β-blockers are indicated in all patients with medium or large varices and no history of bleeding. An endoscopic variceal ligation (EVL) can be used if nonselective β-blockers are contraindicated.

(f) Mechanism of nonselective β-blockers: Blockade of β_1-receptors reduces cardiac output, whereas blockade of β_2-receptors prevents splanchnic vasodilation; unopposed α_1-mediated constriction of the splanchnic circulation also leads to reductions in portal pressure.

(g) Therapy should aim for an HR of 55–60 beats/minute or a 25% reduction from baseline.

(h) Nonselective β-blockers are associated with a significant reduction in the incidence of first bleed.

(i) Long-acting nitrates (isosorbide mononitrate or dinitrate) should not be used for primary prophylaxis. These agents are believed to decrease intrahepatic resistance and are considered as effective as propranolol; however, there is an increased incidence of mortality in some studies when they are used as monotherapy.

(j) Shunt surgery or endoscopic sclerotherapy should not be used for primary prophylaxis.

ii. Secondary prophylaxis

(a) All patients with a history of variceal bleeding should receive secondary prophylaxis to prevent recurrent bleeding.

(b) A combination of endoscopic variceal band ligation and nonselective β-blockers is considered the most effective regimen.

(c) Nonselective β-blockers are associated with approximately a 20% reduction in the incidence of variceal rebleeding; reductions in mortality are minimal and inconsistent between trials most studies are of patients with Child-Pugh class A or B cirrhosis; class C patients may be unable to tolerate β-blockers.

(d) Combining nonselective β-blockers with nitrates leads to slightly higher reductions in rebleeding rates; however, no added mortality benefit is observed, and there is a higher incidence of adverse effects with the combination.

(e) Sclerotherapy is no longer recommended for secondary prophylaxis because EVL has been shown to be better, with fewer complications.

(f) The transjugular intrahepatic portosystemic shunt is very effective at preventing recurrent bleeding; however, it is associated with a 30%–40% incidence of encephalopathy; reserve for medically unresponsive patients

(g) Contraindications to nonselective β-blockers: asthma, insulin-dependent diabetes with frequent hypoglycemia, peripheral vascular disease

(h) Adverse effects of nonselective β-blockers: light-headedness, fatigue, shortness of breath, sexual dysfunction, bradycardia

(i) Adverse effects of EVL: transient dysphagia, chest discomfort

D. Spontaneous Bacterial Peritonitis (SBP)
1. Background
   a. Definition: Infection of previously sterile ascitic fluid without an apparent intra-abdominal source. SBP is considered a primary, as opposed to secondary, peritonitis.
   b. May be present in 10%–30% of hospitalized patients with cirrhosis and ascites
   c. Associated with 20%–40% of in-hospital mortality; poor prognosis after recovery, with 2-year survival after initial episode reported as about 30%
2. Pathophysiology
   a. Principal theory is seeding of the ascitic fluid from an episode of bacteremia.
   b. The bacteria present are usually enteric pathogens; thus, they may enter the blood because of increases in gut permeability secondary to portal hypertension, suppression of hepatic reticuloendothelial cells, or translocation of the gut wall and dissemination through the mesenteric lymph system.
   c. Reduced opsonic activity of the ascitic fluid and alterations in neutrophil function may also be contributing factors.
   d. Enteric gram-negative pathogens are most commonly involved, and more than 90% of cases involve a single bacterial species.

Table 20. Most Commonly Isolated Bacteria Responsible for Spontaneous Bacterial Peritonitis

Gram-negative Bacilli (50%)	Gram-positive Bacilli (17%)
Escherichia coli, 37%	Streptococcus pneumoniae, 10%
Klebsiella spp., 6%	Other streptococci, 6%
Other, 7%	*Staphylococcus aureus,* 1%

3. Clinical and laboratory features
   a. Clinical presentation may be variable, but common symptoms include fever, abdominal pain, nausea, vomiting, diarrhea, rebound tenderness, and exacerbation of encephalopathy; about 33% of patients may present with renal failure, which is associated with significant increases in mortality. Although GI bleeding and septic shock or hypotension occur, they are rare.
   b. Laboratory
      i. May see systemic leucocytosis or increases in serum creatinine (SCr)
      ii. Abdominal paracentesis must be performed
         (a) The presence of more than 250 polymorphonuclear cells/mm^3 is diagnostic for SBP.

   (b) Lactate dehydrogenase, glucose, and protein values may help distinguish it from secondary peritonitis.

  iii. Blood cultures positive in 50%–70% of cases; ascitic fluid cultures positive in 67% of cases

  iv. Gram stain of ascitic fluid is typically low yield.

4. Treatment of acute SBP

 a. Because of the high associated mortality, treatment should be initiated promptly in patients with clinical and laboratory features consistent with SBP. If ascitic fluid polymorphonuclear cells are less than 250 cells/mm^3, empiric antibiotic therapy can be initiated if other signs of infection are present.

 b. Up to 86% of ascitic fluid cultures may be negative if one dose of an antibiotic is given before cultures are drawn.

 c. Predictors of poor outcomes include bilirubin more than 8 mg/dL, albumin less than 2.5 g/dL, creatinine more than 2.1 mg/dL, hepatic encephalopathy, hepatorenal syndrome (HRS), and upper GI bleeding.

 d. Antibiotic therapy plus albumin if patient meets criteria for use (see below)

  i. Empiric therapy targeting enteric gram-negative organisms should be instituted.

  ii. Third-generation cephalosporins have been studied the most and are considered first line: cefotaxime (2 g every 8–12 hours) or ceftriaxone (2 g/day intravenously).

  iii. Other agents such as fluoroquinolones may be used. Ofloxacin 400 mg orally twice daily can be considered in patients without prior exposure to fluoroquinolones and no evidence of shock, vomiting, grade II or higher encephalopathy, or SCr greater than 3 mg/dL.

  iv. Avoid aminoglycosides because of the high risk of renal failure in patients with cirrhosis and SBP.

  v. Treatment duration: 5–10 days; most studies suggest that a 5-day treatment period is as effective as a 10-day period

 e. Albumin

  i. Rationale: The hemodynamics of patients with cirrhosis reflect a state of intravascular hypovolemia and organ hypoperfusion; SBP is thought to exacerbate this effect, resulting in progressive renal hypoperfusion and precipitation of renal failure or HRS.

  ii. The regimen most commonly used is based on one study (N Engl J Med 1999;341:403-9).

   (a) Albumin dosing: 1.5 g/kg on admission; 1 g/kg on hospital day 3

   (b) In addition, should give antibiotic treatment; cefotaxime was used in this study

   (c) The incidence of renal failure was 10%, compared with 33% for placebo (p=0.002).

   (d) In-hospital mortality was 10% for albumin, 29% for placebo (p=0.01).

   (e) Thirty-day mortality was reduced to 21% with albumin, compared with 41% for placebo (p=0.03).

   (f) Guidelines suggest using this albumin regimen with antibiotics if SCr is more than 1 mg/dL, BUN more than 30 mg/dL, or total bilirubin more than 4 mg/dL.

5. Prevention

 a. Prophylactic oral antibiotics are used to prevent SBP in high-risk patients to reduce the number of enteric organisms in the GI tract (GI decontamination), with the hope of reducing the chance of bacterial translocation.

 b. Antibiotic regimens are similar for both primary and secondary prevention:

  i. Fluoroquinolones: Norfloxacin or ciprofloxacin

  ii. Trimethoprim/sulfamethoxazole 1 double-strength tablet five times/week (Monday through Friday)

    c. Primary prevention
        i. For acute upper GI bleeding (7-day course during hospitalization only), give ceftriaxone or norfloxacin 400 mg twice daily.
        ii. May also consider for indefinite use in patients without GI bleeding if ascitic fluid protein concentration is less than 1.5 g/dL and at least one of the following is present: SCr more than 1.2 mg/dL, BUN more than 25 mg/dL, sodium less than 130 mg/dL, or Child-Pugh score more than 9 with bilirubin more than 3 mg/dL
        iii. Use norfloxacin 400 mg once daily or trimethoprim/sulfamethoxazole.
    d. Secondary prevention
        i. All patients recovering from an initial episode of SBP should be treated with oral prophylactic antibiotics (norfloxacin or trimethoprim/sulfamethoxazole) indefinitely.
        ii. Consider patient for liver transplantation because 2-year survival is 25%–30% after recovery.

E. Hepatorenal Syndrome (HRS)
    1. Criteria in patients with cirrhosis and ascites: SCr greater than 1.5 mg/dL, no improvement in SCr to less than 1.5 mg/dL after withdrawal of diuretics and administration of albumin, absence of shock, no current nephrotoxins, absence of parenchymal kidney disease and microhematuria, and a normal renal ultrasound
    2. Subtypes
        a. Type 1: Doubling of SCr to greater than 2.5 mg/dL or a 50% reduction in CrCl to less than 20 mL/minute in less than 2 weeks
        b. Type 2: Nonrapid progression of worsening of renal function. Associated with high mortality
    3. Treatment: Albumin in combination with octreotide (200 mcg subcutaneously three times daily) or midodrine (12.5 mg three times daily maximum) may be considered for type 1 HRS. Albumin plus norepinephrine may also be tried if the patient is in the ICU.

F. Alcoholic Liver Disease
    1. Subset of chronic liver disease. Patients may develop steatosis and eventually progress to cirrhosis. About 10%–35% of patients may develop severe alcoholic hepatitis.
    2. Prognosis of alcoholic hepatitis may be initially evaluated by the Maddrey discriminant function (MDF) score, calculated as 4.6 × (patient's PT − control PT) + total bilirubin (mg/dL), where PT is prothrombin time. Patients whose score is greater than 32 are believed to have a poor prognosis. Patients with a model for end-stage liver disease (MELD) score greater than 18 can also be considered for drug therapy.
        a. Patients with an MDF greater than 32, with or without encephalopathy, or a MELD score greater than 18 should be considered for a 4-week course of prednisolone 40 mg/day, followed by a 2-week taper. This may lead to a 30% decrease in the risk ratio of short-term death.
        b. Patients with an MDF greater than 32 can be considered for treatment with pentoxifylline 400 mg three times/day, especially if there are contraindications to corticosteroids. This has shown to lower hospital mortality by 14% compared with placebo.
    3. Long-term treatment of alcoholic liver disease with propylthiouracil or colchicine is not recommended.

Patient Cases

6. A 47-year-old woman with a history of alcoholic cirrhosis (Child-Pugh class C) is admitted to the hospital with nausea, abdominal pain, and fever. Physical examination reveals a distended abdomen with shifting dullness, a positive fluid wave, and the presence of diffuse rebound tenderness. She also has 1+ lower extremity edema. Current medications include furosemide 80 mg twice daily and spironolactone 200 mg once daily. A diagnostic paracentesis reveals turbid ascitic fluid, which was sent for culture. Laboratory analysis of the fluid revealed an albumin concentration of 0.9 g/dL and the presence of 1×10^3 white blood cells (45% polymorphonuclear neutrophils). Serum laboratory studies reveal an SCr of 1.2 mg/dL, BUN 37 mg/dL, aspartate aminotransferase AST 60 IU/mL, alanine aminotransferase (ALT) 20 IU/mL, serum albumin 2.5 g/dL, and total bilirubin 3.2 mg/dL. Which is the best course of action?

   A. Initiate intravenous albumin and await culture results.

   B. Initiate intravenous vancomycin plus tobramycin.

   C. Initiate intravenous cefotaxime plus albumin therapy.

   D. Initiate oral trimethoprim/sulfamethoxazole double strength.

7. A 56-year-old man with a history of Child-Pugh class B cirrhosis secondary to alcohol abuse is admitted with a 2-day history of confusion, disorientation, somnolence, and reduced oral intake. On examination, he is afebrile, with abdominal tenderness, reduced reflexes, dry mucous membranes, and asterixis. Paracentesis is negative for infection. He takes propranolol 40 mg three times/day. Which recommendation is best for treating this patient's hepatic encephalopathy?

   A. Initiate rifaximin 550 mg orally twice daily.

   B. Initiate lactulose 30 mL orally every 2 hours.

   C. Initiate PEG-3350 17 g orally twice daily.

   D. Initiate ceftriaxone 1 g intravenously daily.

VI. VIRAL HEPATITIS

A. Definitions: For all hepatitis virus infections, acute hepatitis is defined as infection for less than 6 months, whereas chronic infection is infection for more than 6 months.

B. Hepatitis A Virus (HAV)
   1. Background
      a. An RNA virus that is associated with the development of self-limited hepatitis
      b. Transmission occurs mainly through the fecal-oral route.
         i. Areas of poor sanitation; also associated flooding leading to increased spread
         ii. Foodborne: shellfish, water, milk, vegetables
         iii. Person-to-person contact: sexual, day care, intravenous drug use, household, restaurant workers
      c. After exposure, incubation for 14–50 days takes place; patients may have general, nonspecific symptoms such as nausea, vomiting, diarrhea, myalgia, fever, abdominal pain, and jaundice.
      d. Most patients have self-limited disease lasting less than 2 months; death of the hepatocyte results in elimination of the virus.
      e. HAV is associated with very low mortality (less than 1%) and is not associated with the development of chronic hepatitis. Fulminant hepatitis may occur in some instances.

2. Diagnosis
   a. Clinical signs and symptoms such as nausea, abdominal pain, jaundice, fever, malaise, or anorexia. Some patients may have mild asymptomatic disease.
   b. Recent possible exposures
   c. Laboratory data
      i. Immunoglobulin M (IgM) antibody to HAV (anti-HAV): Detectable in the serum 5–10 days before the onset of symptoms; once the infection clears, the IgM antibody is replaced by IgG antibodies during a 2- to 6-month period; these antibodies confer lifelong protective immunity against subsequent infection.
      ii. Elevation of aminotransferases
   d. Management of acute HAV infection is mainly supportive; avoid hepatotoxic medications such as acetaminophen.
3. Preexposure prophylaxis
   a. Active (vaccination) or passive (immune globulin) prophylaxis can be used.
   b. Havrix (GlaxoSmithKline) and Vaqta (Merck) are the two available HAV vaccines; Twinrix is a combination HAV and HBV product (GlaxoSmithKline).
   c. Populations requiring preexposure prophylaxis with HAV vaccine
      i. All children older than 1 year
      ii. Children living in areas where rates of hepatitis are above twice the national average
      iii. People working in or traveling to countries with high or intermediate endemicity (may take up to 4 weeks for full protection)
      iv. Men who have sex with men
      v. Illegal drug users
      vi. Those with occupational risk of exposure (exposure to sewage)
      vii. Patients with chronic liver disease
      viii. Patients with clotting factor disorders
      ix. Optional: Food handlers, workers in institutions
   d. Populations requiring preexposure prophylaxis with HAV immune globulin
      i. Travelers to endemic countries
      ii. Children younger than 1 year (vaccine not approved for this age group)
      iii. Doses: 0.02 mL/kg intramuscularly (3 months' coverage or more); 0.06 mL/kg intramuscularly (3–5 months' coverage); repeat every 5 months if travel or exposure is prolonged
4. Postexposure prophylaxis
   a. Immune globulin can be given at a dose of 0.02 mL/kg intramuscularly within 2 weeks of exposure. HAV vaccine may also be used. Efficacy approaches that of immune globulin, but it is recommended only in patients 12 months to 40 years of age.
   b. Offer to those not previously vaccinated in the following situations:
      i. Close personal contact with a documented infected person
      ii. Staff or attendees of day care centers if one or more cases are recognized in children or employees or if cases are recognized in two or more households of attendees
      iii. Common source of exposures
         (a) If a food handler receives a diagnosis of HAV, vaccine or immune globulin should be administered to other food handlers at the same establishment. Administration of HAV vaccine or immune globulin to patrons typically is not indicated but may be considered if:
            (1) Although the food handler was probably infectious, he or she both directly handled uncooked or cooked food and had diarrhea or poor hygienic practices.
            (2) Patrons can be identified and treated in 2 weeks or less after exposure.

(b) In settings where repeated exposures to HAV may have occurred, stronger consideration of HAV vaccine or immune globulin use could be warranted. In a common-source outbreak, postexposure prophylaxis should not be provided to exposed individuals after cases have begun to occur because the 2-week period after exposure during which immune globulin or HAV vaccine is known to be effective will have been exceeded.

C. Hepatitis B Virus
   1. Background
      a. HBV is a DNA virus; there are more than 350 million infected patients worldwide.
      b. Transmission routes
         i. Parenteral: intravenous drug abuse, needlestick, transfusion, ear or body piercing
         ii. Bodily fluids: saliva, semen, vaginal fluid
         iii. Sexual contact: heterosexual and homosexual; prostitution
         iv. Perinatal: mother to child at birth
      c. Associated with both acute and chronic disease. Natural history of HBV is age-dependent. Risk of developing chronic infection after an acute infection is 90% in neonates, 25%–30% in children younger than 5 years, and 10% in adults.
      d. Chronic infection with HBV increases the risk of developing hepatocellular carcinoma.
      e. Diagnosis
         i. Clinical signs and symptoms: nausea, vomiting, diarrhea, myalgia, fever, abdominal pain, jaundice (30% may have no symptoms)
         ii. Serologic diagnosis
         iii. Combinations of serologic markers must be reviewed to distinguish acute from chronic infections.
         iv. Eight different HBV genotypes (A–H) exist. Routine genotype testing is not endorsed by the guidelines.

Table 21. HBV Serologies

Serologic Marker	Abbreviation	Comment
Surface antigen	HBsAg	First detectable serum antigen during acute infection; also present in chronic infection
Core antigen	HBcAg	Present early after cell damage during acute infection; typically unable to measure this in the serum
E antigen	HBeAg	Denotes ongoing active viral replication
Anti–surface antigen antibody	Anti-HBs	Confers protective immunity; present after recovery from acute infection or after vaccination
Anticore antigen antibody (IgG)	Anti-HBc	Appears at onset of symptoms Denotes prior exposure to HBV Cannot use to distinguish acute from chronic infection
Anti-E antibody	Anti-HBe	May indicate peak replication has passed
HBV DNA	HBV DNA	Marker of active HBV replication

HBcAg = hepatitis B core antigen; HBeAg = hepatitis B early antigen; HBsAg = hepatitis B surface antigen; HBV = hepatitis B virus; IgG = immunoglobulin G.

(a) Most patients have hepatitis B early antigen (HBeAg)-positive disease.

(b) HBeAg-negative disease: Mutation in the precore or core promoter regions. These variants are known as precore mutants; these mutations do not allow monitoring of loss of E antigen as a clinical marker of suppressed replication. Monitor reduction in HBV DNA in these patients; patients infected with these variants also tend to have lower serum HBV DNA and more fluctuating liver function tests.

(c) Centers for Disease Control and Prevention guidelines for screening for HBV infection indicate that the serologic assay for HBV surface antigen (HBsAg) should be the serologic screening test used for the following populations. Additional HBVs are needed in combination with the HBsAg for select populations as listed below.

(1) People born in geographic regions with HBsAg prevalence greater than 2% regardless of vaccination history

(2) Men who have sex with men; also test for anti-HBc or anti-HBs

(3) Past or current intravenous drug users; also test for anti-HBc or anti-HBs

(4) Patients receiving cytotoxic chemotherapy or immunosuppressive therapy related to organ transplantation or rheumatologic or GI disorders. In addition, test for anti-HBc or anti-HBs.

(5) U.S.-born people not vaccinated as infants whose parents were born in regions with HBV endemicity greater than 8%

(6) People with elevated ALT and AST of unknown etiology

(7) Donors of blood, plasma, organs, tissues, or semen. In addition, test for anti-HBc and HBV DNA.

(8) Pregnant women (during each pregnancy, preferably in the first trimester)

(9) Infants born to HBsAg-positive mothers

(10) Household, needle sharing, or sex contacts of people known to be HBsAg positive. In addition, test for anti-HBc or anti-HBs.

(11) People who are the sources of blood or bodily fluid for exposures that might require postexposure prophylaxis

(12) People who are human immunodeficiency virus (HIV) positive. In addition, test for anti-HBc or anti-HBs.

v.   Clinical definitions

Table 22. Clinical Definitions of HBV

Chronic HBV Infection	Inactive HBV Carrier State
• HBsAg positive >6 months	• HBsAg positive >6 months
• Serum HBV DNA 20,000 IU/mL (105 copies/mL), lower values 2000–20,000 IU/ mL (104–105 copies/mL) are often observed in HBeAg-negative chronic HBV	• HBeAg negative, anti-HBeAg positive
• Persistent/intermittent elevation of AST and ALT	• Serum HBV DNA <2000 IU/mL (104 copies/mL)
• Chronic hepatitis and moderate–severe necroinflammation on biopsy	• Persistently normal AST and ALT; absence of significant hepatitis on biopsy

ALT = alanine aminotransferase; AST = aspartate aminotransferase; HBcAg = hepatitis B core antigen; HBeAg = hepatitis B early antigen; HBsAg = hepatitis B surface antigen; HBV = hepatitis B virus; LFT = liver function test.

2. Treatment of chronic infection
   a. Treatment recommendations
      i. Patients who are HBeAg positive with elevated ALT concentrations and compensated liver disease should be observed for 3–6 months for spontaneous conversion from HBeAg positive to anti-HBeAg negative before initiating treatment. Antiviral treatment should be considered in patients whose ALT remains greater than two times the ULN and whose HBV DNA is more than 20,000 IU/mL.
      ii. Patients who are HBeAg negative with positive anti-HBe as well as normal ALT and HBV less than 2000 IU/mL should be monitored every 3 months for 1 year and then every 6–12 months if they remain in the inactive carrier state.
   b. Patients who meet the criteria for chronic infection as outlined previously should be treated. Choice of initial therapy is based on patient profile, prior treatments, contraindications to drug therapy, and medication and monitoring costs.
   c. Monitoring for efficacy should be based on the following responses:
      i. Biochemical: ↓ Liver function tests to within the normal range
      ii. Virologic: ↓ HBV DNA to undetectable concentrations and loss of HBeAg if HBeAg positive
         (a) A primary nonresponse is considered a decrease in HBV DNA of less than 2 log/mL after at least 24 weeks of therapy. Patients *NOT* meeting these criteria should receive an alternative treatment.
         (b) Response should be assessed by reductions in HBV DNA for HBeAg-negative patients.

3. Drug therapies
   a. Interferon alfa (IFNα)/PEG-IFN
      i. Cytokine with antiviral, antiproliferative, and immunomodulatory effects
      ii. Best predictors of response to treatment are high pretreatment ALT, low-serum HBV DNA, presence of active inflammation on biopsy, and acquisition of infection because an adult HBeAg-negative disease responds less favorably to interferon (IFN).
      iii. Dosing
         (a) Traditional agents: HBeAg positive: Typical dose is 5 million units/day subcutaneously × 16–24 weeks or 10 million units subcutaneously three times/week × 16–24 weeks; patients with HBeAg-negative disease should be treated for 12 months.
         (b) PEG-α-2a (Pegasys): 180 mcg subcutaneously once weekly × 48 weeks (duration is the same for HBeAg-negative and HBeAg-positive disease)
      iv. In general, response to traditional IFN is poor; 37% loss of HBsAg, 33% loss of HBeAg with 12–24 weeks of treatment; this equates to about 20% better than placebo. Some trials suggest that PEG-IFN has only slightly better efficacy in HBeAg-positive disease, with 25% loss of HBV DNA and 30% loss of HBeAg at 48 weeks. Adherence may be better because of less-frequent dosing.
      v. If a response is obtained, it is usually long lasting (more than 4 years).
      vi. Treatment with IFN typically results in an increase in ALT 4–8 weeks into treatment. This is an expected response; it should not be viewed as an adverse effect of therapy.

Table 23. Available IFNα Products

Product	IFN Subtype	Route of Administration	Dosage Forms
Roferon-A[a]	α-2a	SC or IM	Single-dose vial (36 MU/mL)
			Multidose vial (18 MU/vial)
			Prefilled syringe (3, 6, 9 MU/0.5 mL)
Infergen	Acon-1	SC	Single-dose vials
			9 mcg (0.3 mL), 15 (0.5 mL)
Intron[a]	α-2b	SC or IM	Powder, solution, multidose pen
PEG-Intron	PEG-α-2b	SC	Single-dose vials (2 mL) + diluent 50, 80, 120, 150 mcg/0.5 mL
			Single-use Redipen 50, 80, 120, 150 mcg/0.5 mL
Pegasys[a,b]	PEG-α-2a	SC	Single-dose vial (1 mL) 180 mcg/mL
			Prefilled 180 mcg syringes (4/pack)
			Autoinjector 180 mcg

[a]Preferred for HBV.

[b]FDA approved for HBV.

HBV = hepatitis B virus; IFNα = interferon alfa; IM = intramuscular; PEG = pegylated; SC = subcutaneous.

      vii. Adverse effects
         (a) IFN is associated with many serious adverse effects, including bone marrow suppression.
            (1) Leukopenia: May use filgrastim (granulocyte colony-stimulating factor) for support
            (2) Thrombocytopenia: Minimal data with oprelvekin (interleukin-11). Not used because of many adverse effects including pulmonary hypertension
         (b) Predisposition to infections
         (c) CNS: Depression, psychosis, anxiety, insomnia, seizures. Adverse CNS effects occur in 22%–31% of patients.
         (d) Flulike symptoms (tolerance usually develops after a few weeks)
         (e) Anorexia, alopecia, thyroid dysfunction, neuropathy
         (f) Exacerbation of underlying autoimmune disorders (i.e., thyroid)
         (g) Ischemic or hemorrhagic cerebrovascular disorders
         (h) Serious hypersensitivity and rash formation
         (i) Manufacturers give recommendations for dose reductions in patients who develop bone marrow suppression and depression while on therapy.
         (j) Contraindicated in patients with current psychosis, a history of severe depression, neutropenia, thrombocytopenia, symptomatic heart disease, decompensated liver disease, and uncontrolled seizures; also, use caution in patients with autoimmune disorders
    b. Reverse transcriptase inhibitors
      i. In general, lamivudine and telbivudine are not preferred as first-line therapies because of high rates of resistance.
      ii. All reverse transcriptase inhibitors carry a black box warning for the development of lactic acidosis and severe hepatomegaly with steatosis. Monitor for worsening liver function tests, and periodically assess renal function. Female and obese patients are at higher risk. Reductions in bone mineral density (BMD) have been associated with long-term use. Assess baseline BMD in patients older than 12 years with a history of pathologic fracture or osteoporosis.

    iii. Lamivudine (Epivir-HBV)

      (a) Reduces HBV DNA by 3–4 log

      (b) Dose: 100 mg/day orally (tablets or solution) for at least 1 year (HBeAg negative and positive); dose is 150 mg orally twice daily for patients with HIV coinfection; doses require adjustment for reduced renal function

      (c) Efficacy: 17%–32% loss of HBeAg and 41%–72% normalization of ALT at 52 weeks; may be used for IFN failures and in patients with decompensated liver disease

      (d) Toxicity: Well tolerated (headache, nausea, vomiting, fatigue), rare lactic acidosis

      (e) Resistance: Prolonged use is associated with the development of mutations in the YMDD sequence of the HBV polymerase (20% at 1 year, 70% at 4 years). Risk factors for lamivudine resistance include elevated pretherapy HBV DNA or ALT, male sex, increased body mass index, previous exposure to lamivudine or famciclovir, and inadequate suppression on HBV DNA after 6 months of treatment.

      (f) Therapy discontinuation is often accompanied by rebound liver function test elevations; viral breakthrough may also be evident during treatment.

    iv. Adefovir (Hepsera)

      (a) Reduces HBV DNA by 24 log

      (b) Indicated in HBeAg-positive and HBeAg-negative disease, as well as in decompensated liver disease; also effective in lamivudine-resistant YMDD mutants and IFN failures

      (c) Dose: 10 mg orally every day for at least 1 year in HBeAg-negative and HBeAg-positive disease

      (d) Efficacy: Up to 72% normalization of ALT and 12% loss of HBeAg at 48 weeks

      (e) Toxicity: Renal dysfunction (3%), headache, nausea, vomiting, fatigue, rare lactic acidosis

      (f) Therapy discontinuation is often accompanied by rebound liver function test elevations; viral breakthrough may also be evident during treatment. Resistance reported as 29% at 5 years

    v. Entecavir (Baraclude)

      (a) Indicated for HBeAg-negative and HBeAg-positive patients with persistently elevated AST or ALT or histologically active disease. Effective in lamivudine-resistant YMDD mutants

      (b) Reduces HBV DNA by up to 6.86 log in HBeAg-positive, naive patients and by 5.2 log in HBeAg-negative patients or those with lamivudine resistance

      (c) Dose: 0.5 mg orally once daily for patients older than 16 years and nucleoside naive; 1 mg orally once daily for patients older than 16 years with HBV viremia while receiving lamivudine or in lamivudine-resistant HBV

      (d) Dose adjustments required for renal impairment

      (e) Toxicity: Similar to lamivudine with headache, cough, upper respiratory infection, abdominal pain; possibly fewer ALT flares. Rare lactic acidosis. Resistance reported as similar to 1% at 5 years.

    vi. Telbivudine (Tyzeka)

      (a) Indicated for HBeAg-negative and HBeAg-positive patients with persistently elevated AST or ALT or histologically active disease

      (b) Not effective in lamivudine-resistant YMDD mutants

      (c) A direct comparison with lamivudine (GLOBE trial) showed greater efficacy in both HBeAg-negative and HBeAg-positive patients. Reduces HBV DNA by up to 6.45 log in HBeAg-positive, naive patients and by 5.2 log in HBeAg-negative patients. Dose: 600 mg orally once daily. Dose adjustments required for renal impairment

(d) Toxicity: Similar to lamivudine; small incidence of myopathy. Creatine kinase elevations greater than 7 times the ULN; for telbivudine, 9% versus 3% with lamivudine in the GLOBE study. Rare lactic acidosis. Resistance reported as 25% at 2 years

  vii. Tenofovir (Viread)

    (a) Nucleotide analog, formulated as tenofovir disoproxil fumarate, indicated for chronic HBV infection

    (b) Effective for lamivudine-resistant HBV

    (c) Dose adjustments required for renal impairment

    (d) Toxicity: Overall, well tolerated. Headache, nausea, and nasopharyngitis most commonly reported. Potential renal toxicity, so periodic monitoring of SCr recommended. Potential ALT flares on withdrawal. Rare lactic acidosis

Table 24. Summary of Treatment Recommendations for Chronic HBV Infection in Adults

HBV Population	Preferred Treatment Options	Duration	Comments
HBeAg positive	Entecavir and tenofovir are preferred oral agents Use of the other oral reverse transcriptase inhibitors is possible but not preferred	Minimum of 1 year	Preferred if contraindications or nonresponse to IFNα
	IFNα PEG-IFNα	16 weeks 48 weeks	If contraindication or no response, use entecavir and tenofovir
HBeAg negative	Entecavir and tenofovir are preferred oral agents Use of the other oral reverse transcriptase inhibitors is possible but not preferred	>1 year	Preferred if contraindications or no response to IFNα
	IFNα PEG-IFNα	≥1 year	If contraindication or nonresponse, use entecavir and tenofovir
Development of resistant HBV	Lamivudine or telbivudine resistance: Add adefovir or tenofovir or change to entecavir Adefovir resistance: Add lamivudine Entecavir resistance: Change to tenofovir	N/A	Confirm resistance with genotypic testing Reinforce adherence to therapy

HBeAg = hepatitis B early antigen; HBV = hepatitis B virus; IFNα = interferon alfa; N/A = not applicable; PEG = pegylated.

4. Preventive strategies

  a. Vaccination (preexposure); indicated in the following groups:

    i. All infants born to HBsAg-negative mothers

    ii. Adolescents with high-risk behavior (intravenous drug abuse, multiple sex partners)

    iii. Workers with possible occupational risk of exposure

    iv. Staff and clients at institutions for the developmentally disabled

    v. Hemodialysis patients

    vi. Patients receiving clotting factor concentrates

    vii. Household contacts and sex partners of infected patients

    viii. Adoptees from countries where HBV infection is endemic

    ix. International travelers (more than 6 months' travel in an endemic area, short-term travel if contact with blood in a medical setting is expected, or sexual contact with residents in areas of intermediate to high endemic disease); series of vaccinations started 6 months before travel

x. Injection drug users

xi. Sexually active homosexual or bisexual men, as well as heterosexual men and women

xii. Patients seeking treatment for a sexually transmitted disease

xiii. Inmates of long-term correctional facilities

xiv. Patients with chronic HIV infection or chronic liver disease

xv. All HCPs whose work-, training-, and volunteer-related activities involving reasonably anticipated risk of exposure to blood or bodily fluids. Recently vaccinated HCPs should, if possible, undergo testing for anti-HBs 1–2 months after finishing the HBV series. If anti-HBs is greater than 10 mIU/mL, no further testing is necessary. If anti-HBs is less than 10 mIU/mL, an additional dose of HBV vaccine should be administered, with repeat testing at 1–2 months.

xvi. All other people seeking protection from HBV infection

b. Available HBV vaccines (dose schedules vary by age)

i. Dose schedules

Table 25. Dose Schedules for Hepatitis B Vaccinations

Patient and Age Groups		Recombivax HB		Engerix-B		Schedule
		Dose (mcg)	Volume (mL)	Dose (mcg)	Volume (mL)	Most common schedule is 3 IM doses at 0, 1, and 6 months
Infants (<1 year)		5	0.5	10	0.5	Variations in schedule may occur, depending on age and medical history
Children (1–10 years)		5	0.5	10	0.5	
Adolescents	11–15 years	10	1	N/A	N/A	
	11–19 years	5	0.5	10	0.5	
Adults	≥20 years	10	1	20	1	
Hemodialysis patients and other immunocompromised people	<20 years	5	0.5	10	0.5	
	>20 years	40	1	40	2	

IM = intramuscular; N/A = not applicable.

ii. Obtain titers 1–2 months after the third dose of the series for HCPs.

iii. HBV vaccines are available as combination products with HAV (Twinrix), DTP/IPV (Pediarix), and Hib (Comvax).

c. Postexposure prophylaxis

i. Exposure may result in the need for HBV vaccine or immune globulin.

ii. Doses of HBV immune globulin are 0.06 mL/kg intramuscularly and must be given within 7 days of exposure.

iii. Patient populations requiring postexposure prophylaxis

(a) Perinatal transmission

(1) Children born to HBsAg-positive mothers should receive vaccine plus HBV immune globulin within 12 hours of birth.

(2) Children born to mothers with unknown HBsAg status (but suspected) should receive vaccine within 12 hours of birth; testing should be performed on child, and if positive, HBV immune globulin should be administered within 1 week.

(3) Infants weighing less than 2 kg at birth whose mothers are documented as HBsAg negative should receive the first dose of vaccine 1 month after birth or at hospital discharge, whichever comes first.

(b) Sexual contact or household contact with an infected person: Should receive HBV immune globulin plus vaccine series if exposed person is previously unvaccinated

(c) Sexual contact or household contact with an HBV carrier: Should receive vaccine series if exposed person was previously unvaccinated

(d) Postexposure recommendations for HCPs

Table 26. Centers for Disease Control and Prevention Recommendations for Management of HBV Postexposure for HCPs

HBV Status of HCP	Postexposure Testing		Postexposure Prophylaxis		Postvaccination Serologic Testing[a]
	Source Patient (HBsAg)	HCP Testing (anti-HBs)	HBIG	Vaccination	
Documented responder[b]	No action needed				
Documented nonresponder after 6 doses[c]	Positive or unknown	—[d]	HBIG × 2 separated by 1 month	—	No
	Negative	No action needed			
Response unknown after 3 doses	Positive or unknown	<10 mIU/mL[d]	HBIG × 1	Initiate revaccination	Yes
	Negative	<10 mIU	None		
	Any result	≥10 mIU	No action needed		
Unvaccinated or incompletely vaccinated or vaccine refusers	Positive or unknown	—[d]	HBIG × 1	Complete vaccination	Yes
	Negative	—	None	Complete vaccination	Yes

[a]1–2 months after last dose of HBV vaccine series.

[b]Anti-Hbs >10 mIU/mL after >3 doses of HBV vaccine.

[c]Anti-Hbs <10 mIU/mL after >6 doses of HBV vaccine.

[d]HCPs who have anti-HBs <10 mIU/mL, or who are unvaccinated or incompletely vaccinated, and sustain an exposure to a source patient who is HBsAg positive or has unknown HBsAg status should undergo baseline testing for HBV infection as soon as possible after exposure and follow-up testing about 6 months later.

HBIG = hepatitis B immune globulin; HBsAg = hepatitis B surface antigen; HBV = hepatitis B virus; HCP = health care provider.

D. Hepatitis C Virus
   1. Background
      a. RNA virus: Six genotypes (50 subtypes)
         i. Genotype 1 (subtypes 1a, 1b, and 1c) accounts for 70%–75% of infections in the United States.
         ii. Genotypes 2 (subtypes 2a, 2b, and 2c) and 3 (3a and 3b) are common in the United States.
         iii. Genotype helps determine therapy duration and likelihood of responding to therapy.
      b. Leading cause of liver disease and liver transplantation in the United States; also a common cause of hepatocellular carcinoma
      c. Viral replication occurs in the hepatocyte (virus is not directly cytopathic).
      d. Transmission: Mainly bloodborne (transfusion, intravenous drug abuse)
         i. High risk: Transfusion, intravenous drug abuse, men who have unprotected sex with men, hemodialysis, incarceration
         ii. Low risk
            (a) Snorting cocaine or other drugs
            (b) Occupational exposure

    (c) Body piercing and acupuncture with unsterilized needle

    (d) Tattooing

    (e) From pregnant mother to child

    (f) Nonsexual household contacts (rare)

    (g) Sharing razors or toothbrushes

    (h) Sexual transmission

  e. Associated with acute and chronic infection; after acute infection, most patients (60%–85%) develop chronic infection

2. Clinical features: About 30% of patients are asymptomatic.

  a. Acute infection: Symptoms present 4–12 weeks after exposure; most patients are asymptomatic and seldom progress to fulminant disease; those who develop symptoms have nonspecific findings such as malaise, weakness, anorexia, and jaundice.

  b. Chronic infection: Defined as the presence of viral RNA in the serum for 6 months or more

    i. May be associated with the long-term development of end-stage liver disease, cirrhosis, hepatocellular carcinoma

    ii. Progression to complications and end-stage liver disease may be accelerated by concurrent alcohol use and coinfection with HIV; younger female patients have slower progression.

  c. Extrahepatic manifestations: rheumatoid symptoms, glomerulonephritis, cryoglobulinemia

3. Diagnosis and monitoring

  a. Clinical signs and symptoms such as nausea, abdominal pain, jaundice, fever, malaise, or anorexia. Many patients have asymptomatic disease.

  b. Populations to test

    i. Suspected exposure

    ii. HIV infection

    iii. Intravenous or intranasal drug abuse

    iv. Receipt of clotting factors before 1987 or blood before 1992

    v. Hemodialysis

    vi. Abnormal ALT

    vii. Those receiving an organ transplant before 1992, including those who were ever incarcerated

    viii. Adults born between 1945 and 1965

    ix. Getting a tattoo in an unregulated setting

    x. Health care, emergency medical, and public safety workers after needlesticks, sharps, or mucosal exposures to HCV-infected blood

    xi. Unexplained chronic liver disease and chronic hepatitis, including elevated ALT

    xii. Annual testing for injection drug users and HIV-positive men who have unprotected sex with men

  c. Laboratory

    i. Serum anti-HCV antibodies: 99% sensitivity and specificity (enzyme immunoassays). Used as an initial screening for HCV; presence of anti-HCV antibody does not confer protective immunity from subsequent infection

    ii. Serum HCV RNA

      (a) Obtain in patients who test positive for anti-HCV antibodies, in patients with negative anti-HCV antibodies who are suspected to have liver disease and have had an HCV exposure in the past 6 months, and in immunocompromised patients.

      (b) Quantitative: Viral load is typically polymerase chain reaction reported in international units per milliliter; obtain for patients who will receive treatment; for use in monitoring treatment response. Preferred assays for diagnosis and monitoring of drug therapy

(c) Qualitative: Typically polymerase chain reaction; lower limit of detection of 50 IU/mL (equivalent to 100 copies/mL) is preferred (specificity is about 98%); typically used to confirm diagnosis in patients who are HCV antibody positive. The American Association for the Study of Liver Diseases (AASLD) guidelines state that there is no longer a need for qualitative assays. Quantitative assays are preferred.

(d) Important 2013 update from the FDA regarding HCV assays

  (1) An HCV assay with a lower limit of quantification of 25 IU/mL or less and a limit of HCV RNA detection of around 10–15 IU/mL should be used for monitoring response to therapy and decision-making during triple therapy (Class 2a, Level A).

  (2) Response-guided therapy should be considered only when no virus is detected by a sensitive assay 4 weeks after initiation of the HCV protease inhibitor (Class 1, Level A).

Table 27. Definitions and Monitoring of Long-term HCV Treatment Based on HCV RNA

Parameter	Definition
Rapid virologic response	Undetectable HCV RNA at week 4 of treatment
Sustained virologic response	Undetectable HCV RNA 12 weeks after finishing treatment

HCV = hepatitis C virus.

  iii. Liver biopsy: Consider if patient and HCP want to obtain information about fibrosis stage or prognosis or to make a decision about treatment. ALT: Nonspecific; may fluctuate with chronic disease (should decrease with treatment)

  iv. Genotyping: Genotype 1 is the most common genotype in the United States; it is also the least responsive to treatment. Genotypes 2 and 3 are the other two most common genotypes in the United States.

  v. Treatment response depends on other factors such as race, age, or coinfection. *IL28B* genotyping can also be considered for genotype 1 infection to help predict response to therapy.

4. Treatment

  a. Acute HCV infection

    i. Preexposure or postexposure prophylaxis is not recommended.

    ii. Monitor HCV RNA every 4–6 weeks for 6–12 months to detect spontaneous clearance. If the decision is to treat, monitor for at least 12 weeks to detect spontaneous clearance.

    iii. The same regimens used for chronic HCV are recommended for treatment. An alternative regimen is PEG ± ribavirin (RIBA) for 16 weeks in genotype 2 or 3 if a rapid virologic response (RVR) is obtained or for 24 weeks if genotype 1.

  b. Chronic infection

    i. Therapy goal is to attain a sustained virologic response (SVR), defined as the absence of detectable HCV RNA 12 weeks after treatment and is considered a clinical cure if obtained.

    ii. Prioritization for treatment should be given to the following patient populations.

      (a) Highest priority

        (1) Advanced fibrosis (Metavir F3) or compensated cirrhosis (Metavir F4)

        (2) Organ transplant

        (3) Type 2 or 3 mixed cryoglobulinemia with end-organ manifestations such as vasculitis

        (4) Proteinuria, nephrotic syndrome, or membranoproliferative glomerulonephritis

      (b) Next highest priority

        (1) Fibrosis (Metavir F2)

        (2) HIV-1 coinfection

        (3) Hepatitis B virus coinfection

   (4) Other coexistent liver disease such as nonalcoholic steatohepatitis

   (5) Debilitating fatigue

   (6) Type 2 diabetes (insulin resistant)

   (7) Porphyria cutanea tarda

  (c) Patients who may be at high risk for transmission and may benefit from prioritized treatment to reduce risk of transmission

   (1) Men who have sex with men

   (2) Active injected drug users

   (3) Incarcerated people

   (4) People on long-term hemodialysis

 c. RIBA in the treatment of HCV infection

  i. Oral nucleoside analog

  ii. Available as 200-mg tablets (Copegus) or capsules (Rebetol) (generic now available)

  iii. Significant adverse effect profile

   (a) Hemolytic anemia: May occur in up to 10% of patients (usually within 1–2 weeks of initiating therapy); may worsen underlying cardiac disease; monitor complete blood cell count (CBC) at baseline, 2 weeks, 4 weeks, and periodically thereafter. In patients with no cardiac history, decrease dose to 600 mg/day when hemoglobin drops to 10 g/dL or less, and discontinue when hemoglobin drops to 8.5 g/dL or less. In patients with a cardiac history, decrease dose to 600 mg/day if hemoglobin drops more than 2 g/dL in any 4-week period during treatment. Discontinue if hemoglobin drops to less than 12 g/dL 4 weeks after dose reduction. May use epoetin or darbepoetin to stimulate red blood cell production, improve anemia and sustain initial starting dose. Also need to confirm iron studies are normal and within range during treatment

   (b) Teratogenicity: Category X drug; requires a negative pregnancy test at baseline and every month up to 6 months after treatment, as well as the use of two forms of barrier contraception during treatment and for 6 months after treatment. Applies to women taking the drug and female partners of male patients taking ribavirin

   (c) Other possible adverse events include pancreatitis, pulmonary dysfunction (dyspnea, pulmonary infiltrate, and pneumonitis), insomnia, irritability or depression (often referred to as "riba rage"), and pruritus.

 d. Protease inhibitors for chronic HCV infection. Telaprevir and boceprevir agents are no longer recommended as first-line therapies for HCV infection.

Table 28. Protease Inhibitors Used to Treat Chronic HCV Infection

	Telaprevir (Incivek)	Boceprevir (Victrelis)	Simeprevir (Olysio)
FDA-approved indication	Long-term HCV therapy (genotype 1) in combination with PEG-IFNα and ribavirin in patients with compensated liver disease Not studied in Child-Pugh class B or C	Chronic HCV genotype 1 infection, in combination with PEG-IFNα and ribavirin, in adult patients (≥18 years) with compensated liver disease, including cirrhosis, who were previously untreated or who have not responded to previous interferon and ribavirin therapy	Chronic HCV genotype 1 infection in combination with PEG/RIBA or sofosbuvir
Dose and formulation	750 mg orally 3 times/day for at least 12 weeks, followed by PEG-IFN and ribavirin for 12 weeks if undetectable HCV RNA at weeks 4 and 12 Give doses 7–9 hours apart; give with meal that has at least 20 g of fat, ingested 20 minutes previously 375-mg tablets Take missed doses if within 4 hours	800 mg orally three times/day Give doses 7–9 hours apart; give with meal or light snack 200-mg capsules Take missed doses if within 2 hours	150 mg once daily with food for 12 weeks, combined with PEG-IFN and ribavirin Dose recommendations cannot be made for patients of East Asian ancestry or those with moderate to severe hepatic impairment
Contraindications	Pregnant women or male partners of pregnant women (category B, but must be used with ribavirin, which is category X) CYP3A4 substrates or inducers Alfuzosin, rifampin, DHE, St. John's wort, atorvastatin, lovastatin, simvastatin, pimozide, sildenafil, tadalafil, oral triazolam, or midazolam Several other drug-drug interactions that may require dose adjustment of interacting drug (see package insert)	Pregnant women or male partners of pregnant women (category B, but must be used with ribavirin, which is category X) CYP3A4 substrates or inducers Alfuzosin, rifampin, DHE, St. John's wort, atorvastatin. lovastatin, simvastatin, pimozide, sildenafil, tadalafil, oral triazolam, or midazolam Several other drug-drug interactions that may require dose adjustment of interacting drug (see package insert)	Pregnant women or male partners of pregnant women (category C, but must be used with ribavirin, which is category X) Screening for the NS3Q80K polymorphism Alternative therapies should be considered in patients with genotype 1a and this polymorphism Administration with substances that are moderate or strong inducers or inhibitors of CYP3A is not recommended Also inhibits OATP1B1/3 and P-glycoprotein Several drug-drug interactions that may require dose adjustment of interacting drug (see package insert)
Adverse effects	Rash (56%), DRESS syndrome, or Stevens-Johnson syndrome Anemia, pruritus, nausea	Anemia, neutropenia, fatigue, dysgeusia	Photosensitivity, rash; contains a sulfonamide moiety but no reports of problems with sulfa allergy

CYP = cytochrome P450; DHE = dihydroergotamine; DRESS = drug reaction/rash with eosinophilia and systemic symptoms; FDA = U.S. Food and Drug Administration; HCV = hepatitis C virus; PEG-IFN = pegylated interferon.

   e. NS5B/A polymerase inhibitors sofosbuvir (Sovaldi) and sofosbuvir/ledipasvir (Harvoni)

      i. Indications

         (a) Sofosbuvir: HCV genotypes 1, 2, 3, and 4, including those with hepatocellular carcinoma meeting Milan criteria and those with HCV/HIV coinfections in combination with PEG/RIBA

         (b) Sofosbuvir/ledipasvir: genotype 1 infection in combination with simeprevir

     ii. Dosing: 400-mg tablet once daily with or without food

         (a) Sofosbuvir renal dosing: No dosing recommendations for glomerular filtration rate (GFR) less than 30 mL/minute

         (b) Dose reductions for ribavirin

            (1) When used with sofosbuvir according to U.S. prescribing information, 600 mg daily is recommended in patients with no cardiac disease if hemoglobin is less than 10 g/dL, and recommendations are to discontinue if hemoglobin is less than 8.5 g/dL. In patients with stable cardiac disease, reduce the ribavirin dose if there is a greater than 2-g/dL decrease in hemoglobin during any 4-week period, and discontinue if hemoglobin is less than 12 g/dL, despite 4 weeks at reduced dose.

            (2) When used with sofosbuvir according to the 2014 AASLD/Infectious Diseases Society of America (IDSA) guidelines: For GFR 30–50 mL/minute, use alternating doses of 200 and 400 mg daily; for GFR less than 30 mL/minute or with end-stage renal disease or hemodialysis, reduce to 200 mg/day

    iii. Adverse effects: fatigue, headache

    iv. Drug interactions

         (a) Avoid use with potent P-glycoprotein inducers.

         (b) Concentrations are significantly affected by anticonvulsants (carbamazepine, phenytoin, phenobarbital, and oxcarbazepine), rifabutin, rifampin, St. John's wort, and tipranavir/ritonavir.

   f. NS5A/B inhibitor combination (ombitasvir/dasabuvir) plus boosted protease inhibitor (paritaprevir/ritonavir); Viekira Pak

      i. Indication: Genotype 1 infection with or without compensated cirrhosis

     ii. Dosing: Two paritaprevir 75 mg/ritonavir 50 mg/ombitasvir 12.5 mg combination tablets once daily in the morning plus one dasabuvir 250 mg tablet twice daily in combination with ribavirin for genotypes 1a and 1b (with cirrhosis); no ribavirin needed for genotype 1b without cirrhosis

    iii. Duration: 12 weeks except for genotype 1a with cirrhosis or patients with liver transplant, who should receive 24 weeks.

    iv. Interactions with CYP3A4 substrates and inducers and CYP2C8 substrates and inhibitors. Contraindicated with ethinyl estradiol–containing products

     v. Adverse effects: fatigue, nausea, pruritus, and those associated with ribavirin. Avoid in Child-Pugh class C liver disease.

   g. Treatment recommendations for chronic HCV infection

Table 29. Treatment Recommendations for Chronic HCV Genotype 1 Infection in Treatment-Naive Patients or Those Who Have Experienced Relapse After Prior PEG-IFN/RBV Therapy

Genotype	Recommended Therapies	Alternative	Not Recommended
1a	LDV (90mg)/SOF (400mg) × 12 weeks SOF (400mg)+ SMV (150mg)[c] ± RBV[a] × 12 weeks[d] PVR/RITON/OMBI/ DAS + RBV[a] × 12 weeks[d]	None	SOF + RBV PEG/RBV +/- SOF, SMV, TVR, BOC PEG, RBV, or DAA Monotherapy
1b	LDV (90mg)/SOF (400mg) × 12 weeks SOF (400mg)+ SMV (150mg)[c] × 12 weeks[d] PVR/RITON/OMBI/ DAS (+/- RBV)[e] × 12 weeks[d]	None	
2	SOF + RBV × 12 weeks; extend to 16 weeks if cirrhosis	None	PEG/RBV × 24 weeks PEG, RBV, DAA monotherapy Any regimen with TVR, BOC, LDV
3	SOF + RBV × 24 weeks	SOF + RBV + PEG × 12 weeks	PEG/RBV × 24–48 weeks PEG, RBV, DAA monotherapy Any regimen with TVR, BOC, SMV
4	LDV (90mg)/SOF (400mg) × 12 weeks SOF (400mg)+ RBV[a] × 24 weeks PVR/RITON/OMBI/ DAS + RBV[a] x 12 weeks[d]	SOF + SMV + RBV[a] + PEG × 12 weeks SOF + SMV +/- RBV[a] × 24–48 weeks	PEG/RBV +/- SMV × 24-48 weeks PEG, RBV, DAA monotherapy Any regimen with TVR or BOC
5	SOF + RBV + PEG × 12 weeks	PEG/RBV × 48 weeks	PEG, RBV, DAA monotherapy Any regimen with TVR or BOC
6	LDV (90mg)/SOF (400mg) × 12 weeks	SOF + RBV[a] + PEG × 12 weeks	

[a]RBV dosing is weight based (1000 mg/day for <75 kg and 1200 mg/day for >75 kg).

[b]Sofosbuvir and simeprevir are FDA approved for use without RBV for genotype 1 infection [c]For genotype 1a, testing for the Q80K polymorphism should be performed and other treatments considered, if present.

[d]12 weeks without cirrhosis; 24 weeks with cirrhosis

[e]RBV only recommended if presence of cirrhosis

BOC = boceprevir; DAA = directly acting agent; DAS = dasabuvir; IFN = interferon; LDV = ledipasvir; PEG = pegylated interferon alfa; PVR = paritaprevir RBV = ribavirin; RIT = ritonavir SMV = simeprevir; SOF = sofosbuvir; TVR = telaprevir.

h. Monitoring
   i. Baseline HCV RNA, genotype, CBC, liver function tests (LFTs), thyroid-stimulating hormone (TSH), and GFR. Pregnancy test for women receiving RIBA
   ii. On therapy: Obtain HCV at 4 weeks to assess for RVR and then again at the end of treatment. Every 4 weeks check CBC, SCr, LFTs; every 12 weeks check TSH.
   iii. After treatment: Check HCV RNA at 12 weeks to assess for SVR
i. Prevention of HCV
   i. No vaccine or immune globulin available
   ii. Risk factor modification
      (a) Intravenous drug abuse: methadone maintenance, syringe exchange
      (b) Sexual contact: appropriate barrier contraception
      (c) Avoid blood exposure: Occupational (universal precautions) or other contact (e.g., sharing toothbrushes or razors or receiving a tattoo)
      (d) The HAV and HBV vaccine to prevent further progression of liver disease

---

Patient Cases

8. A 45-year-old woman with a history of intravenous drug abuse is seen in the clinic for an evaluation of chronic HBV infection. Although she received the HBV diagnosis 8 months ago, she has not yet been treated for it. Laboratory values reported today include HBsAg positive, HBeAg positive, AST 650 IU/mL, ALT 850 IU/mL, HBV DNA 107,000 IU/mL, SCr 0.9 mg/dL, INR 1.3, and albumin 3.9 g/dL. She has no evidence of ascites or encephalopathy. A liver biopsy has revealed severe necroinflammation and bridging fibrosis. Resistance testing reveals the presence of the YMDD mutation. Which is the best course of action?

   A. Withhold drug therapy and recheck HBV DNA in 6 months.

   B. Initiate PEG-IFNα-2a plus ribavirin.

   C. Initiate lamivudine 100 mg/day.

   D. Initiate tenofovir 300 mg/day.

9. A 38-year-old white man is seen today for a new diagnosis of chronic HCV, genotype 1a. Pretreatment laboratory values include AST 350 IU/mL, ALT 420 IU/mL, HCV RNA 950,000 IU/mL, SCr 1 mg/dL, hemoglobin 12 g/dL, and white blood cell count (WBC) 12 ′ 103 cells/mm3. A liver biopsy reveals a Metavir score of F3/A2, and overall he has compensated liver disease. Further testing reveals presence of the NS3 80 QK polymorphism. He weighs 75 kg and is 72 inches tall. He reports no known drug allergies. Which option is best for treating this patient's chronic HCV infection?

   A. Withhold therapy and reassess in 12 months.

   B. Initiate sofosbuvir and simeprevir.

   C. Initiate sofosbuvir and ledipasvir.

   D. Initiate ribavirin and sofosbuvir.

VII. NAUSEA AND VOMITING

A. Definitions and Pathophysiology
1. Definitions
    a. Nausea: Unpleasant sensation of the imminent need to vomit; may or may not lead to the act of vomiting
    b. Vomiting: Forceful expulsion of gastric contents associated with contraction of the abdominal and chest wall musculature
2. Pathophysiology
    a. Stimuli for nausea are processed through several major anatomic areas, each of which has various receptors associated with input to the medullary vomiting center.
        i. Visceral stimuli: Mediated through dopamine and serotonin receptors. Major stimuli include:
            (a) Gastric irritants
            (b) Nongastric stimuli (peritonitis, intestinal or biliary distension, pancreatitis, gastroparesis)
            (c) Abdominal radiation
            (d) Chemotherapeutic agents
            (e) Pharyngeal stimulation
        ii. Chemoreceptor trigger zone (located in the area postrema): Mediated by dopamine (D_2), serotonin, and some histamine (H_1) and muscarinic (M_1) and substance P/neurokinin 1; major stimuli include:
            (a) Medications: Opiates, dopamine agonists, digoxin, chemotherapeutic agents, macrolides, general anesthetics
            (b) Metabolic disturbances (uremia, diabetic ketoacidosis, hypercalcemia, hypoxemia)
            (c) Bacterial toxins
            (d) Radiation therapy
        iii. Vestibular labyrinths: Mediated through H_1 and M_1. Major stimuli include:
            (a) Motion sickness
            (b) Labyrinth infection
        iv. Cerebral cortex: Receptor involvement not well characterized; noxious odors, visions, and tastes

Table 30. Common Clinical Conditions Associated with Nausea and Vomiting

Category	Conditions
Infectious	Viral or bacterial gastritis or gastroenteritis, pyelonephritis
Gastrointestinal	Pancreatitis, gastroparesis, hepatitis
CNS	Migraine, stroke, pain, seizures, motion sickness, meningitis
Endocrine or metabolic	Pregnancy, uremia, DKA, hypercalcemia
Cardiovascular	Myocardial infarction, heart failure
Other	Postoperative, cerebral mass

CNS = central nervous system; DKA = diabetic ketoacidosis.

    b. Clinical consequences of nausea and vomiting include dehydration, electrolyte disturbances, aspiration, and Mallory-Weiss syndrome.

B. Treatment and Prevention Strategies
   1. Removal or treatment of the underlying cause
   2. Correction of dehydration and electrolyte disturbances. Oral rehydration preferred, if possible, with oral rehydration solutions (e.g., Pedialyte, diluted Gatorade)
   3. Drug treatment: Use drugs that target receptors involved with stimuli. May need combination of drugs with different mechanisms. Also may need alternative dose forms (intravenous, subcutaneous, suppository)
      a. Major drug classes of antiemetics: All are antagonists at the respective receptors.
      b. Drugs of choice for different situations include:
         i. General medical use: phenothiazines, serotonin antagonists
         ii. Chemotherapy induced: Serotonin antagonists, phenothiazines, aprepitant, and dronabinol. (See "Oncology Supportive Care" chapter for treatment and prevention.)
         iii. Postoperative: serotonin antagonists, scopolamine
         iv. Motion sickness: antihistamines, scopolamine
         v. Pregnancy: phosphorylated carbohydrate solution, pyridoxine, antihistamines
         vi. Gastroparesis: Metoclopramide

Table 31. Select Antiemetics

Drug	Formulations	Comments
Phenothiazines		
Promethazine (Phenergan)	Tablets Suppositories Injection	Antidopaminergic, anticholinergic, and antihistaminergic activity May cause EPS, injection site irritation (do not use subcutaneously), sedation, anticholinergic effects IV formulation should be diluted because of risk of tissue necrosis
Prochlorperazine (Compazine)	Tablets Syrup Suppositories Injection	Mainly antidopaminergic activity May cause EPS, injection site irritation (do not use subcutaneously)
Serotonin antagonists		
Ondansetron (Zofran)	Tablets ODT Oral solution Injection Oral-soluble film (Zuplenz)	Overall, well tolerated No liquid required for ODT or soluble film Contraindicated with apomorphine Associated with QTc prolongation; correct hypomagnesemia and hypokalemia
Granisetron (Kytril)	Injection Tablet Oral solution Patch	Overall, well tolerated Twice-daily dosing Associated with QTc prolongation
Palonosetron (Aloxi)	Injection	Long duration of action: 24 hours to 5 days Only one dose required
Dolasetron (Anzemet)	Injection Tablets	Typically, a one-time dose Contraindicated with apomorphine Associated with QTc prolongation; correct hypomagnesemia and hypokalemia

Table 31. Select Antiemetics *(continued)*

Drug	Formulations	Comments
Antihistamines		
Dimenhydrinate (Dramamine) Cyclizine (Marezine) Meclizine (Bonine) Doxylamine (Unisom)	Tablets	Take 30–60 minutes before travel Risk of sedation and anticholinergic adverse effects
Butyrophenones		
Haloperidol Droperidol	Injection, tablets Injection	Risk of extrapyramidal adverse effects; risk of QTc prolongation; requirement for baseline ECG and 2- to 3-hour postdose cardiac monitoring
Miscellaneous agents		
Scopolamine (Transderm Scop)	Patch	Apply behind ear 4 hours before travel May wear for up to 72 hours Do not cut patch Risk of anticholinergic adverse effects
Aprepitant Fosaprepitant (Emend) Netupitant/ palonosetron (Akynzeo)	Capsules Injection Capsule	Targets substance P/neurokinin 1 (NK1) receptors Reduces efficacy of warfarin and oral contraceptives Dose-dependent inhibitor of CYP3A4 Targets substance P/neurokinin 1 (NK1) receptors and 5-HT3 Avoid in severe renal or hepatic disease
Dronabinol (Marinol)	Tablets	Delta-9 tetrahydrocannabinol Targets central endogenous cannabinoid receptors Used most often for chemotherapy-induced N/V May cause appetite stimulation, euphoria, cognitive impairment
Phosphorylated carbohydrate solution (Emetrol)	Oral solution	Use undiluted for best effect Do not use for >1 hour (or maximum of 5 doses) Safe in pregnancy Avoid in diabetes and fructose intolerance
Doxylamine/ pyridoxine (Diclegis)	Delayed-release tablet (10 mg/ 10 mg)	Approved for NVP in women who do not respond to conservative management 2–4 tablets daily Pregnancy category A

CYP = cytochrome P450; ECG = electrocardiogram; EPS = extrapyramidal symptoms; IV = intravenous; N/V = nausea and vomiting; NVP = nausea and vomiting of pregnancy; ODT = orally disintegrating tablet; SR = sustained release.

    c. Nondrug therapy for nausea and vomiting: Acupressure wristbands (Sea-Band); work by stimulating the pericardium 6 (P6) point. May be used for preventing all types of nausea

VIII. PANCREATITIS

A. Classification and Pathophysiology
   1. Acute
      a. Characterized by inflammation in the pancreas ranging from mild to severe
      b. An initial insult leads to the release of trypsin in the pancreas, leading to the activation of pancreatic enzymes and intrapancreatic inflammation and complications. May then progress to extrapancreatic complications. Usually reversible once underlying cause is removed
      c. Two distinct phases
         i. Early (within 1 week): Associated with systemic inflammatory response syndrome (SIRS) or organ damage
         ii. Late (more than 1 week): Associated with local complications
      d. Typical signs and symptoms include abdominal pain and distension, nausea, vomiting, jaundice, and fever.
         i. Local complication: necrosis, hemorrhage, pseudocyst, abscess, infection
         ii. Systemic complications: SIRS, acute respiratory distress syndrome, shock, organ failure
      e. Main causes of acute pancreatitis
         i. Long-term alcohol abuse
         ii. Gallstones
         iii. Drugs

Table 32. Common Causes of Drug-Induced Pancreatitis

Didanosine	Pentamidine
Asparaginase	Mesalamine/sulfasalazine
Azathioprine/mercaptopurine	Estrogens
Valproic acid	Tetracycline
Diuretics (furosemide, HCTZ)	Trimethoprim/sulfamethoxazole
Exenatide	Sitagliptin

HCTZ = hydrochlorothiazide.

         iv. Post–endoscopic retrograde cholangiopancreatography
         v. Hypertriglyceridemia (generally greater than 1000 mg/dL)
         vi. Idiopathic
         vii. Structural abnormalities
         viii. Toxins (scorpion venom)
         ix. Trauma
         x. Ischemia
   2. Chronic
      a. Characterized by irreversible structural and functional loss of pancreatic function caused by long-standing inflammation and repeated injury
      b. Repeated injury results in loss of both exocrine and endocrine function.
      c. Typical signs and symptoms include chronic abdominal pain, steatorrhea, weight loss or cachexia, jaundice, and hyperglycemia. Complications: diabetes, pseudocysts, calcification, ascites, biliary stricture

d. Risk factors for chronic pancreatitis are based on the M-ANNHEIM Classification

    M = Multiple risk factors

    A = Alcohol consumption

    N = Nicotine

    N = Nutritional factors (high fat and protein, hyperlipidemia)

    H = Hereditary factors

    E = Efferent duct factors

    I = Immunologic factors

    M = Miscellaneous and rare factors (includes drugs)

B. Diagnosis
1. Acute pancreatitis
    a. Diagnosis is typically made on the basis of two of the three following:
        i. Presence of abdominal pain
        ii. Laboratory diagnosis: Serum lipase (more than 3 times the ULN) is the most sensitive test. Patients may also have hyperglycemia and other electrolyte abnormalities related to vomiting. Patients often have a leukocytosis and a fever.
        iii. Imaging: Abdominal ultrasonography and computed tomography (CT) scan to evaluate pancreas, biliary system, and presence of local complications
    b. Severity and prognosis

Table 33. Common Scoring Systems to Classify Severity and Prognosis of Acute Pancreatitis

Atlanta Symposium Criteria for Acute Pancreatitis	Ranson Criteria for Prognosis[a]	
Mild: Absence of organ failure or local complications **Moderately severe:** Local complications or transient organ failure (<48 hours) **Severe:** Persistent organ failure >48 hours	**At admission:** Age >55 years (older than 70 years) WBC >16,000/L (18,000/L) Blood glucose >200 mg/dL (220 mg/dL) Serum lactate dehydrogenase >350 IU/L (>400 IU/L) Serum AST >250 IU/L (same)	**Within next 48 hours:** Decrease in hematocrit by >10% (same) Estimated fluid sequestration of >6 L (4 L) Serum calcium <8 mg/dL (same) Pao_2 <60 mm Hg (omitted) BUN level increase >5 mg/dL after intravenous fluid hydration (>2 mg/dL) Base deficit of >4 mmol/L (6 mmol/L)

[a]Values in parentheses are for gallstone induced; >3 criteria indicate severe disease.

AST = aspartate transaminase; BUN = blood urea nitrogen; WBC = white blood cell count.

2. Chronic pancreatitis: Diagnosis is typically made on the basis of clinical signs and symptoms plus laboratory and imaging.
    a. Laboratory diagnosis: Serum lipase may be normal; hyperglycemia and low albumin or prealbumin may also be present.
    b. Imaging: CT scan may reveal pancreatic calcification or pseudocyst.

C. Treatment Strategies
1. Acute pancreatitis: Treatment is largely supportive; should include removal or treatment of underlying cause if possible
    a. Temporarily withhold oral intake and provide rehydration with intravenous fluids, typically 250–500 mL/hour of lactated Ringer's. Treat electrolyte disturbances (hypokalemia, hypocalcemia, hyperglycemia).
    b. Pain management: Use of intravenous narcotics (avoid meperidine); patient-controlled analgesia is often used
    c. Antiemetics: intravenous ondansetron, prochlorperazine, or promethazine
    d. Nutrition: If mild pancreatitis, then oral feeding can be resumed if no vomiting is present. If severe pancreatitis is present, use enteral nutrition to prevent infectious complications. Avoid total parenteral nutrition (higher rates of infection, mortality, and length of stay).
    e. Antibiotics: In general, not recommended for routine prophylaxis in severe pancreatitis. Antibiotics may be used if extrapancreatic infection is present. If infected necrosis is present, then carbapenems, fluoroquinolones, or metronidazole may be useful in delaying the need for intervention.
    f. Endoscopic retrograde cholangiopancreatography may be needed for cholangitis or gallstone pancreatitis. This is often followed by cholecystectomy to prevent future episodes.
2. Chronic pancreatitis: Treatment is largely symptomatic.
    a. Abstinence from alcohol is essential. May need pharmacologic intervention and supportive care (e.g., Alcoholics Anonymous)
    b. Pain management: Often requires combination of nonnarcotic and narcotic analgesics (long-acting morphine, oxycodone, or transdermal fentanyl) in combination with pancreatic enzyme replacement. Avoid acetaminophen if long-term alcohol use.
    c. Antiemetics: oral ondansetron, prochlorperazine, or promethazine as needed
    d. Nutrition: Goal is to maximize caloric intake and weight gain and reduce steatorrhea. May need more frequent, lower-fat meals and fat-soluble vitamin supplementation. Long-term enteral or parenteral nutrition may be required.
    e. Use of pancreatic enzyme replacement therapy
3. Pancreatic enzyme replacement therapy
    a. Goal is to simulate the digestion of food that normally occurs with normal pancreatic enzyme release to reduce maldigestion and malabsorption.
    b. Products are enteric-coated microspheres or microtablets that contain lipase, amylase, and protease. Meant to mix with food, they release enzymes at intestinal pH values greater than 5.5. Products should not be crushed or chewed.
    c. Enzyme products were historically considered nutritional supplements. The FDA has now mandated FDA approval of all enzyme products.

Table 34. Pancreatic Enzyme Replacement Products

Brand Name	Lipase (units)	Amylase (units)	Protease (units)	Formulation
Viokace	10,440 20,880	39,150 78,300	39,150 78,300	Immediate-release tablet
Creon	3000 6000 12,000 24,000 36,000	15,000 30,000 60,000 120,000 180,000	9500 19,000 36,000 76,000 114,000	Capsules with enteric-coated microspheres (0.17–1.6 mm)
Ultresa	13,800 20,700 23,000	27,600 41,400 46,000	27,600 41,400 46,000	Capsules with enteric-coated minitablets (2 mm in diameter × 2–4 mm in thickness)
Zenpep	3000 5000 10,000 15,000 20,000 25,000 40,000	16,000 27,000 55,000 82,000 109,000 136,000 218,000	10,000 17,000 34,000 51,000 68,000 85,000 136,000	Capsules with enteric-coated beads (1.8–1.9 mm for 3000/5000 units) (2.2–2.5 mm for all other strengths)
Pancreaze	2600 4200 10,500 16,800 21,000	10,850 17,500 43,750 70,000 61,000	6200 10,000 25,000 40,000 37,000	Capsules with enteric-coated microtablets (2 mm)
Pertzye	8000 16,000	30,250 28,750	28,750 57,500	Capsules with bicarbonate-buffered enteric-coated microspheres (0.8–2 mm)

    d.   Dosing is based on the lipase content (units) of the product.
        i.   Starting adult doses are generally 30,000–40,000 units per meal, with one-half dose for snacks. May also use weight-based dosing of 500–1000 units/kg per meal for those older than 4 years or 1000–2500 units/kg per meal for ages 1–4
        ii. Maximal dose is 2500 units/kg per dose or 10,000 units/kg/day.
        iii. Give enzymes immediately before or during meal.
        iv. Titrate according to weight gain and reduction in steatorrhea.
        v.   May need to add PPI if maximal response is not seen
    e.   Adverse effects of pancreatic enzyme therapy
        i.   Nausea or abdominal cramping
        ii. Enzymes are derived from porcine pancreas, so patients with pork allergy cannot use them.
        iii. Hyperuricosuria, hyperuricemia
        iv. Fibrosing colonopathy (generally seen with doses greater than 10,000 units/kg/day)
        v.   Pregnancy category C

IX. DIARRHEA

A. Classification and Pathophysiology
1. Clinical definition: Alteration in a normal bowel movement characterized by an increase in the water content, volume, or frequency (more than three per day) of stool
   a. Acute is generally considered less than 72 hours to 14 days.
   b. Chronic is generally considered more than 14–30 days.
2. May be classified into several major categories related to underlying cause
   a. Secretory
      i. Secondary to enhanced secretion by intestinal mucosa. Often, large, watery volume with loss of electrolytes
      ii. Common causes: bacterial or viral or bacterial enteritis, gastric hypersecretion, carcinoid, stimulant laxatives, bile acid malabsorption, celiac disease, IBD (mucosal)
   b. Osmotic
      i. Secondary to the presence of hyperosmolar gradient in the intestinal lumen
      ii. Common causes: osmotic laxatives, carbohydrate malabsorption (lactase deficiency), fat malabsorption (pancreatic insufficiency), short bowel syndrome
   c. Exudative or inflammatory
      i. Secondary to inflammation or infiltration or invasion of the intestinal mucosa
      ii. Common causes: IBD, invasive infection (*C. difficile* toxin, enterotoxigenic *Escherichia coli*, cytomegalovirus, *Shigella*), ischemic colitis, radiation enterocolitis, neoplasm
   d. Altered motility or motor
      i. Secondary to autonomic nerve dysfunction
      ii. Common causes: diabetic neuropathy, postvagotomy, hyperthyroidism, irritable bowel syndrome (IBS), Addison disease
3. Drug-induced diarrhea. May occur by a variety of mechanisms

Table 35. Common Causes of Drug-Induced Diarrhea

Antibiotics	NSAIDs
Antineoplastics	Digoxin
Laxatives	Prostaglandins (misoprostol)
Levothyroxine (over-replacement)	Colchicine
Metoclopramide	Orlistat
Acarbose or miglitol	Sorbitol (sugar-free products)

NSAID = nonsteroidal anti-inflammatory drug.

B. Diagnosis
1. Need to evaluate patient history thoroughly
   a. Evaluate for disease- and drug-induced causes (laxative, recent antibiotic use), recent travel history, and temporal relation to food intake.
   b. Assess fluid and electrolyte status.
   c. Assess CBC and stool culture, and evaluate for ova and parasites if infectious cause is suspected. *C. difficile* toxin and culture if recent antibiotic use or hospitalization
   d. Evaluate stool pH, electrolytes, osmolarity, or fat content, if indicated.
   e. Imaging (abdominal CT scan) or endoscopy with biopsy may be indicated, particularly for inflammatory diarrhea or suggestion of neoplasm or celiac disease.
2. Referral to higher level of care or further evaluation may be necessary for some patients.
   a. Immunocompromised
   b. Infants and children
   c. Pregnant women
   d. Presence of fever
   e. Blood in the stool
   f. Weight loss (greater than 5%)
   g. Suspected invasive infection

C. Treatment Strategies
1. Removal or treatment of underlying causes, if possible
2. Rehydration
   a. Intravenous fluids appropriate for hospitalized patients
   b. Oral rehydration appropriate for all patients if no vomiting is present
      i. Sodium and glucose are key ingredients of oral rehydration solutions because they have active uptake into the intestinal mucosa even during active diarrhea. This results in water being pulled back into circulation. Other formulations (popsicles) are also available.
      ii. Gatorade may need to be diluted because it has a large amount of carbohydrates.
3. Dietary modifications
   a. Avoid dairy products because transient lactase deficiency may occur.
   b. "BRAT" diet for adults
   c. May need to interrupt feedings for pediatric patients
4. Drug therapy for diarrhea (see "Infectious Diseases" chapter for management of infectious causes)
   a. Several different agents available for management of diarrhea
   b. Avoid antimotility agents if invasive infection is suspected.

Table 36. Select Therapies for the Management of Diarrhea

Drugs	Mechanism	Role	Adverse Effects and Precautions
Loperamide	μ-Receptor agonist	Mild to moderate noninvasive diarrhea Adjunctive to other nonopiate therapies	Minimal CNS effects Avoid if suspected invasive infection Pregnancy category B
Opiates Tincture of opium Diphenoxylate + atropine	μ-Receptor agonist	Moderate to severe noninvasive diarrhea Suboptimal response to loperamide or bismuth Refractory diarrhea	CNS effects, respiratory depression Constipation, possible anticholinergic effects with atropine Avoid if suspected invasive infection
Bismuth subsalicylate	Antisecretory Binds toxins	Mild–moderate diarrhea Prevention of traveler's diarrhea	Stool discoloration Avoid in salicylate allergy, age <12 years, pregnancy, nursing Caution with anticoagulants May bind other drugs May interfere with some radiographic procedures
Lactase	Enzyme	Lactase deficiency or intolerance	Well tolerated
Probiotics (*Lactobacillus*, *Saccharomyces*)	Competition with pathogenic organisms, production of anti-microbial substances, enhancement of immune response	Prevention of antibiotic-associated diarrhea Adjunctive therapy for treatment of *C. difficile* Small intestinal bacterial overgrowth	Well tolerated Caution if severely immunocompromised
Octreotide	Antisecretory suppression of hormone release	Treatment of tumor-associated diarrhea (VIPoma [Verner-Morrison syndrome], carcinoid) HIV-associated diarrhea	Hyperglycemia Gallstone formation
Teduglutide (Gattex)	GLP-2 analog	Approved for adult patients with short bowel syndrome who are dependent on parenteral support	Colonic neoplasms; colonoscopy recommended every 5 years Intestinal obstruction Biliary/pancreatic disease (bilirubin, amylase, lipase, alkaline phosphatase, every 6 months)

CNS = central nervous system; GLP-2 = glucagon-like peptide-2; HIV = human immunodeficiency virus.

X. CONSTIPATION

A. Definition and Pathophysiology
   1. Bowel symptoms (difficult or infrequent passage of stool, hardness of stool, or a feeling of incomplete evacuation) that may occur in isolation or secondary to another underlying disorder. The 2013 guidelines distinguish between normal-transit constipation and slow-transit constipation. Another definition is "a symptom based disorder defined as unsatisfactory defecation and is characterized by infrequent stools, difficult stool passage, or both"
   2. May also be characterized by difficulty with or incomplete evacuation, straining, or presence of hard, dry stools. Abdominal pain and distension may occur, as well as low back pain and anorexia.
   3. Pathophysiology is related to many different factors. Common causes include:
      a. Altered motility (e.g., ileus)
      b. Neurogenic causes (autonomic neuropathies, Parkinson disease)
      c. Endocrine or metabolic disorders (e.g., hypothyroidism, diabetes, hypokalemia, hypercalcemia, uremia)
      d. Pregnancy
      e. Psychogenic causes
      f. Structural abnormalities or obstruction
      g. Nutritional (e.g., reduced fiber and water intake)
      h. Medications
   4. Constipation that is not due to an underlying organic cause is referred to as chronic idiopathic constipation (CIC) or functional constipation.

Table 37. Common Causes of Drug-Induced Constipation

Opioids	Calcium channel blockers
Antihistamines	Calcium supplements and antacids
Tricyclic antidepressants	Aluminum-containing drugs (antacids, sucralfate)
Scopolamine, benztropine	Iron supplements
Diuretics	Phenothiazines
Bile acid sequestrants	Benzodiazepines

B. Diagnosis
   1. Need to evaluate patient history thoroughly
      a. Need to establish patient baseline and evaluate for disease- and drug-induced causes
      b. Assessment of fluid and electrolyte status, thyroid function
      c. Imaging (abdominal CT scan or radiograph) may be necessary to assess for ileus, obstruction, or dilatation.
   2. Referral for further evaluation may be necessary for some patient populations.
      a. Symptoms for more than 1–2 weeks despite treatment
      b. Considerable pain or cramping
      c. Pregnancy
      d. Presence of fever
      e. Blood in the stool
      f. Reduction in stool caliber
      g. Weight loss
      h. Paraplegia, quadriplegia
   3. Diagnosis of CIC (functional constipation) is based on the ROME III Criteria, which is presence of two or more of the following:
      a. Straining during at least 25% of defecations

   b. Lumpy or hard stools in at least 25% of defecations
   c. Sensation of incomplete evacuation for at least 25% of defecations
   d. Sensation of anorectal obstruction or blockage for at least 25% of defecations
   e. Manual maneuvers to facilitate at least 25 % of defecations (e.g., digital evacuation, support of the pelvic floor)
   f. Fewer than three defecations per week

C. Treatment Strategies
   1. Removal or treatment of underlying causes, if possible
   2. Nonpharmacologic interventions
       a. Increase fluid intake to 6–8 glasses of water per day, although minimal evidence to support efficacy if dehydration is not present
       b. Increase dietary fiber to 20–30 g/day.
       c. Incorporate or increase exercise to 3–5 days/week.
   3. Drug therapy for prevention and treatment of constipation
       a. Choose drug therapy on the basis of desired onset of action, patient preference, presence of potential contraindications, and use in special populations.
       b. Provide patient education on alternative dose forms (enema, suppository).

Table 38. Drug Therapy Options for Treatment and Prevention of Constipation

Drugs	Role	Comments
Saline osmotic laxatives		
Magnesium citrate Magnesium hydroxide Sodium phosphate	Acute or intermittent constipation Preoperative or preprocedure bowel preparation	Fast onset (15 minutes to 3 hours) Avoid in renal impairment, HF, cirrhosis FDA warning regarding oral sodium phosphate and development of acute phosphate nephropathy (avoid use for bowel preparations)
Osmotic laxatives		
Glycerin	Management of acute or intermittent constipation Used in pediatric patients	Suppository Fast onset (within 1 hour)
Lactulose	Management of acute, intermittent, or chronic constipation, including CIC; preferred in chronic liver disease	Onset 1–2 days (may require multiple doses) Associated with gas and bloating Syrup or powder for solution
Polyethylene glycol	Acute or chronic constipation Effective for CIC Preoperative/colon preparation	Onset 1–3 days Safe in renal and hepatic disease and pregnancy Overall, well tolerated; may be used long term
Stimulant laxatives		
Bisacodyl	Short-term relief of acute or intermittent constipation or as part of preoperative or colonoscopy bowel preparation	Oral onset 6–12 hours, suppository within 1 hour Oral tablets are enteric coated
Senna	Short-term relief of acute or intermittent constipation Often used long term for prevention of opioid-induced constipation	Tablets and liquid Onset 6–12 hours May cause abdominal cramping, electrolyte disturbances, melanosis coli

Table 38. Drug Therapy Options for Treatment and Prevention of Constipation *(continued)*

Drugs	Role	Comments
Bulk-forming laxatives		
Psyllium Inulin Wheat dextrin Calcium polycarbophil Methylcellulose	Intermittent or chronic constipation	Onset 12–72 hours; less effective in drug-induced constipation and STC Requires adequate water intake to be effective Several formulations; soluble forms can be incorporated into foods, liquids, and recipes Safe in renal and hepatic disease, pregnancy, geriatrics May cause gas and bloating
Miscellaneous agents		
Docusate sodium Docusate potassium	Prevention of opioid-induced constipation in combination with senna or prevention of straining in post-MI, postsurgical, and pregnant patients	Onset 1–6 days Requires adequate water intake to be effective
Methylnaltrexone (Relistor)	FDA approved for opioid-induced constipation in palliative care patients and for opioid-induced constipation in adult patients with noncancer pain	Peripheral opiate antagonist; will not reverse central analgesia Subcutaneous injection given every other day Based on weight Onset within 4 hours in ~50% of patients
Naloxegol (Movantik)	FDA approved for opioid-induced constipation in adult patients with noncancer pain	Peripheral μ-receptor opioid antagonist 12.5-mg and 25-mg capsules Adjust dose for CrCl <60 mL/minute Contraindicated with use of strong CYP3A4 inhibitors or in patients with obstruction
Lubiprostone (Amitiza)	FDA approved for CIC in adults and for IBS-C in women >18 years	Chloride channel (ClC-2) activator; results in intestinal fluid secretion May reduce bloating and abdominal pain Main adverse effect: Nausea Dose is 24 mcg twice daily for constipation and 8 mcg twice daily for IBS-C Need negative pregnancy test before use
Linaclotide (Linzess)	FDA approved for IBS-C and CIC	Guanylate cyclase-C agonist: Increases fluid secretion and transit time 145- and 290-mcg capsules IBS-C: 290 mcg orally once daily; for CIC: 145 mcg orally once daily Take on empty stomach 30 minutes before meal Common adverse effects: diarrhea, abdominal pain, flatulence, and abdominal distension Contraindicated in pediatric patients <6 years and in mechanical obstruction Avoid in patients 6–17 years of age Pregnancy category C

CIC = chronic idiopathic constipation; CrCl = creatinine clearance; CYP = cytochrome P450; FDA = U.S. Food and Drug Administration; HF = heart failure; IBS-C = constipation-predominant irritable bowel syndrome; MI = myocardial infarction; STC = slow-transit constipation.

XI. IRRITABLE BOWEL SYNDROME

A. Definition and Pathophysiology
   1. IBS is considered a functional GI disorder.
   2. Definition divides IBS into the following subtypes:
      a. Diarrhea predominant (IBS-D)
      b. Constipation predominant (IBS-C)
      c. Mixed IBS (IBS-M): features of both IBS-D and IBS-C
      d. Unclassified (IBS-U)
   3. The pathophysiology is thought to involve alterations in both CNS and intestinal pain perception, alterations in GI motility and secretion, and contributions from current or past psychosocial factors, gas retention, and possibly previous GI infection or bacterial overgrowth.
      a. IBS is more common in women, people in lower socioeconomic groups, and patients younger than 50 years.
      b. Patients experience significant reductions in quality of life and use more health care resources.
      c. Comorbid psychiatric illnesses such as depression and anxiety may be present in a significant percentage of patients.
   4. Symptoms: In addition to diarrhea or constipation, pain is often a component of all subtypes. Other symptoms (e.g., bloating, distension, spasm, urgency) may be present as well.

B. Diagnosis
   1. Typically a diagnosis of exclusion. Need to rule out other GI causes with a thorough workup. Evaluation of a patient's pattern of symptoms may provide insight into subtype, although patients may alternate between forms.
   2. Several diagnostic criteria and scoring systems have been developed, including the Kruis, Manning, and Rome criteria.
      a. Generally the ROME III criteria are used mostly commonly and are as follows: Recurrent abdominal pain or discomfort at least 3 days per month in the past 3 months, associated with one of the following: improvement with defecation, onset with change in frequency of stool, onset in change in form or appearance of stool. Symptoms should have started at least 6 months before diagnosis.
      b. Guidelines recommend that if other GI diseases are excluded and no alarm features (e.g., weight loss, bleeding, anemia) are present, diagnosis of IBS can be made with confidence.
      c. The ACG guidelines also recommend:
         i. Screening for celiac disease in patients with IBS-D and IBS-M
         ii. No endoscopy if younger than 50 years and no alarm symptoms
         iii. No routine food allergy testing
         iv. No routine checking for small intestinal bacterial overgrowth unless lactose intolerance is a concern, despite dietary intervention

C. Treatment Strategies
   1. Treatment involves a mix of drug, diet, and psychosocial interventions. Cognitive behavioral therapy, dynamic psychotherapy, and hypnotherapy have all shown effectiveness in IBS.
   2. Dietary intervention involves avoidance of foods that trigger symptoms.
   3. Drug therapy should target main symptoms and possible psychiatric comorbidities. Combinations of drugs may be necessary for maximal effectiveness.
      a. Antispasmodics: Used mostly for short-term relief of abdominal pain but may also treat diarrhea in patients with IBS-D. May be used on an as-needed or scheduled basis
         i. Dicyclomine (Bentyl): Anticholinergic adverse effects

      ii.   Hyoscyamine (Levsin, Levsin SL), anticholinergic adverse effects

      iii. Peppermint oil: Use enteric-coated products; may worsen GERD but may improve symptoms in IBS and is superior to placebo

  b. Tricyclic antidepressants: Treat pain, improve global symptoms, and slow motility in patient with IBS-D. Can be used in IBS-C but may worsen constipation.

      i.   Amitriptyline, nortriptyline, and imipramine are the most studied.

      ii.   Doses cannot be raised high enough to treat comorbid depression.

      iii. Potential for anticholinergic effects, sedation, CV effects, and drug interactions

  c. Selective serotonin reuptake inhibitors (SSRIs): Treat pain and improve global symptoms similar to tricyclic antidepressants. Used for both IBS-D and IBS-C

      i.   Fluoxetine, sertraline, citalopram, and paroxetine are all viable options.

      ii.   Tend to have a prokinetic effect, so may also improve constipation in IBS-C; however, can also use in IBS-D, especially if comorbid depression or anxiety exists

      iii. Adverse effects include insomnia, sexual dysfunction, and withdrawal.

  d. Laxatives: Used for IBS-C

      i.   Psyllium has best evidence; however, it may cause bloating and gas formation. Calcium polycarbophil may be used as an alternative bulk-forming agent; wheat or corn bran should not be used.

      ii.   PEG-based laxatives (MiraLAX) may increase stool frequency, but they have no effects on reductions in abdominal pain and overall symptoms in IBS. Minimal to no bloating.

      iii. Avoid stimulant laxatives because they may worsen abdominal pain.

  e. Lubiprostone: FDA approved for IBS-C in women older than 18 years

      i.   Chloride channel activator; improves motility and possibly pain

      ii.   Dose is 8 mcg twice daily with meals for IBS-C.

      iii. Nausea and diarrhea are main adverse effects; it is costly as well.

  f. Tegaserod (Zelnorm): Serotonin-4 partial agonist that is FDA approved for IBS-C

      i.   Improves pain, global symptoms, and motility

      ii.   Available on an emergency-use basis only because of its association with the development of CV events in women

  g. Alosetron (Lotronex): Serotonin-3 antagonist that is FDA approved for IBS-D

      i.   Improves global symptoms and reduces motility

      ii.   Associated with the development of colonic ischemia, so available only through manufacturer prescribing program

  h. Loperamide: No effects on global symptoms or pain but reduces motility and increases stool consistency. May be used as an adjunct to other therapies in IBS-D

  i. Probiotics: Some evidence to support improvement in global symptoms, bloating, and flatulence. Not enough evidence exists to recommend specific strains.

  j. Antibiotics: A short course (10–14 days) of nonabsorbable antibiotic may improve global symptoms of IBS, especially bloating in IBS-D.

      i.   Rifaximin 400 mg two or three times daily for 10–14 days has shown some efficacy. This agent is expensive and does not have an FDA-approved indication for IBS.

      ii.   Limited data with neomycin and metronidazole

  k. Linaclotide (Linzess)

      i.   Approved for IBS-C

      ii.   Guanylate cyclase-C agonist: Increases fluid secretion and decreases transit time

      iii. 290 mcg orally once daily taken on an empty stomach 30 minutes before meals

      iv. Common adverse effects: diarrhea, abdominal pain, flatulence, and abdominal distension

Patient Cases

10. A 55-year-old man with a history of chronic alcohol abuse for 25 years is seen in the clinic for an evaluation of chronic pancreatitis. For the past 2 months, he has noticed an increase in the frequency of bowel movements to four or five times daily. He describes his stools as foul smelling and slimy. During this time, he has experienced 14 kg of unintentional weight loss and has intermittent abdominal pain. Quantification of fecal fat indicates an excretion of 20 g every 24 hours. His albumin is 2.1 g/dL, and he weighs 61 kg. He currently takes morphine controlled release 45 mg twice daily and oxycodone 5–10 mg every 4–6 hours as needed. Which is the best course of action for this patient?

    A. Increase MS-Contin to 60 mg twice daily.

    B. Initiate dronabinol to improve appetite.

    C. Initiate pancrelipase 30,000 units per meal.

    D. Add a multivitamin to his regimen.

11. A 32-year-old woman has experienced intermittent crampy abdominal pain 3–5 days/week, bloating, and reduced frequency of bowel movements for the past 6 months. Before this, she had a bowel movement on a daily basis; now, she reports a bowel movement every 2–3 days. She often needs to strain to evacuate her bowels. She reports that her symptoms do not appear related to specific foods. An extensive diagnostic workup is negative, and she is given a diagnosis of IBS-C. She is otherwise healthy and reports no known drug allergies. Which therapeutic intervention is best for this patient?

    A. Amitriptyline 50 mg/day.

    B. VSL #3 three capsules daily.

    C. Tegaserod 6 mg twice daily.

    D. Lubiprostone 8 mcg twice daily.

12. A 30-year-old woman who is 14 weeks pregnant presents with mild myalgias; a low-grade fever (temperature 99.8°F); four or five loose, watery bowel movements; and one episode of vomiting during the past 18 hours. She reports her 3-year-old daughter and several children in her day care class had the same symptoms 3 days ago. A rapid influenza test is negative, her WBC is 8×10^3 cells/mm³, and her SCr is 0.9 mg/dL. She takes a prenatal vitamin and reports no known drug allergies. She is given a diagnosis of a presumed viral gastroenteritis. Which is the best treatment for this patient's diarrhea?

    A. Loperamide.

    B. Bismuth subsalicylate.

    C. Lactase.

    D. Pyridoxine.

REFERENCES

Gastroesophageal Reflux Disease

1. American Gastroenterological Association Institute. Guideline for the diagnosis and management and diagnosis of gastroesophageal reflux disease. Gastroenterology 2013;108:308-28.
2. Haag S, Andrews JM, Katelaris PH, et al. Management of reflux symptoms with over-the-counter proton pump inhibitors: issues and proposed guidelines. Digestion 2009;80:226-34.

Peptic Ulcer Disease

1. ACCF/ACG/AHA. 2008 expert consensus document on reducing the gastrointestinal risks of antiplatelet therapy and NSAID use. Circulation 2008;118:1894-909.
2. ACCF/ACG/AHA 2010 expert consensus document on the concomitant use of proton pump inhibitors and thienopyridines: a focused update of the ACCF/ACG/AHA 2008 expert consensus document on reducing the gastrointestinal risks of antiplatelet therapy and NSAID use. J Am Coll Cardiol 2010;56:2051-66.
3. Chey WD, Wong BVY. American College of Gastroenterology guidelines for the management of *Helicobacter pylori* infection. Am J Gastroenterol 2007;102:1808-25.
4. Lanza FL, Chan FKL, Quigley EMM, et al. Guidelines for the prevention of NSAID-ulcer complications. Am J Gastroenterol 2009;104:728-38.
5. Wilcox CM, Allison J, Benzuly K, et al. Consensus development conference on the use of non-steroidal anti-inflammatory agents, including cyclooxygenase inhibitors and aspirin. Clin Gastroenterol Hepatol 2006;4:1082-9.

Upper GI Bleeding and SRMD

1. American Society of Health-System Pharmacists (ASHP). Therapeutic guidelines on stress ulcer prophylaxis. Am J Health Syst Pharm 1999;56:347-79.
2. Laine L, Jensen DM. Management of patients with ulcer bleeding. Am J Gastroenterol 2012;107:345-60.

Inflammatory Bowel Disease

1. American Gastroenterological Association Institute. Technical review on the use of thiopurines, methotrexate, and anti-TNF-α biologic drugs for the induction and maintenance of remission in Crohn's disease. Gastroenterology 2013;145:1464-78.
2. Kornbluth A, Sachar DB. Ulcerative practice guidelines in adults: American College of Gastroenterology, Practice Parameters Committee. Am J Gastroenterol 2010;105:501-23.
3. Lichtenstein GR, Hanauer SB, Sandborn WJ; the Practice Parameters Committee of the American College of Gastroenterology. Management of Crohn's disease in adults. Am J Gastroenterol 2009;104:465-83.
4. Talley NJ, Abreu MT, Anchkar JP, et al. An evidence-based systematic review on medical therapies for inflammatory bowel disease. Am J Gastroenterol 2011;106:S2-25.
5. Terdiman JP, Gruss CB, Heidelbaugh JJ, et al. American Gastroenterological Association Institute technical review on the use of thiopurines, methotrexate, and anti-TNF-α biologic drugs for the induction and maintenance of remission in Crohn's disease. Gastroenterology 2013;145:1459-63.
6. AGA Institute Guidelines for the Identification, Assessment and Initial Medical Treatment in Crohn's Disease Clinical decision support tool. http://campaigns.gastro.org/algorithms/IBDCarePathway. Accessed October 30, 2014.
7. Gecse KB, Bemelman W, Kamm MA, et al. A global consensus on the classification, diagnosis and multidisciplinary treatment of perianal fistulizing Crohn's disease. Gut 2014;63:1381-92.

Complications of Chronic Liver Disease

1. Vilstrup H, Amodio P, Bajaj J, et al.; Hepatic Encephalopathy in Chronic Liver Disease. 2014 practice guideline by the American Association for the Study of Liver Diseases and the European Association for the Study of the Liver. Hepatology 2014;715-35.

2. Garcia-Tsao G, Lim J; Members of the Veterans Affairs Hepatitis C Resource Center Program. Management and treatment of patients with cirrhosis and portal hypertension: recommendations from the Department of Veterans Affairs Hepatitis C Resource Center Program and the National Hepatitis C. Am J Gastroenterol 2009;104:1802-29.

3. O'Shea RS, Dasarathy S, McCullough AJ. Alcoholic liver disease. Am J Gastroenterol 2010;105:14-32.

4. Runyon BA. Management of adult patients with ascites due to cirrhosis: an update. 2012. Hepatology 2013;57:1651-3.

Viral Hepatitis

1. American Association for the Study of Liver Diseases and Infectious Diseases Society of America. Recommendations for Testing, Managing, and Treating Hepatitis C. Available at www.hcvguidelines.org/full-report-view. Accessed February 20, 2015.

2. Centers for Disease Control and Prevention (CDC). Updated U.S. Public Health Service guidelines for the management of occupational exposures to HBV, HCV, and HIV and recommendations for postexposure prophylaxis. MMWR 2001;50(RR11):1-52.

3. Centers for Disease Control and Prevention (CDC). A comprehensive immunization strategy to eliminate transmission of hepatitis B virus infection in the United States: recommendations of the Advisory Committee on Immunization Practices (ACIP). Part 1. Immunization of infants, children, and adolescents. MMWR 2005;54(RR16):1-23.

4. Centers for Disease Control and Prevention (CDC). A comprehensive immunization strategy to eliminate transmission of hepatitis B virus infection in the United States: recommendations of the Advisory Committee on Immunization Practices (ACIP). Part II. Immunization of adults. MMWR 2006;54(RR16):1-40.

5. Centers for Disease Control and Prevention (CDC). Update: prevention of hepatitis A after exposure to hepatitis A virus and in international travelers. Updated recommendations of the Advisory Committee on Immunization Practices (ACIP). MMWR 2007;56:1080-4.

6. Centers for Disease Control and Prevention (CDC). Recommendations for identification and public health management of persons with chronic hepatitis B virus infection. MMWR 2008;57(RR08):1-20.

7. Centers for Disease Control and Prevention (CDC). Immunization of health-care personnel: recommendations of the Advisory Committee on Immunization Practices (ACIP). MMWR 2011;60(RR07):1-45.

8. Centers for Disease Control and Prevention (CDC). Guidance for evaluating health-care personnel for hepatitis B virus protection and for administering postexposure management. MMWR 2013;62:1-19.

Diarrhea and Constipation

1. Bharucha AE, Dorn SD, Lembo A, et al. American Gastroenterological Association medical position statement: guidelines on constipation. Gastroenterology 2013;144:211-7.

2. Bharucha AE, Pemberton JH, Locke GR. AGA technical review on constipation. Gastroenterology 2013;144:218-38.

3. Ramkumar D, Rao SSC. Efficacy and safety of traditional medical therapies for chronic constipation: systematic review. Am J Gastroenterol 2005;100:936-71.

4. Ford AC, Moayyaedi P, Lacy BE, et al. American College of Gastroenterology Monograph on the Management of Irritable Bowel Syndrome and Chronic Idiopathic Constipation. Am J Gastroenterol 2014;109:S2-26.

Pancreatitis

1. American College of Gastroenterology. Practice guidelines: management of acute pancreatitis. Am J Gastroenterol 2013;108:1400-1.

2. Ferrone M, Raimondo M, Scolapio JS. Pancreatic enzyme pharmacotherapy. Pharmacotherapy 2007;27:910-20.

3. Trivedi CD, Pitchumoni CS. Drug-induced pancreatitis. J Clin Gastroenterol 2005;39:709-16.

4. Waljee AK, Dimagno MJ, Wu BU, et al. Systematic review: pancreatic enzyme treatment of malabsorption associated with chronic pancreatitis. Aliment Pharmacol Ther 2009;29:235-46.

5. Witt H, Apte MV, Kiem V, et al. Chronic pancreatitis: challenges and advances in pathogenesis, genetics, diagnosis, and therapy. Gastroenterology 2007;132:1557-73.

Nausea and Vomiting

1. American College of Obstetrics and Gynecology. Practice bulletin: nausea and vomiting of pregnancy. Obstet Gynecol 2004;103:803-14.

2. American Gastroenterological Association Institute. AGA technical review on nausea and vomiting. Gastroenterology 2001;120:263-86.

3. Flake ZA, Scalley RD, Bailey AG. Practical selection of antiemetics. Am Fam Physician 2004;69:1169-74.

Irritable Bowel Syndrome

1. Ford AC, Moayyaedi P, Lacy BE, et al. American College of Gastroenterology monograph on the management of irritable bowel syndrome and chronic idiopathic constipation. Am J Gastroenterol 2014;109:S2-26.

2. American College of Gastroenterology IBS Task Force. An evidence-based position statement on the management of irritable bowel syndrome. Am J Gastroenterol 2009;104:S1-35.

ANSWERS AND EXPLANATIONS TO PATIENT CASES

1. Answer: B

Patients receiving PPI therapy for GERD should be reassessed for evaluation of efficacy. This patient has had some improvement in frequency of symptoms but is still not optimally controlled despite implementing lifestyle modifications and being adherent. There is no evidence that upper GI dysmotility is the cause of his GERD symptoms, so adding metoclopramide would not be preferred (Answer A). Switching to an alternative PPI such as omeprazole (Answer C) could be attempted, but typically this would be considered in the case of intolerance to another agent. Sucralfate (Answer D) has no role in GERD treatment. The GERD guidelines do endorse increasing the PPI frequency to twice daily in patients with continued symptoms, making Answer B correct.

2. Answer: C

The two most common causes of PUD are *H. pylori* and NSAID use. This patient has a gastric ulcer with evidence of a clot (indicating recent bleeding) in the setting of multiple NSAID use (aspirin plus ketoprofen). In addition, she is older than 60 years, which is another risk factor for an NSAID-induced ulcer. This is probably contributing to her upper GI problems and anemia. The rapid urease test performed on the biopsy specimen is negative, indicating the absence of *H. pylori*. First, the patient should discontinue NSAID use. NSAID use can markedly delay healing; therefore, it should be continued only if necessary. Healing of the ulcer should be facilitated by appropriate acid-suppressive therapy. Histamine-2 receptor antagonists, although effective in some instances, are less efficacious in the healing of gastric ulcers than are the PPIs, making Answer A incorrect. Because the patient has tested negative for *H. pylori,* use of an *H. pylori* eradication regimen is not necessary; therefore, Answer B is incorrect. Misoprostol, which is effective in preventing and healing ulcers, is not preferred because of the need for several daily doses, and it is very poorly tolerated because of a high incidence of abdominal pain, cramping, and diarrhea. The dose should also be at least 600 mcg/day. PPIs are the preferred drugs for healing NSAID-induced ulcers because of their excellent efficacy and favorable adverse effect profile, and they are better tolerated, making Answer C correct.

3. Answer: C

The test-and-treat approach is appropriate in dyspeptic patients thought to have *H. pylori* infections. Patients older than 45–55 years, or those with alarm features, should be referred for endoscopic evaluation to rule out the possibility of a more complicated disease. Ambulatory patients can be tested for *H. pylori* using various diagnostic approaches (e.g., UBT). The eradication of *H. pylori* leads to high rates of ulcer healing and minimizes ulcer recurrence. According to treatment guidelines, eradication regimens for *H. pylori* infection should include at least two antibiotics plus an antisecretory agent given for 10–14 days. This can be accomplished with triple-drug therapies containing amoxicillin (or metronidazole) plus clarithromycin in addition to a PPI. Likewise, quadruple therapy with bismuth, tetracycline, metronidazole, and a PPI can be used first line in penicillin-allergic patients or as a second-line treatment of initial failures of triple-drug therapy. This patient requires treatment secondary to a positive test. Answer A would be appropriate if the duration were at least 10 days. Answer B is not correct because cephalosporins are not recommended in *H. pylori* treatment regimens. Answer D is incorrect because fluoroquinolone-based regimens should be reserved as salvage therapy for patients whose triple and quadruple therapy has failed and the duration of 21 days is too long, making Answer C correct; quadruple therapy offers similar efficacy and is a viable first line. Patient adherence should be reinforced to maximize efficacy.

4. Answer: D

Treatment with topical aminosalicylate therapy (e.g., a suppository or enema) (Answer D) is a more effective option for patients with mild–moderate UC with distal disease compared with oral therapies such as balsalazide (Answer A). Methotrexate (Answer B) has a limited role in maintaining corticosteroid-induced remission in patients with CD. Infliximab would be indicated for moderate–severe UC when aminosalicylate therapy or budesonide has failed.

5. Answer: B

This patient is experiencing moderate to severe to CD involving the terminal ileum and colon. Mesalamine

(Answer A), though well tolerated, is minimally effective in CD and would not be indicated for moderate to severe disease. Budesonide (Answer C) is effective in mild–moderate CD affecting the terminal ileum and proximal colon, so the disease severity and location of the disease would not fit this regimen. Adalimumab would be appropriate, but the dose is for maintenance and would need to be 160 mg initially for induction. Combining infliximab and azathioprine (Answer B) has been shown to result in the highest rates of remission in moderate to severe CD compared with use of either agent alone.

6. Answer: C

Patients with cirrhosis and ascites are at risk of developing SBP, an infection of the ascitic fluid usually caused by an enteric gram-negative organism. Typical signs of infection include fever, abdominal pain, nausea, and rebound tenderness. Diagnosis is made on the basis of clinical symptoms plus laboratory evidence. The laboratory diagnosis is by paracentesis, with identification of more than $250/mm^3$ neutrophils (polymorphonuclear neutrophils) in the ascitic fluid. This patient's value is $450/mm^3$. Should clinical and laboratory signs and symptoms be present, antibiotic therapy directed against enteric gram-negative bacteria should be initiated. Third-generation cephalosporins such as cefotaxime and ceftriaxone are preferred. Aminoglycosides should be avoided because of their potential to cause nephrotoxicity. Vancomycin should be reserved for resistant gram-positive organisms. In addition to antibiotic therapy, use of intravenous albumin reduces the incidence of renal failure and improves in-hospital and 30-day mortality; it is indicated given that the patient's SCr is greater than 1.0 mg/dL and her BUN is greater than 30 mg/dL. Use of oral antibiotics to treat acute SBP is not well studied; however, an oral regimen (e.g., norfloxacin or trimethoprim/sulfamethoxazole daily) should be instituted and continued indefinitely after recovery to reduce the incidence of subsequent infections.

7. Answer: B

Management of overt hepatic encephalopathy should initially involve removal and treatment of precipitating factors and use of therapies aimed at reducing ammonia concentration. Recent guidelines recommend use of lactulose (Answer B) to rapidly reduce ammonia concentrations in the short term. Therapy can also be continued as prophylaxis against subsequent episodes if needed. Nonabsorbable antibiotics such as rifaximin can be used, but rifaximin 550 mg twice daily (Answer A) is indicated for use in prevention of recurrent hepatic encephalopathy and is effective when combined with lactulose. Ceftriaxone (Answer D) would not as effective as rifaximin and is indicated in patients with cirrhosis who present with upper GI bleeding. Although PEG-3350 (Answer C) has been shown to have some efficacy in treatment of hepatic encephalopathy, the dose used in recent trials was 4 L administered over 4 hours.

8. Answer: D

This patient has evidence of a chronic HBV infection on the basis of elevations in ALT and AST, the presence of HBsAg, and high concentrations of circulating HBV DNA, as well as evidence of severe necroinflammation on biopsy. The patient has HBeAg positivity, and a YMDD mutation is present. She appears to have compensated liver disease on the basis of her albumin, INR, and lack of ascites or encephalopathy. Given her persistently elevated liver function tests, biopsy results, and high viral load, she should receive treatment. Treatment with an oral reverse transcriptase inhibitor is preferred first-line therapy. Interferon and ribavirin are preferred for chronic HCV infection (Answer B). Given that the patient has a lamivudine-resistant organism, as evidenced by the presence of the YMDD mutation, a drug therapy that treats lamivudine-resistant pathogens (e.g., tenofovir) is recommended as initial therapy (Answer D).

9. Answer: C

This patient has newly diagnosed chronic HCV infection. Withholding therapy (Answer A) at this time would not be optimal because the patient is considered high priority for treatment because of advanced fibrosis and has no contraindications to treatment. Sofosbuvir and simeprevir (Answer B) could be used for genotype 1a, but the NS3 80 QK polymorphism significantly reduces the effectiveness of simeprevir, making this the less preferred choice. The combination of sofosbuvir and ledipasvir (Answer C) is another first line option and would be preferred. Sofosbuvir and ribavirin (Answer D) is the recommended regimen for genotypes 2 and 3.

10. Answer: C

This patient has signs and symptoms of maldigestion and malabsorption secondary to the loss of pancreatic exocrine function. This is manifested by the presence of steatorrhea, weight loss, and an elevated fecal fat concentration. Management should include replacement of exogenous pancreatic enzymes to facilitate nutrient digestion and absorption. Oral pancrelipase products are pork derived and contain lipase, amylase, and protease. A typical starting dose for an adult patient should deliver 30,000–40,000 lipase units per meal, with titration based on reduction in steatorrhea and evidence of weight gain. Although chronic abdominal pain is a typical symptom of chronic pancreatitis, increasing the patient's morphine dose will not help with the symptoms related to the lack of enzymes. Likewise, using appetite stimulants such as dronabinol will not be beneficial if enzyme therapy is not initiated. Finally, this patient is malnourished, and use of a multivitamin would beneficial; however, patients with chronic pancreatitis may need extra supplementation of fat-soluble vitamins after enzyme therapy is initiated and increased caloric intake to facilitate weight gain.

11. Answer: D

This patient meets the criteria for IBS-C on the basis of a negative diagnostic workup and the presence of abdominal pain, bloating, and constipation for more than 3 months. Drug therapy should target the predominant symptoms. The agents most beneficial in IBS-C are bulk-forming laxatives, which improve the frequency of bowel movements and may reduce bloating, and SSRIs, which provide relief from abdominal pain, improve global symptoms of IBS, and improve motility in most patients. The tricyclic antidepressants have effects similar to those of the SSRIs but are associated with anticholinergic effects, which may worsen constipation. Thus, amitriptyline would not be preferred in this case. Lubiprostone is approved for IBS-C in women older than 18 years and improves motility and possibly abdominal pain. It is the best choice presented, given the patient's symptoms. Probiotics such as VSL #3 may improve global symptoms of IBS, but they would not improve bowel frequency, so use would be best with another therapy that would increase stool frequency. Though effective for IBS-C when it was available, tegaserod is available only on an emergency basis because of its association with the development of CV events.

12. Answer: A

Diarrhea is caused by a variety of conditions, with viral pathogens being one of the most common causes. This patient probably developed diarrhea through contact with her daughter, who is in day care and had similar symptoms a few days earlier. In addition, her low-grade fever, myalgias, watery diarrhea, and vomiting point to a potential viral cause. Although most episodes of viral gastroenteritis are self-limited, symptomatic relief may be necessary prevent dehydration. Selection of antidiarrheal therapy should be based on patient preference and the presence of any precautions or contraindications. If this patient desires therapy, a therapy should be chosen that minimizes risk to the patient and the fetus given that she is pregnant. Loperamide is an effective agent for short-term relief of diarrhea and carries an FDA pregnancy category B rating, so it would be the best choice in this case. Use of bismuth, although effective, should be avoided in pregnant and nursing patients because of the risk of potential toxicity. Lactase would be indicated only if the patient's diarrhea were secondary to lactose intolerance. Pyridoxine is used for the treatment and prevention of nausea and vomiting in pregnancy, but it has no effect on the treatment of diarrhea related to viral gastroenteritis.

ANSWERS AND EXPLANATIONS TO SELF-ASSESSMENT QUESTIONS

1. Answer: B

This patient has signs of dysphagia, an alarm symptom that may be associated with a more complicated case of GERD. The patient has tried antacids with minimal relief and has a history of NSAID use. The patient is older than 45 years, which increases his risk of developing gastric cancer. Therefore, he should be referred for endoscopic evaluation to rule out a more complicated disease. Using either H2RAs or a PPI as initial therapy would be appropriate if the patient did not respond to antacids; however, a twice-daily dosing of PPIs is not necessary as initial dosing. Changing medications that reduce LES tone (e.g., calcium channel antagonists) is an appropriate recommendation for reducing GERD symptoms; this should be considered after invasive testing is performed.

2. Answer: C

For patients beginning long-term NSAID therapy, a thorough assessment of patient- or drug-related factors that may predispose them to the development of GI toxicity is necessary. Likewise, an evaluation of the patient's level of CV risk is necessary. Based on the use of low-dose aspirin for preventing CV events, this patient would be considered at high risk of CV events. Efforts to avoid GI toxicity should include the use of the least GI-toxic agent at the lowest effective therapeutic dose. A GI-protective agent should be considered to minimize NSAID-induced erosions and ulcers. Indomethacin and piroxicam are more likely to cause GI complications than naproxen. Use of COX-2 inhibitors is acceptable in patients with rheumatoid arthritis because these agents reduce GI complications and effectively treat pain. However, this patient has CV risk factors including diabetes, hypertension, and dyslipidemia. Recent findings of increased CV events, especially with high doses of COX-2 inhibitors, would preclude their use. Therapy with an acid-suppressive agent is also an acceptable choice for GI prevention in users of nonselective NSAIDs. Proton pump inhibitors are effective for this indication. The H2RAs are ineffective in preventing serious NSAID-induced GI complications. Misoprostol, although effective, is associated with a high incidence of diarrhea and abdominal pain, as well as the need for multiple daily dosing. Given that this patient is considered at moderate risk of

GI complications because of the patient's use of aspirin and need for high-dose NSAIDs, the use of naproxen plus a PPI would be preferred, according to the recent ACG guidelines.

3. Answer: D

This patient presents with signs and symptoms consistent with an NSAID-induced upper GI bleed. He has several risk factors for NSAID-induced GI bleeding, including age older than 60 years, use of aspirin, and long duration of NSAID use. The presence of underlying CV disease, although not a direct risk factor, may also contribute to increases in NSAID GI toxicity. He also has many criteria that place him at high risk of rebleeding. On the basis of the consensus recommendations for nonvariceal bleeding, he should receive an intravenous PPI by bolus and subsequent continuous infusion for 72 hours. Note that in the guidelines provided, it states that this therapeutic approach can be extrapolated to patients with NSAID-induced ulcers and bleeding, even though most of the data included in the guidelines pertain to non–NSAID-induced causes of upper GI bleeding. He will then require treatment with an appropriate dose of an oral PPI for at least 8 weeks; after that, he should be assessed for possible continued prophylactic use. Histamine-2 receptor antagonists are less efficacious for the treatment and prevention of rebleeding for NSAID-induced ulcers. Sucralfate has minimal efficacy in the setting of acute GI bleeding; more often, it is used in preventing SRMD in critically ill patients. Oral PPIs are effective in preventing and healing NSAID-induced ulcers; however, in this case, the dose of lansoprazole is inadequate for treatment. Oral PPIs should be used at an appropriate dose after intravenous therapy.

4. Answer: D

On the basis of this patient's presenting symptoms, she would probably be classified in the mild to moderate active disease category. First-line therapy for active extensive disease would consist of an oral aminosalicylate at a dose equivalent to mesalamine 4.8 g/day. A product such as Asacol is formulated to release mesalamine in the colon, which would be appropriate in this case. Sulfasalazine has reported efficacy for this indication and is activated in the colon; however, this patient reports a life-threatening allergy to sulfonamide-containing medications. Topical therapy with hydrocortisone enema would be appropriate if the patient had disease distal to the splenic flexure. Immune modulators such as 6-MP have a long onset of action (3–15 months) and are not appropriate for acute active disease.

5. Answer: B

Primary prophylaxis of bleeding should be instituted in patients with large varices and cirrhosis. Nonselective β-blockers are appropriate as first-line therapy. Therapy should be targeted to achieve an HR of 55 beats/minute or a 25% reduction from baseline. The patient has taken propranolol for 1 month and has not met these goals. Because he is tolerating propranolol, the dose should be increased, and he should be observed to reassess the need for further dosage adjustments. Adding a nitrate would increase the reduction in portal pressures; however, nitrates have not been shown to improve mortality. Most patients experience an increased risk of adverse effects with this combination. Nonselective β-blockers are preferred to β-selective agents because antagonism of the β-receptor prevents splanchnic vasodilation.

6. Answer: C

The sensitivity of a test can be thought of as the proportion of patients with a disease who have a positive test, whereas specificity deals with the proportion of patients without the disease who have a negative test. Calculating these values is accomplished by establishing a 2 × 2 table representing the results of the test. The sensitivity can be calculated by dividing the number of patients having the disease using the new test who were also positive using a gold standard test (true positives), which in this case is 850, by the number of patients receiving a diagnosis of having the disease using the gold standard, which in this case is 900. The 900 represents the true positives as well as the 50 patients with the disease but without the diagnosis of it, according to the new test (false negatives). Specificity can be calculated by taking the number of patients not having the disease using the gold standard who tested negative with the new test (true negatives = 85). Then, divide this by the number of patients who truly had no disease using the gold standard, 100, which incorporates the 15 patients who tested positive with the new test but truly had no disease (i.e., false positives). Sensitivity = 850/(850 + 50) = 94%; specificity = 85/(85 + 15) = 85%.

Result	Infection	No Infection	Total
Positive	850	15	865
Negative	50	85	135
Total	900	100	1000

7. Answer: C

Postexposure therapy for HAV may be offered to restaurant patrons if a food handler at a restaurant is documented to have HAV and is considered infectious while handling food. The most effective therapies for postexposure prophylaxis are administration of HAV immune globulin or vaccine. The efficacy of the vaccine approaches that of immune globulin but only in patients younger than 40, according to the Centers for Disease Control and Prevention guidelines. The period for administration should be within 14 days of exposure; therefore, this patient does not meet the criteria for receiving HAV immune globulin or vaccine. She should be observed for signs and symptoms of active disease. Hepatitis A vaccine should be offered to patients as pre-exposure therapy if they are considered at risk of exposure to HAV. The combination of vaccine and immune globulin for postexposure therapy is unnecessary.

8. Answer: C

This patient is presenting with elevated aminotransferases, consistent with alcoholic hepatitis. Prognosis of alcoholic hepatitis may be initially evaluated by the Maddrey discriminant function (MDF) score, calculated as 4.6 × (patient's PT − control PT) + total bilirubin (mg/dL), where PT is prothrombin time. Patients whose score is greater than 32 are believed to have a poor prognosis. This patient's MDF score is 42.5, so she would qualify for treatment with a 4-week course of prednisolone 40 mg/day, followed by a 2-week taper (Answer C). This may lead to a 30% decrease in the risk ratio of short-term death. Naproxen (Answer A), though having anti-inflammatory activity, has no role in the treatment of alcoholic hepatitis and may precipitate acute kidney injury in patients with liver disease and therefore should be avoided. Octreotide (Answer B) would be indicated in the setting of acute variceal bleeding, and midodrine (Answer D) is indicated for hepatorenal syndrome. This patient has no evidence of either condition.

9. Answer: D

The treatment of chronic HCV is PEG-IFN in combination with ribavirin. Genotypes 2 and 3 respond well to therapy. Although this patient appears to be responding to treatment, as evidenced by reductions in aminotransferases and HCV RNA, the earliest that HCV RNA should be evaluated is 4 weeks, not 2 weeks. Interferon therapy is associated with many adverse effects (e.g., flulike symptoms, CNS effects, leukopenia, thrombocytopenia). This patient does not appear to be experiencing these types of symptoms or those consistent with extrahepatic manifestations of HCV (e.g., glomerulonephritis or rheumatologic disorders). The patient does have evidence of hemolysis, including scleral icterus, rapid decline in hematocrit, fatigue, and elevated indirect bilirubin, probably representing hemolytic anemia secondary to ribavirin, which commonly occurs within the first 2 weeks of therapy. Furthermore, there is no evidence that the decrease in hematocrit is secondary to bleeding.

10. Answer: A

Infliximab is an appropriate agent for the treatment of fistulizing CD. Because of its effects on TNF, latent infections such as tuberculosis may become reactivated during therapy. Therefore, patients should have a purified protein derivative or QuantiFERON-TB test to rule out underlying tubercular disease before treatment is initiated. Although infliximab therapy is associated with infusion-related reactions, administering a test dose is not routinely recommended. Infliximab may be administered in a clinic setting; it does not require admission to the hospital for monitoring. Infliximab therapy is associated with exacerbations of underlying heart failure and is contraindicated in patients with New York Heart Association class III or IV disease. This patient is young, with no history of heart failure, and has no clinical signs of heart failure. Therefore, a baseline echocardiogram is not necessary to assess cardiac function.

11. Answer: C

Treatment of nausea and vomiting in medical inpatients may be accomplished by administering a variety of antiemetics. Nausea and vomiting are common symptoms associated with pyelonephritis and will subside once appropriate antibiotic therapy adequately treats the infection. However, patients will need symptomatic relief until the antibiotics take effect. Agents typically used for medical inpatients include phenothiazines and serotonin antagonists. Use of intravenous or rectal formulations is usually preferred for patients with severe nausea, such as this patient. Ondansetron is a serotonin antagonist that can be administered as needed intravenously and is effective in treating nausea caused by a variety of medical conditions. Despite its effects on serotonin, it should not cause any significant interaction with the patient's sertraline dose. Prochlorperazine, a commonly used antiemetic, would be a viable option; however, using the oral product in this case would not be preferred, given that the patient has severe vomiting. In addition, prochlorperazine is a dopamine antagonist, and the patient is receiving a high dose of risperidone. This combination may lead to the development of EPS and, in severe cases, QTc prolongation. Metoclopramide is typically used as an antiemetic when gastroparesis is present or as an adjunctive therapy for patients whose other therapies have failed. Metoclopramide also has dopamine antagonist effects and may lead to the development of EPS. Diphenhydramine is more effective for nausea related to motion sickness, but it would not effectively treat severe short-term nausea or the other options.

12. Answer: B

This patient presents with acute constipation given his symptoms of abdominal pain, both by complaints and on examination; reduced frequency of bowel movements; and radiographic evidence of a large quantity of stool in the colon. Contributing factors include the use of verapamil and oxycodone without the use of a drug regimen to prevent constipation. Therapy should be instituted to provide a quick onset to initiate a bowel movement and provide symptom relief. Saline laxatives such as sodium phosphate provide quick results, especially when given by enema. The oral formulation of sodium phosphate results in phosphate absorption and is problematic in patients with chronic kidney disease caused by the development of hyperphosphatemia and phosphate nephropathy. This patient's CrCl is about 34 mL/minute, so saline laxatives should be avoided. Bisacodyl suppositories provide rapid stimulation of the lower intestinal tract without the risk of electrolyte absorption, so they would be preferred in this case. Methylcellulose is a bulk-forming laxative that would not treat the patient's acute constipation, but it would be an option for preventing constipation on a long-term basis in this patient once the short-term episode is resolved. Although methylnaltrexone is indicated for opioid-induced constipation, it would generally not be used as first-line agent given the need for injection and the added cost compared with traditional laxatives.

13. Answer: D
Stress-related mucosal disease develops in critically ill patients and may lead to significant upper GI bleeding. Therapy initiation to prevent SRMD is based on the presence of risk factors. Independent risk factors include mechanical ventilation and coagulopathy. This patient is currently on a ventilator and has other risk factors such as sepsis, hypotension, and acute renal insufficiency, so he would meet criteria for initiating pharmacologic prophylaxis. Both H2RAs and PPIs are viable first-line options. Cimetidine carries an FDA-approved indication for the prevention of SRMD; however, the dosing provided is incorrect because 50 mg/hour is the approved dose. Likewise, cimetidine would need to be dose adjusted for the patient's CrCl, which can be assumed less than 10 mL/minute. Pantoprazole would be a better choice in this case, and it does not require adjustment for the CrCl. Sucralfate has been historically used to prevent SRMD, but it has fallen out of favor because of the need for multiple daily dosing and the risk of aluminum accumulation in patients with kidney disease. Antacids are not as effective as H2RAs, require multiple daily dosing, and are associated with electrolyte accumulation in patients with kidney injury.

14. Answer: D
Several different forms of bias exist that may adversely affect the validity or results of a trial. Errors in sampling or measurement, incorrect patient enrollment methods, or differences in patient populations studied in a trial are examples of areas of study design and conduction that may introduce bias. When evaluating drug literature, an important aspect of deciding whether the reported results are valid is to recognize important causes of bias. A retrospective cohort design typically uses medical records to evaluate events that occurred in the past after exposure to a drug. Recall bias pertains to study outcomes or events that patients are asked to recall, with results differing depending on the ability of patients to remember an event. For this study, objective documentation of ulceration or bleeding was performed to make

comparisons between groups, eliminating patient recall as a potential bias. Misclassification bias is typically problematic in case-control studies, in which patients may be entered in the case study group but have not actually been exposed to the drug in question, which would not be applicable in this case. Interviewer bias, also known as observer bias, is typically problematic in direct patient survey studies and pertains to variation in the way different investigators collect data within a trial. To eliminate this bias, everyone involved in data collection in a study should be appropriately trained in the same manner of data collection to maintain consistency. Again, because an objective measure of GI toxicity was recorded by endoscopy, the possibility of interviewer bias is minimized. Channeling bias is a form of allocation bias in which medications with similar therapeutic indications are administered to patients with differing prognoses or risk levels. Should claims be made that a new drug introduced to a therapeutic class has particular advantages—in this case, a safer GI toxicity profile—then the chance that use will be channeled to high-risk patients is much greater. Given that the drug may be studied in higher-risk patients rather than the comparator group, the development of more events in this newer drug group may mask potential differences in safety and cause these events to be attributed to drug-induced toxicity.

Result	Infection	No Infection	Total
Positive	190	24	214
Negative	10	276	286
Total	200	100	500

15. Answer: B
Positive predictive value tells you the proportion of patients with a disease when the presence of the disease is indicated by a diagnostic test. It is affected by disease prevalence; thus, as disease prevalence falls, so does the positive predictive value of the test. Using the sensitivity, specificity, and prevalence, a 2×2 table can be constructed. The positive predictive value is calculated by dividing the true positives by the sum of the true and false positives. In this case, that would be $190/(190 + 24) \times 100 = 89\%$.

Ambulatory Care

Ila M. Harris, Pharm.D., FCCP, BCPS

University of Minnesota
Minneapolis, Minnesota

AMBULATORY CARE

ILA M. HARRIS, PHARM.D., FCCP, BCPS

UNIVERSITY OF MINNESOTA
MINNEAPOLIS, MINNESOTA

Learning Objectives

1. Classify patients, assess control, and select and monitor appropriate acute and preventive treatments for pediatric and adult patients with asthma and for adult patients with chronic obstructive pulmonary disease, depending on patient-specific factors.

2. Assess, classify, and select appropriate acute and chronic pharmacotherapy (including nonpharmacologic therapy), and monitor, reassess, and adjust therapy in patients with gout.

3. Determine appropriate immunizations for an adult given his or her age and medical conditions and apply cautions, contraindications, and drug interactions with immunizations to adult patients.

Self-Assessment Questions

Answers and explanations to these questions can be found at the end of this chapter.

1. A 20-year-old woman is admitted to the hospital for an asthma exacerbation. She states that she has been using her boyfriend's albuterol inhaler on a regular basis for the past 2 years. During the past few months, she has been using the inhaler throughout the day on a daily basis and sometimes at night. Which best classifies her asthma severity?

   A. Mild intermittent.
   B. Mild persistent.
   C. Moderate persistent.
   D. Severe persistent.

2. Which is the best maintenance therapy for her asthma?

   A. Fluticasone low dose.
   B. Montelukast.
   C. Fluticasone medium dose plus salmeterol.
   D. Theophylline.

3. Which type of measurement best classifies the number of times a short-acting β_2-agonist (SABA) is used in 1 month?

   A. Nominal.
   B. Ordinal.
   C. Interval.
   D. Ratio.

4. You are designing a study in which you will compare the percentage of patients with an asthma-related hospitalization receiving fluticasone/salmeterol with those receiving fluticasone alone. Which statistical test is best for analyzing this comparison?

   A. Analysis of variance (ANOVA).
   B. Chi-square.
   C. Mann-Whitney U test.
   D. Student unpaired t test.

5. A 22-year-old woman with asthma is taking an albuterol metered dose inhaler (MDI) 2 puffs as needed and fluticasone (Flovent) 110 mcg/puff MDI 2 puffs twice daily. She received the influenza vaccine during last year's influenza season, and her last tetanus vaccine (tetanus, diphtheria, and pertussis [Tdap]) was at age 17; there is no documentation of her having received a pneumococcal vaccine. Which is the best vaccine for her to receive at her next family medicine clinic appointment scheduled in July?

   A. Influenza.
   B. Pneumococcal.
   C. Td (tetanus and diphtheria).
   D. Herpes zoster.

6. A 60-year-old man with chronic obstructive pulmonary disease (COPD) has been using albuterol HFA 2 puffs four times per day as needed. His symptoms have worsened during the past year, and now he has persistent symptoms and shortness of breath, even while walking around his one-level house. His Modified Medical Research Council (mMRC) score is 2. His spirometry shows a forced expiratory volume in 1 second (FEV_1) of 70% of predicted and an FEV_1/forced vital capacity (FEV_1/FVC) of 60% of predicted. He has had no previous COPD exacerbations. Which medication is best to initiate?

   A. Fluticasone.
   B. Tiotropium.
   C. Fluticasone/salmeterol combination inhaler.
   D. Omalizumab.

7. A patient with severe polyarticular gout and three tophi, uric acid 12.3 mg/dL, and stage 4 chronic kidney disease (CKD) (glomerular filtration rate [GFR] 25 mL/minute/1.73 m^2) requires urate-lowering therapy (ULT). Which is the most appropriate drug and starting dose?

A. Probenecid 500 mg twice daily.

B. Probenecid 250 mg twice daily.

C. Allopurinol 100 mg once daily.

D. Allopurinol 50 mg once daily.

I. ASTHMA

Guidelines:

National Institutes of Health (NIH) National Heart Lung and Blood Institute (NHLBI). National Asthma Education and Prevention Program Guidelines (NAEPP). NAEPP Expert Panel Report 3. NIH Publication 08-5846. July 2007. Available at www.nhlbi.nih.gov/guidelines/asthma/. Accessed September 1, 2014. *(main guidelines presented in this chapter)*

Global Initiative for Asthma (GINA): Global Strategy for Asthma Management and Prevention 2014. Available at www.ginasthma.org/. Accessed October 15, 2014. *(for reference; these largely mirror the NHLBI guidelines)*

A. Definition: Asthma is a chronic inflammatory disorder of the airways causing recurrent episodes of wheezing, breathlessness, cough, and chest tightness, particularly at night or early in the morning. During episodes, there is variable airway obstruction, often reversible spontaneously or with treatment. There is also increased bronchial hyperresponsiveness to a variety of stimuli.

B. Diagnosis
   1. Episodic symptoms of airflow obstruction are present.
   2. Airway obstruction is reversible (FEV_1 improves by 12% or more after short-acting β_2-agonists [SABAs]).
   3. Alternative diagnoses are excluded. Asthma versus COPD:
      a. Cough is usually nonproductive with asthma and productive with COPD.
      b. FEV_1 is reversible with asthma but is irreversible with COPD.
      c. Cough is worse at night and early in the morning with asthma; occurs throughout the day with COPD.
      d. Asthma is often related to allergies and environmental triggers; patients with COPD have a common history of smoking or exposure to other irritants.
      e. Asthma can be reversible; lung damage from COPD is irreversible.
   4. Asthma-COPD overlap syndrome (ACOS)
      a. Persistent airflow limitation with features of both asthma and COPD.
      b. If three or more features favor asthma, use diagnosis/treatment for asthma.
      c. If three or more features favor COPD, use diagnosis/treatment for COPD.
      d. If a similar number of features exist for both asthma and COPD, consider a diagnosis of ACOS (Table 1).
   5. Exercise-induced bronchospasm
      a. Presents with cough, shortness of breath, chest pain or tightness, wheezing, or endurance problems during exercise.
      b. Diagnosis is made by an exercise challenge in which a 15% decrease in FEV_1 or peak expiratory flow occurs before and after exercise, measured at 5-minute intervals for 20–30 minutes.

Table 1. Syndromatic Diagnosis in Adults: Asthma vs. COPD vs. ACOS

Feature	Asthma	COPD
Age of onset	☐ Before age 20 years	☐ After age 40 years
Pattern of symptoms	☐ Variation in symptoms over minutes, hours, or days ☐ Worse during the night or early morning ☐ Triggered by exercise, emotions, dust, or exposure to allergens	☐ Persistence of symptoms despite treatment ☐ Good and bad days but always daily symptoms and exertional dyspnea ☐ Chronic cough and sputum precede onset of dyspnea, unrelated to triggers
Lung function	☐ Record of variable airflow limitation (spirometry or peak flow), showing reversibility	☐ Record of persistent airflow limitation (postbronchodilator FEV_1/FVC <0.7)
Lung function between symptoms	☐ Normal	☐ Abnormal
Past history or family history	☐ Previous diagnosis of asthma ☐ Family history of asthma and other allergic conditions (allergic rhinitis or eczema)	☐ Previous diagnosis of COPD, chronic bronchitis, or emphysema ☐ Heavy exposure to a risk factor: tobacco smoke, biomass fuels
Time course	☐ No worsening of symptoms over time; symptoms vary either seasonally or from year to year ☐ May improve spontaneously or have an immediate response to bronchodilators or to ICS over weeks	☐ Symptoms slowly worsen over time (progressive course over years) ☐ Rapid-acting bronchodilator provides only limited relief
Chest radiograph	☐ Normal	☐ Severe hyperinflation
Syndromatic Diagnosis Instructions:		
1. Check each box in both columns that pertains to the patient. 2. Count the number of check boxes in each column. 3. If three or more boxes are checked for either asthma or COPD, that diagnosis is suggested. 4. If similar number of boxes are checked in each column, consider a diagnosis of ACOS.		

COPD = chronic obstructive pulmonary disease; ACOS = asthma COPD overlap syndrome; ICS = inhaled corticosteroids; FEV_1/FVC = forced expiratory volume in 1 second/forced vital capacity.

From: Global Initiative for Asthma (GINA) and Global Initiative for Chronic Obstructive Lung Disease (GOLD). Diagnosis of diseases of chronic airflow limitation: Asthma, COPD and Asthma-COPD overlap syndrome (ACOS). Available at www.ginasthma.org/. Accessed October 15, 2014.

Table 2. Interpreting Spirometry

Component	What It Measures	Normal Values
FEV_1	Volume of air exhaled forcefully in the first second of maximal expiration	Normal is ≥80% In asthma, reversibility is shown by an increase in FEV_1 of ≥12% after SABA
FVC	The maximum volume of air that can be exhaled after full inspiration	Reported in liters and percentage predicted Normal adults can empty 80% of air in <6 seconds
FEV_1/FVC ratio	Differentiates between obstructive and restrictive disease	Normal: Within 5% of predicted range, which varies with age; usually 75%–80% in adults Decreased in obstructive disease (asthma, COPD) (<70%) Normal or high in restrictive disease (pulmonary fibrosis)

COPD = chronic obstructive pulmonary disease; FEV_1/FVC = forced expiratory volume in 1 second/forced vital capacity; SABA = short-acting β-agonist.

C. Classification of Asthma Severity and Control

Table 3. Classification of Asthma Severity in Adults and Children[a]

Components	Age Group (years)	Intermittent	Mild Persistent	Moderate Persistent	Severe Persistent
Frequency of symptoms	All ages	≤2 days/week	>2 days/week but not daily	Daily	Throughout the day
Nighttime awakening	≥12	≤2 times/month	3 or 4 times/month	More than once weekly but not nightly	Often 7 times/week
	5–11				
	0–4	0	1 or 2 times/month	3 or 4 times/month	More than once weekly
SABA; used for symptom control	All ages	≤2 days/week	>2 days/week but not daily	Daily	Several times a day
Interference with normal activity	All ages	None	Minor limitation	Some limitations	Extremely limited
FEV$_1$/FVC[b]	≥12	Normal	Normal	Reduced 5%	Reduced >5%
	5–11	>85%	>80%	75%–80%	<75%
	0–4	N/A			
FEV$_1$ (% of normal)	≥12	>80% (normal)	>80% (normal)	>60% to <80%	<60%
	5–11				
	0–4	N/A			
Exacerbations requiring oral steroids	≥12	0 or 1/year	≥2/year	≥2/year	≥2/year
	5–11				
	0–4	0 or 1/year	≥2 in 6 months or ≥4 wheezing episodes per year[c]		
Recommended step for initiating treatment (see Table 5)	≥12	Step 1	Step 2	Step 3[d] and consider short course of oral steroids	Step 4 or 5 and consider short course of oral steroids
	5–11				Step 3[d] or 4 and consider short course of oral steroids
	0–4				Step 3 and consider short course of oral steroids

[a]The patient is classified according to the sign or symptom that is in the most severe category.

[b]Normal FEV$_1$/FVC: 8–19 years old, 85%; 20–39 years old, 80%; 40–59 years old, 75%; 60–80 years old, 70%.

[c]Episodes lasting >1 day and risk factors for persistent asthma.

[d]For ages 5–11, initial step 3 therapy should be medium-dose ICS.

FEV$_1$ = forced expiratory volume in 1 second; FVC = forced vital capacity; ICS = inhaled corticosteroid; N/A = not applicable; SABA = short-acting β-agonist.

Adapted from NIH Asthma Guidelines. National Institutes of Health National Heart, Lung and Blood Institute. National Asthma Education and Prevention Program (NAEPP) guidelines. NAEPP Expert Panel Report 3. NIH Publication 08-5846. Available at www.nhlbi.nih.gov/guidelines/index.htm. Accessed September 1, 2014.

Table 4. Assessing Asthma Control in Adults and Children

Component	Age Group (years)	Well Controlled	Not Well Controlled	Very Poorly Controlled
Symptoms	≥12	≤2 days/week	>2 days/week	Throughout the day
	5–11	≤2 days/week but not >1 time each day	>2 days/week or >1 time/day on any day	
	0–4			
Nighttime awakenings	≥12	≤2 times/month	1–3 times/week	≥4 times/week
	5–11	≤1 time/month	≥2 times/month	≥2 times/week
	0–4		>1 time/month	>1 time/week
Interference with normal activity	All ages	None	Some limitations	Extremely limited
SABA use for symptom control[a]	All ages	≤2 days/week	>2 days/week	Several times a day
FEV$_1$ or peak flow	≥12	>80% of predicted/ personal best	60%–80% of predicted/ personal best	<60% of predicted/ personal best
	5–11			
	0–4	N/A	N/A	N/A
Questionnaires ATAQ ACQ ACT	≥12 (N/A if <12)	0 ≤0.75 ≥20	1 or 2 ≥1.5 16–19	3 or 4 N/A ≤15
Exacerbations requiring oral steroids	≥12	0 or 1/year	≥2/year	≥2/year
	5–11			
	0–4		2 or 3 times/year	>3 times/year
Recommended action for treatment	All ages	Maintain current step; regular follow-up every 1–6 months; consider step-down if well controlled ≥3 months	Step-up one step Reevaluate in 2–6 weeks	Consider short course of oral steroids Step-up one or two steps Reevaluate in 2 weeks

[a]Does not include β$_2$-agonist used to prevent exercise-induced asthma.

ACQ = Asthma Control Questionnaire (Juniper et al. Eur Respir J 1999;14:902-7); ACT = Asthma Control Test (Nathan et al. Allergy Clin Immunol 2004;113:59-65); ATAQ = Asthma Therapy Assessment Questionnaire (Vollmer et al. Am J Respir Crit Care Med 1999;160 (5 pt 1):1647-52); FEV$_1$ = forced expiratory volume in 1 second; N/A = not applicable; SABA = short-acting β$_2$-agonist.

Adapted from NIH Asthma Guidelines. National Institutes of Health National Heart Lung and Blood Institute. National Asthma Education and Prevention Program (NAEPP) Guidelines. NAEPP Expert Panel Report 3. NIH Publication 08-5846. Available at www.nhlbi.nih.gov/ guidelines/index.htm. Accessed September 1, 2014.

    D.   Treatment Goals
        1.   Minimal or no chronic symptoms day or night
        2.   Minimal or no exacerbations
        3.   No limitations on activities; no school or work missed
        4.   Maintain (near) normal pulmonary function.
        5.   Minimal use of SABAs
        6.   Minimal or no adverse effects from medications

E. Treatment Guidelines

Table 5. Pharmacologic Treatment of Asthma

Step	Age Group (years)	Long-term Control	Quick Relief
1	All ages	No controller needed	Use SABA PRN SABA >2 times/week (excluding preexercise doses) indicates inadequate control and need to step up treatment
2	≥12	Preferred: Low-dose ICS	
	5–11	Alternatives: LTM, theophylline, or cromolyn[a]	
	0–4	Preferred: Low-dose ICS	
		Alternatives: Montelukast or cromolyn[a]	
3	≥12	Preferred: Low-dose ICS plus LABA OR medium-dose ICS alone	
		Alternative: Low-dose ICS plus LTM or theophylline	
	5–11	Preferred: Low-dose ICS plus LABA, LTM, or theophylline OR medium-dose ICS alone (medium-dose ICS preferred as initial therapy)	
	0–4	Medium-dose ICS	
4	≥12	Preferred: Medium-dose ICS plus LABA	
	5–11	Alternative: Medium-dose ICS plus LTM or theophylline	
	0–4	Preferred: Medium-dose ICS plus LABA or montelukast	
		Alternative: Medium-dose ICS plus other LTM or theophylline	
5	≥12	High-dose ICS plus LABA AND consider omalizumab for patients with allergic asthma	
	5–11	Preferred: High-dose ICS plus LABA	
		Alternative: High-dose ICS plus LTM or theophylline	
	0–4	High-dose ICS plus LABA or montelukast	
6	≥12	High-dose ICS plus LABA plus systemic corticosteroids AND consider omalizumab for patients with allergic asthma	
	5–11	Preferred: High-dose ICS plus LABA plus systemic corticosteroids	
		Alternative: High-dose ICS plus LTM or theophylline plus systemic corticosteroids	
	0–4	High-dose ICS plus LABA or montelukast plus systemic corticosteroids	

[a]Cromolyn and nedocromil are included in the National Asthma Education and Prevention Program guidelines. Cromolyn and nedocromil inhalers have been discontinued by the manufacturer; only generic cromolyn nebulization solution is still available.

ICS = inhaled corticosteroid; LABA = long-acting β_2-agonist; LTM = leukotriene modifier; PRN = as needed; SABA = short-acting β_2-agonist.

Adapted from NIH Asthma Guidelines. National Institutes of Health National Heart, Lung and Blood Institute. National Asthma Education and Prevention Program (NAEPP) guidelines. NAEPP Expert Panel Report 3. NIH Publication 08-5846. Available at www.nhlbi.nih.gov/guidelines/index.htm. Accessed September 1, 2014.

F.   Pharmacologic Therapy for Asthma

Table 6. Pharmacologic Agents Used for Asthma and COPD

Generic	Brand	Dose	Adverse Effects	Comments
Corticosteroid inhalers				
Beclomethasone MDI 40 mcg/puff 80 mcg/puff	QVAR (HFA)	See ICS dosing table	**Inhaled:** Oral candidiasis Hoarseness May slow bone growth in children but similar adult height	ICSs are first line for persistent asthma • Use holding chambers only if needed for technique; not needed or well studied with HFA inhalers; holding chambers are only for MDIs, cannot be used for DPIs; holding chambers with a mask can be used for young children • Rinse mouth with water after inhalations • Use corticosteroid inhaler as scheduled, not as needed • Onset of improvement is 5–7 days; additional benefit may occur over several weeks • Consider calcium and vitamin D supplements in adults, particularly in perimenopausal women • Pulmicort Respules are the only nebulized steroid available Arnuity Ellipta inhalation powder is contraindicated if severe hypersensitivity to milk proteins
Fluticasone MDI 44 mcg/puff 110 mcg/puff 220 mcg/puff	Flovent HFA			
Fluticasone DPI 50 mcg/puff 100 mcg/puff 250 mcg/puff	Flovent Diskus			
Fluticasone furoate (inhalation powder) 100 mcg/puff 200 mcg/puff	Arnuity Ellipta 1 inhalation once daily			
Mometasone DPI 220 mcg/puff	Asmanex Twisthaler Can be used once daily			
Budesonide DPI 90 mcg/dose 180 mcg/dose 0.25-, 0.5-, and 1-mg/2-mL nebs	Pulmicort Flexhaler and Respules			
Ciclesonide MDI 80 mcg/puff 160 mcg/puff	Alvesco (HFA)			
Anticholinergics				
Ipratropium MDI 17 mcg/puff	Atrovent HFA	2–4 puffs TID–QID (up to 12 puffs/ 24 hours)	Headache Flushed skin Blurred vision Tachycardia Palpitations	Used mainly for COPD and for acute asthma exacerbations requiring emergency treatment Duration: 2–8 hours Also available as a solution for nebulization
Tiotropium DPI 18 mcg	Spiriva	Inhale 1 capsule/day		Used for COPD; not currently standard of care for asthma
Tiotropium mist 2.5mcg	Spiriva Respimat	2 puffs once daily		Long acting; not for rapid relief Duration: >24 hours
Aclidinium bromide DPI 400 mcg per puff	Tudorza Pressair	1 puff BID		Long-acting anticholinergic for COPD Dry powder inhaler with counter; does not involve putting capsules into inhaler at each dose
β₂-Agonists (short acting): SABA				
Albuterol MDI 90 mcg/puff	Proventil HFA Ventolin HFA ProAir HFA	2 puffs every 4–6 hours PRN	Tremor Tachycardia Hypokalemia Hypomagnesemia Hyperglycemia Tachyphylaxis	Used for acute bronchospasm; regular use indicates poor control Also available as solution for nebulization Duration of effect (MDI): 3–4 hours (up to 6)
Levalbuterol MDI 45 mcg/puff	Xopenex HFA	2 puffs every 4–6 hours PRN		R-enantiomer of albuterol Also available as a solution for nebulization Duration (MDI): 3–4 hours (up to 6)

Table 6. Pharmacologic Agents Used for Asthma and COPD *(continued)*

Generic	Brand	Dose	Adverse Effects	Comments
β₂-Agonists (long acting): LABA				
Salmeterol DPI 50 mcg/puff	Serevent Diskus	Inhale 1 blister/ puff BID	Tremor Tachycardia Electrolyte effects (rare)	Not for acute symptoms Should not be used as monotherapy for asthma Duration: 8–12 hours
Formoterol DPI 12-mcg capsule Formoterol 20-mcg/ 2-mL nebs Arformoterol 15-mcg/ 2-mL nebs	Foradil Aerolizer Perforomist Brovana	Inhale 1 capsule BID 20-mcg BID nebs 15-mcg BID nebs		Onset of action 1–3 minutes but should not be used as acute therapy Should not be used as monotherapy for asthma Duration of MDI: 8–12 hours Formoterol Aerolizer is indicated to prevent exercise-induced bronchospasm; should be used at least 15 minutes before exercise Arformoterol is the *R,R*-isomer of racemic formoterol
Indacaterol inhalation powder 75-mcg capsule	Arcapta Neohaler	Inhale 1 capsule once daily		Indacaterol is only indicated for COPD Not indicated for use in asthma Duration of action: 24 hours
Combination inhalers				
Albuterol/ ipratropium MDI 100/20 mcg/puff	Combivent Respimat	1 puff QID (Respimat) Maximum dose 6 puffs/day		Used primarily for COPD Combivent MDI is no longer available Combination solution for nebulization is also available as DuoNeb or generic
Fluticasone/ salmeterol DPI 100/50, 250/50, 500/50 mcg/puff	Advair Diskus	1 puff BID		Combination of ICS and LABA Breo: • The only once-daily combination inhaler • Indicated for COPD, not asthma • Contraindicated if severe hypersensitivity to milk proteins
Fluticasone/ salmeterol MDI 45/21, 115/21, 230/21 mcg/puff	Advair HFA	2 puffs BID		
Budesonide/ formoterol MDI 80/4.5, 160/ 4.5 mcg/puff	Symbicort (HFA)	2 puffs BID		
Mometasone/ formoterol MDI 100/5, 200/ 5 mcg/puff	Dulera (HFA)	2 puffs BID		
Fluticasone furoate/ vilanterol inhalation powder 100/25 mcg	Breo Ellipta (double-foil blister strips of powder)	1 inhalation once daily		

Table 6. Pharmacologic Agents Used for Asthma and COPD *(continued)*

Generic	Brand	Dose	Adverse Effects	Comments
Methylxanthine				
Theophylline Extended-release 24-hour capsules 100, 200, 300, 400 mg Extended-release 24-hour tablets 400, 600 mg Oral elixir Oral solution Extended-release 12-hour tablets 100, 200, 300, 450 mg	Theo-Dur Uniphyl Theo-24 Theochron Elixophyllin	**Adults:** 300 mg/day initial dose, divided according to formulation Adjust according to concentration Usual dose 400–600 mg/day **Children:** Start at 10 mg/kg/day Adjust according to concentration Smokers may need higher doses at more frequent intervals	**At high levels:** Nausea Vomiting CNS stimulation Headache Tachycardia, SVT Seizures Hematemesis Hyperglycemia Hypokalemia **At therapeutic levels:** Insomnia GI upset Increased hyperactivity in some children Difficult urination in BPH	Achieve concentrations of 5–15 mcg/mL Beneficial for night symptoms Not for acute relief Duration: variable, up to 24 hours
Leukotriene modifiers (note: FDA Caution*)				
Zafirlukast 10-mg tablet 20-mg tablet	Accolate	10–20 mg BID	Hepatotoxicity (zileuton and zafirlukast only) • Zileuton: monitor LFTs (baseline, every month × 3 months, every 2–3 months for remainder of first year) • Zafirlukast: monitor symptoms, regular LFT monitoring not required; could be considered Headache GI upset	Drug interactions: Warfarin, erythromycin, theophylline FDA approved for children ≥5 years old Bioavailability decreases with food; take 1 hour before or 2 hours after meals
Montelukast Oral 10-mg tablet Chewable 4- and 5-mg tablets Oral granules 4 mg/packet	Singulair	Dose in the evening Adults and children ≥15 years: 10 mg/day Children 6 to <15 years: 5 mg/day Children 1 to <6 years: 4 mg/day		Also indicated in exercise-induced bronchospasm and seasonal and perennial allergic rhinitis Drug interactions: Phenobarbital FDA approved for use in children ≥1 year old; used in children 6 months and older Churg-Strauss syndrome associated with tapering doses of steroids
Zileuton 600-mg CR tablet	Zyflo CR	1200 mg BID	*FDA Caution: Risk of neuropsychiatric events (behavior and mood changes: aggression, agitation, anxiousness, dream abnormalities, hallucinations, depression, insomnia, irritability, restlessness, suicidal thinking and behavior, tremor)	Drug interactions: Warfarin and theophylline Only for those ≥12 years old

Table 6. Pharmacologic Agents Used for Asthma and COPD *(continued)*

Generic	Brand	Dose	Adverse Effects	Comments
Monoclonal antibody/IgE binding inhibitor				
Omalizumab	Xolair	150–375 mg SC every 2–4 weeks Dose and frequency based on baseline IgE and weight in kilograms Do not inject >150 mg per injection site	Injection site reactions • Urticaria • Thrombocytopenia (transient) • Anaphylaxis (rare) • Malignancy	September 2014: New FDA Drug Safety Communication. Slightly increased risk of cardiovascular and cerebrovascular serious adverse events, including MI, unstable angina, TIA, PE/DVT, pulmonary HTN; no increased risk of stroke or CV death Used in severe persistent allergy-related asthma Use in ≥12 years Half-life: 26 days Second-line therapy Expensive

BPH = benign prostatic hyperplasia; BID = twice daily; CNS = central nervous system; COPD = chronic obstructive pulmonary disease; CR = controlled release; CV = cardiovascular; DOC = drug of choice; DPI = dry powder inhaler; DVT = deep vein thrombosis; FDA = US Food and Drug Administration; GERD = gastroesophageal reflux disease; GI = gastrointestinal; HFA = hydrofluoroalkane; HTN = hypertension; ICS = inhaled corticosteroid; IgE = immunoglobulin E; LABA = long-acting β_2-agonist; LFT = liver function test; MDI = metered dose inhaler; MI, myocardial infarction; MOA = mechanism of action; nebs = nebulizers; OTC = over the counter; PE = pulmonary embolism; PRN = as needed; QID = four times daily; SC = subcutaneously; SVT = supraventricular tachycardia; TIA = transient ischemic attack; TID = three times daily.

Table 7. Inhaled Corticosteroid Daily Dosing in Children and Adults

Inhaled Corticosteroids	Low Dose (mcg/day) Steps 2 and 3			Medium Dose (mcg/day) Steps 3 and 4			High Dose (mcg/day) Steps 5 and 6		
Age group (years)	0–4	5–11	≥12	0–4	5–11	≥12	0–4	5–11	≥12
Budesonide Pulmicort DPI 90, 180	N/A	180–400	180–600	N/A	>400–800	>600–1200	N/A	>800	>1200
Fluticasone Flovent HFA 44, 110, 220 Flovent DPI 50, 100, 250 Arnity Ellipta 100, 200[a]	176 N/A	88–176 100–200	88–264 100–300	>176–352 N/A	>176–352 >200–400	>264–440 >300–500	>352 N/A	>352 >400	>440 >500
Beclomethasone QVAR HFA 40, 80	N/A	80–160	80–240	N/A	>160–320	>240–480	N/A	>320	>480
Mometasone Asmanex DPI 110, 220 (delivers 100 and 200 mcg/puff)[a,b]	110 (age 4 only)	110	200	110 (age 4 only)	110	400	110 (age 4 only)	110	>400
Ciclesonide[c] Alvesco HFA 80, 160	N/A	N/A	160	N/A	N/A	320	N/A	N/A	640
Budesonide suspension for nebulization	0.25–0.5 mg	0.5 mg	N/A	>0.5–1 mg	1 mg	N/A	>1 mg	2 mg	N/A

[a]Once daily.

[b]The guidelines state the delivered dose of mometasone, not the actual dose; indicated in ages 4–11 after guidelines were published; doses are estimated from package insert.

[c]Ciclesonide was not available when the National Asthma Education and Prevention Program guidelines were published. The dose ranges are estimated from the package insert.

DPI = dry powder inhaler; HFA = hydrofluoroalkane; N/A = not applicable.

Adapted from NIH Asthma Guidelines. National Institutes of Health National Heart, Lung and Blood Institute. National Asthma Education and Prevention Program (NAEPP) guidelines. NAEPP Expert Panel Report 3. NIH Publication 08-5846. Available at www.nhlbi.nih.gov/guidelines/index.htm. Accessed September 1, 2014.

Patient Cases

1. A 23-year-old woman has been coughing and wheezing about twice weekly, and she wakes up at night about three times per month. She has never received a diagnosis of asthma, and she has not been to a doctor "in years." She uses her boyfriend's albuterol inhaler, but he recently ran out of refills, so she is seeking care. Her activities are not limited by her symptoms. Spirometry is done today, and her FEV_1 is 82% of predicted. From the current NAEPP guidelines, which is the best classification of her asthma?

   A. Intermittent.

   B. Mild persistent.

   C. Moderate persistent.

   D. Severe persistent.

2. Which medication is best to recommend for her, in addition to albuterol metered dose inhaler (MDI) 1 or 2 puffs every 4–6 hours as needed?

   A. No additional therapy needed.

   B. Montelukast 10 mg/day.

   C. Mometasone dry powder inhaler (DPI) 220 mcg/puff 1 puff daily.

   D. Budesonide/formoterol 80/4.5 mcg per puff 2 puffs twice daily.

3. At first, her symptoms were well controlled on your recommended therapy. However, when winter arrived, she started having symptoms and using her albuterol about 3 or 4 days per week during the day. Which is the preferred treatment change?

   A. No change in therapy is needed.

   B. Switch to budesonide/formoterol MDI 160/4.5 mcg per puff 2 puffs twice daily.

   C. Add montelukast orally 10 mg daily.

   D. Increase mometasone DPI to 220 mcg/puff 2 puffs daily.

4. An 8-year-old boy has been having daytime asthma symptoms once or twice weekly and is awakened twice weekly at night with coughing. In addition to albuterol MDI 1 or 2 puffs every 4–6 hours as needed, which is the best initial therapy for him?

   A. Fluticasone 44 mcg/puff 1 puff twice daily.

   B. Montelukast 10 mg/day.

   C. Fluticasone/salmeterol 100/50 mcg per puff 1 puff twice daily.

   D. Fluticasone 110 mcg/puff 1 puff twice daily.

   G. Pharmacologic Treatment of ACOS
      1. Start treatment according to an asthma diagnosis.
      2. Inhaled corticosteroid (ICS) and long-acting β_2-agonist (LABA) combination therapy should be used.
      3. Do not use LABA monotherapy if there are features of asthma.
      4. Do not use ICS monotherapy if there are features of COPD.

H. Long-Acting β₂-Agonists (LABAs): According to a U.S. Food and Drug Administration (FDA) safety announcement, issued because of safety concerns with LABAs:

1. Use of a LABA alone without a long-term asthma control drug such as an ICS is contraindicated.
2. LABAs should not be used in patients whose asthma is adequately controlled on low- or medium-dose ICSs.
3. LABAs should be used only as additional therapy for patients who are currently taking but not adequately controlled on a long-term asthma control agent (e.g., an ICS).
4. Once asthma control is achieved and maintained, patients should be assessed at regular intervals and stepped down (e.g., discontinue the LABA), if possible, and the patients should continue to be treated with a long-term asthma control agent (e.g., an ICS).
5. Pediatric and adolescent patients who require a LABA and an ICS should use a combination product to ensure adherence to both medications.

I. Exercise-Induced Bronchospasm: Prevention and Treatment of Symptoms
1. Long-term control therapy, if otherwise appropriate (initiate or step-up)
2. Pretreatment with a SABA before exercise
3. Leukotriene modifiers (LTMs) can attenuate symptoms in 50% of patients.

J. Monitoring
1. Peak flow monitoring
   a. Symptom-based and peak flow–based monitoring have similar benefits; either is appropriate for most patients. Symptom-based monitoring is more convenient.
   b. May consider daily home peak flow monitoring for moderate to severe persistent asthma if patient has history of severe exacerbations or has poor perception of worsening of asthma symptoms.
   c. Personal best peak expiratory flow rate (PEFR), not predicted PEFR, should be determined if using peak flow–based asthma action plan.
      i. Personal best PEFR is the highest number attained after daily monitoring for 2 weeks twice daily when asthma is under good control.
      ii. Predicted PEFR is based on population norms using sex, height, and age.
2. Spirometry (only used if 5 years or older)
   a. At initial assessment
   b. After treatment is started and symptoms are stabilized
   c. If prolonged or progressive loss of asthma control
   d. At least every 2 years or more often depending on response to therapy

K. Asthma Action Plan: Usually symptom based (equal benefits of symptom-based or peak flow–based monitoring); home treatment of an asthma exacerbation

Table 8. Asthma Action Plan

Zone	Signs and Symptoms	Treatment
Green	Doing well; no or minimal symptoms of coughing, wheezing, or dyspnea PEFR 80%–100% of personal best	Take long-term asthma control agent only (if one is prescribed) Use 2 puffs of SABA 5–15 minutes before exercise if exercise-induced asthma and before known triggers
Yellow	Getting worse; increased frequency of symptoms (e.g., coughing, wheezing, or dyspnea) PEFR 50%–79% of personal best	Use SABA: 2–4 puffs by MDI (up to 6 puffs if needed) or 1 nebulizer treatment; may repeat in 20 minutes if needed; reassess 1 hour after initial treatment If complete response at 1 hour, contact clinician for follow-up instructions and consider OCS burst[a] If incomplete response in 1 hour (still some coughing, wheezing, or dyspnea), repeat SABA and add OCS burst; contact clinician that day for further instructions If poor response in 1 hour (e.g., marked coughing, wheezing, or dyspnea), repeat SABA immediately; add OCS burst; contact clinician immediately; proceed to the ED if the distress is severe and unresponsive to treatment; consider calling 911 May continue to use SABA every 3–4 hours regularly for 24–48 hours
Red	Medical alert (e.g., marked coughing, wheezing, or dyspnea); inability to speak more than short phrases; use of accessory respiratory muscles; drowsiness PEFR <50% of personal best	Begin treatment and consult clinician immediately Use SABA: 2–6 puffs by MDI (higher dose of 4–6 puffs usually recommended) or 1 nebulizer treatment; repeat every 20 minutes up to 3 times; add OCS burst If incomplete or poor response, repeat SABA immediately; proceed to the ED or call 911 if distress is severe and unresponsive to treatment Call 911 or go to the ED immediately if lips or fingernails are blue or gray or if there is trouble walking or talking because of shortness of breath Continue using SABA every 3–4 hours regularly for 24–48 hours

[a]OCS burst: prednisone (or equivalent) 40–60 mg/day for 5–10 days (adults) or 1–2 mg/kg/day (maximum 60 mg/day) for 3–10 days (children).

ED = emergency department; MDI = metered dose inhaler; OCS = oral corticosteroid; PEFR = peak expiratory flow rate; SABA = short-acting beta agonist.

After initial treatment, immediate medical attention is required if patient is at high risk of a fatal attack. Risk factors: Asthma-related (history of severe attack [previous intubation or intensive care unit admission for asthma], 2 or more asthma hospitalizations for asthma in past year, 3 or more ED visits for asthma in past year, hospitalization or ED visit for asthma in past month, using more than 2 canisters of SABA a month, difficulty perceiving asthma symptoms), social (low socioeconomic status or inner-city residence, illicit drug use, major psychosocial problems), and comorbidities (cardiovascular disease, other chronic lung disease, chronic psychiatric disease).

L. Managing Exacerbations: Initial—Emergency Department (ED) or Hospital

Table 9. Classifying Severity of Asthma Exacerbations in the Urgent or Emergency Care Setting[a]

	Symptoms and Signs	**Initial PEF or FEV$_1$[b]**	**Clinical Course**
Mild	Dyspnea only with activity	≥70% of predicted or personal best	Usually cared for at home Prompt relief with an inhaled SABA Possible short course of OCS
Moderate	Dyspnea interferes with or limits usual activity	40%–69% of predicted or personal best	Usually requires office or ED visit Relief from frequently inhaled SABAs and OCS; some symptoms last for 1–2 days after treatment is begun
Severe	Dyspnea at rest; interferes with conversation	<40% of predicted or personal best	Usually requires ED visit and likely hospitalization Partial relief from frequent inhaled SABA Oral systemic corticosteroids; some symptoms last for >3 days after treatment is begun Adjunctive therapies are helpful
Life threatening	Too dyspneic to speak; perspiring	<25% of predicted or personal best	Requires ED or hospitalization, possible ICU Little or no relief from frequent inhaled SABAs IV corticosteroids Adjunctive therapies are helpful

[a]For all ages.

[b]Lung function measures (PEF or FEV$_1$) may be useful for children ≥5 years old but may not be attainable in children during an exacerbation.

ED = emergency department; FEV$_1$ = forced expiratory volume in 1 second; ICU = intensive care unit; IV = intravenous; OCS = oral corticosteroid; PEF = peak expiratory flow; SABA = short-acting β$_2$-agonist.

Adapted from NIH Asthma Guidelines. National Institutes of Health National Heart, Lung and Blood Institute. National Asthma Education and Prevention Program Guidelines (NAEPP). NAEPP Expert Panel Report 3. NIH Publication 08-5846. Available at www.nhlbi.nih.gov/guidelines/asthma/. Accessed September 1, 2014.

1. Mild to moderate exacerbation (FEV$_1$ of 40% or more)
   a. Oxygen to achieve oxygen saturation (Sao$_2$) of 90% or more
   b. An inhaled SABA (MDI with valved holding chamber or nebulizer) up to three doses in the first hour
      i. Adult dose: Albuterol MDI 4–8 puffs every 20 minutes for up to 4 hours, then every 1–4 hours as needed or by nebulizer 2.5–5 mg every 20 minutes for three doses, then 2.5–10 mg every 1–4 hours as needed
      ii. Pediatric dose (12 years or younger): Albuterol MDI 4–8 puffs every 20 minutes for three doses, then every 1–4 hours as needed; use holding chamber (add mask if younger than 4 years) or by nebulizer 0.15 mg/kg (minimal dose 2.5 mg) every 20 minutes for three doses, then 0.15–0.3 mg/kg up to 10 mg every 1–4 hours as needed
   c. Oral corticosteroid (OCS) if no response immediately or if patient recently took an OCS

2. Severe exacerbation (FEV$_1$ less than 40%)
   a. Oxygen to achieve Sao$_2$ of 90% or more
   b. High-dose inhaled SABA plus ipratropium by MDI plus valved holding chamber or nebulizer every 20 minutes or continuously for 1 hour
   c. Oral corticosteroids
      i. Adult dose: Prednisone 40–80 mg/day in one or two divided doses until peak expiratory flow reaches 70% of predicted
      ii. Pediatric dose (12 years or younger): 1–2 mg/kg in two divided doses (maximum 60 mg/day) until peak expiratory flow reaches 70% of predicted
   d. Consider adjunctive therapies (intravenous magnesium or heliox) if still unresponsive.
3. Impending or actual respiratory arrest
   a. Intubation and mechanical ventilation with oxygen 100%
   b. Nebulized SABA plus ipratropium
   c. Intravenous corticosteroids
   d. Consider adjunctive therapies (intravenous magnesium or heliox) if patient is still unresponsive to therapy.
   e. Admit to intensive care.

M. Managing Exacerbations: ED or Hospital After Repeat Assessment
   1. Moderate exacerbation (FEV$_1$ 40%–69%)
      a. Inhaled SABA every 60 minutes
      b. Oral corticosteroid
      c. Continue treatment for 1–3 hours if improving.
   2. Severe exacerbation (FEV$_1$ less than 40%); no improvement after initial treatment
      a. Oxygen
      b. Nebulized SABA plus ipratropium; hourly or continuous
      c. Consider adjunctive therapies.
   3. If good response to above treatment and maintained for at least 60 minutes
      a. Continue inhaled SABA.
      b. Continue OCS course.
      c. Consider initiating an ICS (if not already taking one).
      d. Discharge home.
   4. If incomplete response (FEV$_1$ 40%–69%), admit to hospital ward.
   5. If poor response (FEV$_1$ less than 40%), admit to intensive care.

Patient Case

5. A 25-year-old man presents to the ED with shortness of breath at rest. He is having trouble with conversation. He used 4 puffs of albuterol MDI at home with no resolution of symptoms. His FEV$_1$ is checked, and it is 38% of predicted. Which is the best initial therapy for him in the ED, in addition to oxygen?

   A. Oxygen alone is sufficient.

   B. Give inhaled albuterol MDI 8 puffs every 20 minutes for 1 hour.

   C. Give inhaled albuterol plus ipratropium by nebulizer every 20 minutes for 1 hour plus intravenous corticosteroids.

   D. Give inhaled albuterol plus ipratropium by nebulizer every 20 minutes for 1 hour plus an OCS.

N. Vaccines: Adults with asthma (19–64 years of age) should receive
1. The 23-valent pneumococcal polysaccharide vaccine (PPSV23; Pneumovax) once, then follow U.S. Centers for Disease Control and Prevention (CDC) recommendations for pneumococcal vaccination at age 65 and older
2. Influenza vaccine every fall or winter

O. Asthma in Pregnancy
1. Asthma may worsen, improve, or stay the same during pregnancy.
2. Asthma may increase the risk of perinatal mortality, hyperemesis, vaginal hemorrhage, preeclampsia, complicated labor, neonatal mortality, prematurity, and low-birth-weight infants, especially if uncontrolled. Risks are small and are not shown in all studies.
3. Medications
    a. Preferred controller: Budesonide ICS (only category B ICS); however, if well controlled on other ICS before pregnancy, it may be continued.
    b. Preferred rescue: Albuterol
    c. LABAs are category C; less clinical experience. Use during pregnancy is reasonable if necessary for asthma control. Salmeterol is preferred LABA.
    d. LTMs have limited data; most data are with montelukast (category B), and the data for montelukast are reassuring. Considered an alternative therapy.
    e. Prednisone is category C; potential adverse effects in pregnancy are cleft palate, preeclampsia, gestational diabetes, low birth weight, and prematurity. However, few studies were of patients with asthma, and women might have been exposed to longer-term prednisone use. Prednisone should be used, if necessary, for acute exacerbations in pregnancy.

II. CHRONIC OBSTRUCTIVE PULMONARY DISEASE

Guidelines:

Global Initiative for Chronic Obstructive Lung Disease. Global Strategy for Diagnosis, Management and Prevention of COPD. Global Initiative for Chronic Obstructive Lung Disease (GOLD) 2014 Update. Available at www.goldcopd.org/. Accessed September 1, 2014.

Qaseem A, Wilt TJ, Weinberger SE, et al. Diagnosis and management of stable chronic obstructive pulmonary disease: a clinical practice guideline update from the American College of Physicians, American College of Chest Physicians, American Thoracic Society, and European Respiratory Society (ACP/ACCP/ATS/ERS guidelines). Ann Intern Med 2011;155:179-91.

A. Definition: COPD is a syndrome of chronic limitation in expiratory airflow encompassing emphysema and chronic bronchitis. Airflow obstruction may be accompanied by airway hyperresponsiveness and may be not be fully reversible.
1. Chronic bronchitis consists of persistent cough plus sputum production for most days of 3 months in at least 2 consecutive years.
2. Emphysema is abnormal permanent enlargement of the airspaces distal to the terminal bronchioles, accompanied by destruction of their walls and without obvious fibrosis.

B. Diagnosis and Assessment
   1. The diagnosis of COPD is based on a history of exposure to risk factors and the presence of airflow limitation that is not fully reversible, with or without the presence of symptoms.
      a. Symptoms: Dyspnea (described by patients as "increased effort to breathe," "heaviness," "air hunger," or "gasping"), poor exercise tolerance, chronic cough, sputum production, wheezing
      b. GOLD guidelines: Perform spirometry and consider COPD if a patient is older than 40 years and has any of the following:
         i. Dyspnea that is progressive (worsens over time), persistent (present every day), and worse with exercise or on exertion
         ii. Chronic cough that is present intermittently or every day; often present throughout the day; seldom only nocturnal. May be nonproductive
         iii. Chronic sputum production in any pattern
         iv. History of exposure to risk factors, especially tobacco smoke (most common risk factor), occupational dusts and chemicals, and smoke from home cooking and heating fuels
      c. American College of Physicians, American College of Chest Physicians, American Thoracic Society, and European Respiratory Society (ACP/ACCP/ATS/ERS) guidelines: The single best predictor of airflow obstruction is the presence of all three of the following:
         i. Smoking history of more than 55 pack-years
         ii. Wheezing on auscultation
         iii. Patient self-reported wheezing
   2. For the diagnosis and assessment of COPD, spirometry is the gold standard.
      a. Spirometry showing an FEV_1/FVC less than 70% of predicted is the hallmark of COPD. Bronchodilator reversibility testing is no longer recommended.
      b. Measurement of arterial blood gas tension should be considered for all patients with FEV_1 less than 50% of predicted or clinical signs suggestive of respiratory failure or right heart failure.
   3. Validated symptom scales or questionnaires
      a. Modified Medical Research Council (mMRC) breathlessness scale for assessing severity of breathlessness (Bestall et al. 1999)
      b. COPD Assessment Test (CAT) measures health status impairment in COPD (www.catestonline.org).

C. Factors Determining Severity of COPD
   1. Severity of symptoms
   2. Severity of airflow limitation (FEV_1)
   3. Frequency of exacerbations
   4. Presence of comorbidities that may restrict activity (e.g., heart failure, heart disease, musculoskeletal disorders)

D. Therapy Goals
   1. Relieve symptoms.
   2. Reduce the frequency and severity of exacerbations.
   3. Improve exercise tolerance.
   4. Improve health status.
   5. Minimize adverse effects from treatment.

E. Management of Stable COPD
   1. Description of levels of evidence or grades of recommendations

Table 10. Grades for Strength of Recommendations for COPD Guidelines

GOLD Guidelines	
A	Randomized clinical trials Rich body of data
B	Randomized clinical trials Limited body of data
C	Nonrandomized trials Observational studies
D	Panel judgment consensus
ACP/ACCP/ATS/ERS Guidelines	
Recommendation grade	Strong (S): Benefits clearly outweigh risks and burden, or risks and burden clearly outweigh benefits Weak (W): Benefits finely balanced with risks and burden
Quality of evidence	High (H) Moderate (M) Low (L)

2. Existing medications for COPD have not been shown to modify the long-term decline in lung function, the hallmark of this disease (level of evidence A). Therefore, pharmacotherapy for COPD is used to decrease symptoms, complications, or both.

3. Smoking cessation is a critical component of COPD management.

4. Bronchodilator medications are central to the symptomatic management of COPD (level of evidence A).

   a. They are given on an as-needed basis or on a regular basis to prevent or reduce symptoms.

   b. The principal bronchodilator treatments are β_2-agonists, anticholinergics, or a combination of these drugs. Theophylline is also a bronchodilator but is not recommended unless other long-term bronchodilators are unavailable or unaffordable.

   c. Inhaled therapy is preferred.

   d. The choice between a LABA, anticholinergic, theophylline, and combination therapy depends on availability and individual response in symptom relief and adverse effects.

   e. Regular treatment with a long-acting (LA) bronchodilator is more effective and convenient than regular treatment with SABAs (level of evidence A).

   f. Combining bronchodilators from different pharmacologic classes may improve efficacy with the same or fewer adverse effects compared with increasing the dose of a single bronchodilator (level of evidence A).

   g. Adding tiotropium to a LABA-ICS combination (triple therapy) improves lung function and health-related quality of life and reduces the number of exacerbations (level of evidence B). Retrospective data show decreased mortality, fewer hospital admissions, and fewer OCS bursts. All bronchodilators improve symptoms and exercise capacity.

      i. Treatment with an LA anticholinergic delays first exacerbation, reduces the overall number of COPD exacerbations and related hospitalizations, improves symptoms and health status (level of evidence A), and improves the effectiveness of pulmonary rehabilitation (level of evidence B). LA anticholinergics have no effect on the rate of decline of lung function. Initial studies with tiotropium showed elevated cardiovascular risk, but newer strong evidence shows no increase in risk. Anticholinergics may not significantly improve FEV_1.

ii. LABAs improve health status, quality of life, and FEV$_1$ and decrease COPD exacerbation rate (level of evidence A). LABAs have no effect on mortality and rate of decline of lung function. Salmeterol reduces hospitalization rate (level of evidence B). Indacaterol significantly improves breathlessness, health status, and exacerbation rate (level of evidence B). Indacaterol is a LABA with a significantly greater bronchodilator effect than formoterol and salmeterol and a bronchodilator effect similar to that of tiotropium (level of evidence A). LABAs do not have the same potential safety concerns as with use in asthma.

iii. LA anticholinergic versus LABAs:

(a) POET-COPD study: Tiotropium is more effective than salmeterol as initial LA bronchodilator therapy in moderate to very severe COPD regarding time to first exacerbation and annual number of exacerbations. (Vogelmeier et al. 2011)

(b) Cochrane review concluded that tiotropium is more effective than LABAs in preventing COPD exacerbations and COPD-related hospitalization but not in overall hospitalization or mortality. Symptom and lung function improvement were similar. However, there are only a few studies. Fewer serious adverse events and withdrawals from studies occurred with tiotropium versus LABAs (Chong et al. 2012).

5. ICSs in stable COPD

a. ICSs improve symptoms, lung function, and quality of life and decrease the frequency of exacerbations in patients with FEV$_1$ less than 60% of predicted; they do not modify the progressive decline in FEV$_1$ or decrease mortality (level of evidence A).

b. The dose response with ICS in COPD is unknown (in contrast to asthma treatment). Moderate to high doses have been used in COPD clinical trials.

c. An ICS combined with a LABA is more effective than the individual components (level of evidence A). An ICS/LABA combination reduces the rate of decline of FEV$_1$ and reduces the exacerbation rate; the reduction in mortality compared with placebo fell just short of statistical significance (relative risk reduction 17.5%; absolute risk reduction 2.6%; adjusted p=0.052) (Calverley et al. 2007). A subsequent meta-analysis showed that ICS/LABA might reduce mortality (number needed to treat was 36) (level of evidence B) (Nannini et al. 2007).

d. ICS use is associated with an increased incidence of pneumonia in COPD (Singh et al. 2009; Ernst et al. 2007).

e. Long-term monotherapy with ICSs is not recommended; they are less effective than ICS/LABA combination.

f. Long-term treatment with ICSs should not be used outside their indications because of the risk of pneumonia and possible increased risk of fractures after long-term exposure.

g. Chronic treatment with OCSs should be avoided because of an unfavorable benefit-risk ratio (level of evidence A).

6. Patient assessment and selection of therapy

a. GOLD guidelines combine symptoms (based on symptom scores), airflow limitation (based on postbronchodilator FEV$_1$), and frequency of exacerbations to determine patient risk group and recommended treatment.

b. ACP/ACCP/ATS/ERS guidelines simplify treatment even further on the basis of FEV$_1$ in patients with COPD with symptoms. They do not provide detailed treatment guidelines.

Table 11. GOLD Guidelines: Assessment of COPD Severity and Risk

Patient Group	Characteristic	Spirometric GOLD Classification[a]	Exacerbations per Year[a]	Symptom Score[b]
A	Low risk Fewer symptoms	GOLD 1: Mild (FEV_1 ≥80% of predicted) *or* GOLD 2: Moderate (50% ≤ FEV_1 <80% of predicted)	≤1 and no hospitalization	mMRC 0–1 CAT <10
B	Low risk More symptoms	GOLD 1: Mild (FEV_1 ≥80% of predicted) *or* GOLD 2: Moderate (50% ≤ FEV_1 < 80% of predicted)	≤1 and no hospitalization	mMRC ≥2 CAT ≥10
C	High risk Fewer symptoms	GOLD 3: Severe (30% ≤ FEV_1 < 50% of predicted) *or* GOLD 4: Very severe (FEV_1 <30% of predicted)	≥2 or ≥1 with hospitalization	mMRC 0–1 CAT <10
D	High risk More symptoms	GOLD 3: Severe (30% ≤ FEV_1 < 50% of predicted) *or* GOLD 4: Very severe (FEV_1 < 30% of predicted)	≥2 or ≥1 with hospitalization	mMRC ≥2 CAT ≥10

[a]Postbronchodilator FEV_1 should be used. To determine the risk of exacerbation, either the spirometric GOLD classification or the number of exacerbations per year can be used. If they are both used and the patient would fall into two different categories, always assign patient to the category with the highest risk and symptoms.

[b]CAT score is preferred, but any can be used.

CAT = COPD Assessment Test (validated questionnaire); COPD = chronic obstructive pulmonary disease; FEV_1 = forced expiratory volume in 1 second; GOLD = Global Initiative for Chronic Obstructive Lung Disease; mMRC = Modified Medical Research Council breathlessness scale (validated questionnaire).

Adapted from: Global Initiative for Chronic Obstructive Lung Disease. Global Strategy for Diagnosis, Management and Prevention of COPD. Global Initiative for Chronic Obstructive Lung Disease (GOLD) 2014 Update. Available at www.goldcopd.org/. Accessed September 1, 2014.

Table 12. GOLD Guidelines: Pharmacotherapy for Stable COPD

Patient Group	Recommended First Choice	Alternative Choice	Other Possible Treatments[a]
A	SA anticholinergic PRN *or* SABA PRN	LA anticholinergic *or* LABA *or* SABA + SA anticholinergic	Theophylline[b]
B	LA anticholinergic *or* LABA	LA anticholinergic + LABA	SABA *and/or* SA anticholinergic Theophylline[b]
C	ICS + LABA *or* LA anticholinergic	LA anticholinergic + LABA *or* LA anticholinergic + PDE-4 inhibitor[c] *or* LABA + PDE-4 inhibitor[c]	SABA *and/or* SA anticholinergic Theophylline[b]
D	ICS + LABA *and/or* LA anticholinergic	ICS + LABA + LA anticholinergic *or* ICS + LABA + PDE-4 inhibitor[c] *or* LA anticholinergic + LABA *or* LA anticholinergic + PDE-4 inhibitor[c]	SABA *and/or* SA anticholinergic Theophylline[b]

Note: All medication choices are listed in alphabetical order and are not necessarily in order of preference.

[a]Medications in third column (other possible treatments) can be used alone or in combination with first- and alternative-choice columns.

[b]Theophylline is not recommended unless other long-term bronchodilators are unavailable or unaffordable.

[c]If patient has chronic bronchitis.

COPD = chronic obstructive pulmonary disease; GOLD = Global Initiative for Chronic Obstructive Lung Disease; ICS = inhaled corticosteroid; LA = long-acting; LABA = long-acting β_2-agonist; PDE-4 = phosphodiesterase type-4; PRN = as needed; SA = short-acting; SABA = short-acting β_2-agonist.

Adapted from: Global Initiative for Chronic Obstructive Lung Disease. Global Strategy for Diagnosis, Management and Prevention of COPD. Global Initiative for Chronic Obstructive Lung Disease (GOLD) 2014 Update. Available at www.goldcopd.org/. Accessed September 1, 2014.

Table 13. ACP/ACCP/ATS/ERS Guidelines: Treatment Recommendations for Stable COPD

- For patients with respiratory symptoms and FEV_1 between 60% and 80% of predicted, treatment with LA inhaled bronchodilators is suggested.
  (Grade W, level of evidence L)

- For patients with respiratory symptoms and FEV_1 <60% of predicted, treatment with LA inhaled bronchodilators is recommended.
  (Grade S, level of evidence M)

- Monotherapy using either LA inhaled anticholinergics or LABAs is recommended for symptomatic patients with FEV_1 <60% of predicted. The choice of specific monotherapy should be based on patient preference, cost, and adverse effect profile.
  (Grade S, level of evidence M)

- Combination inhaled therapies (LA inhaled anticholinergics, LABAs, or ICS) may be used for symptomatic patients with FEV_1 <60% of predicted.
  (Grade W, level of evidence M)

COPD = chronic obstructive pulmonary disease; FEV_1 = forced expiratory volume in 1 second; ICS = inhaled corticosteroid; LA = long-acting; LABA = long-acting β-agonist.

Qaseem A et al. ACP/ACCP/ATS/ERS COPD guidelines. Ann Intern Med 2011;155:179-91.

7. Other pharmacologic treatments
   a. Phosphodiesterase-4 inhibitor: Roflumilast (Daliresp)
      i. Indication: As a daily treatment to reduce the risk of COPD exacerbations in patients with severe COPD (FEV_1 less than 50% of predicted) associated with chronic bronchitis and a history of frequent exacerbations. In these patients, studies show a reduction in exacerbations and a reduction in the composite end point of moderate exacerbations treated with oral or systemic corticosteroids or severe exacerbations requiring hospitalization or causing death (level of evidence B). These effects also occur when roflumilast is added to LA bronchodilators (level of evidence B). No trials have assessed the effects of roflumilast on COPD exacerbations when added to an ICS-LA bronchodilator combination. No comparison of adding roflumilast versus ICS to LA bronchodilators is available (currently being studied).
      ii. Mechanism: Reduces inflammation through inhibition of the breakdown of intracellular cyclic adenosine monophosphate; no direct bronchodilator activity.
      iii. Dose: 500 mcg orally once daily
      iv. Contraindications: Moderate to severe liver impairment; use in nursing mothers
      v. Precautions: Weight loss (monitor); psychiatric events including suicidality (monitor; weigh risk-benefit ratio in patients with preexisting psychiatric illness). Twenty percent of patients studied had weight loss of 5%–10% of body weight compared with 7% with placebo; average weight loss was 2 kg.
      vi. Adverse reactions: Diarrhea, weight loss or decreased appetite, nausea, headache, back pain, influenza, insomnia, and dizziness
      vii. Drug interactions: Use with strong cytochrome P450 (CYP) enzyme inducers is not recommended (e.g., rifampin, phenobarbital, carbamazepine, phenytoin); use with CYP3A4 inhibitors or dual inhibitors of CYP3A4 and CYP1A2 (e.g., erythromycin, ketoconazole, fluvoxamine) increases roflumilast exposure and adverse effects (risk-benefit ratio must be weighed).
   b. Smoking cessation therapy (essential for all patient groups A–D)
   c. Influenza vaccine annually (essential for all patient groups A–D)

    d.   The 23-valent pneumococcal polysaccharide vaccine (PPSV23; Pneumovax) once before age 65, then follow CDC recommendations for pneumococcal vaccination at age 65 and older.

    e. α_1-Antitrypsin augmentation therapy (level of evidence C)

        i.   For young patients with severe hereditary α_1-antitrypsin deficiency and established emphysema, but an expensive treatment

        ii.   Patients with α_1-antitrypsin deficiency usually are white, usually develop COPD at a young age (younger than 45 years), and have a strong family history. It may be worthwhile to screen such patients.

Patient Cases

6.   A 62-year-old man was recently diagnosed with COPD. Spirometry shows he has an FEV_1/FVC 60%, prebronchodilator FEV_1 70% of predicted, and postbronchodilator FEV_1 72% of predicted. His symptoms are very bothersome. He reports walking more slowly than others because of shortness of breath and having to stop to catch his breath every so often when walking on level ground (mMRC grade 2). He had one exacerbation in the past year. Which is the most appropriate patient group classification for him, according to the GOLD guidelines?

    A. Patient group A.

    B. Patient group B.

    C. Patient group C.

    D. Patient group D.

7.   In addition to albuterol HFA 2 puffs every 4–6 hours as needed, which pharmacotherapy option is most appropriate to initiate?

    A. No additional therapy needed.

    B. Formoterol: Inhale contents of 1 capsule twice daily.

    C. Salmeterol/fluticasone 50/500 1 puff twice daily.

    D. Salmeterol/fluticasone 50/500 1 puff twice daily plus roflumilast 500 mcg orally once daily.

8.   A 52-year-old woman with COPD reports a gradual worsening in shortness of breath during the past few years. Spirometry shows FEV_1/FVC 55% and FEV_1 63% of predicted. Her CAT score is 10. She has not had a COPD exacerbation or received systemic corticosteroids in the past 2 years. Her current COPD medications are tiotropium inhaler once daily and albuterol HFA as needed. According to the GOLD guidelines, which is the most appropriate course of action?

    A. Add salmeterol 1 puff twice daily.

    B. Add long-term azithromycin 250 mg once daily.

    C. Add fluticasone 110 mcg 2 puffs twice daily.

    D. Discontinue tiotropium and initiate salmeterol/fluticasone 250/50 1 puff twice daily.

8. Nonpharmacologic therapy
   a. Home oxygen therapy
      i. Recommended in patients who have a Pao_2 of 55 mm Hg or less (or 55–60 mm Hg if pulmonary hypertension, peripheral edema, or polycythemia [level of evidence D]) or Sao_2 of 88% or less, with or without hypercapnia, confirmed twice during a 3-week period (level of evidence B)
      ii. Long-term (more than 15 hours/day) use in patients with chronic respiratory failure improves survival.
   b. Pulmonary rehabilitation (essential for patient groups B–D; level of evidence A)
      i. Includes exercise training, nutrition counseling, and education
      ii. Recommended for stage II–IV COPD. Patients should be referred when they have moderate (stage II) COPD; not wait until it is more severe.
      iii. Improves many outcomes in COPD, including quality of life and survival.
9. Newer data in COPD
   a. Chronic azithromycin for prevention of COPD exacerbations (Albert et al. 2011)
      i. Compared with placebo, daily azithromycin significantly lengthened time to first exacerbation, decreased rate of exacerbations, and improved quality of life in patients with COPD at increased risk of exacerbations, at the expense of risk of hearing decrements and increasing macrolide-resistant organism colonization.
      ii. Number needed to treat to prevent one acute exacerbation of COPD is 2.86; number needed to harm for hearing decrements is 20.
      iii. The GOLD guidelines state that the role of treatment with daily antibiotics is unclear and that treatment is currently not recommended because of an unfavorable balance between benefits and adverse effects.
   b. β-Blockers
      i. Observational data suggest that long-term treatment with β-blockers reduces risk of exacerbations and improves survival, even in patients without overt cardiovascular disease (Rutten et al. 2010).
      ii. More than half of the patients studied had cardiovascular risk factors or coronary artery disease. Mostly cardioselective β-blockers were used.
      iii. It is too early to recommend β-blockers for the treatment of COPD, but β-blockers should not be withheld in patients with COPD who also have heart disease, chronic heart failure, or other cardiovascular conditions in which β-blockers are beneficial (Salpeter 2002, update 2005, reviewed 2008)
      iv. Mechanism for benefit in COPD is unknown, but β-blockers can upregulate $β_2$-receptors in the lungs, which may improve the effectiveness of inhaled β-agonists.

F. Management of Acute Exacerbations of Chronic COPD
   1. A COPD exacerbation is an acute worsening of a patient's baseline respiratory symptoms (e.g., dyspnea, cough, and/or an increase in quantity or purulence of sputum) that is worse than normal day-to-day variation and results in a change in medication. Diagnosis is based purely on clinical presentation.
   2. Common precipitating factors include infection of tracheobronchial tree and viral upper respiratory tract infections (most common) and air pollution. However, the cause of one-third of exacerbations cannot be determined.
   3. Spirometry is not accurate during an exacerbation and is not recommended.
   4. Pulse oximetry can be used to determine the need for supplemental oxygen, which should be given in severe exacerbations. In exacerbations requiring hospitalization, an arterial blood gas measurement should be performed.

5. Inhaled bronchodilators (inhaled SABAs with or without short-acting anticholinergics) are the preferred treatment of COPD exacerbations (level of evidence C).
    a. Usual doses of albuterol are 2.5 mg via nebulizer every 1–4 hours as needed or 4–8 puffs by MDI with holding chamber every 1–4 hours as needed.
    b. Short-acting anticholinergics (ipratropium) are generally added for acute exacerbation.
6. Systemic corticosteroids are effective, and they shorten recovery time, improve FEV_1, and improve hypoxemia (level of evidence A). They also lower the risk of treatment failure, early relapse rate, and length of hospital stay. Systemic corticosteroids should be used in most exacerbations. OCS dose for outpatient treatment: 40 mg of oral prednisone once daily for 5 days is recommended in the GOLD guidelines (level of evidence B), but insufficient data are available to provide strong conclusions about the optimal duration.
    a. Higher daily doses or oral prednisone/prednisolone may be used (e.g., 50–60 mg daily).
    b. A recent study showed that in patients with a COPD exacerbation presenting to the hospital, a shorter course of systemic corticosteroids (5 days) was noninferior to a longer (14 days) course with respect to re-exacerbation within 6 months (Leuppi et al. 2013).
7. Antibiotic treatment should be initiated for exacerbations if the criteria below are met. The most common pathogens in COPD exacerbations: *Streptococcus pneumoniae, Haemophilus influenzae,* and *Moraxella catarrhalis.* In patients with GOLD 3 and 4 severity, *Pseudomonas aeruginosa* infection becomes an important pathogen.
    a. The three cardinal symptoms in COPD exacerbations are increased dyspnea, increased sputum volume, and increased sputum purulence.
        i. Antibiotics should be given if all three cardinal symptoms are present (level of evidence B).
        ii. Antibiotics should be given if two of the three cardinal symptoms are present and if increased sputum purulence is one of the symptoms (level of evidence C).
        iii. Antibiotics should be given to patients with a severe exacerbation requiring mechanical ventilation (level of evidence B).
    b. Recommended duration of antibiotic treatment is usually 5–10 days (level of evidence D).
    c. Recommended antibiotics
        i. Optimal antibiotic therapy has not been determined but should be based on local resistance patterns.
        ii. If recent (less than 3 months) antibiotics, use alternative class.
        iii. Usual initial antibiotics for uncomplicated COPD include azithromycin, clarithromycin, doxycycline, trimethoprim/sulfamethoxazole, and amoxicillin, with or without clavulanate.
        iv. In complicated COPD with risk factors: Amoxicillin/clavulanate, levofloxacin, moxifloxacin. Risk factors: Comorbid diseases, severe COPD (FEV_1 less than 50% of predicted), more than 3 exacerbations/year, antibiotic use in past 3 months
        v. If at risk of *Pseudomonas* infection: High-dose levofloxacin (750 mg) or ciprofloxacin; obtain sputum culture. Risk factors: Four or more courses of antibiotics in past year, recent hospitalization (past 90 days), isolation of *Pseudomonas* during past hospitalization, severe COPD (FEV_1 less than 50% of predicted)
        vi. If exacerbation does not respond to initial antibiotic, sputum culture and sensitivity should be performed.

G. Vaccinations: All patients with COPD should receive the influenza vaccine yearly and the polysaccharide pneumococcal vaccine once before age 65; then a one-time revaccination 5 years or more after the first vaccination.

Patient Case

9. A 64-year-old woman with COPD in GOLD patient group A presents for a clinic visit. In the past few days, she has had a worsening in shortness of breath and a productive cough with more "cloudy" and more copious sputum than usual. Pulse oximetry is 95% on room air. She has a nebulizer at home. In addition to regular use of albuterol plus ipratropium by nebulizer every 1–4 hours, which is the best course of action?

   A. No additional therapy is necessary.

   B. Add oral prednisone 40 mg once daily for 5 days

   C. Add trimethoprim/sulfamethoxazole double-strength 1 tablet twice daily for 7 days.

   D. Add oral prednisone 40 mg once daily for 5 days and trimethoprim/sulfamethoxazole double strength 1 tablet twice daily for 7 days.

III. GOUT

Guidelines:

Khanna D, Fitzgerald JD, Khanna PP, et al. 2012 American College of Rheumatology Guidelines for Management of Gout. Part 1. Systematic nonpharmacologic and pharmacologic therapeutic approaches to hyperuricemia. Arthritis Care Res 2012;64:1431-46.

Khanna D, Khanna PP, Fitzgerald JD, et al. 2012 American College of Rheumatology Guidelines for Management of Gout. Part 2. Therapy and antiinflammatory prophylaxis of acute gouty arthritis. Arthritis Care Res 2012;64:1447-61.

A. Definition: A spectrum of clinic and pathologic features caused by hyperuricemia (serum urate level more than 6.8 mg/dL), resulting in tissue deposition of monosodium urate monohydrate crystals in the extracellular fluid of joints and other sites. Most common rheumatic disease of adults; prevalence estimated at 3.9% of adults (around 8.3 million people)

B. Diagnosis
   1. Typically presents as acute episodic arthritis.
   2. Can also present as chronic arthritis of one or more joints.
   3. Tophi may be present: Detected by physical examination or imaging and pathology.
   4. Renal manifestations include urolithiasis.
   5. Features of acute gouty attack
      a. Severe pain, redness, swelling; maximum severity in 12–24 hours; may continue for a few days to several weeks.
      b. Most often occurs in the lower extremities and in a single joint.
         i. Most common joint: First metatarsophalangeal joint (podagra) or knee
         ii. May occur in many other joints, including upper extremity.
         iii. May be polyarticular at first presentation (less than 20% of cases).
   6. Ideally, definitive diagnosis should be made by visualization of monosodium urate crystals by polarized compensated light microscopy in fluid aspirated from the affected joint during an acute gouty attack.
      a. For diagnosis of gout, monosodium urate crystals are negatively birefringent (needle-shaped or rods).
      b. In pseudogout, crystals are calcium pyrophosphate dihydrate and are weakly positively birefringent (rods or rhomboidal).

      c. Diagnosis by joint aspiration is difficult because patients are in severe pain and often refuse joint aspiration during an acute attack. In this case, a provisional diagnosis may be made according to clinical data.

    7. If diagnosis by joint aspiration is not possible, a tentative diagnosis may be made by a combination of presentation or clinical picture and elevated uric acid. Use of hyperuricemia as one of the criteria for diagnosing gout may be difficult during an initial acute attack because serum uric acid may be low during flares. Best time to check uric acid is 2 weeks after a flare.

C. Predisposing Factors (Singh et al. 2011)
    1. Dietary: High meat and seafood consumption, fatty foods, dietary overindulgence, high intake of beer and spirits in men (not wine), sugar-sweetened soft drinks, high-fructose foods
    2. Drugs: Xanthine oxidase inhibitors (XOIs) and uricosuric agents (with initial therapy), thiazides and loop diuretics, niacin, calcineurin inhibitors, low-dose aspirin (325 mg/day or less)
    3. Medical conditions and other factors: Obesity, diabetes, hypertension, dyslipidemia, renal insufficiency, early menopause, trauma, surgery, starvation, dehydration

D. Classification
    1. Three stages of gout:
        a. Acute gouty arthritis
        b. Intercritical gout
        c. Chronic recurrent gout
    2. Severities of chronic tophaceous gouty arthropathy (CTGA)
        a. Mild: One joint, stable disease
        b. Moderate: Two to four joints, stable disease
        c. Severe
            i. Chronic CTGA of more than four joints OR
            ii. One or more unstable, complicated, severe articular tophi
    3. Size of joints
        a. Large joints (e.g., knee, ankle, wrist, elbow, hip, shoulder)
        b. Medium joints (e.g., wrist, ankle, elbow)
        c. Small joints (e.g., interphalangeal)

E. Treatment Goals
    1. Serum urate target: Minimum is less than 6 mg/dL.
    2. Serum urate target of less than 5 mg/dL may be needed to improve gout signs and symptoms. Consider goal of less than 5 mg/dL if tophi present.
    3. Decrease frequency of acute gouty attacks.

F.   Nonpharmacologic Therapy

Table 14. Nonpharmacologic Therapy for Gout

Lifestyle and General Health		
Weight loss if obese Healthy overall diet Exercise Smoking cessation Proper hydration		
Food and Drink to Avoid	**Food and Drink to Limit**	**Food and Drink to Encourage**

Organ meats high in purine (e.g., liver, kidney, sweetbreads)	Serving sizes of:
	  Beef, lamb, pork
	  Seafood with high purine content
	  (e.g., sardines, shellfish)
		Low-fat or nonfat dairy products

High-fructose corn syrup–sweetened sodas, other beverages, foods	Servings of naturally sweet fruit juices Table sugar, sweetened beverages, desserts Table salt	Vegetables
Alcohol overuse (>2 per day for men and >1 per day for women) in all patients with gout Any alcohol use in gout during times of frequent gouty attacks or advanced gout under poor control	Alcohol (particularly beer but also wine and spirits) in all patients with gout	

Adapted from: Khanna D, Fitzgerald JD, Khanna PP, et al. 2012 American College of Rheumatology Guidelines for Management of Gout. Part 1. Systematic nonpharmacologic and pharmacologic therapeutic approaches to hyperuricemia. Arthritis Care Res 2012;64:1431-46.

G.   Pharmacologic Treatment of Hyperuricemia
   1.   Consider discontinuing nonessential medications that cause hyperuricemia.
   2.   Indications for urate-lowering therapy (ULT):
       a.   Tophi by clinical examination or imaging study
       b.   Two or more acute gouty attacks per year
       c.   CKD stage 2 or worse
       d.   Past urolithiasis
   3.   ULT can be initiated during an acute gouty attack as long as concomitant anti-inflammatory therapy is given.
   4.   First-line ULT:
       a.   XOI: Allopurinol or febuxostat
       b.   Can switch to alternative XOI if patient is intolerant of or refractory to first XOI.
   5.   Alternative first-line ULT (uricosuric): Probenecid (if at least one XOI is contraindicated or not tolerated). History of urolithiasis and CrCl less than 50 mL/minute contraindicates first-line use of probenecid.

6. Initiate anti-inflammatory prophylaxis for acute gout concomitantly with or just before ULT in all patients.
   a. Early increase in acute gouty attacks during initiation of ULT
      i. May be caused by rapid decrease in urate concentrations, resulting in remodeling of articular urate crystal deposits
      ii. Often leads to nonadherence to ULT; patient education is critical.
   b. Oral low-dose colchicine is first-line option.
   c. Other first-line option is low-dose nonsteroidal anti-inflammatory drugs (NSAIDs) (lower evidence grade than colchicine). Add concomitant proton pump inhibitor or other agent for suppression of peptic ulcer disease when indicated.
   d. OCS is an alternative for anti-inflammatory gouty attack prophylaxis (level of evidence C).
      i. If colchicine and NSAIDs are contraindicated, not tolerated, or ineffective
      ii. Because of risks associated with prolonged use of OCSs, the risk-benefit ratio of this strategy should be considered and reevaluated with continued ULT therapy because the risk of acute gout decreases in time.
   e. Anti-inflammatory prophylaxis of acute gout should continue for the greater of:
      i. 6 months (level of evidence A)
      ii. 3 months after achieving target serum urate level if no tophi (level of evidence B)
      iii. 6 months after achieving target serum urate level if tophi were previously present but are now resolved (level of evidence C)
      iv. However, continue anti-inflammatory prophylaxis if any clinical evidence of gout disease activity is present (tophi, recent acute gouty attacks, chronic gouty arthritis).
7. Monitor serum urate every 2–5 weeks. After goal is achieved, continue monitoring every 6 months. If serum urate goals are not achieved:
   a. Titrate single-agent XOI to maximum appropriate dose.
   b. Next, add uricosuric to XOI (probenecid, losartan, or fenofibrate). Probenecid is first-line uricosuric; losartan and fenofibrate are off-label but recommended second-line uricosurics.
   c. If goal serum urate still not achieved, add pegloticase only if severe gout disease burden *and* patient is refractory to or intolerant of other ULT options. Pegloticase is not recommended for first-line therapy in any case.
8. Indefinite duration of ULT is recommended.
9. Allopurinol hypersensitivity syndrome (AHS)
   a. Risk of severe morbidity and hospitalization
   b. Mortality rate of 20%–25% in AHS
   c. Manifestations of AHS: Stevens-Johnson syndrome, toxic epidermal necrolysis, clinical constellation of symptoms: eosinophilia, rash, vasculitis, major end-organ disease
   d. Highest risk is during the first few months of therapy.
   e. Risk factors: Concomitant thiazide diuretics, renal impairment, people of Han Chinese or Thai descent (irrespective of renal function), people of Korean descent with stage 3 or worse CKD. Consider testing for *HLA-B*5801* in these ethnic groups (if positive, higher risk of AHS).

H. Treatment of Acute Gout
   1. Assess severity of gouty attack (Table 15) and select treatment according to severity.
   2. Initiate pharmacologic treatment within 24 hours of onset of acute gouty attack. Colchicine is appropriate only if initiated within 36 hours of attack onset.
   3. Continue established ULT without interruption during acute gouty attack (do not discontinue ULT).

Table 15. Severity, Duration, and Extent of Acute Gouty Attacks

Severity (self-reported; based on visual analog scale; 0–10)	
Mild	≤4
Moderate	5–6
Severe	≥7
Duration Since Onset	
Early	<12 hours after attack onset
Well established	12–36 hours after attack onset
Late	>36 hours after attack onset
Extent	
One or a few small joints	
One or two large joints	Large joints: Ankle, knee, wrist, elbow, hip, shoulder
Polyarticular	Four or more joints involving >1 region (regions: forefoot, midfoot, ankle or hindfoot, knee, hip, fingers, wrist, elbow, shoulder)
	Three separate large joints

   a. For mild to moderate pain affecting one or a few small joints or one or two large joints, use *monotherapy.*
   b. For severe pain or polyarticular attack, or if multiple large joints are affected, use *initial combination therapy.*
      i. Monotherapy: NSAID *or* OCSs *or* colchicine (level of evidence A for all choices), supplemented with topical ice (adjunctive therapy) as needed
         (a) No preference for one choice over another; select treatment according to gout flare presentation, comorbidities, previous response, and patient preference.
            (1) Consider intra-articular corticosteroids if one or two large joints; use OCSs for all other presentations; may consider single-dose intramuscular triamcinolone followed by an OCS.
            (2) Concomitant use of colchicine with P-glycoprotein (Pgp) inhibitors or strong CYP3A4 inhibitors is contraindicated in renal or hepatic impairment (fatal toxicity has occurred).
            (3) Colchicine dose should be reduced if normal renal or hepatic function and concomitant use of Pgp inhibitors or moderate to strong CYP3A4 inhibitors.
            (4) If the patient has received acute gout treatment with colchicine in the past 2 weeks, use alternative therapy.
            (5) Colchicine should not be used to treat gouty attacks in patients with renal or hepatic impairment who are taking prophylactic colchicine, according to labeling.
         (b) Celecoxib is an option in certain patients with contraindications or intolerance to NSAIDs; risk-benefit ratio unclear.
         (c) Adrenocorticotropic hormone 20–40 international units subcutaneously is an option if patient is taking nothing by mouth.
      ii. Initial combination therapy: Can use full doses of both agents or, when appropriate, full dose of one agent and prophylactic dose of another agent
         (a) Colchicine plus an NSAID
         (b) OCSs plus colchicine

(c) Intra-articular steroids with all other modalities

(d) Combination of an NSAID and systemic corticosteroids has synergistic GI toxicity.

iii. Continue acute treatment until the gouty attack has resolved.

4. If inadequate response to initial treatment of acute gouty attack:

a. Inadequate response defined as either less than 20% improvement in pain score in 24 hours or less than 50% improvement in 24 hours or more after starting drug therapy for acute attack.

b. If inadequate response, switch to a different monotherapy (level of evidence C) or add a second agent (level of evidence C).

c. Biologic agents that inhibit interleukin-1 (anakinra and canakinumab) are considered investigational for the treatment of acute gout but can be considered when gout flares are frequent and resistant to all other therapies.

5. Educate patients and provide a prescription so that patients can initiate treatment for acute gouty attacks on their own.

Table 16. Medication Dosing for Gout

Drug	Dose	Comments
Acute Gouty Attack Treatment		
Colchicine (Colcrys)	1.2 mg; then 0.6 mg 1 hour later; then 0.6 mg once or twice daily until attack resolves CrCl 30–80 mL/minute: Monitor for adverse effects; dose adjustment not necessary CrCl <30 mL/minute: Dose adjustment not necessary but may be considered; do not repeat course of treatment more than every 2 weeks Dialysis: 0.6-mg single dose; do not repeat course of treatment more than every 2 weeks Severe hepatic impairment: Dose reduction not required but may be considered; do not repeat course of treatment more frequently than every 2 weeks	Concomitant use of colchicine with Pgp inhibitors or strong CYP3A4 inhibitors is contraindicated in renal or hepatic impairment (fatal toxicity has occurred) Colchicine dose should be reduced if renal and hepatic function is normal and if used concomitantly with Pgp inhibitors or moderate to strong CYP3A4 inhibitors
NSAIDs	Naproxen: 750 mg initially, followed by 250 mg every 8 hours Naproxen ER: 1000–1500 mg once daily, followed by 1000 mg once daily Indomethacin: 50 mg 3 times daily until pain tolerable, then reduce dose until attack resolves Sulindac: 200 mg twice daily Use at anti-inflammatory/analgesic doses of other NSAIDs, same as for treatment of acute pain or inflammation	Only FDA-approved NSAIDs are naproxen, indomethacin, and sulindac; however, other NSAIDs may be as effective Continue full dose until attack completely resolves Can taper dose if comorbidities or renal or hepatic impairment is present
Celecoxib (Celebrex)	800 mg once, followed by 400 mg on day 1, then 400 mg twice daily for 1 week	Only in certain patients when NSAIDs are contraindicated or not tolerated

Table 16. Medication Dosing for Gout *(continued)*

Drug	Dose	Comments
Acute Gouty Attack Treatment		
Cortico-steroids	OCSs for all cases of gout (level of evidence B)	Intra-articular corticosteroids can be used in combination with OCSs, NSAIDs, or colchicine (level of evidence B)
	Prednisone 0.5 mg/kg per day for 5–10 days (level of evidence A) OR	
	Prednisone 0.5 mg/kg per day for 2–5 days, then taper for 7–10 days, then discontinue (level of evidence C) OR	
	Methylprednisolone dose pack (level of evidence C)	
	Option for 1 or 2 large joints: Intra-articular corticosteroids (level of evidence B)	
	Dose based on the size of the joint (e.g., triamcinolone 40 mg for large joint, 30 mg for medium joint, 10 mg for small joint or equivalent)	
	IM triamcinolone followed by OCS (level of evidence C)	
	60 mg IM, followed by OCS (dosed as above)	
Urate-Lowering Therapy		
Allopurinol (Zyloprim)[a]	Starting dose: 100 mg daily (50 mg daily in stage 4 CKD)	XOI
	Gradually titrate dose every 2–5 weeks to appropriate maximum dose (800 mg daily with normal renal function) or until goal urate level reached	Low starting dose reduces early gout flares and risk of hypersensitivity syndrome
	Maintenance dose can be higher than 300 mg daily, even in CKD, as long as patient is educated and regular monitoring occurs for hypersensitivity, rash, pruritus, elevated hepatic enzymes, and eosinophilia	Consider keeping dose lower in CKD and not increasing to maximum dose; data with dosing >300 mg/day in CKD are limited
		Dose reduction algorithms in CKD have been developed but are not evidence based; the ACR guidelines do not recommend following them
Febuxostat (Uloric)[a]	Starting dose: 40 mg once daily	XOI
	May increase dose to 80 mg once daily if goal serum urate not reached	More expensive than allopurinol; no generic available
	CrCl <30 mL/minute: Use caution; insufficient data	
Probenecid (generic only)[a]	Starting dose: 250 mg twice daily	Uricosuric; first-line
	May increase weekly in 500-mg/day increments to maximum dose of 1 g twice daily if needed	According to the guidelines, not recommended for first-line or alternative first-line treatment if CrCl < 50 mL/minute or history of urolithiasis
	Avoid if CrCl < 30 mL/minute	Do baseline and periodic urine uric acid; elevated urine uric acid level (uric acid overproduction) contraindicates probenecid
		When initiating, increase fluid intake and consider urine alkalinization (e.g., potassium citrate)

Table 16. Medication Dosing for Gout *(continued)*

Drug	Dose	Comments
Urate-Lowering Therapy		
Losartan	Dose according to other indications and as tolerated	Uricosuric; second-line Off-label use
Fenofibrate	Dose according to other indications and as tolerated	Uricosuric; second line Off-label use
Pegloticase (Krystexxa)[a]	8 mg intravenously every 2 weeks No dosage adjustment for CKD	Use only if severe gout disease burden *and* refractory to or intolerant of other ULT options All other antihyperuricemic agents must be discontinued before initiating pegloticase; do not administer concomitantly Premedicate with antihistamines and corticosteroids
Gouty Attack Prophylaxis		
Colchicine (Colcrys)	0.6 mg once or twice daily CrCl 30–80 mL/minute: Monitor for adverse effects; dose adjustment not required CrCl <30 mL/minute: Initial dose 0.3 mg/day; use caution and monitor if dose titrated further Dialysis: 0.3 mg twice weekly; monitor for adverse effects Severe hepatic impairment: Dose reduction not required necessary but may be considered; do not repeat course of treatment more often than every 2 weeks	First-line Concomitant use of colchicine with Pgp inhibitors or strong CYP3A4 inhibitors is contraindicated in renal or hepatic impairment (fatal toxicity has occurred) Colchicine dose should be reduced if renal and hepatic function is normal and if used concomitantly with Pgp inhibitors or moderate to strong CYP3A4 inhibitors
NSAIDs	Lower doses than used for acute attacks (e.g., naproxen 250 mg twice daily, indomethacin 25 mg twice daily)	Alternative first-line; less strong evidence than with colchicine Consider concomitant proton pump inhibitor or other agent for suppression of PUD when indicated
OCSs	Prednisone or prednisolone ≤10 mg daily	Alternative Only if colchicine and NSAIDs are both contraindicated, ineffective, or not tolerated

[a]Always initiate concomitant prophylactic therapy.

ACR = American College of Rheumatology; CKD = chronic kidney disease; CrCl = creatinine clearance; CYP = cytochrome P450; ER = extended release; FDA = U.S. Food and Drug Administration; IM = intramuscular(ly); NSAID = nonsteroidal anti-inflammatory drug; OCS = oral corticosteroid; Pgp = P-glycoprotein; PUD = peptic ulcer disease; ULT = urate-lowering therapy; XOI = xanthine oxidase inhibitor.

Patient Cases

10. A 60-year-old man presents with his third gouty attack in the past year. His last attack was 10 days ago, for which he took colchicine with good response. His pain is in his left knee and in the third and fourth proximal interphalangeal joints on his left hand. The pain started about 10 hours ago. He rates his pain as 6/10. He has COPD and dyslipidemia, his renal function is normal, and his weight is 80 kg. His uric acid level from 1 month ago is 10 mg/day. He has no tophi. His only medications are inhaled tiotropium, albuterol, and simvastatin. Which is most appropriate for treatment of this acute gouty attack?

    A. Naproxen 750 mg, then 250 mg every 8 hours.

    B. Colchicine 1.2 mg, then 0.6 mg in 1 hour, then 0.6 mg every 12 hours.

    C. Intra-articular triamcinolone injection of all affected joints.

    D. Prednisone 40 mg daily plus naproxen 750 mg, then 250 mg every 8 hours.

11. Which is most appropriate regarding ULT in this patient?

    A. Probenecid should be started, but treatment should be delayed until after the acute attack is resolved.

    B. Probenecid should be started and can be initiated during the acute attack.

    C. Allopurinol should be started, but treatment should be delayed after the acute attack has resolved.

    D. Allopurinol should be started and can be initiated during the acute attack.

12. Which regimen for anti-inflammatory prophylaxis with ULT therapy is most appropriate in this patient, once the acute attack has resolved?

    A. Colchicine 0.6 mg once daily.

    B. Prednisone 10 mg daily.

    C. Colchicine 0.6 mg once daily plus naproxen 250 mg twice daily.

    D. Pegloticase 8 mg intravenously every 2 weeks.

13. What is the initial goal uric acid level and duration of anti-inflammatory prophylaxis in this patient?

    A. Goal <6 mg/dL; continue for a total of 6 months.

    B. Goal <6 mg/dL; continue for 3 months after achieving goal serum urate for at least 6 months total.

    C. Goal <5 mg/dL; continue for a total of 6 months.

    D. Goal <5 mg/dL; continue for 3 months after achieving goal serum urate for at least 6 months total.

IV. ADULT IMMUNIZATIONS

VACCINE ▼ AGE GROUP ►	19-21 years	22-26 years	27-49 years	50-59 years	60-64 years	≥ 65 years
Influenza*,2	1 dose annually					
Tetanus, diphtheria, pertussis (Td/Tdap)*,3	Substitute 1-time dose of Tdap for Td booster; then boost with Td every 10 yrs					
Varicella*,4	2 doses					
Human papillomavirus (HPV) Female*,5	3 doses					
Human papillomavirus (HPV) Male*,5	3 doses					
Zoster6					1 dose	
Measles, mumps, rubella (MMR)*,7	1 or 2 doses					
Pneumococcal 13-valent conjugate (PCV13)*,8						1-time dose
Pneumococcal polysaccharide (PPSV23)8	1 or 2 doses					1 dose
Meningococcal*,9	1 or more doses					
Hepatitis A*,10	2 doses					
Hepatitis B*,11	3 doses					
Haemophilus influenzae type b (Hib)*,12	1 or 3 doses					

*Covered by the Vaccine Injury Compensation Program

For all persons in this category who meet the age requirements and who lack documentation of vaccination or have no evidence of previous infection; zoster vaccine recommended regardless of prior episode of zoster

Recommended if some other risk factor is present (e.g., on the basis of medical, occupational, lifestyle, or other indication)

No recommendation

Report all clinically significant postvaccination reactions to the Vaccine Adverse Event Reporting System (VAERS). Reporting forms and instructions on filing a VAERS report are available at www.vaers.hhs.gov or by telephone, 800-822-7967.

Information on how to file a Vaccine Injury Compensation Program claim is available at www.hrsa.gov/vaccinecompensation or by telephone, 800-338-2382. To file a claim for vaccine injury, contact the U.S. Court of Federal Claims, 717 Madison Place, N.W., Washington, D.C. 20005; telephone, 202-357-6400.

Additional information about the vaccines in this schedule, extent of available data, and contraindications for vaccination is also available at www.cdc.gov/vaccines or from the CDC-INFO Contact Center at 800-CDC-INFO (800-232-4636) in English and Spanish, 8:00 a.m. - 8:00 p.m. Eastern Time, Monday - Friday, excluding holidays.

Use of trade names and commercial sources is for identification only and does not imply endorsement by the U.S. Department of Health and Human Services.

The recommendations in this schedule were approved by the Centers for Disease Control and Prevention's (CDC) Advisory Committee on Immunization Practices (ACIP), the American Academy of Family Physicians (AAFP), the America College of Physicians (ACP), American College of Obstetricians and Gynecologists (ACOG) and American College of Nurse-Midwives (ACNM).

Figure 1. Recommended adult immunization schedule, by vaccine and age group,[1] United States, 2015.

Centers for Disease Control and Prevention (CDC). Advisory Committee on Immunization Practices (ACIP). Recommended Immunization Schedule for Adults Aged 19 Years and Older: —United States, 2015. Available at www.cdc.gov/vaccines/schedules/downloads/adult/adult-combined-schedule.pdf. Accessed February 12, 2015.

VACCINE ▼ INDICATION ►	Pregnancy	Immuno-compromising conditions (excluding human immunodeficiency virus [HIV]) 4,6,7,8,13	HIV infection CD4+ T lymphocyte count 4,6,7,8,13 < 200 cells/μL	HIV infection CD4+ T lymphocyte count ≥ 200 cells/μL	Men who have sex with men (MSM)	Kidney failure, end-stage renal disease, receipt of hemodialysis	Heart disease, chronic lung disease, chronic alcoholism	Asplenia (including elective splenectomy and persistent complement component deficiencies) 8,12	Chronic liver disease	Diabetes	Healthcare personnel
Influenza*,2	1 dose IIV annually	1 dose IIV annually	1 dose IIV annually	1 dose IIV or LAIV annually	1 dose IIV annually	1 dose IIV annually	1 dose IIV annually	1 dose IIV annually	1 dose IIV annually	1 dose IIV annually	1 dose IIV or LAIV annually
Tetanus, diphtheria, pertussis (Td/Tdap)*,3	1 dose Tdap each pregnancy	Substitute 1-time dose of Tdap for Td booster; then boost with Td every 10 yrs									
Varicella*,4	Contraindicated	Contraindicated		2 doses							
Human papillomavirus (HPV) Female*,5	3 doses through age 26 yrs				3 doses through age 26 yrs						
Human papillomavirus (HPV) Male*,5	3 doses through age 26 yrs				3 doses through age 21 yrs						
Zoster6	Contraindicated	Contraindicated		1 dose							
Measles, mumps, rubella (MMR)*,7	Contraindicated	Contraindicated		1 or 2 doses							
Pneumococcal 13-valent conjugate (PCV13)*,8		1 dose									
Pneumococcal polysaccharide (PPSV23)8		1 or 2 doses									
Meningococcal*,9		1 or more doses									
Hepatitis A*,10		2 doses									
Hepatitis B*,11		3 doses									
Haemophilus influenzae type b (Hib)*,12		post-HSCT recipients only		1 or 3 doses							

*Covered by the Vaccine Injury Compensation Program

For all persons in this category who meet the age requirements and who lack documentation of vaccination or have no evidence of previous infection; zoster vaccine recommended regardless of prior episode of zoster

Recommended if some other risk factor is present (e.g., on the basis of medical, occupational, lifestyle, or other indications)

No recommendation

Figure 2. Vaccines that might be indicated for adults, based on medical and other indications, [1, a] United States, 2015.

aThe above recommendations must be read together with the footnotes on the following pages of this schedule.

Centers for Disease Control and Prevention (CDC). Advisory Committee on Immunization Practices (ACIP). Recommended Immunization Schedule for Adults Aged 19 Years and Older: United States, 2015. Available at www.cdc.gov/vaccines/schedules/downloads/adult/adult-combined-schedule.pdf. Accessed February 12, 2015.

Footnotes—Recommended Immunization Schedule for Adults Aged 19 Years or Older: United States, 2015

1. Additional information
- Additional guidance for the use of the vaccines described in this supplement is available at www.cdc.gov/vaccines/hcp/acip-recs/index.html.
- Information on vaccination recommendations when vaccination status is unknown and other general immunization information can be found in the General Recommendations on Immunization at www.cdc.gov/mmwr/preview/mmwrhtml/rr6002a1.htm.
- Information on travel vaccine requirements and recommendations (e.g., for hepatitis A and B, meningococcal, and other vaccines) is available at wwwnc.cdc.gov/travel/destinations/list.
- Additional information and resources regarding vaccination of pregnant women can be found at www.cdc.gov/vaccines/adults/rec-vac/pregnant.html.

2. Influenza vaccination
- Annual vaccination against influenza is recommended for all persons aged 6 months or older.
- Persons aged 6 months or older, including pregnant women and persons with hives-only allergy to eggs can receive the inactivated influenza vaccine (IIV). An age-appropriate IIV formulation should be used.
- Adults aged 18 years or older can receive the recombinant influenza vaccine (RIV) (FluBlok). RIV does not contain any egg protein and can be given to age-appropriate persons with egg allergy of any severity.
- Healthy, nonpregnant persons aged 2 to 49 years without high-risk medical conditions can receive either intranasally administered live, attenuated influenza vaccine (LAIV) (FluMist) or IIV.
- Health care personnel who care for severely immunocompromised persons who require care in a protected environment should receive IIV or RIV; health care personnel who receive LAIV should avoid providing care for severely immunosuppressed persons for 7 days after vaccination.
- The intramuscularly or intradermally administered IIV are options for adults aged 18 through 64 years.
- Adults aged 65 years or older can receive the standard-dose IIV or the high-dose IIV (Fluzone High-Dose).
- A list of currently available influenza vaccines can be found at www.cdc.gov/flu/protect/vaccine/vaccines.htm.

3. Tetanus, diphtheria, and acellular pertussis (Td/Tdap) vaccination
- Administer 1 dose of Tdap vaccine to pregnant women during each pregnancy (preferably during 27 to 36 weeks' gestation) regardless of interval since prior Td or Tdap vaccination.
- Persons aged 11 years or older who have not received Tdap vaccine or for whom vaccine status is unknown should receive a dose of Tdap followed by tetanus and diphtheria toxoids (Td) booster doses every 10 years thereafter. Tdap can be administered regardless of interval since the most recent tetanus or diphtheria-toxoid containing vaccine.
- Adults with an unknown or incomplete history of completing a 3-dose primary vaccination series with Td-containing vaccines should begin or complete a primary vaccination series including a Tdap dose.
- For unvaccinated adults, administer the first 2 doses at least 4 weeks apart and the third dose 6 to 12 months after the second.
- For incompletely vaccinated (i.e., less than 3 doses) adults, administer remaining doses.
- Refer to the ACIP statement for recommendations for administering Td/Tdap as prophylaxis in wound management (see footnote 1).

4. Varicella vaccination
- All adults without evidence of immunity to varicella (as defined below) should receive 2 doses of single-antigen varicella vaccine or a second dose if they have received only 1 dose.
- Vaccination should be emphasized for those who have close contact with persons at high risk for severe disease (e.g., health care personnel and family contacts of persons with immunocompromising conditions) or are at high risk for exposure or transmission (e.g., teachers; child care employees; residents and staff members of institutional settings, including correctional institutions; college students; military personnel; adolescents and adults living in households with children; nonpregnant women of childbearing age; and international travelers).
- Pregnant women should be assessed for evidence of varicella immunity. Women who do not have evidence of immunity should receive the first dose of varicella vaccine upon completion or termination of pregnancy and before discharge from the health care facility. The second dose should be administered 4 to 8 weeks after the first dose.
- Evidence of immunity to varicella in adults includes any of the following:
  — documentation of 2 doses of varicella vaccine at least 4 weeks apart;
  — U.S.-born before 1980, except health care personnel and pregnant women;
  — history of varicella based on diagnosis or verification of varicella disease by a health care provider;
  — history of herpes zoster based on diagnosis or verification of herpes zoster disease by a health care provider; or
  — laboratory evidence of immunity or laboratory confirmation of disease.

5. Human papillomavirus (HPV) vaccination
- Two vaccines are licensed for use in females, bivalent HPV vaccine (HPV2) and quadrivalent HPV vaccine (HPV4), and one HPV vaccine for use in males (HPV4).
- For females, either HPV4 or HPV2 is recommended in a 3-dose series for routine vaccination at age 11 or 12 years and for those aged 13 through 26 years, if not previously vaccinated.

- For males, HPV4 is recommended in a 3-dose series for routine vaccination at age 11 or 12 years and for those aged 13 through 21 years, if not previously vaccinated. Males aged 22 through 26 years may be vaccinated.
- HPV4 is recommended for men who have sex with men through age 26 years for those who did not get any or all doses when they were younger.
- Vaccination is recommended for immunocompromised persons (including those with HIV infection) through age 26 years for those who did not get any or all doses when they were younger.
- A complete series for either HPV4 or HPV2 consists of 3 doses. The second dose should be administered 4 to 8 weeks (minimum interval of 4 weeks) after the first dose; the third dose should be administered 24 weeks after the first dose and 16 weeks after the second dose (minimum interval of at least 12 weeks).
- HPV vaccines are not recommended for use in pregnant women. However, pregnancy testing is not needed before vaccination. If a woman is found to be pregnant after initiating the vaccination series, no intervention is needed; the remainder of the 3-dose series should be delayed until completion or termination of pregnancy.

6. Zoster vaccination
- A single dose of zoster vaccine is recommended for adults aged 60 years or older regardless of whether they report a prior episode of herpes zoster. Although the vaccine is licensed by the U.S. Food and Drug Administration for use among and can be administered to persons aged 50 years or older, ACIP recommends that vaccination begin at age 60 years.
- Persons aged 60 years or older with chronic medical conditions may be vaccinated unless their condition constitutes a contraindication, such as pregnancy or severe immunodeficiency.

7. Measles, mumps, rubella (MMR) vaccination
- Adults born before 1957 are generally considered immune to measles and mumps. All adults born in 1957 or later should have documentation of 1 or more doses of MMR vaccine unless they have a medical contraindication to the vaccine or laboratory evidence of immunity to each of the three diseases. Documentation of provider-diagnosed disease is not considered acceptable evidence of immunity for measles, mumps, or rubella.

Measles component:
- A routine second dose of MMR vaccine, administered a minimum of 28 days after the first dose, is recommended for adults who:
  — are students in postsecondary educational institutions,
  — work in a health care facility, or
  — plan to travel internationally.
- Persons who received inactivated (killed) measles vaccine or measles vaccine of unknown type during 1963–1967 should be revaccinated with 2 doses of MMR vaccine.

Mumps component:
- A routine second dose of MMR vaccine, administered a minimum of 28 days after the first dose, is recommended for adults who:
  — are students in a postsecondary educational institution,
  — work in a health care facility, or
  — plan to travel internationally.
- Persons vaccinated before 1979 with either killed mumps vaccine or mumps vaccine of unknown type who are at high risk for mumps infection (e.g., persons who are working in a health care facility) should be considered for revaccination with 2 doses of MMR vaccine.

Rubella component:
- For women of childbearing age, regardless of birth year, rubella immunity should be determined. If there is no evidence of immunity, women who are not pregnant should be vaccinated. Pregnant women who do not have evidence of immunity should receive MMR vaccine upon completion or termination of pregnancy and before discharge from the health care facility.

Health care personnel born before 1957:
- For unvaccinated health care personnel born before 1957 who lack laboratory evidence of measles, mumps, and/or rubella immunity or laboratory confirmation of disease, health care facilities should consider vaccinating personnel with 2 doses of MMR vaccine at the appropriate interval for measles and mumps or 1 dose of MMR vaccine for rubella.

8. Pneumococcal (13-valent pneumococcal conjugate vaccine [PCV13] and 23-valent pneumococcal polysaccharide vaccine [PPSV23]) vaccination
- General information
  — When indicated, only a single dose of PCV13 is recommended for adults.
  — No additional dose of PPSV23 is indicated for adults vaccinated with PPSV23 at or after age 65 years.
  — When both PCV13 and PPSV23 are indicated, PCV13 should be administered first; PCV13 and PPSV23 should not be administered during the same visit.
  — When indicated, PCV13 and PPSV23 should be administered to adults whose pneumococcal vaccination history is incomplete or unknown.
- Adults aged 65 years or older who
  — Have not received PCV13 or PPSV23: Administer PCV13 followed by PPSV23 in 6 to 12 months.
  — Have not received PCV13 but have received a dose of PPSV23 at age 65 years or older: Administer PCV13 at least 1 year after the dose of PPSV23 received at age 65 years or older.

Footnotes—Recommended Immunization Schedule for Adults Aged 19 Years or Older: United States, 2015 (continued)

8. Pneumococcal vaccination (continued)

— Have not received PCV13 but have received 1 or more doses of PPSV23 before age 65: Administer PCV13 at least 1 year after the most recent dose of PPSV23; administer a dose of PPSV23 6 to 12 months after PCV13, or as soon as possible if this time window has passed, and at least 5 years after the most recent dose of PPSV23.

— Have received PCV13 but not PPSV23 before age 65 years: Administer PPSV23 6 to 12 months after PCV13 or as soon as possible if this time window has passed.

— Have received PCV13 and 1 or more doses of PPSV23 before age 65 years: Administer PPSV23 6 to 12 months after PCV13, or as soon as possible if this time window has passed, and at least 5 years after the most recent dose of PPSV23.

• Adults aged 19 through 64 years with immunocompromising conditions or anatomical or functional asplenia (defined below) who

— Have not received PCV13 or PPSV23: Administer PCV13 followed by PPSV23 at least 8 weeks after PCV13; administer a second dose of PPSV23 at least 5 years after the first dose of PPSV23.

— Have not received PCV13 but have received 1 dose of PPSV23: Administer PCV13 at least 1 year after the PPSV23; administer a second dose of PPSV23 at least 8 weeks after PCV13 and at least 5 years after the first dose of PPSV23.

— Have not received PCV13 but have received 2 doses of PPSV23: Administer PCV13 at least 1 year after the most recent dose of PPSV23.

— Have received PCV13 but not PPSV23: Administer PPSV23 at least 8 weeks after PCV13; administer a second dose of PPSV23 at least 5 years after the first dose of PPSV23.

— Have received PCV13 and 1 dose of PPSV23: Administer a second dose of PPSV23 at least 5 years after the first dose of PPSV23.

• Adults aged 19 through 64 years with cerebrospinal fluid leaks or cochlear implants: Administer PCV13 followed by PPSV23 at least 8 weeks after PCV13.

• Adults aged 19 through 64 years with chronic heart disease (including congestive heart failure and cardiomyopathies, excluding hypertension), chronic lung disease (including chronic obstructive lung disease, emphysema, and asthma), chronic liver disease (including cirrhosis), alcoholism, or diabetes mellitus: Administer PPSV23.

• Adults aged 19 through 64 years who smoke cigarettes or reside in nursing home or long-term care facilities: Administer PPSV23.

• Routine pneumococcal vaccination is not recommended for American Indian/Alaska Native or other adults unless they have the indications as above; however, public health authorities may consider recommending the use of pneumococcal vaccines for American Indians/Alaska Natives or other adults who live in areas with increased risk for invasive pneumococcal disease.

• Immunocompromising conditions that are indications for pneumococcal vaccination are: Congenital or acquired immunodeficiency (including B- or T-lymphocyte deficiency, complement deficiencies, and phagocytic disorders excluding chronic granulomatous disease), HIV infection, chronic renal failure, nephrotic syndrome, leukemia, lymphoma, Hodgkin disease, generalized malignancy, multiple myeloma, solid organ transplant, and iatrogenic immunosuppression (including long-term systemic corticosteroids and radiation therapy).

• Anatomical or functional asplenia that are indications for pneumococcal vaccination are: Sickle cell disease and other hemoglobinopathies, congenital or acquired asplenia, splenic dysfunction, and splenectomy. Administer pneumococcal vaccines at least 2 weeks before immunosuppressive therapy or an elective splenectomy, and as soon as possible to adults who are newly diagnosed with asymptomatic or symptomatic HIV infection.

9. Meningococcal vaccination

• Administer 2 doses of quadrivalent meningococcal conjugate vaccine (MenACWY [Menactra, Menveo]) at least 2 months apart to adults of all ages with anatomical or functional asplenia or persistent complement component deficiencies. HIV infection is not an indication for routine vaccination with MenACWY. If an HIV-infected person of any age is vaccinated, 2 doses of MenACWY should be administered at least 2 months apart.

• Administer a single dose of meningococcal vaccine to microbiologists routinely exposed to isolates of *Neisseria meningitidis*, military recruits, persons at risk during an outbreak attributable to a vaccine serogroup, and persons who travel to or live in countries in which meningococcal disease is hyperendemic or epidemic.

• First-year college students up through age 21 years who are living in residence halls should be vaccinated if they have not received a dose on or after their 16th birthday.

• MenACWY is preferred for adults with any of the preceding indications who are aged 55 years or younger as well as for adults aged 56 years or older who a) were vaccinated previously with MenACWY and are recommended for revaccination, or b) for whom multiple doses are anticipated. Meningococcal polysaccharide vaccine (MPSV4 [Menomune]) is preferred for adults aged 56 years or older who have not received MenACWY previously and who require a single dose only (e.g., travelers).

• Revaccination with MenACWY every 5 years is recommended for adults previously vaccinated with MenACWY or MPSV4 who remain at increased risk for infection (e.g., adults with anatomical or functional asplenia, persistent complement component deficiencies, or microbiologists).

10. Hepatitis A vaccination

• Vaccinate any person seeking protection from hepatitis A virus (HAV) infection and persons with any of the following indications:

— men who have sex with men and persons who use injection or noninjection illicit drugs;

— persons working with HAV-infected primates or with HAV in a research laboratory setting;

— persons with chronic liver disease and persons who receive clotting factor concentrates;

— persons traveling to or working in countries that have high or intermediate endemicity of hepatitis A; and

— unvaccinated persons who anticipate close personal contact (e.g., household or regular babysitting) with an international adoptee during the first 60 days after arrival in the United States from a country with high or intermediate endemicity. (See footnote 1 for more information on travel recommendations.) The first dose of the 2-dose hepatitis A vaccine series should be administered as soon as adoption is planned, ideally 2 or more weeks before the arrival of the adoptee.

• Single-antigen vaccine formulations should be administered in a 2-dose schedule at either 0 and 6 to 12 months (Havrix), or 0 and 6 to 18 months (Vaqta). If the combined hepatitis A and hepatitis B vaccine (Twinrix) is used, administer 3 doses at 0, 1, and 6 months; alternatively, a 4-dose schedule may be used, administered on days 0, 7, and 21 to 30 followed by a booster dose at month 12.

11. Hepatitis B vaccination

• Vaccinate persons with any of the following indications and any person seeking protection from hepatitis B virus (HBV) infection:

— sexually active persons who are not in a long-term, mutually monogamous relationship (e.g., persons with more than 1 sex partner during the previous 6 months); persons seeking evaluation or treatment for a sexually transmitted disease (STD); current or recent injection drug users; and men who have sex with men;

— health care personnel and public safety workers who are potentially exposed to blood or other infectious body fluids;

— persons with diabetes who are younger than age 60 years as soon as feasible after diagnosis; persons with diabetes who are age 60 years or older at the discretion of the treating clinician based on the likelihood of acquiring HBV infection, including the risk posed by an increased need for assisted blood glucose monitoring in long-term care facilities, the likelihood of experiencing chronic sequelae if infected with HBV, and the likelihood of immune response to vaccination;

— persons with end-stage renal disease, including patients receiving hemodialysis, persons with HIV infection, and persons with chronic liver disease;

— household contacts and sex partners of hepatitis B surface antigen–positive persons, clients and staff members of institutions for persons with developmental disabilities, and international travelers to countries with high or intermediate prevalence of chronic HBV infection; and

— all adults in the following settings: STD treatment facilities, HIV testing and treatment facilities, facilities providing drug abuse treatment and prevention services, health care settings targeting services to injection drug users or men who have sex with men, correctional facilities, end-stage renal disease programs and facilities for chronic hemodialysis patients, and institutions and nonresidential day care facilities for persons with developmental disabilities.

• Administer missing doses to complete a 3-dose series of hepatitis B vaccine to those persons not vaccinated or not completely vaccinated. The second dose should be administered 1 month after the first dose; the third dose should be given at least 2 months after the second dose (and at least 4 months after the first dose). If the combined hepatitis A and hepatitis B vaccine (Twinrix) is used, give 3 doses at 0, 1, and 6 months; alternatively, a 4-dose Twinrix schedule, administered on days 0, 7, and 21 to 30 followed by a booster dose at month 12 may be used.

• Adult patients receiving hemodialysis or with other immunocompromising conditions should receive 1 dose of 40 mcg/mL (Recombivax HB) administered on a 3-dose schedule at 0, 1, and 6 months or 2 doses of 20 mcg/mL (Engerix-B) administered simultaneously on a 4-dose schedule at 0, 1, 2, and 6 months.

12. *Haemophilus influenzae* type b (Hib) vaccination

• One dose of Hib vaccine should be administered to persons who have anatomical or functional asplenia or sickle cell disease or are undergoing elective splenectomy if they have not previously received Hib vaccine. Hib vaccination 14 or more days before splenectomy is suggested.

• Recipients of a hematopoietic stem cell transplant (HSCT) should be vaccinated with a 3-dose regimen 6 to 12 months after a successful transplant, regardless of vaccination history; at least 4 weeks should separate doses.

• Hib vaccine is not recommended for adults with HIV infection since their risk for Hib infection is low.

13. Immunocompromising conditions

• Inactivated vaccines generally are acceptable (e.g., pneumococcal, meningococcal, and inactivated influenza vaccine) and live vaccines generally are avoided in persons with immune deficiencies or immunocompromising conditions. Information on specific conditions is available at www.cdc.gov/vaccines/hcp/acip-recs/index.html.

Figure 3. Footnotes from adult immunization schedule, United States, 2015.

Centers for Disease Control and Prevention (CDC). Advisory Committee on Immunization Practices (ACIP). Recommended Immunization Schedule for Adults Aged 19 Years and Older: United States, 2015. Available at www.cdc.gov/vaccines/schedules/downloads/adult/adult-combined-schedule.pdf. Accessed February 12, 2015.

Table 17. Contraindications and Precautions to Commonly Used Vaccines in Adults: United States, 2015

Vaccine	Contraindications	Precautions
Influenza, inactivated (IIV)[2]	• Severe allergic reaction (e.g., anaphylaxis) after previous dose of any influenza vaccine; or to a vaccine component, including egg protein	• Moderate or severe acute illness with or without fever • History of Guillain-Barré Syndrome within 6 weeks of previous influenza vaccination • Adults who experience only hives with exposure to eggs may receive RIV or, with additional safety precautions, IIV[2]
Influenza, recombinant (RIV)	• Severe allergic reaction (e.g., anaphylaxis) after previous dose of RIV or to a vaccine component. RIV does not contain any egg protein[2]	• Moderate or severe acute illness with or without fever • History of Guillain-Barré Syndrome within 6 weeks of previous influenza vaccination
Influenza, live attenuated (LAIV)[2,3]	• Severe allergic reaction (e.g., anaphylaxis) to any component of the vaccine, or to a previous dose of any influenza vaccine • In addition, ACIP recommends that LAIV not be used in the following populations: — pregnant women — immunosuppressed adults — adults with egg allergy of any severity — adults who have taken influenza antiviral medications (amantadine, rimantadine, zanamivir, or oseltamivir) within the previous 48 hours; avoid use of these antiviral drugs for 14 days after vaccination	• Moderate or severe acute illness with or without fever. • History of Guillain-Barré Syndrome within 6 weeks of previous influenza vaccination • Asthma in persons aged 5 years and older • Other chronic medical conditions, e.g., other chronic lung diseases, chronic cardiovascular disease (excluding isolated hypertension), diabetes, chronic renal or hepatic disease, hematologic disease, neurologic disease, and metabolic disorders
Tetanus, diphtheria, pertussis (Tdap); tetanus, diphtheria (Td)	• Severe allergic reaction (e.g., anaphylaxis) after a previous dose or to a vaccine component • For pertussis-containing vaccines: encephalopathy (e.g., coma, decreased level of consciousness, or prolonged seizures) not attributable to another identifiable cause within 7 days of administration of a previous dose of Tdap, diphtheria and tetanus toxoids and pertussis (DTP), or diphtheria and tetanus toxoids and acellular pertussis (DTaP) vaccine	• Moderate or severe acute illness with or without fever • Guillain-Barré Syndrome within 6 weeks after a previous dose of tetanus toxoid-containing vaccine • History of Arthus-type hypersensitivity reactions after a previous dose of tetanus or diphtheria toxoid-containing vaccine; defer vaccination until at least 10 years have elapsed since the last tetanus toxoid-containing vaccine • For pertussis-containing vaccines: progressive or unstable neurologic disorder, uncontrolled seizures, or progressive encephalopathy until a treatment regimen has been established and the condition has stabilized
Varicella[3]	• Severe allergic reaction (e.g., anaphylaxis) after a previous dose or to a vaccine component • Known severe immunodeficiency (e.g., from hematologic and solid tumors, receipt of chemotherapy, congenital immunodeficiency, or long-term immunosuppressive therapy,[4] or patients with human immunodeficiency virus [HIV] infection who are severely immunocompromised) • Pregnancy	• Recent (within 11 months) receipt of antibody-containing blood product (specific interval depends on product)[5] • Moderate or severe acute illness with or without fever • Receipt of specific antivirals (i.e., acyclovir, famciclovir, or valacyclovir) 24 hours before vaccination; avoid use of these antiviral drugs for 14 days after vaccination
Human papillomavirus (HPV)	• Severe allergic reaction (e.g., anaphylaxis) after a previous dose or to a vaccine component	• Moderate or severe acute illness with or without fever • Pregnancy
Zoster[3]	• Severe allergic reaction (e.g., anaphylaxis) to a vaccine component • Known severe immunodeficiency (e.g., from hematologic and solid tumors, receipt of chemotherapy, or long-term immunosuppressive therapy,4 or patients with HIV infection who are severely immunocompromised) • Pregnancy	• Moderate or severe acute illness with or without fever • Receipt of specific antivirals (i.e., acyclovir, famciclovir, or valacyclovir) 24 hours before vaccination; avoid use of these antiviral drugs for 14 days after vaccination
Measles, mumps, rubella (MMR)[3]	• Severe allergic reaction (e.g., anaphylaxis) after a previous dose or to a vaccine component • Known severe immunodeficiency (e.g., from hematologic and solid tumors, receipt of chemotherapy, congenital immunodeficiency, or long-term immunosuppressive therapy,[4] or patients with HIV infection who are severely immunocompromised) • Pregnancy	• Moderate or severe acute illness with or without fever • Recent (within 11 months) receipt of antibody-containing blood product (specific interval depends on product)[5] • History of thrombocytopenia or thrombocytopenic purpura • Need for tuberculin skin testing[6]
Pneumococcal conjugate (PCV13)	• Severe allergic reaction (e.g., anaphylaxis) after a previous dose or to a vaccine component, including to any vaccine containing diphtheria toxoid	• Moderate or severe acute illness with or without fever
Pneumococcal polysaccharide (PPSV23)	• Severe allergic reaction (e.g., anaphylaxis) after a previous dose or to a vaccine component	• Moderate or severe acute illness with or without fever
Meningococcal, conjugate (MenACWY); meningococcal, polysaccharide (MPSV4)	• Severe allergic reaction (e.g., anaphylaxis) after a previous dose or to a vaccine component	• Moderate or severe acute illness with or without fever
Hepatitis A	• Severe allergic reaction (e.g., anaphylaxis) after a previous dose or to a vaccine component	• Moderate or severe acute illness with or without fever
Hepatitis B	• Severe allergic reaction (e.g., anaphylaxis) after a previous dose or to a vaccine component	• Moderate or severe acute illness with or without fever
Haemophilus influenzae Type b (Hib)	• Severe allergic reaction (e.g., anaphylaxis) after a previous dose or to a vaccine component	• Moderate or severe acute illness with or without fever

1. Vaccine package inserts and the full ACIP recommendations for these vaccines should be consulted for additional information on vaccine-related contraindications and precautions and for more information on vaccine excipients. Events or conditions listed as precautions should be reviewed carefully. Benefits of and risks for administering a specific vaccine to a person under these circumstances should be considered. If the risk from the vaccine is believed to outweigh the benefit, the vaccine should not be administered. If the benefit of vaccination is believed to outweigh the risk, the vaccine should be administered. A contraindication is a condition in a recipient that increases the chance of a serious adverse reaction. Therefore, a vaccine should not be administered when a contraindication is present.

2. For more information on use of influenza vaccines among persons with egg allergies and a complete list of conditions that CDC considers to be reasons to avoid receiving LAIV, see CDC. Prevention and control of seasonal influenza with vaccines: recommendations of the Advisory Committee on Immunization Practices (ACIP) — United States, 2014–15 Influenza Season. MMWR 2014;63(32):691–97.

3. LAIV, MMR, varicella, or zoster vaccines can be administered on the same day. If not administered on the same day, live vaccines should be separated by at least 28 days.

4. Immunosuppressive steroid dose is considered to be >2 weeks of daily receipt of 20 mg of prednisone or the equivalent. Vaccination should be deferred for at least 1 month after discontinuation of such therapy. Providers should consult ACIP recommendations for complete information on the use of specific live vaccines among persons on immune-suppressing medications or with immune suppression because of other reasons.

5. Vaccine should be deferred for the appropriate interval if replacement immune globulin products are being administered. See CDC. General recommendations on immunization: recommendations of the Advisory Committee on Immunization Practices (ACIP). MMWR 2011;60(No. RR-2). Available at www.cdc.gov/vaccines/pubs/pinkbook/index.html.

6. Measles vaccination might suppress tuberculin reactivity temporarily. Measles-containing vaccine may be administered on the same day as tuberculin skin testing. If testing cannot be performed until after the day of MMR vaccination, the test should be postponed for at least 4 weeks after the vaccination. If an urgent need exists to skin test, do so with the understanding that reactivity might be reduced by the vaccine.

* Adapted from CDC. Table 6. Contraindications and precautions to commonly used vaccines. General recommendations on immunization: recommendations of the Advisory Committee on Immunization Practices. MMWR 2011;60(No. RR-2):40–41 and from Atkinson W, Wolfe S, Hamborsky J, eds. Appendix A. Epidemiology and prevention of vaccine preventable diseases. 12th ed. Washington, DC: Public Health Foundation, 2011. Available at www.cdc.gov/vaccines/pubs/pinkbook/index.html.

† Regarding latex allergy, consult the package insert for any vaccine administered.

Centers for Disease Control and Prevention (CDC). Advisory Committee on Immunization Practices (ACIP). Recommended Immunization Schedule for Adults Aged 19 Years and Older: United States, 2015. Available at www.cdc.gov/vaccines/schedules/downloads/adult/adult-combined-schedule.pdf. Accessed February 12, 2015.

A. Major Changes in the 2015 Adult Immunization Schedule from the 2014 Schedule
    1. Pneumococcal vaccination
        a. PCV13 (Prevnar) should now be used for adult pneumococcal vaccination in people age 65 years and older, in addition to PPSV23 (Pneumovax).
        b. In pneumococcal vaccine-naive patients 65 years or older: PCV13 at age 65 years or older, followed by PPSV23 6–12 months later.
        c. In patients who previously received PPSV23 at age 65 years or older: Vaccinate with PCV13 1 year or more after PPSV23.
        d. In patients who previously received PPSV23 before age 65 years who are now aged 65 years or older: Vaccinate with PCV13 1 year or more after receipt of PPSV23 and revaccinate with PPSV23 6–12 months after PCV13, as long as 5 or more years has passed since the previous PPSV23.
    2. Influenza vaccination
        a. All adults aged 18 and older can receive recombinant hemagglutinin influenza vaccine, trivalent (RIV3) [previously was adults aged 18 – 49]
        b. There are changes to the contraindications and precautions section for LAIV
            i.   Influenza antiviral use within the last 48 hours is now a contraindication (was previously a precaution)
            ii. Asthma and chronic lung diseases; cardiovascular, renal and hepatic diseases; and diabetes and other conditions are now precautions (were previously contraindications)

B. Newer Issues with Influenza Vaccine
    1. Trivalent inactivated influenza vaccine (TIV) is now called inactivated influenza vaccine, trivalent (IIV3) (all egg-based); several brands available, including one that is high-dose.
    2. Quadrivalent IIV vaccines (IIV4) are available (all egg-based); several brands available.
    3. A trivalent cell culture–based IIV3 is available (not egg-based) (ccIIV3) (Flucelvax), indicated for age 18 and older.
        – Egg amount is very low but is not considered egg-free.
    4. A recombinant hemagglutinin influenza vaccine, trivalent (RIV3) (FluBlok) is available, indicated for age 18 and older.
        – Eggs not used in development; is completely egg-free.
    5. LAIV is still available as a nasal spray and is now quadrivalent, indicated for healthy, nonpregnant patients age 2–49 years.
        a. LAIV should not be used in:
            i.   Patients aged less than 2 or more than 49 years
            ii.   Children aged 2–17 years who are receiving aspirin or aspirin-containing products
            iii. Pregnant women
            iv.   Immunocompromised patients
            v.   Patients with an egg allergy or with history of a severe allergic reaction to the vaccine
            vi.   Children aged 2–4 years who have asthma or who have had a wheezing episode in the past 12 months
                  – Use with caution in patients of any age who have asthma, because they are at greater risk of wheezing after receipt of LAIV.
            vii. Patients who have taken influenza antiviral medications in past 48 hours
            viii. Patients who care for immunocompromised people should not receive LAIV or should avoid contact for 7 days after receiving the vaccine.

6. Egg allergy
    a. If a patient has experienced only hives after eating eggs or egg-containing foods, he or she should receive influenza vaccine, either IIV3, IIV4, ccIIV3, or RIV3. Avoid LAIV.
        i.   If IIV3, IIV4, or ccIIV3 is used, the health care provider administering the vaccine should be familiar with manifestations of egg allergy.
        ii. The vaccine recipient should be observed for at least 30 minutes after each vaccine dose.
        iii. If RIV3 is used, no special precautions are necessary.
    b. If a patient has experienced a severe reaction to eggs, such as angioedema, respiratory distress, lightheadedness, or recurrent emesis, or required epinephrine or emergency treatment, he or she may receive RIV3 (if age 18–49 years).
        i.   If RIV3 is not available or the recipient is outside the age range, any of the IIVs can be used but should be administered by a physician with experience in recognition and management of severe allergic conditions.
        ii. The vaccine recipient should be observed for at least 30 minutes after each vaccine dose.
    c. Some people who report egg allergies may not actually be allergic to eggs. Those who are able to eat lightly cooked egg (e.g., scrambled egg) without a reaction are not likely to be allergic and can receive any influenza vaccine.

C. Current Issues with Herpes Zoster Vaccine (HZV): The HZV package insert states not to give HZV and PPSV concurrently but to separate them by at least 4 weeks because of decreased immunologic response to HZV. Their conclusion is based on a Merck-sponsored, unpublished study. The ACIP states that the clinical relevance of this recommendation is unknown, and a subsequent study showed no compromise in HZV efficacy. The Advisory Committee on Immunization Practices/Centers for Disease Control and Prevention (ACIP/CDC), which reviewed the data, continues to recommend that HZV and PPSV be administered at the same visit if the person is eligible for both vaccines.

Patient Cases

14. A 71-year-old woman with COPD is taking tiotropium (Spiriva) inhaled 1 capsule/day. She received the influenza vaccine last October, her last tetanus and diphtheria (Td) vaccine was at age 65, and her PPSV23 was given at age 60. She has not previously received the zoster vaccine, but she had an episode of severe zoster infection 5 years ago. Which is the most appropriate choice of vaccines that should be given at her October internal medicine clinic appointment?

    A. Only the influenza vaccine should be given.

    B. Influenza and PPSV23 vaccines should be given.

    C. Influenza, PPSV23, and zoster vaccines should be given.

    D. Influenza, PPSV23, zoster, and tetanus, diphtheria, and pertussis [Tdap] vaccines should be given.

15. A 20-year-old woman who is going away to college presents for a physical examination in July. She will be living in the dormitory. She smokes 1/2 pack/day but has no other medical conditions. She is up to date with all of her routine childhood vaccines, but she has not received any vaccines in the past 11 years. She is not sexually active. Which is the most appropriate choice for vaccines that should be given today?

    A. Td and human papillomavirus (HPV) vaccines.

    B. Tdap, quadrivalent meningococcal conjugate vaccine (MenACWY), and HPV vaccines.

    C. MenACWY, PPSV23, and Td vaccines.

    D. MenACWY, PPSV23, Tdap, and HPV vaccines.

16. A 21 year-old man with type 1 diabetes presents for an influenza vaccine. He has an egg allergy. After further questioning, you find out that when he has eaten scrambled eggs, he has experienced hives. Which is the most appropriate regarding influenza vaccination in this patient?

    A. Either IIV3, IIV4, ccIIV3, RIV3, or LAIV can be used; observe patient for 30 minutes.

    B. Either IIV3, IIV4, ccIIV3, or RIV3 can be used; observe patient for 30 minutes.

    C. Only RIV3 should be used; observe patient for 30 minutes.

    D. He should not receive any type of influenza vaccine.

REFERENCES

Asthma

1. Agency for Healthcare Research and Quality. Module 4: measuring quality of care for asthma. Available at www.ahrq.gov/qual/asthmacare/asthmod4.htm. Accessed September 1, 2014.

2. Global Initiative for Asthma (GINA). Global Strategy for Asthma Management and Prevention 2014. Available at www.ginasthma.org. Accessed October 15, 2014.

3. Global Initiative for Asthma (GINA) and Global Initiative for Chronic Obstructive Lung Disease (GOLD). Diagnosis of diseases of chronic airflow limitation: asthma, COPD and asthma-COPD overlap syndrome (ACOS). Available at www.ginasthma.org. Accessed October 15, 2014.

4. Martinez FD, Chinchilli VM, Morgan WJ, et al. Use of beclomethasone dipropionate as rescue treatment for children with mild persistent asthma (TREXA): a randomized, double-blind, placebo-controlled trial. Lancet 2011;377:650-7.

5. National Institutes of Health National Heart, Lung and Blood Institute. National Asthma Education and Prevention Program (NAEPP) guidelines. NAEPP Expert Panel Report 3. NIH Publication 08-5846. July 2007. Available at www.nhlbi.nih.gov/guidelines/index.htm. Accessed September 1, 2014.

6. Nelson HS, Weiss ST, Bleecker ER, et al. The Salmeterol Multicenter Asthma Research Trial (SMART): a comparison of usual pharmacotherapy for asthma or usual pharmacotherapy plus salmeterol. Chest 2006;129:15-26.

7. Perera BJ. Salmeterol Multicentre Asthma Research Trial (SMART): interim analysis shows increased risk of asthma-related deaths. Ceylon Med J 2003;48:99.

8. Peters SP, Kunselman SJ, Icitovic N, et al. Tiotropium bromide step-up therapy for adults with uncontrolled asthma (TALC study). N Engl J Med 2010;363:1715-26.

9. Price D, Musgrave SD, Shepstone L, et al. Leukotriene antagonists as first-line or add-on asthma-controller therapy. N Engl J Med 2011;364:1695-707.

Chronic Obstructive Pulmonary Disease

1. Albert RK, Connett J, Bailey WC, et al. Azithromycin for prevention of exacerbations of COPD. N Engl J Med 2011;365:689-98.

2. Bestall JC, Paul EA, Garrod R, et al. Usefulness of the Medical Research Council (MRC) dyspnea scale as a measure of disability in patients with chronic obstructive pulmonary disease. Thorax 1999;54:581-6.

3. Calverley PMA, Anderson JA, Celli B, et al. Salmeterol and fluticasone propionate and survival in chronic obstructive pulmonary disease (the TORCH study). N Engl J Med 2007;356:775-89.

4. Chong J, Karner C, Poole P. Tiotropium versus long-acting beta-agonists for stable chronic obstructive pulmonary disease. Cochrane Database Syst Rev 2012;9:CD009157.

5. Ernst P, Gonzalez AP, Brassard P, et al. Inhaled corticosteroid use in chronic obstructive pulmonary disease and the risk of hospitalization for pneumonia. Am J Respir Crit Care Med 2007;176:162-6.

6. Fiore MC, Jaen CR, Baker TB, et al. Treating Tobacco Use and Dependence: 2008 Update. Rockville, MD: U.S. Department of Health and Human Services, Public Health Service, 2008. Available at www.ncbi.nlm.nih.gov/bookshelf/br.fcgi?book=hsahcpr&part=A28163. Accessed September 26, 2011.

7. Global Initiative for Chronic Obstructive Lung Disease Workshop Executive Summary: Global Strategy for the Diagnosis, Management, and Prevention of Chronic Obstructive Pulmonary Disease, 2014 Update. Available at www.goldcopd.org. Accessed October 1, 2014.

8. Global Initiative for Asthma (GINA) and Global Initiative for Chronic Obstructive Lung Disease (GOLD). Diagnosis of diseases of chronic airflow limitation: asthma, COPD and asthma-COPD overlap syndrome (ACOS). Available at www.ginasthma.org. Accessed October 15, 2014.

9. Heffner JE, Mularski RA, Calverley PM. COPD performance measures: missing opportunities for improving care. Chest 2010;137:1181-9.

10. Leuppi JD, Schuetz P, Bingisser R, et al. Short-term vs conventional glucocorticoid therapy in acute exacerbations of chronic obstructive pulmonary disease: the REDUCE randomized clinical trial. JAMA 2013;309:2223-31.

11. McEvoy CE, Neiwoehner DE. Adverse effects of corticosteroid therapy for COPD: a critical review. Chest 1997;111:732-43.

12. Nannini LJ, Cates CJ, Lasserson TJ, et al. Combined corticosteroid and long-acting beta-agonist in one inhaler versus placebo for chronic obstructive pulmonary disease. Cochrane Database Syst Rev 2007;4:CD003794.

13. Rutten FH, Zuithoff NP, Hak E, et al. Beta-blockers may reduce mortality and risk of exacerbations in patients with chronic obstructive pulmonary disease. Arch Intern Med 2010;170:880-7.

14. Salpeter SR, Ormiston T, Salpeter E, et al. Cardioselective beta-blockers for chronic obstructive pulmonary disease [review]. Cochrane Database Syst Rev 2002;2:CD003566. Update in: Cochrane Database Syst Rev 2005;4:CD003566.

15. Singh S, Amin AV, Loke YK. Long-term use of inhaled corticosteroids and the risk of pneumonia in chronic obstructive pulmonary disease. Arch Intern Med 2009;169:219-29.

16. VanDerMolen T, Willemse BW, Schokker S, et al. Development, validity and responsiveness of the Clinical COPD Questionnaire. Health Qual Life Outcomes 2003;1:13.

17. van Grunsven PM, van Schayck CP, Dereene JP, et al. Long-term effects of inhaled corticosteroids in chronic obstructive pulmonary disease: a meta-analysis. Thorax 1999;54:7-14.

18. Vogelmeier C, Hederer B, Glaab T, et al. Tiotropium versus salmeterol for the prevention of exacerbations of COPD (POET-COPD study). N Engl J Med 2011;364:1093-103.

19. Welte T, Miravitlles M, Hernandez P, et al. Efficacy and tolerability of budesonide/formoterol added to tiotropium in patients with chronic obstructive pulmonary disease. Am J Respir Crit Care Med 2009;180:741-50.

Gout

1. Khanna D, Fitzgerald JD, Khanna PP, et al. 2012 American College of Rheumatology Guidelines for Management of Gout. Part 1. Systematic non-pharmacologic and pharmacologic therapeutic approaches to hyperuricemia. Arthritis Care Res 2012;64:1431-46.

2. Khanna D, Khanna PP, Fitzgerald JD, et al. 2012 American College of Rheumatology Guidelines for Management of Gout. Part 2. Therapy and anti-inflammatory prophylaxis of acute gouty arthritis. Arthritis Care Res 2012;64:1447-61.

3. Singh JA, Reddy SG, Kundukulam J. Risk factors for gout and prevention: a systematic review of the literature. Curr Opin Rheumatol 2011;23:192-202.

Immunizations

1. Centers for Disease Control and Prevention (CDC). Advisory Committee on Immunization Practices (ACIP). Recommended Immunization Schedule for Adults Aged 19 Years and Older: United States, 2015. Available at www.cdc.gov/vaccines/schedules/downloads/adult/adult-combined-schedule.pdf. Accessed February 11, 2015.

2. Use of 13-valent pneumococcal conjugate vaccine and 23-valent pneumococcal polysaccharide vaccine among adults aged $\geq$ 65 years: Recommendations of the Advisory Committee on Immunization Practices (ACIP). MMWR Morb Mortal Wkly Rep 2014;63(37):822–5. Available at www.cdc.gov/mmwr/preview/mmwrhtml/mm6337a4.htm. Accessed October 10, 2014.

ANSWERS AND EXPLANATIONS TO PATIENT CASES

1. Answer: B

Her symptom frequency of twice weekly, her FEV_1 of more than 80% of predicted (normal), and the lack of interference with activity are consistent with intermittent asthma. However, her night awakenings for asthma symptoms occur three times per month, which is consistent with mild persistent asthma. In addition, mild persistent asthma still has normal spirometry. The specific level of persistent asthma is based on the most severe category met, so even though only one of her signs and symptoms falls under mild persistent and the rest under intermittent, she would be categorized as mild persistent.

2. Answer: C

Because she has mild persistent asthma, step 2 is recommended for initial treatment. In addition to an inhaled SABA as needed, she would need to use a low-dose ICS (preferred treatment); mometasone 220 mcg once daily is a low-dose ICS. Montelukast is an alternative therapy (not first line) for step 2. Budesonide/formoterol, in the dose listed, is a low-dose ICS plus a LABA, which is a step 3 therapy.

3. Answer: D

Her asthma is not well controlled because the frequency of her daytime symptoms and albuterol use is greater than 2 days/week. Recommended action for treatment is to step up to step 3: a low-dose ICS plus a LABA or a medium-dose ICS alone. The budesonide/formoterol MDI is incorrect because it is a medium-dose ICS plus a LABA (a step 4 treatment). Adding montelukast to low-dose ICS is an alternative therapy.

4. Answer: D

This patient has moderate persistent asthma because of his nighttime symptoms twice weekly and requires step 3 therapy. A medium-dose ICS alone is preferred as initial therapy in this age group (5–11 years). Fluticasone 44 mcg 1 puff twice daily is a low-dose ICS for this age group. Montelukast is not recommended as monotherapy for moderate persistent asthma in this age group; montelukast is recommended only in combination with a low-dose ICS. Fluticasone/salmeterol 100/50 twice daily is a medium-dose ICS plus a LABA, which is step 4 in this age group.

5. Answer: D

Because he is experiencing shortness of breath at rest, has trouble with conversation, and has an FEV_1 less than 40%, his asthma exacerbation is classified as severe. For severe asthma exacerbations in the ED setting, the recommended treatment is oxygen to achieve an Sao_2 of 90% or greater, high-dose inhaled SABA plus ipratropium by either nebulizer or MDI with valved holding chamber every 20 minutes for 1 hour or continuously, and OCSs.

6. Answer: B

He is in GOLD guidelines patient group B because his postbronchodilator FEV_1 is between 50% and 80%, he has had 1 or no exacerbations in the past year, and his mMRC score is 2 or more. If the CAT were being used, the score would be 10 or greater.

7. Answer: B

According to the GOLD guidelines, the recommended treatment for patient group B is regular treatment with an LA bronchodilator (either a LABA or LA anticholinergic), in addition to an SA bronchodilator as needed. Inhaled corticosteroids are recommended only in groups C and D. Roflumilast is recommended only if FEV_1 is less than 50% of predicted with chronic bronchitis and the patient has a history of frequent exacerbations.

8. Answer: A

This patient is in GOLD risk group B, according to spirometry and CAT score, and is on the first-choice therapy. Because her control is worsening, she should go to the second-choice therapy, for which combined LA bronchodilators can be used. Inhaled corticosteroids are recommended only in risk groups C and D. Although a recent study showed benefits with chronic azithromycin, the guidelines do not recommend regular treatment with long-term antibiotics. In addition, the study showing the benefits of azithromycin included only patients at a higher risk of exacerbations (on continuous oxygen therapy or using systemic corticosteroids, plus a history of exacerbation requiring an ED visit or hospitalization). She does not meet these criteria.

9. Answer: D

According to the latest GOLD guidelines, OCSs are indicated in most exacerbations. The recommended dose is oral prednisone 40 mg daily for 5 days. Antibiotic treatment is also indicated because the patient has all three cardinal symptoms of airway infection: increased sputum purulence, increased sputum volume, and increased dyspnea. Trimethoprim/sulfamethoxazole is one of the recommended antibiotics.

10. Answer: A

NSAIDs (in anti-inflammatory or acute pain doses), colchicine, or corticosteroids are all appropriate for first-line therapy for acute gout. However, colchicine would not be recommended for this patient because he took acute colchicine doses in the past 2 weeks. Intra-articular corticosteroids are recommended only if only one or two large joints are affected. This patient is having an acute gouty attack of moderate severity. Combination therapy is recommended for initial therapy only if the patient has a severe attack. Oral prednisone alone would also be appropriate; however, this was not a choice.

11. Answer: D

Urate-lowering therapy is indicated in this patient because he has had two or more attacks in the past year. Allopurinol and febuxostat (XOIs) are first-line ULTs; probenecid is an alternative first-line ULT only if XOIs are contraindicated or not tolerated. Urate-lowering therapy can be initiated during an acute gouty attack, according to the American College of Rheumatology guidelines, as long as anti-inflammatory prophylaxis is instituted.

12. Answer: A

Oral corticosteroids are associated with significant risks in long-term therapy; they should not be used for anti-inflammatory prophylaxis unless both colchicine and NSAIDs are contraindicated, not tolerated, or ineffective. Combination therapy is not recommended for anti-inflammatory prophylaxis. Pegloticase is ULT, not anti-inflammatory prophylaxis.

13. Answer: B

If no tophi are present, the initial goal serum urate is <6 mg/dL; if gouty signs and symptoms are still present, then a secondary goal urate is <5 mg/dL. Anti-inflammatory prophylaxis if no tophi are present should continue for 3 months after goal serum urate is achieved, as long as the total duration is at least 6 months.

14. Answer: D

The CDC recommends that the influenza vaccine be given every year in every person 6 months and older. People 65 years and older should have a one-time pneumococcal (PPSV23) revaccination if they were vaccinated 5 or more years previously and were younger than 65 years at the time of primary vaccination. Zoster vaccination is recommended in all adults 60 years and older, regardless of previous zoster infection. The Tdap vaccine is recommended in all people, now including those 65 years and older.

15. Answer: D

First-year college students up to age 21 who live in dormitories, if not previously vaccinated on or after age 16, should receive the meningococcal vaccine (MenACWY; Menactra, Menevo). The PPSV23 is recommended for smokers 19–64 years of age, and this patient is a smoker. The Td vaccine should be given every 10 years. In adults younger than 65, a one-time dose of Tdap should be given, regardless of the time interval since the most recent tetanus vaccination. The HPV vaccine is for girls and women 11–26 years of age. Ideally, it should be given before the start of sexual activity, but it should still be administered to sexually active girls and women.

16. Answer: B

In people with an egg allergy who have only hives, either IIV3, IIV4, ccIIV3, or RIV3 can be used; LAIV should be avoided. The vaccine should be administered by a health professional with knowledge of the manifestations of egg allergy, and the patient should be observed for 30 minutes after administration.

ANSWERS AND EXPLANATIONS TO SELF-ASSESSMENT QUESTIONS

1. Answer: D

That she uses her inhaler throughout the day, every day, and sometimes at night indicates she has daily symptoms. "Severe persistent" means that frequency of symptoms is throughout the day, nighttime symptoms are often 7 times/week, a SABA several times a day, normal activity is extremely limited, FEV_1 is less than 60% of predicted, FEV_1/FVC is reduced more than 5%.

2. Answer: C

"Severe persistent" initial treatment is step 4 or 5. Step 4 preferred: inhaled steroid (medium dose) plus a LABA. Alternative: inhaled steroid (medium dose) plus either an LTM or sustained-release theophylline or zileuton. Step 5 preferred: inhaled steroid (high dose) plus a LABA.

3. Answer: D

Ratio data are ranked in a specific order with a consistent level of magnitude difference between units, with an absolute zero.

4. Answer: B

The percentage of patients receiving fluticasone/salmeterol who have an asthma-related hospitalization will be compared with the percentage of patients receiving fluticasone who have an asthma-related hospitalization. We assume that these two groups are normally distributed. These data are considered nominal. Chi-square test is appropriate to analyze nominal or categoric data. Analysis of variance is appropriate when there are more than two treatment groups. The Student unpaired t-test is used for continuous data that are normally distributed. The Mann-Whitney U test is appropriate when continuous data are not normally distributed.

5. Answer: B

Pneumococcal vaccine is recommended in persons 19–64 years of age with asthma. This patient falls into this category. Influenza vaccine is recommended in persons with chronic cardiovascular or pulmonary diseases such as asthma. However, usually, the influenza vaccine is given in the fall or early winter to offer protection when the risk of infection is highest. The tetanus booster (Td) is recommended every 10 years, and it has not been 10 years since this patient's last Td, which was given as Tdap. The HZV (Zostavax) is recommended at 60 years and older by the CDC; however, it is indicated at 50 years and older in the manufacturer's package insert.

6. Answer: B

This patient is in GOLD patient group B. A single LA bronchodilator is first choice for medication treatment. Tiotropium (Spiriva) is an LA bronchodilator (anticholinergic) that would be appropriate to initiate in this patient. A LABA would also be appropriate, but it was not one of the choices. Omalizumab is recommended for asthma, not COPD. An ICS is recommended only in patient group C or D and should never be used as monotherapy in COPD.

7. Answer: D

The starting allopurinol dose is 50 mg/day in stage 4 (GFR 15–29 mL/minute/1.73 m^2) or worse CKD; the dose should be gradually titrated every 2–5 weeks. Probenecid is not recommended as first-line ULT if CrCl is less than 50 mL/minute.

CRITICAL CARE

CHRISTOPHER A. PACIULLO, PHARM.D., BCPS, FCCM

EMORY UNIVERSITY HOSPITAL
ATLANTA, GEORGIA

CRITICAL CARE

CHRISTOPHER A. PACIULLO, PHARM.D., BCPS, FCCM

EMORY UNIVERSITY HOSPITAL
ATLANTA, GEORGIA

Learning Objectives

1. Interpret hemodynamic parameters and acid-base status in critically ill patients.

2. Differentiate between presentation of and treatment strategies for hypovolemic, obstructive, and distributive shock.

3. Discuss the appropriate use of fluids, vasopressors, antibiotics, and corticosteroids in patients with sepsis, severe sepsis, or septic shock.

4. Discuss strategies to optimize the safety and efficacy of therapeutic hypothermia for patients after cardiac arrest.

5. Recommend therapeutic options to minimize delirium and provide optimal analgesia, sedation, neuromuscular blockade, and nutritional support in critically ill patients.

6. Recommend therapeutic options to prevent stress ulcers, venous thromboembolism, hyperglycemia, and ventilator-associated pneumonia in critically ill patients.

Self-Assessment Questions

Answers and explanations to these questions can be found at the end of this chapter.

1. A 58-year-old woman remains intubated in the intensive care unit (ICU) after a recent abdominal operation. In the operating room, she receives more than 10 L of fluid and blood products but has received aggressive diuresis with furosemide postoperatively. In the past 3 days, she has generated 12 L of urine output, and her blood urea nitrogen (BUN) and serum creatinine (SCr) have steadily increased to 40 and 1.5 mg/dL, respectively. Her urine chloride (Cl) concentration was 9 mEq/L (24 hours after her last dose of furosemide). This morning, her arterial blood gas (ABG) reveals pH 7.50, $Paco_2$ 46 mm Hg, and bicarbonate (HCO_3^-) 34 mEq/L. Her vital signs include a blood pressure (BP) of 85/40 mm Hg and a heart rate (HR) of 110 beats/minute. Which action is best to improve her acid-base status?

    A. 0.9% sodium chloride (NaCl) bolus.

    B. 5% dextrose (D_5W) bolus.

    C. Hydrochloric acid infusion.

    D. Acetazolamide intravenously.

2. A 21-year-old, 80-kg man admitted 1 day ago after a gunshot wound to the abdomen is receiving mechanical ventilation and is thrashing around in bed and pulling at his endotracheal tube. On the Richmond Agitation–Sedation Scale (RASS), he is rated a +3 (very agitated; pulls or removes tubes or catheters; aggressive). The patient is negative for delirium according to the Confusion Assessment Method for the ICU (CAM-ICU). His pulmonary status precludes him from extubation, and the attending physician estimates that he will remain intubated for at least 48 more hours. The medical team has decided that his RASS goal should be −1 (i.e., drowsy; not fully alert but with sustained awakening to voice). He is receiving a morphine 4-mg/hour infusion for pain control, which has been adequately controlling his pain. Vital signs include BP 110/70 mm Hg and HR 110 beats/minute. His baseline QT interval is 480 milliseconds. In addition to nonpharmacologic interventions to treat delirium, which is the best intervention for achieving this patient's RASS goal?

    A. Initiate a dexmedetomidine 1-mcg/kg loading dose over 10 minutes, followed by 0.2 mcg/kg/hour.

    B. Initiate lorazepam 3-mg intravenous load, followed by a lorazepam 3-mg/hour infusion.

    C. Initiate propofol at 5 mcg/kg/minute, and titrate by 5 mcg/kg/minute every 5 minutes as needed.

    D. Initiate haloperidol 1 mg intravenously and double the dose every 20 minutes as needed.

3. A patient is admitted to the ICU after a motor vehicle accident for traumatic brain injury and several abdominal injuries. He is initiated on propofol, morphine, and vecuronium for sedation, analgesia, and neuromuscular blockade to help control his intracranial pressure. On day 3 of hospitalization, the patient develops peritonitis with severe sepsis and is treated with vancomycin, piperacillin/tazobactam, and tobramycin. His train-of-four is 0/4. Which intervention would be best to recommend at this time?

    A. Sedation should be assessed using the RASS.

    B. Change tobramycin to levofloxacin because it can enhance the effects of vecuronium.

C. The patient should be initiated on parenteral nutrition.

D. Morphine can be discontinued because the patient is sedated with propofol.

4. A 62-year-old woman is admitted to your ICU for respiratory dysfunction requiring mechanical ventilation. Her medical history is nonsignificant, and she is taking no medications at home. Her chest radiograph shows bilateral lower lobe infiltrates, her white blood cell count (WBC) is 21×10^3 cells/m^3, her temperature is 39.6°C, her BP is 82/45 mm Hg (normal for her is 115/70 mm Hg), and her HR is 110 beats/minute. After she receives a diagnosis of community-acquired pneumonia, she is empirically initiated on ceftriaxone 2 g/day and levofloxacin 750 mg/day intravenously. After fluid resuscitation with 6 L of lactated Ringer's solution, her BP is unchanged. Dopamine is initiated and titrated to 9 mcg/kg/minute, with a resulting BP of 96/58 mm Hg, and her HR is 138 beats/minute. She has made less than 100 mL of urine during the past 6 hours, and her creatinine (Cr) has increased from 0.9 mg/dL to 1.3 mg/dL. Her serum albumin concentration is 2.1 g/dL. Which therapy is best for this patient at this time?

A. Administer 5% albumin 500 mL intravenously over 1 hour and reassess mean arterial pressure (MAP).

B. Initiate hydrocortisone 50 mg intravenously every 6 hours.

C. Change dopamine to norepinephrine 0.01 mcg/kg/minute to maintain an MAP greater than 65 mm Hg.

D. Reduce the dopamine infusion to 1 mcg/kg/minute to maintain urine output of at least 1 mL/kg/hour.

5. A 92-year-old woman is admitted to the ICU with urosepsis and septic shock. She lives in a long-term care facility and has a medical history significant for coronary artery disease and hypertension. Her BP is 72/44 mm Hg, central venous pressure (CVP) is 5 mm Hg, HR 120 beats/minute, and oxygen saturation is 99%; her laboratory values are normal, except for a BUN of 74 mg/dL and Cr of 2.7 mg/dL (baseline of 1.5 mg/dL according to old records). Her urine output is about 20 mL/hour. Appropriate empiric antibiotics were initiated. Which therapy is most appropriate to initiate next?

A. Norepinephrine 0.05 mcg/kg/minute.

B. Lactated Ringer's 500-mL bolus.

C. Normal saline 500-mL bolus.

D. Albumin 5% 500-mL bolus.

6. A 46-year-old man had a witnessed cardiac arrest in an airport terminal. After about 5 minutes, emergency medical services arrived, and defibrillator pads were applied. The cardiac monitor showed ventricular tachycardia (VT), and the patient had no discernible pulse. He was defibrillated with 200 J without return of spontaneous circulation. He received an additional two shocks of 200 J with no improvement. Between shocks, the patient received cardiopulmonary resuscitation (CPR). An intravenous line was obtained, and an epinephrine 1-mg intravenous push was given; chest compressions and artificial respirations were initiated. Within 1 minute, the patient was reassessed. The cardiac monitor still showed VT, and he remained pulseless; therefore, another shock of 200 J, followed by an amiodarone 300-mg intravenous push, was administered. After this, the patient was converted to a normal sinus rhythm with an HR of 100 beats/minute. The patient was then transported to the hospital, intubated and unresponsive. Which recommendation is most likely to improve this patient's outcomes?

A. Administer sodium bicarbonate intravenously.

B. Administer vasopressin 40 units intravenously.

C. Administer a continuous infusion of heparin.

D. Initiate a targeted temperature management protocol.

7. A 22-year-old man is admitted to the trauma ICU after a motor vehicle accident. He has several rib fractures, a ruptured spleen, and a small brain contusion. He is rushed to the operating room for an emergency splenectomy, and the trauma team places an orogastric feeding tube (OGT) before returning to the ICU. The patient is unresponsive

and mechanically ventilated, with no plans for extubation. Which is most cost-effective for stress ulcer prophylaxis (SUP)?

A. Pantoprazole intravenous push.

B. Famotidine by OGT.

C. Sucralfate by OGT.

D. No SUP indicated.

8. A 45-year-old man is admitted to the ICU with H1N1 causing respiratory failure. He is intubated and sedated with fentanyl 200 mcg/hour and propofol 25 mcg/kg/minute. He has received 4 L of plasmalyte and 1 L of albumin and is currently receiving norepinephrine 0.15 mcg/kg/minute and vasopressin 0.03 units/minute for hemodynamic support. His current vital signs are BP 85/58 mm Hg, HR 99 beats/minute, and respiratory rate (RR) 18 breaths/minute. Which of the following is the best plan for steroid therapy in this patient?

A. Begin hydrocortisone 50 mg every 6 hours intravenously.

B. Steroids are not indicated at this time.

C. Check a random cortisol and begin hydrocortisone 50 mg every 6 hours intravenously if the result is less than 10 mcg/dL.

D. Perform a cosyntropin stimulation test and begin hydrocortisone 50 mg every 6 hours intravenously if the patient does not have an increase greater than 9 mcg/dL from baseline.

9. The patient in question 8 continued to decline and was placed on cisatracurium overnight for hypoxemia. He is currently on cisatracurium 3 mcg/kg/minute, fentanyl 500 mcg/hour, propofol 40 mcg/kg/minute, and ketamine 10 mg/hour. His ABG shows a pH of 7.32, P_{CO_2} of 45 mm Hg, Pa_{O_2} of 60 mm Hg (O_2 saturation 93%), and HCO_3 of 27 mEq/L on 70% Fi_{O_2}. All laboratory values are normal except for a sodium of 148 mEq/L and creatinine of 1.4 mg/dL. His vasopressor doses have increased to norepinephrine 1 mcg/kg/minute and vasopressin 0.03 units/minute. An Scv_{O_2} is measured and found to be 45%. His skin is mottled, and urine output has decreased to 0.1 mL/kg/hour for the last 12 hours. Other pertinent vital signs are BP 100/64 mm Hg, HR 95 beats/minute, and

RR 26 breaths/minute. Which of the following is the best recommendation to optimize the patient's hemodynamics?

A. Start dobutamine 5 mcg/kg/minute.

B. Decrease norepinephrine to 0.5 mcg/kg/minute.

C. Decrease propofol to 20 mcg/kg/minute.

D. Start epinephrine 0.05 mcg/kg/minute.

10. A 69-year-old man has a seizure on postoperative day (POD) 0 after four-vessel coronary bypass and maze procedure. On POD 2, he develops hypotension and an increase in lactate to 3.5 mmol/L. His pulmonary artery catheter shows a cardiac index of 1.5 L/minute/m², pulmonary capillary wedge pressure 34 mm Hg, CVP 24 mm Hg, and systemic vascular resistance of 1240 dynes·s·cm⁻⁵. Other vital signs are HR 110 beats/minute and BP 95/45 mm Hg. Which of the following is the best intervention for the patient's shock?

A. Administer 500 mL of 5% albumin.

B. Start dobutamine 5 mcg/kg/minute.

C. Call surgical attending for immediate pericardiocentesis.

D. Start norepinephrine at 0.05 mcg/kg/minute.

11. A 19-year-old man is admitted to the ICU after ingesting an unknown quantity of acetaminophen. He is 180 cm tall and weighs 68 kg. After initial resuscitation and treatment with acetylcysteine, the patient remains unresponsive and intubated. The intensivist would like to start enteral nutrition as soon as possible. Which of the following is the best way to calculate the patient's caloric and protein requirements?

A. Calculate caloric needs based on the modified Penn State equation and estimate protein needs at 1.2 g/kg.

B. Perform indirect calorimetry to estimate caloric and protein needs.

C. Estimate caloric needs at 14 kcal/kg and protein at 2 g/kg.

D. Calculate caloric needs based on the Mifflin equation and order a prealbumin level to assess protein needs.

12. A 57-year-old woman is admitted to the ICU with injuries sustained after a fall from 12 feet. She has traumatic brain injury and has been intubated for airway protection. Which of the following is the best intervention to prevent ventilator-associated pneumonia in this patient?

    A. Initiate pantoprazole 40 mg intravenously daily.

    B. Perform selective digestive decontamination with enteral polymyxin B sulfate, neomycin sulfate, and vancomycin hydrochloride.

    C. Maintain head of bed elevation at 20° at all times.

    D. Start chlorhexidine 0.12% oral swabs twice daily.

13. You are the critical care pharmacist for a 300-bed hospital. The critical care committee wants to institute an evidence-based glucose control protocol for the ICU. Which of the following goals should be implemented for patients who present with septic shock?

    A. Check blood glucose every 6 hours and treat with sliding scale protocol when greater than 180 mg/dL.

    B. Initiate insulin infusion with a target of 110–140 mg/dL for two blood glucose values greater than 140 mg/dL.

    C. Initiate insulin infusion with a target of 110–180 mg/dL for two blood glucose values greater than 180 mg/dL.

    D. Initiate insulin infusion with a target blood glucose of 80–110 mg/dL for two blood glucose values greater than 150 mg/dL.

I. INTERPRETATION OF HEMODYNAMIC PARAMETERS

A. Hemodynamics

1. Arterial blood pressure is the product of cardiac output and resistance to flow (systemic vascular resistance [SVR]).

   a. Cardiac output (milliliters of blood pumped per minute) consists of stroke volume (milliliters of blood ejected from the left ventricle per beat) and heart rate (HR).

   b. Stroke volume is determined by preload (amount of blood available to eject), afterload (resistance to ejection), and contractility (amount of force generated by the heart). These will be discussed in more detail below.

2. Arterial blood pressure can be described by systolic blood pressure (SBP), diastolic blood pressure (DBP), or mean arterial pressure (MAP). This is the driving pressure for organ perfusion and oxygen delivery. MAP = [SBP + (2 × DBP)]/3. Note that MAP is based largely on DBP because most of the cardiac cycle is spent in diastole.

   a. Normal MAP is 70–100 mm Hg.

   b. MAP is an indication of global perfusion pressure; a MAP of at least 60 mm Hg is necessary for adequate cerebral perfusion.

   c. MAP can be calculated using the above equation, but direct measurement from an arterial line provides more timely and accurate measurements.

3. Preload is defined as ventricular end diastolic volume, and it increases proportionally with stroke volume (Frank-Starling mechanism). Commonly used measures of preload include central venous pressure (CVP), pulmonary capillary wedge pressure (PCWP) or pulmonary artery occlusion pressure (PAOP), and newer measures such as stroke volume variation (SVV) and pulse pressure variation (PPV).

   a. CVP is the pressure in the vena cava at the point of blood returning to the right atrium and may reflect volume status, although its utility in assessing volume responsiveness (whether or not a patient's low blood pressure will improve with an increase in intravascular volume) is poor. A CVP of 8–12 mm Hg (12–16 mm Hg if mechanically ventilated due to increases in thoracic pressure) has been suggested as being optimal for a patient with hypoperfusion from sepsis, but data on the use of CVP are lacking. CVP values at the extremes (less than 2 mm Hg, greater than 18 mm Hg) usually reflect hypovolemia and hypervolemia, respectively.

   b. PCWP or PAOP is the pressure when a balloon is inflated (wedged) in one of the pulmonary artery branches. Because the measurement is taken closer to the left ventricle than CVP, it may be a more accurate marker of volume status, but controversy remains. Its utility is diminished because the use of pulmonary artery catheters has severely declined.

   c. So-called dynamic markers (SVV, PPV) are increasingly used to determine a patient's volume responsiveness when given a fluid challenge. These measurements consider other variables and provide a better assessment of an individual patient's position on the Starling curve. Further information about dynamic markers can be found in the references.

B. Indicators of Oxygen Delivery

1. Assessment of end organ function is perhaps the simplest measurement of adequate oxygen delivery. Changes in mental status, decreased urine output (less than 0.5 mL/kg/hour), and cold extremities may be the first markers of organ hypoperfusion.

2. Blood pressure is the driving force behind oxygen delivery. Every organ is able to autoregulate blood flow, but this ability is generally lost at MAP values lower than 65 mm Hg.

3. Lactic acid

   a. Lactic acid is formed during anaerobic metabolism.

   b. During states of hypoperfusion, the tissues receive less blood and therefore less oxygen.

c. If there is less oxygen for the tissues, they will use anaerobic metabolism, with the subsequent production of lactic acid.

d. Lactate clearance may be used as a therapeutic end point in shock states.

4. Venous oxygen saturation

a. The oxyhemoglobin saturation of venous blood returning to the right atrium is normally 70%–75% (with a normal [99%–100%] arterial oxygen saturation, Sao$_2$), indicating that the normal oxygen extraction ratio is approximately 25%–30%.

b. In times of decreased oxygen delivery (caused by anemia, a decrease in Sao$_2$, CO, or tissue perfusion), more oxygen is extracted from the blood that is being perfused to tissues, causing an increased extraction ratio and thus a decrease in venous oxygen saturation.

c. Central venous oxygen saturation (Scvo$_2$) and mixed venous oxygen saturation (Svo$_2$) are measurements of venous oxygen saturation. These values are similar, but Scvo$_2$ is slightly higher than Svo$_2$ because it has not mixed with venous blood from the coronary sinus. Scvo$_2$ is measured in the superior vena cava, and Svo$_2$ is measured from the pulmonary artery (therefore, Svo$_2$ is about 5% lower than Scvo$_2$).

d. A normal Svo$_2$ does not rule out hypoperfusion in patients with impaired extraction (e.g., sepsis). An elevated lactate concentration may indicate hypoperfusion in this scenario.

Table 1. Hemodynamic Parameters and Normal Values

Parameter	Calculation (if applicable)	Normal Range
Systolic blood pressure (SBP)		90–140 mm Hg
Diastolic blood pressure (DBP)		60–90 mm Hg
Mean arterial blood pressure (MAP)	[SBP + (2·DBP)]/3	70–100 mm Hg
Systemic vascular resistance (SVR)	80 [(MAP – CVP)/CO]	800–1200 dynes·s·cm^{-5}
Heart rate (HR)		60–80 beats/minute
Cardiac output (CO)	HR·SV	4–7 L/minute
Cardiac index (CI)	CO/BSA	2.5–4.2 L/minute/m^2
Stroke volume (SV)	CO/HR	60–130 mL/beat
Pulmonary capillary wedge pressure (PCWP) or pulmonary arterial occlusion pressure (PAOP)		5–12 mm Hg
Central venous pressure (CVP)		2–6 mm Hg
Lactic acid		<1 mmol/L
Central venous oxygen saturation (Scvo$_2$)		70%–75%

BSA= body surface area

II. TREATMENT OF SHOCK

A. Diagnosis of Shock Based on Hemodynamic Parameters. Many patients may have more than one type of shock.

Table 2. Definitions of Shock

Hemodynamic Subset	CI	CVP/PCWP	SVR	Description
Distributive or vasodilatory	High (early) Low (late)	Low (early) Normal to high (late)	Low (early and late)	Patients with distributive shock are typically hyperdynamic (high CI), with vasodilation (low SVR) and increased vascular permeability ("leaky capillaries"), causing intravascular fluid to shift into the interstitial spaces (thus, low PCWP) The vasodilation and vascular permeability are attributable to cytokines and inflammatory mediators
Hypovolemic	Low	Low	High	To understand why patients with hypovolemia have a low CI, the Starling curve illustrates reduced cardiac function as intravascular volume is reduced. The reduced intravascular volume is indicated by a low PCWP, with a reflex increase in SVR to maintain tissue perfusion Remember that resistance (SVR) is inversely related to flow (CI)
Obstructive	Low	Low (impaired ejection) High (impaired filing)	High	Impairment in diastolic filling (caused by tamponade) or systolic contraction (massive pulmonary embolus, aortic stenosis) lead to the same hemodynamic status Differentiation can usually be made by patient history
Cardiogenic	Low	High	High	Patients with cardiogenic shock have acute heart failure (low CI) The insufficient forward flow of blood causes venous congestion (high PCWP) and an underfilled arterial blood volume The subsequent reduced tissue perfusion causes a reflex vasoconstriction (which, although it can improve blood flow to vital organs, can worsen heart function by increasing afterload) and reduced renal excretion of Na^+ and water

CI = cardiac index; CVP = central venous pressure; Na^+ = sodium; PCWP = pulmonary capillary wedge pressure; SVR = systemic vascular resistance.

B. Treatment of Hypovolemic Shock
  1. Treatment centers on restoring intravascular volume and oxygen-carrying capacity as indicated. Crystalloids and colloids are discussed in the chapter titled "Fluids, Electrolytes, and Nutrition."
  2. Blood products (packed red blood cells and coagulation factors) should be administered in hypovolemic shock, if clinically indicated.
     a. A hemoglobin less than 7 g/dL is defined as a transfusion threshold in general ICU patients. It is reasonable to have higher hemoglobin targets in selected patients (symptomatic cardiovascular disease).
     b. Actively bleeding patients should have blood products administered regardless of hemoglobin level.
  3. Patients may require vasopressors if hypotension is not rapidly reversed with fluid resuscitation. See below for vasopressor options.
     a. The efficacy of vasopressors is reduced in patients who have not received adequate intravascular volume resuscitation.
     b. The risk associated with vasopressors (e.g., arrhythmias, ischemia) are greater in patients who have not received adequate fluid resuscitation.

C. Treatment of Obstructive Shock
  1. Fluids and vasopressors may be used temporarily to improve end organ perfusion but may not improve outcomes.
  2. Treatment of the actual obstruction is the only way to reverse the shock state.
     a. Massive pulmonary embolism: Thrombectomy or administration of systemic or catheter-directed thrombolytics may be indicated if the patient has a high risk of death.
     b. Cardiac tamponade: Drainage or removal of fluid in the pericardial sac is the only definitive treatment.

Table 3. Classification of Sepsis Syndromes

	Definition	Criteria
Sepsis	Documented or suspected infection plus some of the criteria on the right	Temperature >38.3°C or <36°C[a] Heart rate >90 beats/minute[a] Respiratory rate greater than 20 breaths/minute or $Paco_2$ <32 mm Hg[a] WBC >12 × 10³ cells/m³ or <4 × 10³ cells/mm³[a] Altered mental status Hyperglycemia (BG >120 mg/dL without diabetes) Immature leukocytes (bands) >10% Significant edema or positive fluid balance (>20 mL/kg over 24 hours)

Table 3. Classification of Sepsis Syndromes *(continued)*

	Definition	Criteria
Severe sepsis	Sepsis complicated by organ dysfunction or hypoperfusion	SBP <90 mm Hg (or a >40–mm Hg drop) or MAP <70 mm Hg Venous saturation (Svo_2) <70% Need for mechanical ventilation Hypoxemia (Pao_2/Fio_2 <300) CI >3.5 Lactate >1 mmol/L Decreased capillary refill (press finger until turns white; time for color to return is refill time and normally less than 2 seconds) Mottling Creatinine increase >0.5 mg/dL Urine output <0.5 mL/kg/hour for ≥2 hours Coagulopathy (INR >1.5 or aPTT >60 seconds) Thrombocytopenia (platelet count <100,000/mm^3) Ileus Hyperbilirubinemia (total bilirubin >4 mg/dL)
Septic shock	Sepsis-induced hypotension	Persistent hypotension or a requirement for vasopressors after the administration of an intravenous fluid bolus

[a]Criteria including temperature, heart rate, respiratory rate, and WBC make up the original definition of systemic inflammatory response syndrome.

aPTT = activated partial thromboplastin time; BG = blood glucose; CI = cardiac index; INR = international normalized ratio; MAP = mean arterial pressure; SBP = systolic blood pressure; WBC = white blood cell count.

Table 4. Organ Dysfunction

Organ System	Signs of Dysfunction
Central nervous system	Altered mental status (Glasgow coma score <15)
Cardiovascular	SBP <90 or MAP <70 mm Hg Positive biomarkers (troponin, CK MB) Persistently hypotensive despite adequate fluid resuscitation Metabolic acidosis
Pulmonary	Need for mechanical ventilation because of respiratory failure
Kidney	Abrupt decrease in urine output (i.e., less than 0.5 mL/kg/hour for at least 2 hours) or increased creatinine
Liver	Elevated liver function tests, prothrombin time, INR, bilirubin
Hematologic or coagulation	Reduced platelet count or white blood cell count or an increase in INR

CK MB = creatinine kinase myocardial band; INR = international normalized ratio; MAP = mean arterial pressure; SBP = systolic blood pressure.

D. Treatment of Vasodilatory and Distributive Shock
1. Septic shock is the most common cause of vasodilatory shock. Other causes such as anaphylaxis, vasoplegia, intoxication, pancreatitis, and neurogenic and endocrine causes will not be discussed in this section.
2. The hallmark treatment of septic shock is rapid antibiotic administration, ideally within the first hour of hypotension.

3. The Surviving Sepsis Campaign (SSC) is an initiative to reduce mortality from severe sepsis and septic shock.

4. SSC "bundles"

   a. The SSC bundles are selected elements of care taken from evidence-based practice guidelines that, when implemented as a group, have a greater effect on outcomes than any individual element.

   b. The SSC recommends the following bundle for patients presenting with severe sepsis or septic shock.

      i. To be completed within 3 hours:

         (a) Measure lactate level.

         (b) Obtain blood cultures before administering antibiotics.

         (c) Administer broad-spectrum antibiotics.

         (d) Administer 30 mL/kg crystalloid for hypotension or lactate 4 mmol/L or more.

            (1) Albumin can be considered when patients require a substantial amount of crystalloids. There is no evidence that colloids are superior to crystalloids in improving outcomes, and they are more costly.

            (2) Hydroxyethyl starches (e.g., hetastarch) are not recommended for fluid resuscitation because of an increased risk of acute kidney injury and mortality.

            (3) The use of "balanced crystalloids" (solutions with electrolyte concentrations similar to extracellular fluid, such as lactated Ringer's, PlasmaLyte) for volume replacement may lead to less acute kidney injury than the use of other fluids (normal saline or 5% albumin).

      ii. To be completed within 6 hours:

         (a) Apply vasopressors (for hypotension that does not respond to initial fluid resuscitation) to maintain MAP 65 mm Hg or greater (see Table 5).

            (1) The goal MAP of 65 mm Hg should be individualized. A higher goal may be appropriate in patients with atherosclerosis or a history of hypertension. The individualized target MAP should correlate with improvement in other clinical parameters (e.g., lactate level, mental status, urine output, capillary refill).

            (2) Ideally, vasopressors should be used after restoration of intravascular volume, but in patients with septic shock and hypoperfusion, vasopressors may be necessary during fluid resuscitation to optimize perfusion of vital organs. Once intravascular volume is optimized with fluid resuscitation, vasopressors should be weaned if possible.

            (3) Vasopressors improve tissue perfusion by increasing BP or CO. Very few studies have evaluated an improvement in clinical outcomes, but differences in safety profile have been observed. Therefore, drug selection is based largely on expert opinion, practitioner experience, and patient response.

            (4) Norepinephrine is the initial vasopressor of choice.

            (5) Epinephrine can be added to or substituted for norepinephrine if needed.

            (6) Vasopressin (0.03 unit/minute) can be added to norepinephrine if needed. The efficacy of vasopressin when added to norepinephrine is similar to that of norepinephrine alone. Vasopressin can have a vasopressor-sparing effect, although mortality is not improved with the combination. The addition of vasopressin earlier (at norepinephrine doses of less than 15 mcg/minute) may be associated with an improvement in outcomes.

            (7) Dopamine is an alternative to norepinephrine, but it is associated with a higher incidence of arrhythmias compared with norepinephrine. Dopamine use should be limited to patients with a low risk of tachyarrhythmias and absolute or relative bradycardia. Low-dose dopamine should not be used for renal protection.

       (8) Phenylephrine is an alternative to consider in patients with vasopressor-induced serious tachyarrhythmias or persistent hypotension.

       (9) Use of an arterial catheter for BP measurements is preferred in patients requiring vasopressors because it is a more accurate measurement of arterial pressure (compared with a BP cuff) and allows continuous monitoring.

      (10) Vasopressors should be administered through a central line as soon as possible to reduce the risk of extravasation and subsequent tissue ischemia. If extravasation occurs, phentolamine (an α-receptor antagonist) can be used to reduce tissue necrosis. In a phentolamine shortage, other options include nitroglycerin ointment (applied around the site of extravasation every 6 hours) or subcutaneous terbutaline (peripheral vasodilation is mediated through β_2-receptors).

      (11) Use caution with calculations and avoid unit errors.

  (b) In the event of persistent arterial hypotension despite volume resuscitation (septic shock) or initial lactate 4 mmol/L or more (see below for updated information):

       (1) Measure CVP. Goal of CVP 8 mm Hg or higher (nonintubated) or 12–15 mm Hg (intubated patients)

       (2) Measure central venous oxygen saturation ($Scvo_2$). Goal of $Scvo_2$ of 70%. If $Scvo_2$ target is not achieved despite restoration of intravascular volume and MAP, consider additional fluid resuscitation, packed red blood cells (to hematocrit of more than 30%), or dobutamine infusion.

       (3) Remeasure lactate if initial lactate was elevated. Goal is normalization of lactate.

c. The use of early goal-directed therapy (similar to the bundle above) was found to reduce mortality by 16% when compared with standard therapy in a single-center study of patients with severe sepsis or septic shock who presented to an emergency department.

  i. Two subsequent multicenter studies of early goal-directed therapy have not replicated these results.

  ii. In response, the SSC Executive Committee released a statement about portions of the SSC guidelines:

    (a) CVP and $Scvo_2$ monitoring does not confer a survival benefit in patients who receive timely antibiotics and fluid resuscitation.

    (b) Measurement of CVP and $Scvo_2$ in patients with lactate greater than 4 mmol/L or persistent hypotension after initial fluid challenge and those who have received timely antibiotics is not necessary but has not shown to be harmful.

Table 5. Vasopressors and Inotropes

Drug	Dose	α_1	β_1	β_2	DA	Notes
Norepinephrine	0.01–3 mcg/kg/minute	++++	+++	0	0	↓ Renal perfusion ↑ SVR, ↑ BP 0 – ↓ CO (at high doses) Peripheral ischemia Can induce tachyarrhythmias and myocardial ischemia
Epinephrine	0.04–1 mcg/kg/minute for refractory hypotension	+++	+++	++	0	Positive inotropic and chronotropic effects can induce arrhythmias and myocardial ischemia Low doses primarily β-adrenergic; escalating doses primarily α-adrenergic Some evidence of reduced splanchnic circulation, which can lead to gut ischemia Increases blood glucose and lactate concentrations (type B lactic acidosis)
Vasopressin	0.03–0.04 unit/minute (physiologic replacement dose)	0	0	0	0	Direct stimulation of smooth muscle V1 vasopressin receptors; peripheral vasoconstriction, no adrenergic activity Theoretically beneficial because of an apparent relative vasopressin deficiency in septic shock but no evidence of efficacy over other vasopressors Effective during acidosis and hypoxia because it does not rely on adrenergic receptors Doses ≥0.04 unit/minute are associated with coronary vasoconstriction and peripheral necrosis Not titrated like traditional vasopressors Prone to dosing errors because of "unit/minute"
Phenylephrine	0.5–8 mcg/kg/minute for septic shock (or a common maximum amount is 300 mcg/minute)	++++	0	0	0	↓ Renal perfusion Pure α-adrenergic agonist with minimal cardiac activity Rapid ↑ SBP and DBP can cause a reflex bradycardia and reduction in CO Can be administered as a rapid bolus for acute hypotension (e.g., intraoperative) or as a continuous infusion. Extravasation produces ischemic necrosis and sloughing

Table 5. Vasopressors and Inotropes *(continued)*

Drug	Dose	α_1	β_1	β_2	DA	Notes
Dopamine	1–3 mcg/kg/minute	+/–	++	+/–	++++	Lower doses cause renal, coronary, mesenteric, and cerebral arterial vasodilation and a natriuretic response Lower "inotropic" doses can complement the vasoconstrictive effects of norepinephrine Do not use low-dose dopamine for renal protection because evidence does not support this practice
	3–10 mcg/kg/minute	++	+++	+	++	Moderate doses can ↑ contractility and SVR Any dose can induce arrhythmias
	10–20 mcg/kg/minute	++++	+++	0	+	Any dose can cause endocrine changes (e.g., decreased prolactin, growth hormone, thyroid hormone); however, the clinical significance is unknown Immediate precursor of norepinephrine Prolonged infusions can deplete endogenous norepinephrine stores, resulting in a loss of vasopressor response Effects on renal blood flow may be lost at higher doses because of predominant α_1-vasoconstrictive effects
Dobutamine	2–20 mcg/kg/minute	+	+++	+	0	Positive inotrope to ↑ CO Can cause hypotension because of β_2-stimulation Higher doses can cause tachyarrhythmias and changes in BP, which can lead to myocardial ischemia
Milrinone	50-mcg/kg load over 10 minutes, followed by 0.375–0.75 mcg/kg/minute	0	0	0	0	Noncatecholamine, phosphodiesterase inhibitor Positive inotrope Vasodilation or hypotension, arrhythmias possible Use lower doses in renal failure Loading doses often omitted especially if patient hypotensive

BP = blood pressure; CO = cardiac output; DA = dopamine; DBP = diastolic blood pressure; SBP = systolic blood pressure; SVR = systemic vascular resistance.

E. Appropriate Use of Antimicrobials in Patients with Sepsis
    1. Empiric antimicrobials should cover likely pathogens according to suspected location of infection and risk of multidrug-resistant pathogens. Common sources of infection are lung, abdomen, blood, and urinary tract.
    2. Consider empiric fungal therapy with either triazoles such as fluconazole, an echinocandin, or a lipid formulation of amphotericin B if patients have several risk factors, including recent abdominal surgery, chronic parenteral nutrition, indwelling central venous catheters, or recent treatment with broad-spectrum antibiotics or if patients are immunocompromised (e.g., chronic corticosteroids or other immunosuppressants, neutropenia, malignancy, organ transplant). An echinocandin is preferred in patients recently treated with antifungal agents or if *Candida glabrata* or *krusei* infection is suspected.
    3. Other considerations in choosing appropriate antimicrobials include the patient's history of drug allergy or intolerance, recent antibiotic use, comorbidities, and antimicrobial susceptibility patterns in the community and hospital.
    4. Begin intravenous antimicrobials as early as possible, at least within the first hour but preferably after at least two sets of blood cultures (one drawn percutaneously) are obtained. Quantitative cultures of other potential sites of infection (e.g., urine, sputum) should also be obtained before the administration of antimicrobials if possible.
    5. If several antibiotics are prescribed, administer the broadest coverage first and infuse as quickly as possible.
    6. Mortality increases by 7.9% for each 1-hour delay in administering appropriate antimicrobials.
    7. Appropriate antimicrobials do not reduce the importance of emergency source control by drainage, debridement, or device removal as needed.
    8. De-escalation should occur with respect to culture data or clinical judgment. Empiric use of combination therapy should not be administered for longer than 3–5 days if de-escalation to a single agent is appropriate.
    9. Consider discontinuing antimicrobials in 7–10 days unless there is slow response, undrainable foci, immunosuppression, or multidrug-resistant pathogens. Blood cultures will be negative in most patients, despite a bacterial or fungal origin of sepsis. Clinical judgment is needed when considering discontinuation of antimicrobials.
    10. Procalcitonin, a biomarker for bacterial infections, can be used as a guide for antibiotic therapy.
    11. Discontinue antimicrobials if no infectious cause is found.
    12. Consider empiric antiviral therapy with oseltamivir for patients presenting with flulike symptoms during flu season.

F. Indication for and Use of Corticosteroids
    1. Adrenal function in critically ill patients may be suppressed by endotoxins produced by bacteria and by the body's immune response to stress.
    2. Early studies showed a relationship between vasopressor responsiveness and glucocorticoid administration.
    3. To determine a patient's adrenal function during critical illness, a corticotropin stimulation test ("stim test") may be performed, although it is no longer recommended.
        a. A corticotropin stimulation test is performed by administering 250 mcg of cosyntropin (synthetic adrenocorticotropic hormone) and measuring cortisol levels at baseline, 30 minutes, and 60 minutes after.
        b. A cortisol increase of more than 9 mcg/dL is said to be an appropriate response (responders), perhaps indicating appropriate adrenal function. Changes of less than 9 mcg/dL may indicate corticosteroid insufficiency. A random cortisol level of less than 10 mcg/dL may also indicate corticosteroid insufficiency.

c. The corticotropin stimulation test has come under criticism because of the high dose of cosyntropin administered, the inability to measure free (active) cortisol, and lack of data on outcomes of responders versus nonresponders, and it is not indicated for use in the general ICU population.

4. Clinical trials of steroids in septic shock

    a. In a study published in 2002, adult patients with septic shock were given a corticotropin stimulation test and then randomly assigned to intravenous hydrocortisone combined with oral fludrocortisone or placebo. In the entire patient population, steroid therapy improved 28-day survival; however, this occurred because of a marked improvement in nonresponders to the corticotropin stimulation test. Responders showed no improvement with steroid therapy.

    b. The CORTICUS trial, published in 2008, had a similar method to the study above but omitted fludrocortisone. In this study, corticosteroids were not associated with a mortality benefit; however, they were associated with a higher risk of hyperglycemia, new sepsis, or septic shock. For this reason, corticosteroids are not recommended in patients with septic shock who have been stabilized with fluid and vasopressor therapy.

5. Evidence-based guidelines

    a. SSC guidelines

        i. The SSC recommends against using hydrocortisone to treat adults with septic shock if adequate fluid resuscitation and vasopressor therapy are able to restore hemodynamic stability. If this is not achievable, the SSC suggests intravenous hydrocortisone alone at a dose of 200 mg per day.

        ii. The SSC recommends against using the corticotropin stimulation test to identify the subset of adults with septic shock who should receive hydrocortisone.

    b. American College of Critical Care Medicine corticosteroid insufficiency guidelines recognize that although hypothalamic-pituitary-adrenal (HPA) axis dysfunction is common in some critically ill patients (sepsis), diagnosis and management of this disorder are complicated.

        i. The expert panel's recommendations for septic shock are similar to the SSC guidelines, that hydrocortisone should be considered in the management strategy for patients with septic shock, particularly those who have responded poorly to fluid resuscitation and vasopressor agents.

        ii. Furthermore, the corticotropin stimulation test should not be used to identify patients with septic shock or acute respiratory distress syndrome (ARDS) who should receive glucocorticoids.

        iii. Patients should be weaned off steroid therapy once vasopressors are no longer necessary.

III. INTERPRETATION OF ACID-BASE DISTURBANCES

A. Normal Arterial Blood Gas Values

pH	7.40 (range 7.35–7.45)
P_{CO_2}	35–45 mm Hg
P_{O_2}	80–100 mm Hg
HCO_3^-	22–26 mEq/L (or mmol/L)
S_{aO_2}	95%–100%

B. Acidosis: Any pH less than 7.35 indicates a primary acidosis.

C. Alkalosis: Any pH greater than 7.45 indicates a primary alkalosis.

D. Metabolic Disorders
   1. Acidosis: Decreased HCO_3^-
   2. Alkalosis: Increased HCO_3^-

E. Respiratory Disorders
   1. Acidosis: Increased P_{CO_2}
   2. Alkalosis: Decreased P_{CO_2}

F. Compensation: Occurs in an attempt to normalize the pH in response to the primary problem
   1. Respiratory compensation occurs immediately with changes in respiratory rate.
      a. The compensation for metabolic acidosis is respiratory alkalosis (i.e., decrease in P_{CO_2}). This is achieved by increasing the respiratory rate to eliminate more CO_2, thus making pH more basic (i.e., higher pH).
      b. The compensation for metabolic alkalosis is a respiratory acidosis (i.e., increase in P_{CO_2}). This is achieved by slowing the respiratory rate to retain more CO_2, thus making pH more acidic (i.e., lower pH).
   2. Metabolic compensation occurs slowly in the kidneys by regulating the excretion and reabsorption of HCO_3^- and H^+.
      a. The compensation for a respiratory acidosis is metabolic alkalosis (i.e., an increase in HCO_3^-).
      b. The compensation for a respiratory alkalosis is metabolic acidosis (i.e., a decrease in HCO_3^-).

Table 6. Predicted Degrees of Compensation in Acid-Base Disturbances

Normal Values $HCO_3^- = 24$ mmol/L $P_{CO_2} = 40$ mm Hg	Primary Disturbance	Compensation
Metabolic acidosis	↓ HCO_3^- by 1 mmol/L	↓ P_{CO_2} by 1.2 mm Hg
Metabolic alkalosis	↑ HCO_3^- by 1 mmol/L	↑ P_{CO_2} by 0.7 mm Hg

Respiratory acidosis
  Chronic (>3 days)
  Acute
	↑ P_{CO_2} by 10 mm Hg
	↑ P_{CO_2} by 10 mm Hg
		↑ HCO_3^- by 3.5 mmol/L
		↑ HCO_3^- by 1 mmol/L

Respiratory alkalosis
  Chronic (>3 days)
  Acute
	↓ P_{CO_2} by 10 mm Hg
	↓ P_{CO_2} by 10 mm Hg
		↓ $HCO_3^- = 4$ mmol/L
		↓ $HCO_3^- = 2$ mmol/L

G. Steps to Evaluate Acid-Base Disorders
   1. Assess pH, P_{CO_2}, and HCO_3^-.
      a. Acidosis if pH less than 7.35
         i. If P_{CO_2} is elevated, the primary disorder is respiratory acidosis.
         ii. If HCO_3^- is decreased, the primary disorder is metabolic acidosis.
      b. Alkalosis if pH is greater than 7.45
         i. If P_{CO_2} is decreased, the primary disorder is respiratory alkalosis.
         ii. If HCO_3^- is elevated, the primary disorder is metabolic alkalosis.
   2. Calculate the anion gap (AG) = $[Na^+] - [Cl^- + HCO_3^-]$.
      a. Normal range is 6–12 mEq/L.
      b. If AG is more than 12, there is a primary metabolic acidosis regardless of pH or HCO_3^-. Some patients have a mixed acid-base disorder in which they have more than one primary disorder.
      c. Hypoalbuminemia decreases the AG by 2.5–3 mEq/L for every 1-g/dL decrease in serum albumin less than 4 g/dL.

3. Calculate the excess AG = total AG − normal AG. Add excess AG to serum bicarbonate.
    a. If the sum is greater than a normal serum bicarbonate (i.e., more than 30 mEq/L), there is also an AG metabolic alkalosis (this can occur in addition to other primary disorders).
    b. If the sum is less than a normal serum bicarbonate (i.e., less than 23 mEq/L), there is an underlying non-AG metabolic acidosis.

Table 7. Causes of Acid-Base Disturbances

	Respiratory Acidosis	Respiratory Alkalosis	Metabolic Acidosis	Metabolic Alkalosis
Etiology	Pulmonary edema Cardiac arrest CNS depression Stroke Pulmonary embolus Pneumonia Bronchospasm Spinal cord injury Sedatives	Anxiety Pain CNS tumor Stroke Head injury Hypoxia Stimulant drugs Reduced oxygen-carrying capacity Reduced alveolar oxygen extraction Respiratory rate stimulation Extracorporeal removal	**Anion gap** (MUDPILES) Methanol Uremia DKA Propylene glycol Intoxication or infection Lactic acidosis Ethylene glycol Salicylate **Non–anion gap** (F-USED CARS) Fistula (pancreatic) Uteroenteric conduits Saline excess Endocrine (hyperparathyroid) Diarrhea Carbonic anhydrase inhibitors Arginine, lysine, Cl^- Renal tubular acidosis Spironolactone	**Urine Cl^- >25** (Chloride resistant) Hyperaldosteronism ↑ Mineralocorticoid **Urine Cl^- <25** (Chloride responsive) Vomiting NG suction Diuretic
Treatment	Correct cause Invasive/ noninvasive ventilation	Correct cause Oxygen supplementation Invasive/ noninvasive ventilation Hypoventilation Sedation	Correct cause Use of bases (sodium bicarbonate or THAM) may be considered in non-AG metabolic acidosis Base use in AG metabolic acidosis is controversial (Sodium bicarbonate and THAM have traditionally been used, but evidence of clinical benefit is lacking)	Correct cause **If urine Cl^- < 25** 0.9% NaCl Consider HCl (if severe) Consider acetazolamide **If urine Cl^- > 25** Potassium Aldosterone antagonist Acetazolamide

AG = anion gap; Cl^- = chloride; CNS = central nervous system; DKA = diabetic ketoacidosis; GI = gastrointestinal; HCl = hydrochloric acid; NaCl = sodium chloride; NG = nasogastric; THAM = tromethamine or tris-hydroxymethyl aminomethane.

Patient Cases

1. A 62-year-old woman has been hospitalized in the ICU for several weeks. Her hospital stay has been complicated by aspiration pneumonia and sepsis, necessitating prolonged courses of antibiotics. For the past few days, she has been having high temperatures again, and her stool output has increased dramatically. Her most recent stool samples have tested positive for *Clostridium difficile* toxin, and her laboratory tests reveal serum sodium 138 mEq/L, potassium (K) 3.5 mEq/L, Cl 115 mEq/L, HCO_3^- 15 mEq/L, albumin 4.4 g/dL, pH 7.32, $Paco_2$ 30 mm Hg, and HCO_3^- 15 mEq/L. Which is most consistent with this patient's primary acid-base disturbance?

    A. AG metabolic acidosis.

    B. Non-AG metabolic acidosis.

    C. Chloride-responsive metabolic alkalosis.

    D. Acute respiratory acidosis.

2. A 27-year-old man with no medical history is admitted to the hospital after being "found down" at a party, where he reportedly ingested a handle of whiskey during a 60-minute period. On arrival at the emergency department, he was neurologically unresponsive, with the following ABG values: pH 7.23, $Paco_2$ 58 mm Hg, Pao_2 111 mm Hg, HCO_3^- 24 mEq/L, and Sao_2 88% on 2 L/minute of oxygen by nasal cannula. Which action is most appropriate?

    A. Administer tromethamine 500 mL over 30 minutes.

    B. Administer 100% oxygen by face mask.

    C. Give $NaHCO_3^-$ 100 mEq intravenous push.

    D. Urgent intubation.

3. A 55-year-old woman is admitted to the hospital after several days of worsening shortness of breath. Recently, she was discharged from the hospital after a similar episode and was doing fine until 3 days before admission, when she developed a productive cough, necessitating an increase in her home oxygen and more frequent use of her metered dose inhalers. On admission to the medical ICU, she was anxious and markedly distressed, with rapid, shallow breaths. She was hypertensive (160/80 mm Hg), tachycardic (140 beats/minute), and tachypneic (respiratory rate 28 breaths/minute). Her ABG showed a pH of 7.30, $Paco_2$ 59 mm Hg, Pao_2 50 mm Hg, HCO_3^- 28 mEq/L, and Sao_2 83% on 6 L/minute of oxygen by face mask, and she was immediately intubated. Which primary acid-base disturbance is most consistent with this patient's presentation and laboratory data?

    A. Metabolic acidosis.

    B. Metabolic alkalosis.

    C. Respiratory acidosis.

    D. Respiratory alkalosis.

Patient Cases *(continued)*

4. A 65-year-old woman is admitted to the cardiac surgery after an aortic valve replacement. On the fourth day of hospitalization, she is hypotensive (BP 80/50 mm Hg), tachycardic (HR 125 beats/minute), tachypneic (respiratory rate 30 breaths/minute), hypoxemic (Pao_2 40 mm Hg), febrile (39.5°C), and confused. The patient is given two 1000-mL boluses of normal saline and then is reintubated and initiated on piperacillin/tazobactam 4.5 g intravenous piggyback every 6 hours and vancomycin 1000 mg intravenous piggyback every 12 hours for possible nosocomial pneumonia. After fluid boluses fail to improve her hemodynamic and clinical status, a pulmonary artery catheter is placed, which reveals a PCWP of 18 mm Hg, CI of 4.8 L/minute/m², and SVR of 515 dynes/second/cm². Her chest radiograph shows a left lower lobe consolidation, and she still requires 100% Fio_2. Which action is best?

   A. Add clindamycin 600 mg intravenous piggyback every 8 hours.

   B. Administer dobutamine infusion titrated to achieve a MAP of at least 65 mm Hg.

   C. Administer norepinephrine infusion titrated to achieve a MAP of at least 65 mm Hg.

   D. Administer hydrocortisone 50 mg intravenously every 6 hours.

5. A 70-kg patient is to be started on a continuous infusion of epinephrine for BP support after return of spontaneous circulation after a cardiac arrest. The nurse has a 250-mL bag of D_5W containing 4 mg of epinephrine. Which rate is most appropriate to infuse the epinephrine drip at a dose of 0.03 mcg/kg/minute?

   A. 8 mL/hour.

   B. 13 mL/hour.

   C. 31.5 mL/hour.

   D. 79 mL/hour.

6. A 42-year-old man was found unresponsive at his group home covered in vomit. He was intubated by the paramedics. On arrival at the emergency department, his BP is 72/30 mm Hg and HR is 122 beats/minute. During the next few hours, he receives 5 L of normal saline, 500 mL of 5% albumin, and norepinephrine infusing at 20 mcg/minute. With these interventions, his BP is 87/56 mm Hg and HR is 95 beats/minute. Pertinent laboratory values include a WBC of 20 × 10³ cells/mm³, lactic acid 1.5 mmol/L, aspartate aminotransferase 78 units/L, Cr 2.2 (baseline 1) mg/dL, platelet count 118,000 cells/mm³, INR 1.4, and urine output about 45 mL/hour since arrival. Which is most appropriate intervention at this time?

   A. Add hydrocortisone 50 mg intravenously every 6 hours.

   B. Add enoxaparin 40 mg subcutaneously every 24 hours.

   C. Add low-dose dopamine.

   D. Add heparin 5000 units subcutaneously every 8 hours.

IV. ACUTE RESPIRATORY FAILURE

A. Causes of Respiratory Failure

Table 8. Respiratory Failure

Indication for Mechanical Ventilation	Examples
Hypoventilation (hypercapnic respiratory failure)	Drug overdose Neuromuscular disease Cardiopulmonary resuscitation Central nervous system injury or disease
Hypoxemia (hypoxic respiratory failure)	Pulmonary injury or disease Pneumonia Pulmonary edema Pulmonary embolus Acute respiratory distress syndrome
Inability to maintain airway	Loss of airway patency (mechanical obstruction, tracheal or chest wall injury) Loss of gag or cough reflex with large-volume aspiration risk (e.g., central nervous system injury, central nervous system depression, cardiovascular accident, seizures, cardiac arrest)

B. Complications Associated with Mechanical Ventilation (see individual sections later in text for prevention of these complications)
   1. Ventilator-associated pneumonia
   2. Stress ulcers
   3. Venous thrombosis

V. CARDIAC ARREST

A. Training: Any pharmacist who participates in codes should complete basic life support (BLS) and advanced cardiac life support (ACLS) training. In general, BLS training takes 3–5 hours to complete, and ACLS training takes 2 days. The information presented in this section consists of selected highlights from these training sessions; it should not be used in place of a comprehensive training program.

B. 2010 American Heart Association (AHA) Guidelines
   1. Medications used during ACLS: See "Cardiology I" chapter for information on drugs, indications, and dosages.
   2. CAB (compressions, airway, breathing): In an unresponsive patient or patient who is not breathing, one rescuer should initiate a cycle of 30 chest compressions as soon as possible, followed immediately by 2 rescue breaths any delays in chest compressions.
   3. Emphasis is on high-quality cardiopulmonary resuscitation (CPR), with a compression rate of at least 100/minute at a depth of at least 2 inches.
   4. Electrical therapy (via an automated external defibrillator [AED] or defibrillator) should be initiated as soon as it is available.
   5. Interruptions in chest compressions should be minimal and last less than 10 seconds. Chest compressions and defibrillation should not be interrupted for vascular access, medication administration, or airway placement.

6. Medication administration
   a. Central venous administration is preferred.
   b. Intraosseous administration is preferred to endotracheal administration if intravenous administration is not possible because of its more predictable drug delivery and pharmacologic effect.
   c. Endotracheal drug administration can be performed by administering 2–2.5 times the standard intravenous dose and diluting in 5–10 mL of sterile water. The following drugs can be administered through an endotracheal tube: naloxone, atropine, vasopressin, epinephrine, lidocaine (NAVEL).
   d. If medications are administered through a peripheral vein, it is important to follow the medication with 20 mL of intravenous fluid to facilitate drug flow from the extremity to the central circulation.

C. Post–Cardiac Arrest Care
   1. After return of spontaneous circulation, systematic postarrest care can improve survival and quality of life.
   2. Initial therapy should be to optimize ventilation, oxygenation, and blood pressure.
      a. Oxygen saturation should be maintained at 94% or higher.
         i. Insertion of an advanced airway may be necessary.
         ii. Hyperventilation and excess oxygen delivery are harmful and should be avoided.
      b. Hypotension (SBP 90 mm Hg or lower) should be treated with fluid boluses and vasopressors if necessary (AHA recommends epinephrine, dopamine, or norepinephrine).
   3. Target temperature management (therapeutic hypothermia)
      a. Induction of hypothermia (32°C–34°C) for 12–24 hours beginning as soon as possible after cardiac arrest can improve neurologic recovery and mortality. Although most evidence of benefit involves patients with an initial rhythm of ventricular fibrillation, hypothermia is recommended by AHA for adult survivors of cardiac arrest regardless of the initial rhythm. One study has shown that a standard target temperature (33°C) did not confer a benefit over a higher target temperature (36°C); however, most centers still target a lower (32°C–34°C) temperature.
      b. Consider hypothermia in patients who have been successfully resuscitated after a cardiac arrest but who remain comatose (usually defined as a lack of meaningful response to verbal commands).
      c. No single method for inducing hypothermia is recommended over another. Surface cooling devices, endovascular catheters, cooling blankets, ice packs, and cold intravenous fluids may be used.
      d. Core temperature should be continuously monitored.
      e. Many patients will need sedation and analgesia during periods of hypothermia.
      f. Rewarming should be done slowly (0.3–0.5°C every hour).
      g. Complications
         i. Shivering
            (a) Shivering causes excess heat production, increased oxygen consumption, and a general stress response and thus should be treated and prevented.
            (b) Shivering can be treated with sedatives (dexmedetomidine, ketamine), anesthetics, analgesics (e.g., meperidine, fentanyl, tramadol), dexamethasone, clonidine, magnesium (Mg), ondansetron, buspirone, and paralytics (see meta-analysis in Park SM, Mangat HS, Berger K, Rosengart AJ. Efficacy spectrum of antishivering medications: Meta-analysis of randomized controlled trials. Crit Care Med. 2012;40:3070–82 for study references for individual drugs and doses).
            (c) Note that shivering can be treated without the use of paralytics in many patients. Thus, paralytics are not mandatory and should be avoided if possible (see disadvantages of paralytics below). Paralytics may be most beneficial during the induction of hypothermia and during rewarming (when risk of shivering is greatest); however, they should be continually reevaluated and discontinued, if possible, once goal temperature is achieved.

   ii. Altered drug metabolism

     (a) Drug clearance is typically reduced during hypothermia, including a depressed activity of cytochrome P450 (CYP) 3A4 and 3A5 hepatic enzymes. Hypothermia can also affect the distribution of drugs to their site of action (e.g., propofol).

     (b) Use bolus dosing during the induction of hypothermia.

     (c) Reduce maintenance doses of sedatives (e.g., midazolam, propofol), opiates (fentanyl, remifentanil), phenobarbital, phenytoin, paralytics, and other drugs as needed (see review article Tortorici MA, Kochanek PM, Poloyac SM. Effects of hypothermia on drug disposition, metabolism, and response: A focus of hypothermia-mediated alterations on the cytochrome P450 enzyme system. Crit Care Med. 2007;35:2196–204).

   iii. Coagulopathy

   iv. Increased renal excretion of water and subsequent volume depletion

   v. Arrhythmia and hypotension

     (a) Usually bradycardia

     (b) Discontinue or slightly warm patient if life-threatening arrhythmias or persistent hemodynamic instability develops.

   vi. Hyperglycemia and hypoglycemia

     (a) Hyperglycemia during hypothermia, hypoglycemia during rewarming.

     (b) Monitor blood glucose frequently (i.e., every 1–2 hours) and adjust insulin accordingly.

   vii. Infection

   viii. Electrolyte disturbances

     (a) Reductions in K, Mg, and phosphate during cooling

     (b) Hyperkalemia during rewarming

     (c) Special electrolyte replacement protocols should be used to ensure patients do not receive too much potassium during cooling such that they are hyperkalemic during rewarming.

Patient Case

7. A 61-year-old woman collapsed in front of her family, who called 911 and began CPR. The paramedics arrive and find the victim unresponsive, with an electrocardiogram showing ventricular fibrillation, and administer two additional rounds of CPR and two defibrillations, which are successful. In the emergency department, the patient's MAP is 68 mm Hg after fluids and norepinephrine, but the patient remains unresponsive. She is initiated on the hypothermia protocol. After 24 hours of hypothermia (temperature 33°C), the patient is in the ICU, and the rewarming process has recently begun. The pharmacist arrives in the ICU about 30 minutes into the rewarming process. The patient has been receiving a continuous infusion of insulin throughout the period of hypothermia at an average rate of 4 units/hour, with blood glucose testing every 3 hours. The patient has been sedated with a continuous infusion of propofol and fentanyl and is on cisatracurium for neuromuscular blockade. The patient's vital signs are stable, and her laboratory values are normal. Which pharmacist recommendation is most appropriate at this time?

A. Increase BG testing to now and every 1–2 hours during rewarming.

B. Adjust cisatracurium infusion to achieve a train-of-four (TOF) of 0/4 impulses.

C. Discontinue propofol infusion to facilitate extubation.

D. Increase insulin infusion to prevent hyperkalemia.

VI. PAIN, AGITATION, DELIRIUM, AND NEUROMUSCULAR BLOCKADE

A. General Considerations
   1. Nonpharmacologic strategies to improve patient comfort include lighting, music, massage, verbal reassurance, avoidance of sleep deprivation, and patient positioning based on patient preferences.
   2. Determine patient goals using validated scales and routinely assess pain and sedation.
       a. Routine assessment of pain and sedation should be performed in every ICU patient.
           i. Self-reporting is preferred to pain scales for assessing pain in patients who are able to communicate.
           ii. To assess pain in patients unable to communicate, the Behavioral Pain Scale (BPS) and the Critical-Care Pain Observation Tool (CPOT) are recommended because, compared with other scores, they are more valid and reliable for monitoring pain in adult ICU patients (except those with brain injury).
               (a) The BPS score can range from 3 (no pain) to 12 (maximum pain). A score of 6 or higher is generally considered to reflect unacceptable pain.
               (b) The CPOT score can range from 0 to 8.

Table 9. The Behavioral Pain Scale

Item	Description	Score
Facial expression	Relaxed	1
	Partially tightened (e.g., brow lowering)	2
	Fully tightened (e.g., eyelid closing)	3
	Grimacing	4
Upper limb movements	No movement	1
	Partially bent	2
	Fully bent with finger flexion	3
	Permanently retracted	4
Compliance with mechanical ventilation	Tolerating movement	1
	Coughing but tolerating ventilation for most of the time	2
	Fighting ventilator	3
	Unable to control ventilation	4

Adapted from Payen JF, Bru O, Bosson JL, Lagrasta A, Novel E, Deschaux I, Lavagne P, Jacquot C. Assessing pain in critically ill sedated patients by using a behavioral pain scale. Crit Care Med. 2001 Dec;29(12):2258-63.

Table 10. Critical Care Pain Observation Tool

Indicator	Description	Score
Facial expression	No muscular tension observed	Relaxed, neutral: 0
	Presence of frowning, brow lowering, orbit tightening, and levator contraction	Tense: 1
	All the above facial movements plus eyelids tightly closed	Grimacing: 2
Body movements	Does not move at all (does not necessarily mean absence of pain)	Absence of movement: 0
	Slow, cautious movements; touching or rubbing the pain site; seeking attention through movements	Protection: 1
	Pulling tube, attempting to sit up, moving limbs or thrashing, not following commands, striking at staff, trying to climb out of bed	Restlessness: 2
Muscle tension	No resistance to passive movements	Relaxed: 0
	Resistance to passive movements	Tense, rigid: 1
	Strong resistance to passive movements, inability to complete them	Very tense or rigid: 2
Compliance with the ventilator *or* Vocalization (extubated patients)	Alarms not activated, easy ventilation	Tolerating ventilator or movement: 0
	Alarms stop spontaneously	Coughing but tolerating: 1
	Asynchrony: blocking ventilation, alarms frequently activated	Fighting ventilator: 2
	Talking in normal tone or no sound	Talking in normal tone or no sound: 0
	Sighing, moaning	Sighing, moaning: 1
	Crying out, sobbing	Crying out, sobbing: 2

Adapted from Gélinas C, Fillion L, Puntillo KA, Viens C, Fortier M. Validation of the critical-care pain observation tool in adult patients. Am J Crit Care. 2006 Jul;15(4):420-7.

iii. Vital signs (e.g., elevated HR or BP) are cues that indicate further assessment of pain is necessary (i.e., using a scale described earlier).

iv. To assess sedation, the Richmond Agitation-Sedation Scale (RASS) and Sedation-Agitation Scale (SAS) are recommended because, compared with other sedation scores, they are more valid and reliable for monitoring the quality and depth of sedation in adult ICU patients. Goal sedation scores should be individualized for each patient, but generally an SAS score of 3 to 4 or a RASS score of 0 to –1 is recommended.

Table 11. Richmond Agitation-Sedation Scale (RASS)

Scale	Term	Description
+4	Combative	Combative, violent, immediate danger to staff
+3	Very agitated	Pulls to remove tubes or catheters; aggressive
+2	Agitated	Frequent nonpurposeful movement, fights ventilator
+1	Restless	Anxious but movements not aggressive
0	Alert and calm	Spontaneously pays attention to caregiver
−1	Drowsy	Not fully alert but has sustained awakening to voice (eye opening and eye contact for ≥10 seconds)
−2	Light sedation	Briefly (<10 seconds) awakens with eye contact to voice
−3	Moderate sedation	Movement or eye opening to voice but no eye contact
−4	Deep sedation	No response to voice but movement or eye opening to physical stimulation
−5	Unarousable	No response to voice or physical stimulation

Table 12. Sedation-Agitation Scale (SAS)

Score	Term	Description
7	Dangerous agitation	Pulling at endotracheal tube, trying to remove catheters, climbing over bedrail, striking at staff, thrashing side to side
6	Very agitated	Requiring restraint and frequent verbal reminding of limits, biting endotracheal tube
5	Agitated	Anxious or physically agitated, calms to verbal instructions
4	Calm and cooperative	Calm, easily roused, follows commands
3	Sedated	Difficult to arouse but awakens to verbal stimuli or gentle shaking, follows simple commands but drifts off again
2	Very sedated	Arouses to physical stimuli but does not communicate or follow commands, may move spontaneously
1	Unarousable	Minimal or no response to noxious stimuli, does not communicate or follow commands

    b.   Pain and discomfort are primary causes of agitation; thus, treat pain first and add a sedative if needed.

         i.   Use bolus dose analgesics or nonpharmacologic interventions before potentially painful procedures.

         ii.   Opioid analgesics are considered first line for the treatment of nonneuropathic pain (gabapentin or carbamazepine can be considered for neuropathic pain).

         iii.   Nonopioid analgesics (e.g., acetaminophen, ketamine) can be used in conjunction with opioids to optimize pain control and avoid dose-related adverse effects.

         iv.   Nonsteroidal anti-inflammatory drugs are usually avoided because of the risk of bleeding and kidney injury in critically ill patients.

         v.   Nonbenzodiazepine sedatives may be preferred to benzodiazepines to improve clinical outcomes in mechanically ventilated patients.

c. Dosing strategies for analgesics and sedatives

   i. Analgesics and sedatives should be dosed to achieve pain and sedation goals. Adjust sedative medications to achieve a light level of sedation (i.e., capable of being roused and able to follow simple commands). Light sedation is needed for evaluating pain and delirium and for early patient mobility.

   ii. Goals may be achieved using intermittent dosing administered routinely or as needed.

   iii. If unable to achieve goals with intermittent dosing, use a combination of bolus dosing with a continuous infusion.

     (a) In patients receiving a continuous infusion, use a bolus dose before or instead of increasing the infusion rate (a bolus dose has a faster onset and can eliminate the need for an increase in the infusion rate). Exception is with drugs such as propofol or dexmedetomidine, which can cause hypotension or bradycardia when bolused.

     (b) Use bolus dosing proactively (e.g., before dressing changes, suctioning, repositioning).

   iv. Daily awakening involves an interruption of continuous infusion opioid or sedatives until the patient is awake (SAS at least 4 or RASS at least 0) or shows discomfort or pain requiring reinitiation. Although evidence is mixed, a scheduled daily interruption of continuous infusions is associated with several important benefits:

     (a) Assess the patient's neurologic function.

     (b) Reevaluate lowest effective opioid or sedative dose.

     (c) Prevent drug accumulation and overdose.

     (d) Reduce time on the ventilator (although one randomized study contradicts this by finding no reduction in the duration of mechanical ventilation or ICU stay with sedation interruption; Mehta S, Burry L, Cook D, et al. Daily Sedation Interruption in Mechanically Ventilated Critically Ill Patients Cared for With a Sedation Protocol: A Randomized Controlled Trial. JAMA. 2012;308(19):1985-1992.).

     (e) Reduces mortality and ICU length of stay when combined with a spontaneous breathing trial.

     (f) Reduce symptoms of posttraumatic stress disorder.

B. Analgesics

Table 13. Analgesics

	Morphine	**Fentanyl**	**Hydromorphone**
Pharmacokinetics			
Onset (minutes)	5–10	1–2	5–10
Duration of effect (hours)	2–4	1–5	2–6
Prolonged in renal failure	Yes	No	No
Prolonged in hepatic failure	Yes	Yes	Yes
Elimination half-life (hours)	1–4	2–5	2–3
Active metabolites	Yes	No	No
Adverse effects			
Hypotension	Yes	No	Yes
Flushing	Yes	No	Yes
Bronchospasm	Yes	No	No
Constipation	Yes	Yes	Yes

C. Sedatives
1. Benzodiazepines should be titrated or avoided to prevent adverse outcomes, including prolonged duration of mechanical ventilation, increased ICU length of stay, and development of delirium.
2. Lorazepam
    a. Intermittent dosing 1–4 mg every 2–6 hours
    b. Continuous infusion: Start at 1 mg/hour and titrate to goal (e.g., RASS, SAS). Total daily doses as low as 1 mg/kg can cause propylene glycol toxicity. Monitor for an osmolal gap greater than 10–12 mOsm/L, indicating propylene glycol toxicity.
    c. Lorazepam is the preferred benzodiazepine in severe hepatic dysfunction due because of metabolism.
    d. Midazolam
        i. Intermittent dosing 1–4 mg every 15 minutes to 1 hour
        ii. Continuous infusion: Start at 1 mg/hour and titrate to goal (e.g., RASS, SAS).
        iii. Frequently used for procedural sedation or daily dressing changes because of its rapid onset and short duration
        iv. Prolonged infusions of midazolam may accumulate because of its greater lipophilicity compared with lorazepam, especially in patients with renal dysfunction.

Table 14. Benzodiazepines

	Diazepam	Lorazepam	Midazolam
Pharmacokinetics			
Onset (minutes)	2–5	5–20	2–5
Duration of effect (hours)	2–4	4–6	1–2
Prolonged in renal failure	Yes	No	Yes
Prolonged in hepatic failure	Yes	No	Yes
Elimination half-life (hours)	24–120	10–20	1–10
Active metabolite	Yes	No	Yes
CYP3A4 interactions	Yes	No	Yes
Adverse effects			
Hypotension	Yes	No	No
Thrombophlebitis	Yes	Maybe	No
Propylene glycol toxicity	No	Yes	No

CYP = cytochrome P450.

3. Propofol
    a. Rapid onset (1–2 minutes) and short duration (3–5 minutes or longer if prolonged infusion)
    b. Initiate at 5 mcg/kg/minute and titrate to achieve sedation goals by 5 mcg/kg/minute every 5 minutes. Avoid prolonged infusions greater than 50 mcg/kg/minute.
    c. Avoid loading doses because of the risk of hypotension.
    d. In general, used in intubated patients because of the risk of respiratory depression
    e. Propofol has no significant analgesic activity. If a patient has pain, will need to combine propofol with an analgesic
    f. Monitoring
        i. Blood pressure
        ii. Triglycerides
        iii. Calories provided from 10% lipid emulsion (1 kcal/mL). May need to adjust lipid or calories provided by nutrition support (i.e., enteral nutrition [EN] or parenteral nutrition [PN])

        iv. Propofol-related infusion syndrome is more likely to occur with prolonged infusions greater than 50 mcg/kg/minute and is associated with metabolic acidosis, cardiac failure, arrhythmias (e.g., bradycardia), cardiac arrest, rhabdomyolysis, hyperkalemia, and kidney failure.

    g. Propofol is more commonly used than benzodiazepines, probably because it has a shorter duration, is easily titratable, and is more predictable.

  4. Dexmedetomidine

    a. Sedative properties through central and peripheral α_2-receptor agonist activity

    b. Extent of analgesic activity in ICU patients is not well described.

    c. Does not cause respiratory depression

    d. Rapid onset (5–15 minutes if bolus, longer without bolus) and short duration (2-hour half-life). Longer duration in patients with severe hepatic dysfunction

    e. A loading dose is suggested for patients undergoing surgery; however, loading doses are *NOT* recommended for ICU patients because of the risk of bradycardia and hypotension.

    f. Maintenance dose of 0.2–0.7 mcg/kg/hour is approved by the U.S. Food and Drug Administration for a maximum of 24 hours; however, there is evidence showing the safety and efficacy of prolonged infusions at doses of up to 1.5 mcg/kg/hour, and this is most commonly used in practice.

    g. Compared with benzodiazepines, dexmedetomidine is associated with a lower prevalence of ICU delirium in some studies.

    h. Results from the MIDEX and PRODEX studies show that dexmedetomidine is noninferior to midazolam and propofol in maintaining light to moderate sedation. Dexmedetomidine reduced the duration of mechanical ventilation compared with midazolam (Jakob SM, Ruokonen E, Grounds R, et al. Dexmedetomidine vs Midazolam or Propofol for Sedation During Prolonged Mechanical Ventilation: Two Randomized Controlled Trials. JAMA. 2012;307(11):1151-1160.)

    i. Monitoring: Primary adverse effects are dose-related bradycardia and hypotension.

    j. Does not cause drug dependency, but withdrawal symptoms (e.g., nausea, vomiting, agitation) have occurred after prolonged use (1 week).

D. Assessment and Management of Delirium

  1. Delirium is an acute change in cognitive function characterized by disorganized thought, altered level of consciousness, and inattentiveness.

  2. Delirium is associated with increased mortality and prolonged length of stay in the ICU.

  3. Validated tools to proactively identify and assess delirium include the CAM-ICU and the Intensive Care Delirium Screening Checklist (ICDSC). The CAM-ICU is designed to detect delirium at the time of testing, whereas the ICDSC detects delirium during a nursing shift.

  4. Nonpharmacologic interventions are preferred to pharmacologic treatment. These include maintaining communication with the patient, reorienting the patient (to person, place, and time), maximizing uninterrupted sleep (e.g., control light and noise, cluster patient care activities, decrease stimuli at night), providing access to natural lighting (rooms with windows), removing unnecessary equipment from room, correcting sensory deficits (e.g., hearing aids, glasses), removing unneeded invasive devices (e.g., urinary catheters, intravenous lines, endotracheal tubes, enteral feeding tubes), minimizing physical restraint, and encouraging patient autonomy and early mobility.

  5. Correctable causes of delirium include hypotension, hypoxia, and electrolyte disturbances.

  6. There are minimal interventions that have been shown to improve delirium-related outcomes, so a strong focus should be put on minimizing or treating reversible risk factors such as avoiding or minimizing the dose of benzodiazepines and other medications that may cause delirium (e.g., opioids, anticholinergic medications).

E. Pharmacologic Treatment of Delirium
  1. Haloperidol
     a. Although commonly used, there is no evidence that haloperidol reduces the duration of delirium.
     b. Monitoring
        i. Hypotension
        ii. Assess QT interval at baseline and daily during haloperidol administration. In addition, monitor for other drugs that could prolong QT interval.
        iii. Extrapyramidal effects, including laryngeal dystonia and dysphagia, are more common with chronic oral administration than with intravenous administration.
     c. Lower initial doses of haloperidol (1–2.5 mg) should be used in older adults. Doses of haloperidol for acute agitation may be doubled every 20 minutes until an effective dose is reached.
  2. Atypical antipsychotics
     a. Atypical or second-generation antipsychotics may reduce the duration of delirium in critically ill patients.
     b. Atypical antipsychotics are associated with a lower incidence of extrapyramidal side effects (EPS) compared with haloperidol.
     c. Differences between agents are half-life, the risk of QT prolongation, sedation and risk of EPS.
        i. Sedative effects may or may not be beneficial (i.e., hyperactive vs. hypoactive delirium).
        ii. Agents with a shorter half-life (quetiapine) will generally act faster and have the ability to be quickly titrated.

Table 15. Medications Used to Treat Delirium

Medication	Initial Dosing	Dosage Forms	Half-life	Side Effects
Haloperidol	2.5 mg every 6 hours	Tablet, IM, IV	18 hours	QT prolongation EPS
Quetiapine	25 mg twice daily	Tablet	6 hours	Sedation QT prolongation
Olanzapine	5 mg daily	Tablet, ODT, IM	33 hours	Sedation
Risperidone	0.5 mg twice daily	Tablet, ODT, Solution, IM[a]	24 hours	EPS (doses >6 mg/day)
Ziprasidone	5 mg daily	Oral, IM	7 hours	QT prolongation

[a]IM formulation of risperidone is a long-acting formulation that is not indicated for acute delirium management.

EPS = extrapyramidal side effects; IM = intramuscular; IV = intravenous; ODT = orally disintegrating tablet;

F. Neuromuscular Blockade in ICU Patients
  1. Neuromuscular blockade is typically indicated for intubated patients with severe respiratory failure (e.g., ARDS, status asthmaticus) despite optimization of analgesia, sedation, and ventilator management. Recent data suggest that early empiric neuromuscular blockade in patients with severe ARDS may be beneficial. Neuromuscular blockers are also used as adjunctive agents to control severe intracranial hypertension in patients with neurologic injury (e.g., traumatic brain injury). A 48-hour infusion of cisatracurium (15-mg bolus followed by 37.5 mg/hour × 48 hours) in patients with severe acute respiratory distress syndrome (defined as Pao_2/Fio_2 less than 150) decreased the adjusted 90-day mortality. Note that in this study, the cisatracurium infusion was a fixed dose and was not adjusted on the basis of the monitoring parameters described later (e.g., TOF).
  2. Neuromuscular blockers are typically used once efforts to facilitate ventilation have failed (e.g., poor oxygenation, dyssynchrony, high intrathoracic pressures that put the patient at risk for barotrauma) using a combination of high-dose opioids and sedatives have failed (i.e., patient continues to have poor oxygenation).

3. *NEVER* use neuromuscular blockers in a patient who is not completely sedated or does not have adequate pain control.

4. Neuromuscular blockers should be used only in conjunction with a continuously infused sedative. Of importance, sedatives should have amnestic properties (e.g., benzodiazepines, propofol). Analgesics can also be used as needed in patients with pain. Many practitioners insist on the combination of a sedative and an analgesic in paralyzed patients. Patients should be provided with lubricating eye drops while paralyzed.

Table 16. Neuromuscular Blocking Agents

Recommendation	Pancuronium	Vecuronium	Atracurium	Cisatracurium
Duration of effect (hours)	0.75–1.5	0.5–0.75	0.25–0.5	0.5–1
Prolonged in renal failure	Yes	Yes	No	No
Prolonged in hepatic failure	Yes	Yes	No	No
Loading dose	0.08 mg/kg	0.1 mg/kg	0.4 mg/kg	0.1 mg/kg
Maintenance dose	0.02–0.04 mg/kg/hour	0.02–0.04 mg/kg/hour	0.4 mg/kg/hour	2–10 mcg/kg/minute
Adverse effects Tachycardia	Yes	No	No	No
Hypotension	No	No	Dose dependent	No

5. Concerns with neuromuscular blockade
   a. May mask seizure activity
   b. Prolonged use is associated with critical illness polyneuromyopathy, characterized by prolonged muscle weakness.
   c. Can mask insufficient analgesia and sedation.
   d. Increased risk of venous thromboembolism (VTE)
   e. Increased risk of skin breakdown and decubitus
   f. Corneal abrasions caused by eye dryness and lack of blinking; prevent by applying ophthalmic ointment or drops to eyes every 6–8 hours

6. Monitoring
   a. Neuromuscular blockers must be monitored to prevent an excessive degree of blockade and prolonged paralysis.
   b. The goal of neuromuscular blockade is to facilitate safe and optimal mechanical ventilation strategies using the minimal degree of neuromuscular blockade needed.
   c. Even with appropriate individualized dosing and monitoring of neuromuscular blockade, a principal adverse effect is prolonged muscle weakness after discontinuation. This can dramatically slow patient recovery, increasing the need for health care resources (e.g., physical therapy, rehabilitation). For this reason, it must be emphasized that the need for therapeutic paralysis must be carefully considered and reevaluated every day.
   d. A simple way to assess the appropriateness of the paralytic is as follows: Regularly (e.g., once daily) but temporarily discontinue the drug to determine the time needed for the patient to move or breathe spontaneously. Although not applicable to all patients, this "drug holiday" can be useful for the following reasons:
      i. Assess sedation and adjust sedatives as needed (i.e., if the patient is agitated after the drug is discontinued, he or she is not receiving adequate sedation or analgesia).
      ii. Assess the need for continued blockade (i.e., if the patient is able to maintain oxygenation, then perhaps the drug is no longer necessary).

      iii. Assess the dose of the paralytic (i.e., did the paralysis wear off within the expected time according to the expected drug duration?); this is especially important for drugs such as vecuronium and pancuronium because of the long half-life and dependence on end organ clearance.

      iv. Note: The study listed above used cisatracurium continuously (without a holiday) for 48 hours without an increased incidence of prolonged weakness.

    e. A peripheral nerve stimulator can be used in conjunction with drug holidays to assess the level of neuromuscular blockade and guide drug dosing.

    f. The TOF refers to peripheral nerve stimulation using four electrical impulses, usually applied to the ulnar or facial nerves.

    g. Obtain a baseline TOF before initiation to determine patient sensitivity to impulses. Patients who are not blocked should exhibit 1 twitch for each impulse (for 4/4 twitches).

    h. During neuromuscular blockade infusions for respiratory failure, patients should typically be maintained at 1–2 twitches, which indicate the extent of receptor blockade.

    i. Technical problems that limit the accuracy of TOF monitoring include the presence of perspiration or tissue edema.

7. In addition to the monitoring described, clinical assessment involves adjusting the neuromuscular blocker dose to prevent patient-ventilator dyssynchrony (e.g., "bucking" the ventilator, elevated peak airway pressures).

8. Avoid other medications or electrolyte abnormalities that can potentiate or inhibit paralysis.

Table 17. Interactions with Neuromuscular Blockers

	Potentiate Block	**Antagonize Block**
Drugs	Corticosteroids Aminoglycosides Clindamycin Tetracyclines Polymyxins Calcium channel blockers Type Ia antiarrhythmics Furosemide Lithium	Aminophylline Theophylline Carbamazepine Phenytoin (chronic)
Electrolyte disorders	Hypermagnesemia Hypocalcemia Hypokalemia	Hypercalcemia Hyperkalemia

Patient Cases

8. An older woman is admitted to the ICU for acute decompensated heart failure and acute kidney injury with an ejection fraction of less than 30%. She is administered a continuous infusion of bumetanide; however, the benefit is limited because of her acute on chronic kidney disease. She is intubated on ICU day 2 because of worsening pulmonary edema and hypoxia. After intubation, she scores a zero on the RASS, but her CAM-ICU is positive for delirium. Her BPS score is 4. Her BP is 120/70 mm Hg, and HR is 88 beats/minute. Which is the best recommendation for achieving her analgesia, sedation, and delirium goals?

    A. Initiate propofol at 5 mcg/kg/minute and titrate as needed.

    B. Administer haloperidol 5 mg intravenously and double the dose every 20 minutes as needed.

    C. Initiate morphine 4 mg intravenously every 4 hours as needed.

    D. Offer the patient verbal reassurance.

Questions 9–11 pertain to the following case:
A 42-year-old woman with acute respiratory distress syndrome and a significant history of alcohol and tobacco abuse is transferred to the medical ICU from an outside hospital. She presented to the outside hospital after 1 week of productive cough, fever, chills, and increased shortness of breath. On admission to the medical ICU, she is hypotensive (80/60 mm Hg), tachycardic (130 beats/minute), and febrile (39.0°C). Her ABG shows pH 7.1, $Paco_2$ 56 mm Hg, Pao_2 49 mm Hg, HCO_3^- 16 mEq/L, and Sao_2 76% on 100% Fio_2. The only other significant laboratory results are a SCr of 2.1 mg/dL and a WBC of 16×10^3 cells/mm³. She is achieving her sedation goals with continuous infusions of midazolam 3 mg/hour and fentanyl 250 mcg/hour.

9. After several nonpharmacologic attempts to improve her oxygenation fail, she is paralyzed, and her ventilator settings are adjusted accordingly. Which statement about neuromuscular blockade in this patient is most appropriate?

    A. Opioids should be discontinued to avoid prolonged neuromuscular weakness.

    B. Vecuronium is the agent of choice.

    C. Sedatives should be titrated to maintain a RASS goal of 0 to –2 during neuromuscular blockade.

    D. Neuromuscular blockers should be titrated to the minimal dose necessary to achieve ventilator synchrony.

10. The patient was initiated on neuromuscular blockade as instructed and appeared to being doing well until about 8 hours later, when she began to move around violently in her bed. At this time, she was tachycardic (120 beats/minute) and appeared very agitated; her Sao_2 dropped to 80%. Which action is best?

    A. Double the rate of the neuromuscular blocker every 5 minutes as needed until the patient stops moving.

    B. Administer a midazolam bolus and increase the infusion rate as needed to achieve sedation goals.

    C. Increase the fentanyl infusion rate as needed to achieve sedation goals.

    D. Check the TOF.

Patient Cases *(continued)*

11. After that event, the patient did poorly the rest of the night. The patient was initiated on a norepinephrine infusion at 0.02 mcg/kg/minute to maintain an adequate BP. Other medications initiated overnight included piperacillin/tazobactam, vancomycin, and gentamicin. By morning, her SCr has increased to 2.8 mg/dL, and the night shift nurse reports that the patient has had 0/4 twitches on TOF for the past 8 hours. Pertinent electrolyte values include K^+ 4.9 mEq/L, calcium (Ca^{++}) 9 mg/dL, and Mg^{++} 2 mg/dL. Which is most likely to potentiate the effects of cisatracurium?

    A. Piperacillin/tazobactam.

    B. Gentamicin.

    C. Norepinephrine.

    D. K value of 4.9 mEq/L.

VII. GLUCOSE CONTROL

A. History of Blood Glucose Control
    1. 2001: Study by van den Berghe et al. of surgical ICU patients showed a significant morbidity and mortality benefit of maintaining blood glucose in the range of 80–110 mg/dL, despite an increased risk of hypoglycemia (5.1% vs. 0.8%).
    2. 2006: Study by van den Berghe et al. of primarily medical ICU patients showed no mortality benefit associated with maintaining blood glucose in the range of 80–110 mg/dL in the entire study population. The study did show a reduction in ventilator time and length of stay, as well as a reduction in mortality in patients with an ICU length of stay of 3 days or more. The incidence of hypoglycemia (18%) was higher than previously reported.
    3. Subsequent investigations of tight glycemic control (80–110 mg/dL) never replicated the mortality benefit seen in the 2001 study. Studies did show much higher rates of hypoglycemia with tight glycemic control.
    4. 2009: Results of a large, international, randomized study (NICE-SUGAR) involving more than 6000 critically ill medical and surgical patients showed higher mortality and higher risk of hypoglycemia in patients receiving intensive blood glucose control (goal glucose 81–108 mg/dL) compared with patients having a goal of 180 mg/dL or less (mean blood glucose 142 mg/dL).
    5. The 2012 SSC guidelines recommend initiating insulin when two consecutive blood glucose readings are greater than 180 mg/dL. The target blood glucose concentration is 180 mg/dL or less for patients with sepsis.
    6. The 2012 Society of Critical Care Medicine guidelines for using an insulin infusion to manage hyperglycemia in general critically ill patients suggest using a blood glucose of 150 mg/dL or higher as a trigger for insulin therapy, adjusted to keep blood glucose less than 150 mg/dL, and maintaining values less than 180 mg/dL using an insulin protocol that achieves a low rate of hypoglycemia (blood glucose 70 mg/dL or less).

B. Treatment Strategies to Achieve Glycemic Control in Critically Ill Patients
    1. For a continuous insulin infusion approach, use a validated dosing protocol that considers blood glucose concentration, rate of change, and insulin infusion rate.
    2. Intravenous insulin is preferred for patients with type 1 diabetes mellitus, for patients with hyperglycemia who are hemodynamically unstable, and for patients in whom long-acting basal insulin should not be initiated because of changing clinical status. Once stable, patients can be considered for transitioning to a protocol-driven subcutaneous insulin regimen.

3. Regularly scheduled subcutaneous administration of basal or rapid-acting insulin can prevent hyperglycemia in clinically stable patients who do not require an intravenous infusion of insulin. The use of subcutaneous insulin is not recommended in patients on vasopressors, patients with significant peripheral edema, or patients for whom rapid correction of blood glucose is warranted.

4. A sliding-scale or correctional insulin regimen can be used in conjunction with the regularly scheduled subcutaneous doses; however, the baseline of insulin administered should be adjusted daily to prevent hyperglycemia and the need for additional doses of insulin. Subcutaneous sliding-scale or correctional insulin should not be the sole method of glucose control in critically ill patients.

C. Monitoring Blood Glucose
1. For a continuous insulin infusion approach, monitoring blood glucose every 1–2 hours is typically needed to provide safe and effective therapy.
2. Interpret point-of-care testing of capillary blood with caution because it can overestimate plasma glucose values. Overestimation of blood glucose is more common in patients with anemia, hypotension, or hypoperfusion. It is also more common when blood glucose is in the hypoglycemic or hyperglycemic range.
3. Arterial or venous whole blood sampling is recommended instead of fingerstick capillary blood glucose testing in patients with shock or severe peripheral edema and for patients on a prolonged insulin infusion.

VIII. PREVENTING STRESS ULCERS

A. Mucosal Bleeding in Critically Ill Adults
1. The incidence of stress-related mucosal bleeding in critically ill adults is estimated to be about 6%.
2. Signs and symptoms of stress ulcers include hematemesis, gross blood in gastric tube aspirates, "coffee ground" emesis or aspiration from gastric tube, and melena. Clinically significant stress ulcers are defined as those that cause hemodynamic compromise or necessitate blood transfusion.

B. Prophylactic therapy for stress ulcers
1. Prophylactic medications are recommended for any one of the following major risk factors:
   a. Respiratory failure necessitating mechanical ventilation (probably for more than 48 hours).
   b. Coagulopathy defined as platelet count less than 50,000/mm³, international normalized ratio (INR) greater than 1.5, or activated partial thromboplastin time more than 2 times control. (Note: Prophylactic or treatment doses of anticoagulants do not constitute coagulopathy.)
2. Prophylactic medications or continuing home acid suppressive regimens are also recommended for any patient with a history of GI ulceration or bleeding within 1 year before ICU admission.
3. Prophylactic medications are recommended for patients with two or more of the following risk factors (though data on this approach are lacking):
   a. Head or spinal cord injury
   b. Severe burn (more than 35% of body surface area)
   c. Hypoperfusion
   d. Acute organ dysfunction
   e. High doses of corticosteroids (>250 mg/day of hydrocortisone or equivalent)
   f. Liver failure with associated coagulopathy
   g. Postoperative transplantation
   h. Acute kidney injury
   i. Major surgery
   j. Multiple trauma

C. Strategies for Stress Ulcer Prophylaxis (see Table 18 for specific medications)

1. Efficacy of intravenous histamine-2 (H_2)-blockers in preventing stress-related upper GI bleeding has been shown in multiple clinical trials. These are commonly administered enterally when possible because of excellent bioavailability; however, evidence of efficacy is primarily with the intravenous administration of H_2-blockers.

2. Despite limited evidence in preventing stress-related mucosal bleeding, intravenous or enterally administered proton pump inhibitors (PPIs) are often used.

3. Regardless of the drug choice or route, it is important to discontinue therapy when risk factors are no longer present to avoid unnecessary drug interactions, adverse effects (pneumonia), and increased costs. This step is easily overlooked, with the result that patients are discharged from hospitals and continued on acid suppressive therapy with no indication.

4. Not recommended for prevention

   a. Antacids are not used to prevent stress ulcers.

   b. Sucralfate has been found to be inferior to H_2-blockers and is therefore not recommended for preventing stress ulcers. In addition, it can cause obstruction of enteral feeding tubes and aluminum toxicity in patients with renal failure.

   c. Safety: The benefits of preventing stress ulcers by increasing the stomach pH must be weighed against an increased risk of infection, including *C. difficile*, hospital-acquired pneumonia, and community-acquired pneumonia (for patients discharged on a PPI).

Table 18. Medications for Stress Ulcer Prophylaxis

Class	Examples and Dosing	Adverse Effects	Notes
H_2-receptor blockers	Ranitidine 150 mg PO every 12 hours or 50 mg IV every 8 hours Famotidine 20 mg IV or PO every 12 hours Nizatidine 150 mg PO every 12 hours Cimetidine 300 mg PO or IV every 6 hours or continuous infusion 37.5–50 mg/hour	Mental status changes, thrombocytopenia (cimetidine)	Cimetidine not routinely used because of drug interactions (strong P450 inhibitor) and side effects Excellent bioavailability Low cost Potential for reduced efficacy over time (tachyphylaxis) Dose adjustment for renal dysfunction Low risk of nosocomial pneumonia

Table 18. Medications for Stress Ulcer Prophylaxis *(continued)*

Class	Examples and Dosing	Adverse Effects	Notes
Proton pump inhibitors	Omeprazole 20 mg PO daily Powder for oral suspension available Esomeprazole 20–40 mg PO or IV daily Lansoprazole 30 mg PO or IV daily Delayed-release orally disintegrating tablets and oral suspension available Pantoprazole 40 mg PO or IV daily Granules available for oral or tube administration	Headache, diarrhea, constipation, abdominal pain, nausea	Solutions of certain PPIs may be compounded; refer to individual package inserts for instructions No adjustment needed for renal or liver dysfunction Higher cost than H$_2$-blockers Administration problems when given via NG tube Risk of ventilator-associated pneumonia increased Risk of *Clostridium difficile* infection (nosocomial or community acquired)

H$_2$ = histamine-2; IV = intravenously; PO = orally; NG = nasogastric; PPI = proton pump inhibitor.

Patient Cases

Questions 12 and 13 pertain to the following case:
A 73-year-old woman weighing 84 kg is admitted to the ICU after a pneumonectomy. Her BP is 104/65 mm Hg, HR is 88 beats/minute, and oxygen saturations are 98% on 40% F$_{IO_2}$ and PEEP 5; her Glasgow Coma Scale score is 11. Other laboratory values are normal. A small-bore feeding tube is in place, she is being fed enterally at goal rate, and she has no gastric residuals. Her medications include simvastatin 20 mg every night, aspirin 81 mg/day, metoprolol 25 mg twice daily, heparin 5000 units subcutaneously every 8 hours, and 0.9% NaCl intravenously at 75 mL/hour.

12. The surgeon would like to initiate stress ulcer prophylaxis (SUP). Which of the following is the best recommendation for this patient?

    A. Famotidine 20 mg per tube every 12 hours.

    B. Esomeprazole 40 mg intravenously daily.

    C. Sucralfate 1 g per tube four times daily.

    D. Ranitidine 50 mg intravenously every 8 hours.

13. One week later, the patient is extubated but still in the ICU. Her Glasgow Coma Scale score is 15, BP 112/70 mm Hg, and HR 75 beats/minute, but her appetite is poor. Which statement is most appropriate regarding SUP for this patient?

    A. SUP should continue until the patient is discharged from the ICU.

    B. SUP should be discontinued now.

    C. Continue SUP until patient is eating.

    D. SUP should be discontinued at hospital discharge.

IX. PHARMACOLOGIC THERAPY FOR PREVENTING VENOUS THROMBOEMBOLISM

A. General Overview: Venous thromboembolism (VTE) is a common complication of critical illness, with an incidence of deep vein thrombosis (DVT) of 8%–40% and pulmonary embolism (PE) of up to 12%.

B. Risk Factors for VTE
   1. All critically ill patients are usually at high risk of VTE.
   2. Additional risk factors include surgery, major trauma, lower extremity injury, immobility, malignancy, sepsis, heart failure, respiratory failure, venous compression, previous VTE, increasing age, pregnancy, erythropoiesis-stimulating agents, obesity, and central venous catheterization.

C. Nonpharmacologic Prevention of VTE
   1. Early mobility is the ideal nonpharmacologic therapy.
   2. Mechanical prophylaxis with intermittent pneumatic compression or graduated compression stockings is recommended for medical patients at risk of VTE who have a contraindication to pharmacologic anticoagulation (e.g., thrombocytopenia, severe coagulopathy, active bleeding, recent intracerebral hemorrhage).
   3. Mechanical prophylaxis can be used in combination with pharmacologic treatment.

D. Recommendations for Critically Ill Patients
   1. American College of Chest Physicians (ACCP) Ninth Edition
      a. Recommends low-molecular-weight heparin or low-dose unfractionated heparin over no prophylaxis
      b. For patients who are bleeding or at high risk for major bleeding, the guidelines recommend mechanical thromboprophylaxis and institution of pharmacologic prophylaxis when the bleeding risk decreases.
      c. The guidelines provide separate postoperative recommendations. A detailed assessment is beyond the scope of this text, and readers are encouraged to see the guideline for more information.
   2. SSC also provides recommendations that are identical to those above.

E. Pharmacologic Prophylaxis (see Table 19 for dosage)
   1. Unfractionated heparin
      a. Low cost
      b. Twice- versus three-times-daily administration: No head-to-head comparison has been completed. Two meta-analyses have been completed on the subject. The first, in 2007, concluded that there was no difference in efficacy, but three-times-daily administration was associated with a slightly higher risk of bleeding. The second, in 2011, found no difference in efficacy or safety with either regimen.
      c. Risk of heparin-induced thrombocytopenia (HIT) lower than full anticoagulation doses
   2. LMWHs
      a. All considered therapeutically equivalent
      b. Dalteparin is renally eliminated but may be considered in patients with CrCl <30 mL/minute due to low accumulation.
      c. Low risk of HIT
   3. Fondaparinux
      a. May be safe in patients with a history of HIT
      b. Data on reversal of fondaparinux are lacking.
      c. Contraindicated for CrCl <30 mL/minute
      d. Very limited data in critically ill patients

4. New oral anticoagulants
    a. Rivaroxaban was evaluated against enoxaparin in a study of acutely ill medical patients requiring hospitalization. Although rivaroxaban was as efficacious as enoxaparin at study day 10, there was an excess risk of bleeding in the rivaroxaban group. Of note, patients with cardiogenic or septic shock with the need for vasopressors were excluded. Rivaroxaban is renally eliminated and is not recommended in patients with renal insufficiency.
    b. Apixaban was evaluated against enoxaparin in a study of acutely ill medical patients requiring hospitalization. There were no difference in rates of VTE but a higher bleeding rate with apixaban. Patients with septic shock were also excluded from this trial.
    c. Compared with heparins, there is limited experience in reversal of anti-Xa inhibitors in clinical practice.
    d. No data exist for dabigatran in this patient population.
    e. At this time, new oral anticoagulants cannot be recommended for routine use in VTE prophylaxis in critically ill patients.

F. Special Populations
    1. Impaired kidney function
        a. If estimated CrCl is less than 30 mL/minute, LMWH dosage reduction is usually necessary. If creatinine clearance is less than 20 mL/minute or patient is on dialysis, dosing information is limited for LMWH; anti-Xa monitoring may not be reliable in dialysis patients.
        b. Alternatively, if estimated CrCl is less than 30 mL/minute, dalteparin can be used because it has minimal renal metabolism.
        c. Fondaparinux is contraindicated in patients with an estimated creatinine clearance less than 30 mL/minute.
        d. Low-dose unfractionated heparin is minimally renally eliminated and is safe to use in patients with reduced kidney function.
    2. Overweight or underweight adults: For obese patients, some experts recommend increasing LMWH prophylaxis doses by 30% if body mass index is greater than 40 kg/m^2; a peak (4 hours postdose) anti-Xa of 0.2–0.4 IU/mL is recommended. Note that these recommendations have not been validated in controlled trials and are considered expert opinion only (see Nutescu, Edith A., et al. "Low-molecular-weight heparins in renal impairment and obesity: available evidence and clinical practice recommendations across medical and surgical settings." Annals of Pharmacotherapy 43.6 (2009): 1064-1083.).

G. Antithrombotic Therapy and Regional Anesthesia
    1. Critically ill patients often have their spinal meninges accessed for either therapeutic (epidural anesthesia, lumbar drains) or diagnostic (lumbar puncture) purposes.
    2. The combination of antithrombotic medications with these techniques is associated with an elevated risk of spinal or epidural hematoma, which may lead to ischemia and paralysis.
    3. The American Society of Regional Anesthesia and Pain Medicine has released guidelines on regional anesthesia in the patient receiving antithrombotic or thrombolytic therapy.
        a. There is no contraindication to low-dose unfractionated heparin at daily doses of less than 10,000 units (i.e., 5,000 units every 12 hours). It is unknown whether subcutaneous heparin at doses greater than 10,000 units daily (i.e., 5,000 units every 8 hours) carries a higher risk of complication than lower doses. If patients receive subcutaneous heparin at doses greater than 10,000 units daily, enhanced monitoring for neurodeficits should take place.
        b. For patients receiving LMWH, needle placement should occur 10–12 hours after the last LMWH dose (longer in patients with renal disease).

      c. Indwelling catheters should be removed before initiation of twice-daily LMWH postoperatively but may be maintained for patients on once-daily regimens.

         i. The first dose of LMWH should be at least 2 hours after catheter removal.

        ii. Catheter removal should be at least 10–12 hours after the last LMWH dose (longer in patients with renal disease).

      d. Because of a lack of data and early clinical trial data, the use of fondaparinux should be avoided.

  H. Prevention of VTE: Pharmacologic Options in Critically Ill Patients

Table 19. Prevention of VTE Pharmacologic Options

Medication	Mechanism	Dosing	Adjustment for Renal Dysfunction
Unfractionated heparin	Factor Xa and indirect thrombin inhibition	5000 units SC 2 or 3 times daily	None
Low-molecular-weight heparins	Factor Xa inhibition and some indirect thrombin inhibition	Enoxaparin 40 mg SC daily Dalteparin 5000 units SC daily	CrCl <30: enoxaparin 30 mg SC daily
Fondaparinux	Factor Xa inhibition	2.5 mg SC daily	Contraindicated for CrCl <30 mL/minute

SC = subcutaneously.

X. PREVENTING VENTILATOR-ASSOCIATED PNEUMONIA

  A. The Institute for Healthcare Improvement has developed a ventilator bundle with the following elements that directly target ventilator-associated pneumonia (VAP) and complications arising from VAP.

    1. Head of the bed elevation: Maintain the head of the bed elevated (about 30–45°).

    2. Daily sedation interruptions and assessment of readiness to extubate

    3. Stress ulcer prophylaxis

    4. VTE prophylaxis

    5. Daily oral care with chlorhexidine (0.12% oral rinse)

  B. Additional Methods

    1. Selective decontamination of the digestive tract (SDD)

      a. SDD is a short course of antimicrobial therapy aimed at eradicating potential pathogens to minimize ICU-acquired infections.

      b. Despite three decades of research, SDD is still not routinely performed.

    2. Endotracheal tubes coated in an antimicrobial (silver) reduce infection but are cost prohibitive in many centers.

XI. NUTRITION SUPPORT IN CRITICALLY ILL PATIENTS

A. General Overview

1. Many critically ill patients have increased caloric and protein needs, and increasing caloric deficit in these patients leads to excess morbidity (length of stay, infection) and mortality.

2. Skeletal muscle wasting and weakness occurring during critical illness may lead to prolonged mechanical ventilation and rehabilitation.

3. Ideally, nutrition should be provided within 24–48 hours of admission to the ICU.

4. Route of delivery (EN vs. PN)

   a. In general, EN is preferred to PN in patients with a functional GI tract who are not malnourished.

   b. American and Canadian guidelines allow hypocaloric feeding during the first 7 days in previously well-nourished patients before consideration of PN.

   c. The SSC guidelines recommend intravenous glucose and EN rather than total PN alone or PN in conjunction with EN in the first 7 days after a diagnosis of severe sepsis or septic shock.

   d. PN is recommended for patients who have extensive small bowel resection, chronic malabsorption, high-output enterocutaneous fistulas, severe malnutrition at baseline, suspected or confirmed GI ischemia, mechanical bowel obstruction, or persistent, severe hemodynamic instability.

B. Estimating Nutrition Needs

1. Traditional biomarkers of nutrition (albumin, prealbumin, nitrogen balance) are not well validated in critically ill patients.

2. Indirect calorimetry and predictive equations may be used to determine energy needs in critically ill patients.

   a. Indirect calorimetry measures the metabolic rate, but it requires special equipment and trained staff, and is subject to inaccuracies in some patient populations. Indirect calorimetry also provides a respiratory quotient (RQ), indicating substrate metabolism and allowing modification of macronutrient delivery (e.g., carbohydrates, fats, protein).

      i. RQ 1.0–1.3: Lipogenesis (overfeeding), hyperventilation, or system "leak"

      ii. RQ 0.9–1.0: Primary carbohydrate oxidation, metabolic acidosis

      iii. RQ 0.82–0.85: Normal, "mixed" substrate oxidation

      iv. RQ 0.80: Primary protein oxidation

      v. RQ 0.70: Primary fat oxidation, systemic inflammatory response syndrome, metabolic alkalosis, or ethanol oxidation

      vi. RQ less than 0.67 or greater than 1.3: Outside range; question test validity

   b. Several predictive equations for determining caloric goals have been used (e.g., Harris-Benedict, Penn State and modified Penn State, Ireton-Jones, Mifflin, and Swinamer equations). See the references for a review of the usefulness of predictive equations in critically ill patients.

   c. Some guidelines recommend a 25-kcal/kg target, but this approach may be too simplistic for the majority of critically ill patients.

3. Hypocaloric feeding

   a. The SSC recommends avoiding mandatory full caloric feeding in the first week, but rather suggests low-dose feeding (i.e., up to 500 kcal per day), advancing only as tolerated.

   b. One study showed that intentional underfeeding (60%–70% of target) of critically ill patients while providing 90%–100% of protein needs showed a significant reduction in hospital mortality.

   c. It is recommended that obese patients (BMI >30) can be fed at 60%–70% of target energy requirements or 11–14 kcal/kg actual body weight per day. Protein should be delivered in the range of 2–2.5 g/kg ideal body weight per day.

4. Protein needs
   a. The stress response in critical illness increases gluconeogenesis, which cannot be fully suppressed by exogenous glucose.
   b. Protein intake of 1.2–2 g/kg of actual body weight is recommended in most critically ill patients.
      i. Patients on continuous renal replacement therapy may require up to 2.5 g/kg per day.
      ii. Patients with acute kidney injury who are not on renal replacement may require as little as 0.6–0.8 g/kg per day.
      iii. Patients with extensive burn injury may require up to 3 g/kg per day.

C. Enteral Nutrition
   1. It is important to recognize that the prescribed dose of enteral nutrition is often not delivered to patients because of interruptions, intolerance or many other reasons. Use of an enteral nutrition protocol with guidance on initiation, advancement, and interruptions is essential.
   2. "Trophic" feeding, or low-dose enteral feeding with the intent of maintaining GI tract function, is commonly used despite limited evidence.
   3. EN may be safely delivered to patients on low-dose vasopressors.
   4. Gastric versus small bowel (postpyloric) feeding delivery
      a. Delivery of EN directly into the small bowel may be associated with a reduction in pneumonia.
      b. In units where small bowel access is readily available, routine use of small bowel feeding is recommended.
      c. If small bowel access is not readily available, then small bowel feedings should be considered only for patients at high risk of intolerance to EN (on inotropes, continuous infusion of sedatives, or paralytic agents, or patients with high nasogastric drainage) or at high risk for regurgitation and aspiration (nursed in supine position) or who have repeatedly demonstrated intolerance of gastric feeds.
   5. Gastric residual volumes
      a. There are no data indicating that interruption of gastric feeding for a specific residual volume prevents morbidity (aspiration pneumonia) in critically ill patients.
      b. A residual volume of 250–500 is recommended as a point where intervention (prokinetic agents, tube feeding interruption, small bowel tube placement) should take place.

D. Parenteral Nutrition
   1. PN should be administered by central vein whenever possible. Peripheral administration is possible but must be dilute and may cause problems with the volume of the solution.
   2. Intravenous catheters intended for PN should not be used for any other purpose.
   3. Blood glucose measurements should be taken at least every 4–6 hours for patients on PN during initiation and changes in carbohydrate content.

E. Supplemental Antioxidants and Immunomodulation: The use of supplemental antioxidants and immuno-modulating micronutrients (vitamin E, selenium, fish oils, arginine, glutamine, zinc) are not recommended for general critically ill patients.
   1. Use of glutamine in burn or trauma patients without multisystem organ failure may be considered.
   2. Addition of fish oils and antioxidants in patients with acute lung injury or acute respiratory distress syndrome may be considered.

F. Further Guidance: See chapter titled "Fluids, Electrolytes, and Nutrition."

Patient Cases

Questions 14 and 15 pertain to the following case:

A 75-year-old woman (height 165 cm, weight 68 kg) who is intubated requires mechanical ventilation for an acute exacerbation of chronic obstructive pulmonary disease. She has a past medical history of heart failure and hypertension. Her laboratory values are normal except for a Cr of 1.9 mg/dL.

14. Which is the most appropriate recommendation to prevent VTE in this patient?

    A. Initiate intermittent pneumatic compression.

    B. Administer fondaparinux 2.5 mg subcutaneously once daily.

    C. Administer enoxaparin 30 mg subcutaneously once daily.

    D. Administer heparin continuous intravenous infusion to maintain an aPTT of 40–60 seconds.

15. Three days later, the patient continues to require mechanical ventilation. Enteral nutrition has been initiated through her nasogastric feeding tube and gradually increased to 45 mL/hr. Her gastric residuals are consistently 150–200 mL. Which statement is most appropriate to optimize nutrition support for this patient?

    A. Switch to PN.

    B. Add metoclopramide 5 mg intravenously every 6 hours.

    C. Switch feeds to a more concentrated formula.

    D. Continue tube feedings at the current infusion rate.

REFERENCES

Acid Base

1. Adrogue HJ, Madias NE. Management of life-threatening acid-base disorders. Part I. N Engl J Med 1998;338:26-34.

2. Adrogue HJ, Madias NE. Management of life-threatening acid-base disorders. Part II. N Engl J Med 1998;338:107-11.

3. Haber RJ. A practical approach to acid-base disorders. West J Med 1991;155:146-51.

4. Berend K, de Vries AP, Gans RO. Physiological approach to assessment of acid-base disturbances. N Engl J Med 2014;371:1434-45.

Shock and Sepsis

1. Vincent JL, De Backer D. Circulatory shock. N Engl J Med 2013;369:1726-34.

2. Annane D, Sebille V, Charpentier C, et al. Effect of treatment with low doses of hydrocortisone and fludrocortisone on mortality in patients with septic shock. JAMA 2002;288:862-70.

3. DeBacker D, Biston P, Devriendt J, et al. Comparison of dopamine and norepinephrine in the treatment of shock. N Engl J Med 2010;362:779-89.

4. Dellinger RP, Levy MM, Rhodes A, et al. Surviving Sepsis Campaign: international guidelines for management of severe sepsis and septic shock: 2012. Crit Care Med 2013;41:580-637.

5. Finfer S, Bellomo R, Boyce N, et al. A comparison of albumin and saline for fluid resuscitation in the intensive care unit. N Engl J Med 2004;350:2247-56.

6. Rivers E, Nguyen B, Havstad S, et al. Early goal-directed therapy in the treatment of severe sepsis and septic shock. N Engl J Med 2001;345:1368-77.

7. Russell JA. Management of sepsis. N Engl J Med 2006;355:1699-713.

8. Russell JA, Walley KR, Singer J, et al. Vasopressin versus norepinephrine infusion in patients with septic shock. N Engl J Med 2008;358:877-87.

9. Sprung CL, Annane D, Keh D, et al. Hydrocortisone therapy for patients with septic shock. N Engl J Med 2008;358:111-4.

10. Sprung CL, Brezis M, Goodman S, et al. Corticosteroid therapy for patients in septic shock: some progress in a difficult decision. Crit Care Med 2011;39:571-4.

11. Angus DC, van der Poll T. Severe sepsis and septic shock. N Engl J Med 2013;369:840-51.

12. Zarychanski R, Abou-Setta AM, Turgeon AF, et al. Association of hydroxyethyl starch administration with mortality and acute kidney injury in critically ill patients requiring volume resuscitation: a systematic review and meta-analysis. JAMA 2013;309(7):678-88.

13. Yunos N, Bellomo R, Hegarty C, et al. Association between a chloride-liberal vs chloride-restrictive intravenous fluid administration strategy and kidney injury in critically ill adults. JAMA 2012;308(15):1566-72.

14. The ARISE Investigators and the ANZICS Clinical Trials Group. Goal-directed resuscitation for patients with early septic shock. N Engl J Med 2014;371:1496-1506.

15. Chew MS, Åneman A. Haemodynamic monitoring using arterial waveform analysis. Curr Opin Crit Care 2013;19(3):234-41.

16. Marik PE, Pastores SM, Annane D, et al. Recommendations for the diagnosis and management of corticosteroid insufficiency in critically ill adult patients: consensus statements from an international task force by the American College of Critical Care Medicine. Crit Care Med 2008;36(6):1937-49.

Cardiac Arrest

1. American Heart Association. American Heart Association guidelines for cardiopulmonary resuscitation and emergency cardiovascular care. Available at http://circ.ahajournals.org/cgi/content/full/122/18_suppl_3/S640. Accessed November 21, 2014.

2. Peberdy MA, Callaway CW, Neumar RW, et al.; American Heart Association. Part 9: post-cardiac arrest care: 2010 American Heart Association guidelines for cardiopulmonary resuscitation and emergency cardiovascular care. Circulation 2010;122(18 suppl 3):S768-86.

3. Nunnally ME, Jaeschke R, Bellingan GJ, et al. Targeted temperature management in critical care: a report and recommendations from five professional societies. Crit Care Med 2011;39:1113-25.

4. Nielsen N, Wetterslev J, Cronberg T, et al. Targeted temperature management at 33°C versus 36°C after cardiac arrest. N Engl J Med 2013;369:2197-2206.

Sedation

1. Barr J, Fraser GL, Puntillo K, et al. Clinical practice guidelines for the management of pain, agitation, and delirium in adult patients in the intensive care unit. Crit Care Med 2013;41:263-306.

2. Kress JP, Pohlman AS, O'Connor MF, et al. Daily interruption of sedative infusions in critically ill patients undergoing mechanical ventilation. N Engl J Med 2000;342:1471-7.

3. Pun B, Dunn J. The sedation of critically ill adults: part 1. Assessment. Am J Nurs 2007;107:40-8.

4. Sessler CN, Varney K. Patient-focused sedation and analgesia in the ICU. Chest 2008;133:552-65.

Delirium

1. Ely EW, Shintani A, Truman B, et al. Delirium as a predictor of mortality in mechanically ventilated patients in the intensive care unit. JAMA 2004;291:1753-62.

2. ICU Delirium and Cognitive Impairment Study Group. Brain dysfunction in critically ill patients. Vanderbilt Medical Center. Available at www.icudelirium.org/delirium. Accessed September 30, 2009.

3. Neil A. Gilchrist NA, Asoh I, Greenberg B. Atypical antipsychotics for the treatment of ICU delirium. J Intensive Care Med 2012;27:354-61.

Neuromuscular Blockade

1. Baumann MH, McAlpin BW, Brown K, et al. A prospective randomized comparison of train-of-four monitoring and clinical assessment during continuous ICU cisatracurium paralysis. Chest 2004;126:1267-73.

2. Murray MJ, Cowen J, DeBlock H, et al. Clinical practice guidelines for sustained neuromuscular blockade in the adult critically ill patient. Crit Care Med 2002;30:142-56.

3. Papazian L, Forel JM, Gacouin A, et al. Neuromuscular blockers in early acute respiratory distress syndrome. N Engl J Med 2010;363:1107-16.

Glucose Control

1. Jacobi J, Bircher N, Krinsley J, et al. Guidelines for the use of an insulin infusion for the management of hyperglycemia in critically ill patients. Crit Care Med 2012;40:3251-76.

2. NICE-SUGAR Study Investigators; Finfer S, Chittock DR, Su SY, et al. Intensive versus conventional glucose control in critically ill patients. N Engl J Med 2009;360:1283-97.

3. Kavanagh BP, McCowen KC. Glycemic control in the ICU. N Engl J Med 2010;363:2540-6.

Stress Ulcer Prophylaxis

1. Allen ME, Kopp BJ, Erstad BL. Stress ulcer prophylaxis in the postoperative period. Am J Health Syst Pharm 2004;61:588-96.

2. ASHP Commission on Therapeutics. ASHP therapeutic guidelines on stress ulcer prophylaxis. Am J Health Syst Pharm 1999;56:347-79.

3. Cook D, Guyatt G, Marshall J, et al. A comparison of sucralfate and ranitidine for the prevention of upper gastrointestinal bleeding in patients requiring mechanical ventilation. N Engl J Med 1998;338:791-7.

4. Herzig SJ, Howell MD, Ngo LH, et al. Acid-suppressive medication use and the risk for hospital-acquired pneumonia. JAMA 2009;301:2120-8.

5. Sessler JM. Stress-related mucosal disease in the intensive care unit: an update on prophylaxis. AACN Adv Crit Care 2007;18:199-26.

6. Stevens AM, Thomas Z. The case against stress ulcer prophylaxis in 2007. Hosp Pharm 2007;42:995-1002.

Preventing VTE

1. Alhazzani W, Lim W, Jaeschke RZ, et al. Heparin thromboprophylaxis in medical-surgical critically ill patients: a systematic review and meta-analysis of randomized trials. Crit Care Med 2013;41:2088-98.

2. Cook D, Meade M, Guyatt G, et al. Dalteparin versus unfractionated heparin in critically ill patients. N Engl J Med 2011;364:1305-14.

3. Guyatt GH, Akl EA, Crowther DD, et al. Executive summary: antithrombotic therapy and prevention of thrombosis, 9th ed. American College of Chest Physicians evidence-based clinical practice guidelines. Chest 2012;141(2 suppl):7S-47S.

4. Nutescu EA. Assessing, preventing, and treating venous thromboembolism: evidence-based approaches. Am J Health Syst Pharm 2007;64 (suppl 7):5-13.

5. Gould MK, Garcia DA, Wren SM, et al. Prevention of VTE in nonorthopedic surgical patients. Chest 2012;141(2 suppl):e227S-77S.

6. Cohen AT, Spiro TE, Buller HR, et al. Rivaroxaban for thromboprophylaxis in acutely ill medical patients. N Engl J Med 2013;368:513-23.

7. Phung OJ, Kahn SR, Cook DJ, et al. Dosing frequency of unfractionated heparin thromboprophylaxis. Chest 2011;140(2):374-81.

Prevention of Ventilator-Associated Pneumonia

1. IHI ventilator bundle. Available at http://www.ihi.org/resources/Pages/Changes/Implementthe VentilatorBundle.aspx. Accessed November 21, 2014.

Nutrition

1. Casaer MP, Mesotten D, Hermans G, et al. Early versus late parenteral nutrition in critically ill adults. N Engl J Med 2011;365:506-17.

2. Martindale RG, McClave SA, Vanek VW, et al. Guidelines for the provision and assessment of nutrition support therapy in the adult critically ill patient: Society of Critical Care Medicine and American Society for Parenteral and Enteral Nutrition: executive summary. Crit Care Med 2009;37:1757-61.

3. Walker RN, Heuberger RA. Predictive equations for energy needs for the critically ill. Respir Care 2009;54:509-21.

4. Ziegler TR. Parenteral nutrition in the critically ill patient. N Engl J Med 2009;361:1088-97.

5. Casaer MP, Van den Berghe G. Nutrition in the acute phase of critical illness. N Engl J Med 2014;370:1227-36.

6. Arabi YM, Tamim HM, Dhar GS, et al. Permissive underfeeding and intensive insulin therapy in critically ill patients: a randomized controlled trial. Am J Clin Nutr 2011;93(3):569-77.

7. Dickerson RN, Boschert KJ, Kudsk KA, et al. Hypocaloric enteral tube feeding in critically ill obese patients. Nutrition 2002;18:241-6.

8. Dhaliwal R, Cahill N, Lemieux M, et al. The Canadian critical care nutrition guidelines in 2013: an update on current recommendations and implementation strategies. Nutr Clin Pract 2014;29(1):29-43.

ANSWERS AND EXPLANATIONS TO PATIENT CASES

1. Answer: B
This ABG is consistent with a metabolic acidosis. The pH is less than 7.40 (indicating a primary acidosis), and the HCO_3^- and $Paco_2$ are lower than normal. In a metabolic acidosis, the decrease in HCO_3^- is the primary disorder. When a metabolic acidosis is present, the AG should be calculated to provide additional insight about the potential cause of the disorder. The AG is calculated by subtracting the sum of measured anions (Cl^- and HCO_3^-) from cations (Na^+). This patient's AG (8 mEq/L) is within the reference range of 6–12 mEq/L; therefore, it is referred to as a normal anion gap metabolic acidosis or non–anion gap metabolic acidosis. *C. difficile*–induced diarrhea is the most likely cause of this patient's acid-base disorder.

2. Answer: D
Given this patient's neurologic status and his elevated $Paco_2$, he should be intubated and transferred to the ICU. In patients without chronic obstructive pulmonary disease, a $Paco_2$ greater than 50 mm Hg is usually an indication for mechanical ventilation, regardless of oxygenation status (this patient was oxygenating well: Pao_2 111 mm Hg, Sao_2 100%). Oxygen (Answer B) therapy alone is unlikely to correct this patient's cause of respiratory failure (i.e., hypoventilation). Likewise, his acid-base disturbance is consistent with a pure acute respiratory acidosis (elevated $Paco_2$, normal HCO_3^-) and is therefore unlikely to respond to HCO_3^- (Answer C), or tromethamine (Answer A), which is usually reserved for a severe metabolic acidosis.

3. Answer: C
This ABG is consistent with a respiratory acidosis. The pH is below 7.40 (indicating acidosis), and the $Paco_2$ is higher than normal (about 40 mm Hg). In chronic respiratory acidosis, the kidneys conserve HCO_3^- (a base) in an attempt to maintain a normal pH. This compensatory metabolic alkalosis is obvious in this patient, whose serum HCO_3^- is 28 mEq/L (which is about 4 mEq/L higher than normal). The elevated HCO_3^- concentration in this patient confirms the diagnosis of respiratory acidosis (because the HCO_3^- would be expected to be less than 24 mEq/L if the acidemia were attributable to a metabolic cause).

4. Answer: C
This patient's hemodynamic profile is most consistent with sepsis (i.e., high CI, low SVR). Her PCWP is consistent with an adequate volume challenge. Because she remains hypotensive despite receiving an adequate fluid load, an α-adrenergic agent such as norepinephrine (Answer C) should be initiated. The goals of treatment are to improve BP (typically MAP) and restore adequate organ perfusion. Norepinephrine is a more potent vasoconstrictor than phenylephrine and provides less β-stimulation than dopamine. If she became more tachycardic while receiving norepinephrine, phenylephrine could be tried. Dobutamine (Answer B) is an inotropic agent that increases CI, which is adequate in this patient. Piperacillin/tazobactam and vancomycin will provide adequate gram-positive, gram-negative, and anaerobic coverage for nosocomial pneumonia, eliminating the need for clindamycin (Answer A). If the patient continues to be hypotensive despite adequate fluid resuscitation and use of vasopressors, then hydrocortisone (Answer D) can be considered.

5. Answer: A
Calculating an infusion rate is a very important role for the pharmacist in code situations. The infusion pump is set to run in milliliters per hour, so the answer should always be in these units. To determine the rate (in milliliters per hour) needed to achieve a 0.03-mcg/kg/minute dose, use the following calculation:

$$\text{concentration of epinephrine drip: } 4 \text{ mg}/250 \text{ mL} = 0.016 \text{ mg/mL or } 16 \text{ mcg/mL}$$

Therefore, 70 kg × 0.03 mcg/kg/minute × 60 minutes/1 hour × 1 mL/16 mcg = 7.875 mL/hour, which is then rounded to 8 mL/hour.

6. Answer: D
This patient is at high risk of developing a VTE and should receive prophylaxis with unfractionated heparin (Answer D). An elevated INR of 1.4, probably caused by temporary hypoperfusion of the liver, is no reason to withhold prophylaxis for VTE. Hydrocortisone (Answer A) is not necessary in this case because the patient is responding to fluid resuscitation and the infusion of norepinephrine, as evidenced by the increase in MAP from 44 mm Hg on arrival to the emergency

department to 66 mm Hg after initial resuscitation. Enoxaparin is appropriate for DVT prophylaxis (Answer B), but his serum creatinine has more than doubled, and because enoxaparin is renally cleared it would not be the preferred answer in this case. Adding dopamine (Answer C) is not necessary at this time because the MAP is greater than 65 mm Hg, thus allowing global organ perfusion. In addition, there is no evidence that a low dose of dopamine will prevent acute kidney injury, and it increases the risk of arrhythmias compared with norepinephrine.

7. Answer: A

During rewarming, patients can become hypoglycemic. Therefore, a reduction in the insulin infusion is likely, and the blood glucose should be monitored more often (Answer A). Neuromuscular blockade assessment can include titrating to a TOF goal; however, a more applicable goal would be the absence of shivering in this patient when the paralytic is briefly interrupted. If the patient is not shivering, consideration should be given to discontinuing the paralytic. Of note, the TOF goal is 2/4 twitches, rather than 0/4 (Answer B), to avoid over-paralysis. Although discontinuing propofol (Answer C) can facilitate extubation, this should not be done until the patient is no longer paralyzed, is at a normal body temperature, and is ready for ventilator weaning. Finally, although rewarming can cause hyperkalemia, it is appropriate to monitor K concentrations and treat as needed. It is not appropriate to increase the infusion of insulin (Answer D) to prevent hyperkalemia because this could precipitate hypoglycemia during rewarming.

8. Answer: D

Using a nonpharmacologic approach such as offering verbal reassurance to the patient is the most logical starting point for this patient with delirium. Although propofol (Answer A) is an effective sedative that does not worsen delirium, a sedative is not needed in this patient with a RASS of 0 (alert and calm). Haloperidol (Answer B) is an option; however, nonpharmacologic strategies should be tried first. Morphine (Answer C) is incorrect because her BPS score is 4. This score ranges from 3 (no pain) to 12 (maximum pain). Furthermore, although opioids can be effective sedatives, morphine should be avoided, if possible, in patients with kidney injury because of active metabolites that are renally eliminated.

9. Answer: D

Neuromuscular blocking agents should be titrated to the minimal effective dose. Although a peripheral nerve stimulator may provide information on the level of blockade, the true therapeutic end point in all patients is ventilator synchrony (Answer D). It is imperative for clinicians to recognize that neuromuscular blocking agents do not cross the blood-brain barrier and are not useful as sedatives or analgesics. For this reason, sedatives and analgesics should be optimized before initiation of neuromuscular blockade, because titrating to a RASS goal while on neuromuscular blockers is not possible (Answer C). Adequate sedation and analgesia must be achieved before initiating a neuromuscular blocker and should continue throughout the treatment. Vecuronium, though inexpensive, accumulates in renal disease and should be avoided (Answer B). Answer A is incorrect because analgesics and sedatives should be continued during paralysis.

10. Answer: B

Although this patient is no longer paralyzed, it would be inappropriate to reparalyze an obviously agitated patient (Answer A) because he or she should first be adequately sedated. Likewise, performing a TOF test using a peripheral nerve stimulator (Answer D) is unnecessary because it is obvious from the patient's movement that she is not adequately blocked. It is possible that the patient is agitated and tachycardic because she was on neuromuscular blockers without adequate sedation or analgesia. Before the paralytic is adjusted, the patient should be given a sedative bolus (Answer B). In patients on neuromuscular blockade, it is generally better to err on the side of oversedation than undersedation, so an increase in the sedative drip rates would also be appropriate in this patient. Answer C is incorrect because increasing the infusion rate of fentanyl will not have an immediate effect. It would be an acceptable option if the increased infusion rate were accompanied by a fentanyl bolus.

11. Answer: B

Gentamicin (Answer B) has pharmacodynamic effects (i.e., inhibits the release of acetylcholine at the nicotinic receptor), which may potentiate the action of neuromuscular-blocking agents. Piperacillin/tazobactam and norepinephrine (Answer A and Answer C) will not prolong the effects of cisatracurium. Although hypokalemia can prolong the effects of neuromuscular blocking agents, a K level of 4.9 mEq/L (Answer D) will not.

12. Answer: A

Although this patient had hypotensive episodes during her resuscitation period, she currently has a functioning GI system, as noted by her tolerance of tube feeds. Therefore, SUP should be administered via her feeding tube, making the best choice for this patient famotidine administered enterally (Answer A). Ranitidine (Answer D) is incorrect because it is administered intravenously. Esomeprazole (Answer B) is incorrect because no data show a benefit of PPIs over histamine receptor antagonists; they are usually more expensive and may have more side effects. Sucralfate (Answer C) is incorrect because it has been shown to be inferior to histamine receptor antagonists.

13. Answer: B

This patient's risk factors for SUP (mechanical ventilation and hypoperfusion) are no longer present, so SUP should be discontinued (Answer B). There is no reason to continue SUP until ICU (Answer A) or hospital (Answer D) discharge, and this practice just increases the risk of continuing the SUP in an outpatient without an appropriate indication. Answer C is incorrect because a poor appetite is not a risk factor for developing stress-related mucosal disease (SRMD).

14. Answer: C

This patient has several risk factors for VTE, including age, respiratory failure, and a history of heart failure. For this reason, intermittent pneumatic compression (Answer A) is insufficient prophylaxis. Fondaparinux (Answer B) is contraindicated in patients with an estimated creatinine clearance less than 30 mL/minute. Enoxaparin 30 mg subcutaneously once daily (Answer C) is an appropriate dose for this patient, considering her reduced kidney function. A continuous infusion of heparin (Answer D) is not an appropriate administration method for preventing a VTE, but it would be appropriate as a treatment strategy for a known or suspected VTE.

15. Answer D

The EN can be continued (Answer D) unless gastric residuals exceed 250 mL. Parenteral nutrition (Answer A) is not indicated in patients with a functional GI tract. Metoclopramide (Answer B) could be considered if gastric residuals increase or if the patient experiences abdominal distention. Switching to a more concentrated feed would not be indicated unless the patient is volume overloaded (Answer C).

ANSWERS AND EXPLANATIONS TO SELF-ASSESSMENT QUESTIONS

1. Answer: A

This patient's ABG and urine Cl are consistent with a saline-responsive metabolic alkalosis. In critically ill patients, the most common cause of metabolic alkalosis is volume contraction. In this case, the volume contraction is probably caused by overly aggressive diuresis. In patients receiving diuretics, the urine Cl should be measured at least 12–24 hours after the last dose. Additionally, the patient is hypotensive with an elevated heart rate, which probably represents hypovolemia. This patient should receive a normal saline infusion. Hydrochloric acid infusions (Answer C) are typically reserved for more severe alkalosis (pH more than 7.55) that is not responding to conventional therapy. Administering D_5W (Answer B) will provide hydration but will not correct intravascular volume depletion. Acetazolamide (Answer D) would be a consideration if the metabolic alkalosis persisted after correcting the underlying problem (i.e., volume contraction).

2. Answer: C

Assuming that analgesia with morphine is adequate, this patient requires a sedative to achieve the RASS goal. Propofol is a sedative that is easily titrated and cost-effective. Dexmedetomidine (Answer A) is another option that is safe and effective, even when used for longer than 24 hours, but it has not been shown superior to propofol in randomized controlled trials. Furthermore, the cost of dexmedetomidine is greater than that of propofol. Lorazepam (Answer B) should be avoided in patients with (or at high risk of) delirium. Use of benzodiazepines is associated with an increased risk of delirium. Haloperidol (Answer D) is incorrect because the patient is CAM-ICU negative. Haloperidol can cause further prolongation of the QT interval and could lead to torsades.

3. Answer: B

Aminoglycosides can potentiate the effect of neuromuscular blockers; therefore, they should be avoided if possible (Answer B). This could be the reason for the TOF score of 0/4, which can indicate overparalysis. A reasonable goal for the TOF is 2/4 twitches. It is important to note that the study of untitrated neuromuscular blockade was with cisatracurium in ARDS, which does not fit this patient case. The level of sedation cannot

be assessed using the RASS (Answer A) or other sedation scales because the patient is under neuromuscular blockade. Parenteral nutrition (Answer C) can be withheld until the patient is hemodynamically stable. Furthermore, late initiation (after 1 week) of PN support is associated with improved outcomes. Opioids such as morphine (Answer D) should not be withheld in paralyzed trauma patients. Propofol has minimal analgesic properties and will not be sufficient in a trauma patient with several injuries.

4. Answer: C

This patient meets the criteria for severe sepsis. Treatment with 5% albumin (Answer A) is unlikely to offer additional benefit because the patient's MAP is at goal (more than 65 mm Hg). Furthermore, colloids are no more effective than crystalloids for fluid resuscitation, and a serum albumin concentration does not predict the efficacy of albumin administration. Hydrocortisone (Answer B) is incorrect because the patient is not persistently hypotensive after receiving fluids and vasopressors. Although this patient's BP is responding to the infusion of dopamine, the HR has increased. Norepinephrine (Answer C) is correct because it has similar efficacy but with fewer tachyarrhythmias than dopamine. The dopamine should not be reduced (Answer D) because lower doses are not renal-protective.

5. Answer: D

The Surviving Sepsis Campaign guidelines recommend adequate fluid resuscitation with either crystalloids or colloids before the addition of vasopressor agents in patients with severe sepsis. This patient's CVP, BP, HR, and BUN/Cr ratio indicate that she has intravascular volume depletion and needs immediate volume replacement. Therefore, intravenous fluids with either crystalloid or colloid should be the next therapy added to this patient's regimen. Answer A is incorrect because fluid resuscitation should be attempted before addition of vasopressors. When deciding between a balanced crystalloid such as lactated Ringer's and a hyperchloremic fluid such as normal saline, many experts would choose Answer B (lactated Ringer's) because of a slight improvement in renal morbidity when used compared with Answer C (normal saline), especially in a patient who already has Acute kidney injury (AKI). There are no data that favor colloids over crystalloids, and the substantial increase in cost associated with colloids precludes it from being first line, so Answer D (albumin) is incorrect.

6. Answer: D

Targeted temperature management (i.e., therapeutic hypothermia) improves neurologic recovery and mortality in patients who have suffered a cardiac arrest. Although the patient probably has a metabolic acidosis, administering sodium bicarbonate (Answer A) does not improve outcomes. Vasopressin (Answer B) is an acceptable option during a cardiac arrest for patients with ventricular fibrillation or pulseless VT, but it has no role after cardiac arrest or in a patient who has returned to normal sinus rhythm. Although acute coronary syndrome is a common cause of cardiac arrest, anticoagulation with heparin (Answer C) would be a consideration after initiation of targeted temperature management. A continuous infusion of heparin does not improve mortality in patients with an acute coronary syndrome. Of note, the induction of hypothermia does not necessarily interfere with treatment plans for acute coronary syndrome (e.g., percutaneous coronary intervention).

7. Answer: B

Mechanical ventilation for more than 48 hours and coagulopathy are independent risk factors for stress ulcers; therefore, Answer D is incorrect because the patient has a high risk of developing a stress ulcer. This patient is critically ill and may be intubated for an extended time; therefore, he is at risk of stress ulcers, and he will require SUP. The patient has an OGT, meaning that EN and medications administered by the tube will go directly into the stomach. Sucralfate (Answer C) was inferior to H_2-receptor antagonists in preventing clinically significant bleeding from SRMD in a large randomized controlled trial, and it is generally not recommended for SUP. Proton pump inhibitors such as intravenous pantoprazole (Answer A) do not prevent SRMD better than H_2-receptor antagonists and have been associated with an increased risk of hospital-acquired pneumonia. Therefore, famotidine (Answer B) administered enterally is the most cost-effective agent for SUP in this patient.

8. Answer: A

The SSC suggests hydrocortisone at a dose of 200 mg per day if fluids and vasopressors cannot restore hemodynamic stability (Answer A, so Answer B is incorrect). Although low random cortisol concentrations predict worse outcomes, there are no data supporting treatment of low cortisol levels (Answer C). Because of the results of the most recent clinical trial and increased health care costs, a cosyntropin stimulation test is no longer recommended for patients with septic shock (Answer D).

9. Answer: A

The patient has an adequate MAP but has poor oxygen delivery to peripheral tissues. Because the MAP is at goal (more than 65 mm Hg), norepinephrine should be continued at the current dose (Answer B). Although decreasing propofol may increase blood pressure and allow a reduction in norepinephrine, this would not be recommended while the patient is on neuromuscular blockade, and the patient is not having problems maintaining an adequate blood pressure (Answer C). The patient needs an increase in oxygen delivery. The arterial oxygen saturation and hemoglobin are adequate, meaning that cardiac output is low. This can be achieved by addition of an inotrope. Dobutamine is the preferred inotrope in septic patients (Answer A) over epinephrine (Answer D), which may cause an unwanted increase in MAP, as well as hyperglycemia and lactic acidosis.

10. Answer: C

The patient's hemodynamics are most consistent with obstructive shock (due to tamponade) and an inability to properly fill the ventricles. Prompt drainage of fluid surrounding the heart is the only definitive therapy (Answer C). Fluid boluses would worsen this condition (Answer A). An intrope may temporize the reduction in cardiac output but will not correct the underlying cause (Answer B). The patient's MAP and SVR are high, so vasopressors would not be indicated (Answer D).

11. Answer: A

There are a number of ways to estimate nutritional needs in critically ill patients. The modified Penn State equation has been found to closely predict caloric needs. The recommended protein intake for medically ill ICU patients is 1.2–1.5 g/kg (Answer A). Indirect calorimetry will most closely calculate caloric needs but does not provide information on the amount of protein required (Answer B). Feeding at 11–14 kcal/kg is recommended for obese patients, but this patient's BMI is less than 30 kg/m^2 (Answer C). Prealbumin levels have not shown good correlation with nutritional deficits in critically ill patients and are not recommended (Answer D).

12. Answer: D

PPIs have been associated with an increase in ventilator-associated pneumonia (Answer A). Selective digestive decontamination has been shown effective, but side effects and increases in resistant bacteria have not led to widespread use, and it is not part of the Institute for Healthcare Improvement ventilator bundle (Answer B). Head elevation prevents ventilator-associated pneumonia but should be between 30° and 45° (Answer C). Chlorhexidine is inexpensive, carries few side effects, is easy to administer, and has been shown effective in the prevention of ventilator-associated pneumonia (Answer D).

13. Answer: C

Sliding scale protocol is inappropriate as the sole therapy for hyperglycemia in the ICU (Answer A). The Surviving Sepsis Campaign recommends an insulin infusion for two blood glucose values greater than 180 mg/dL (Answer C). The ideal blood glucose range for critically ill adults has yet to be determined, but a goal of 80–110 mg/dL has not been found to improve outcomes and may increase mortality (Answer D). A target of 110–180 mg/dL prevents hyperglycemia, but without an excess risk of hypoglycemia (Answer C).

Nephrology

John M. Burke, Pharm.D., FCCP, BCPS

St. Louis College of Pharmacy
St. Louis, Missouri

NEPHROLOGY

JOHN M. BURKE, PHARM.D., FCCP, BCPS

ST. LOUIS COLLEGE OF PHARMACY
ST. LOUIS, MISSOURI

Learning Objectives

1. Categorize acute kidney injury (AKI) as prerenal, intrinsic, or postrenal, based on patient history, physical examination, and laboratory values.
2. Identify risk factors for AKI.
3. Formulate preventive strategies to decrease the risk of developing AKI in specific patient populations.
4. Formulate a therapeutic plan to manage AKI.
5. Identify medications and medication classes associated with acute and chronic kidney damage.
6. Describe characteristics that determine the efficiency of removal of drugs by dialysis.
7. Classify the stage or category of chronic kidney disease (CKD) based on patient history, physical examination, and laboratory values.
8. Identify risk factors for the progression of CKD.
9. Formulate strategies to slow the progression of CKD.
10. Assess for the presence of common complications of CKD.
11. Develop a care plan to manage the common complications observed in patients with CKD (e.g., anemia, secondary hyperthyroidism).

Self-Assessment Questions

Answers and explanations to these questions can be found at the end of this chapter.

1. A 75-year-old man (weight 92.5 kg, height 73 inches) presents to your institution with abdominal pain and dizziness. He has a brief history of gastroenteritis and has had nothing to eat or drink for 24 hours. His blood pressure (BP) reading while sitting is 120/80 mm Hg, which drops to 90/60 mm Hg when standing. His heart rate is 90 beats/minute. His basic metabolic panel shows sodium (Na) 135 mEq/L, chloride (Cl) 108 mEq/L, potassium (K) 4.7 mEq/L, CO_2 26 mEq/L, blood urea nitrogen (BUN) 40 mg/dL, serum creatinine (SCr) 1.5 mg/dL, and glucose 188 mg/dL. He has no known drug allergies. Which is the best approach to treat this patient?

    A. Administer furosemide 40 mg intravenously × 1.

    B. Insert Foley catheter to check for residual urine.

    C. Administer fluid bolus (500 mL of normal saline solution).

    D. Administer insulin lispro 3 units subcutaneously.

2. A 44-year-old man is admitted with gram-negative bacteremia. He receives 4 days of parenteral aminoglycoside therapy and develops acute tubular necrosis (ATN). Antibiotic therapy is adjusted on the basis of culture and sensitivity results. Which set of laboratory data is most consistent with this presentation?

    A. BUN/SCr ratio greater than 20:1, urine sodium less than 10 mOsm/L, fractional excretion of sodium (FENa) less than 1%, specific gravity more than 1.018, and hyaline casts.

    B. BUN/SCr ratio greater than 20:1, urine sodium more than 20 mOsm/L, FENa more than 3%, specific gravity 1.010, no casts visible.

    C. BUN/SCr ratio of 10–15:1, urine sodium more than 40 mOsm/L, FENa more than 1%, specific gravity less than 1.015, muddy casts.

    D. BUN/SCr ratio of 10–15:1, urine sodium less than 10 mOsm/L, FENa less than 1%, specific gravity more than 1.018, muddy casts.

3. A patient with chronic kidney disease (CKD) category G4 (estimated creatinine clearance [eCrCl] of 25 mL/minute) has received a diagnosis of gram-positive bacteremia, which is susceptible only to drug X. There are no published reports on how to adjust the dose of drug X in patients with impaired kidney function. Review of the drug X package insert shows that it has significant renal elimination, with 40% excreted unchanged in the urine. The usual dose for drug X is 600 mg/day intravenously and is provided as 100 mg/mL in a 6-mL vial. Which is the best dose (in milliliters of drug X) to give this patient?

    A. 3.6.

    B. 4.1.

    C. 4.5.

    D. 5.5.

4. A 45-year-old man (weight 59 kg, height 70 inches) has a long history of both cancer and malnutrition. His SCr is 0.5 mg/dL. He is to be given carboplatin, for which an accurate estimate of kidney function is critical. Which is the best method for assessing kidney function in this patient?

   A. Cockcroft-Gault equation.

   B. Modification of Diet in Renal Disease (MDRD) study equation.

   C. 24-hour urine collection.

   D. Iothalamate study.

5. A 59-year-old patient who has had category G5 CKD for 10 years is maintained on chronic hemodialysis. He has a history of hypertension, coronary artery disease (CAD), mild congestive heart failure (CHF), and type 2 diabetes mellitus. Medications are as follows: epoetin 10,000 units intravenously three times/week at dialysis, renal multivitamin once daily, atorvastatin 20 mg/day, insulin, and calcium acetate 1334 mg three times/day with meals. Laboratory values are as follows: hemoglobin 9.2 g/dL, intact parathyroid hormone (PTH) 300 pg/mL, Na 140 mEq/L, K 4.9 mEq/L, SCr 7.0 mg/dL, calcium 9 mg/dL, albumin 3.5 g/dL, and phosphorus 4.8 mg/dL. He has a serum ferritin concentration of 80 ng/mL and a transferrin saturation (TSAT) of 14%. Mean corpuscular volume, mean corpuscular hemoglobin concentration, and white blood cell count (WBC) are all normal. He is afebrile. Which is the best approach to managing anemia in this patient?

   A. Increase epoetin.

   B. Add oral iron.

   C. Add intravenous iron.

   D. Maintain current regimen; patient is at goal.

6. A 60-year-old (72-kg) patient with a history of diabetes and hypertension is in the intensive care unit after suffering a myocardial infarction about 1 week ago with secondary heart failure. He now has pneumonia. He has been hypotensive for the past 5 days. Before his admission 1 week ago, he had a SCr of 1.0 mg/dL. His urine output has been steadily declining for the past 3 days, despite adequate hydration, with 700 mL of urine output in the past 24 hours. His medications since surgery include intravenous dobutamine, nitroglycerin, and cefazolin. Yesterday, his BUN and SCr were 32 and 3.1 mg/dL, respectively; today, they are 41 and 3.9 mg/dL. His urine osmolality is 290 mOsm/kg. His urine sodium is 40 mEq/L, and there are tubular cellular casts in his urine. Which is the most likely renal diagnosis?

   A. Prerenal azotemia.

   B. ATN.

   C. Acute interstitial nephritis (AIN).

   D. Hemodynamic/functional-mediated acute kidney injury (AKI).

7. You are evaluating a study comparing epoetin and darbepoetin in terms of their efficacy on mean hemoglobin concentrations. Both drugs are initiated at the recommended dose, and the hemoglobin concentration is checked at 4 weeks. Fifty patients are in each group. The mean hemoglobin in the epoetin group is 12.1 g/dL, and in the darbepoetin group, it is 12.2 g/dL. Which statistical test is best for this comparison?

   A. A paired t-test.

   B. An independent (unpaired) t-test.

   C. An analysis of variance.

   D. A chi-square test.

8. A pharmacoeconomic study is performed to compare the use of erythropoiesis-stimulating agents with various hemoglobin concentrations. The primary outcome of this study was cost per quality-adjusted life-year gained. Which is the best description of this economic evaluation?

   A. Cost minimization.

   B. Cost-effectiveness.

   C. Cost-benefit.

   D. Cost-utility.

Patient Cases

1. A 48-year-old African American man is admitted to the intensive care unit after an acute myocardial infarction. He has a history of type 2 diabetes mellitus, hypertension, and tobacco use. Current medications include metformin 500 mg orally twice daily, lisinopril 20 mg/day, nicotine patch 14 mg/day applied each morning, and aspirin 81 mg/daily. Before admission, his kidney function was normal (serum creatinine [SCr] 1.0 mg/dL); however, during the past 24 hours, his kidney function has declined (blood urea nitrogen [BUN] 20 mg/dL, SCr 2.1 mg/dL). His urine shows muddy casts. He has been anuric for 6 hours. His current blood pressure (BP) is 110/70 mm Hg. He has edema and pulmonary congestion. Which is the best assessment of this patient's kidney function?

    A. 26.2 mL/minute (creatinine clearance [CrCl] using the Cockcroft-Gault equation).

    B. 44 mL/minute/1.73 m² (glomerular filtration rate [GFR] using the abbreviated Modification of Diet in Renal Disease [MDRD] study equation).

    C. 23.1 mL/minute/70 kg (CrCl using the Brater equation).

    D. Assumed CrCl of less than 10 mL/minute.

2. Which is the most likely cause of impaired kidney function in this patient?

    A. Prerenal azotemia.

    B. Intrinsic renal disease.

    C. Postrenal obstruction.

    D. Functional acute kidney injury (AKI).

3. Which medication is best to discontinue at this time because of its potential adverse effect on kidney function?

    A. Lisinopril.

    B. Nicotine patch.

    C. Metformin.

    D. Aspirin.

4. Which intervention is most appropriate to add at this time?

    A. Intravenous 0.9% sodium chloride (NaCl).

    B. Hydrochlorothiazide.

    C. Furosemide.

    D. Fluid restriction.

I. ACUTE KIDNEY INJURY OR ACUTE RENAL FAILURE

  A. Definitions and Background
    1. Acute kidney injury (AKI) is defined as an acute decrease in kidney function or glomerular filtration rate (GFR) over hours, days, or even weeks and is associated with an accumulation of waste products and (usually) volume.
      a. Common definitions
        i. An increase in SCr of 0.5 mg/dL or greater
        ii. A decrease of 25% or greater in estimated GFR (eGFR)

      iii. An increase of 1 mg/dL or greater in SCr in patients with chronic kidney disease (CKD)

      iv. Urine output less than 0.5 mL/kg/hour for at least 6 hours

  b. The Acute Kidney Injury Network (AKIN): Diagnostic criteria require one of the following within a 48-hour period:

      i. An absolute increase in SCr of more than 0.3 mg/dL

      ii. An increase in baseline SCr by 50% or more

      iii. Urine output of less than 0.5 mL/kg/hour for more than 6 hours

  c. Can further classify into stages 1–3 on the basis of degree of SCr rise and urine output

  d. Stratifying AKI using risk, injury, failure, loss, and end-stage kidney disease (RIFLE) criteria. Developed by the Acute Dialysis Quality Initiative (ADQI) Group. Uses change in baseline SCr/GFR or urine output (Table 1)

Table 1. Stratification of AKI

RIFLE Classification			Common Criteria	AKIN Criteria	
	Classification	**SCr or GFR Criteria**	**Urine output**	**Stage**	**SCr or GFR Criteria**
R	Risk of renal dysfunction	SCr increase to 1.5 times baseline *or* GFR decrease by more than 25%	Less than 0.5 mL/kg/hour for more than 6 hours	1	SCr increase to more than 0.3 mg/dL or 1.5–1.9 times baseline
I	Injury to kidney	SCr increase to 2 times baseline *or* GFR decrease by more than 50%	Less than 0.5 mL/kg/hour for more than 12 hours	2	SCr increase to 2–2.9 times baseline
F	Failure of kidney function	SCr increase to 3 times baseline *or* GFR decrease by more than 75% *or* SCr greater than 4 mg/dL with acute rise greater than 0.5 mg/dL	Less than 0.3 mL/kg/hour for more than 24 hours *or* anuria × 12 hours	3	SCr increase to 3 times baseline or more or SCr greater than 4 mg/dL with an acute increase of more than 0.5 mg/dL; or on RRT
L	Loss of kidney function	Complete loss of kidney function for more than 4 weeks			
E	End-stage kidney disease	Complete loss of kidney function for more than 3 months			

AKI = acute kidney injury; AKIN = Acute Kidney Injury Network; GFR = glomerular filtration rate; RIFLE = risk, injury, failure, loss, and end-stage kidney disease; RRT = renal replacement therapy; SCr = serum creatinine.

  e. Common complications include fluid overload and acid-base and electrolyte abnormalities.

  f. Urine output classification:

      i. Anuric: Less than 50 mL/24 hours; associated with worse outcomes

      ii. Oliguric: 50–500 mL/24 hours

      iii. Nonoliguric: More than 500 mL/24 hours; associated with better patient outcomes and easier to manage because of fewer problems with volume overload

2. Community-acquired AKI

  a. Low incidence (0.02%) in otherwise healthy patients

  b. As high as 13% incidence among patients with CKD

   c. Usually has a very high survival rate (70%–95%)

   d. Single insult to the kidney, often drug-induced

   e. SCr may return to baseline but may lead to development or progression of CKD

  3. Hospital-acquired AKI

   a. Has a moderate incidence (2%–5%) and moderate survival rate (30%–50%)

   b. Single or multifocal insults to the kidney

   c. Can still be reversible

  4. Intensive care unit–acquired AKI: 5%–6% of patients in intensive care develop AKI during unit stay, and patients who develop this condition have a low survival rate (10%–30%)

  5. Estimating kidney function in AKI

   a. Difficult because commonly used SCr-based equations (Cockcroft-Gault, Modification of Diet in Renal Disease [MDRD], and Chronic Kidney Disease Epidemiology Collaboration [CKD-EPI]) are not appropriate (assume stable SCr)

   b. Equations by Brater and Jeliffe are probably more accurate than the Cockcroft-Gault equation but have not been rigorously tested.

   c. Can do a urine collection in nonoliguria by obtaining a SCr before and after the collection and averaging these values for the calculation

B. Risk Factors Associated with AKI

  1. Preexisting CKD (eGFR less than 60 mL/minute/1.73 m^2)

  2. Volume depletion: Vomiting, diarrhea, poor fluid intake, fever, diuretic use, intravascular or effective volume depletion (e.g., congestive heart failure [CHF], liver disease with ascites)

  3. Use of nephrotoxic agents or medications

   a. Intravenous radiographic contrast

   b. Aminoglycosides and amphotericin

   c. Nonsteroidal anti-inflammatory drugs (NSAIDs) and cyclooxygenase-2 (COX-2) inhibitors

   d. Angiotensin-converting enzyme inhibitors (ACEIs) and angiotensin II receptor blockers (ARBs)

   e. Cyclosporine and tacrolimus

  4. Obstruction of the urinary tract

C. Classifications of AKI (Table 2)

  1. Prerenal AKI

   a. Initially, the kidney is undamaged.

   b. Characterized by hypoperfusion to the kidney

    i. Systemic hypoperfusion: hemorrhage, volume depletion, drugs, CHF

    ii. Isolated kidney hypoperfusion: renal artery stenosis, emboli

   c. Physical examination: hypotension, signs of volume depletion

   d. Urinalysis will initially be normal (no sediment) but concentrated

  2. Functional AKI

   a. Kidney is undamaged; often classified as prerenal azotemia

   b. Caused by reduced glomerular hydrostatic pressure; often without hypotension

   c. In general, medication-related (cyclosporine, ACEIs and ARBs, and NSAIDs) or seen in patients with low effective blood flow (patients with CHF, patients with liver disease, and older adults) who cannot compensate for alterations in afferent and efferent tone

   d. Concentrated urine

  3. Intrinsic AKI

   a. Kidney is damaged, and damage can be linked to the structure involved: small blood vessels, glomeruli, renal tubules, and interstitium

    b. Most common cause is acute tubular necrosis (ATN); other causes include acute interstitial nephritis (AIN), vasculitis, and acute glomerulonephritis

    c. History: identifiable insult, drug use, infections

    d. Physical examination: Normotensive, euvolemic, or hypervolemic depending on the cause; check for signs of allergic reactions or embolic phenomenon

    e. Urinalysis will reflect damage; urine generally not concentrated

4. Postrenal AKI

    a. Kidney is initially undamaged. Bladder outlet obstruction is the most common cause of postrenal AKI. Lower urinary tract obstruction may be caused by calculi. Ureteric obstructions may be caused by clots or intraluminal obstructions. Extrarenal compression can also cause postrenal disease. Increased intraluminal pressure upstream of the obstruction will result in damage if the obstruction is not relieved.

    b. History: trauma, benign prostatic hyperplasia, cancers

    c. Physical examination: distended bladder, enlarged prostate

    d. Urinalysis may be nonspecific.

Table 2. Classifications of Acute Kidney Injury

	Prerenal and Functional	**Intrinsic (ATN and AIN)**	**Postrenal**
History and clinical presentation	Volume depletion Renal artery stenosis CHF Hypercalcemia NSAID, ACEI, and ARB use Cyclosporine	Long-standing renal hypoperfusion Nephrotoxins (e.g., contrast or antibiotics) Vasculitis Glomerulonephritis	Kidney stones BPH Cancers
Physical examination	Hypotension Dehydration Petechia if thrombotic Ascites	Rash, fever (with AIN)	Distended bladder Enlarged prostate
Serum BUN/SCr ratio	Greater than 20:1	15:1	15:1
Urine sodium	Less than 20 mEq/L	Greater than 40 mEq/L	Greater than 40 mEq/L
FENa	Less than 1%	Greater than 2%	Greater than 2%
Urine osmolality	High urine osmolarity	Low urine osmolarity	Low urine osmolarity
Urine sediment	Normal	Muddy brown granular casts; tubular epithelial casts	Variable; may be normal
Urinary WBC	Negative	2–4+	Variable
Urinary RBC	Negative	2–4+	1+
Proteinuria	Negative	Positive	Negative

ACEI = angiotensin-converting enzyme inhibitor; AIN = acute interstitial nephritis; ARB = angiotensin II receptor blocker; ATN = acute tubular necrosis; BPH = benign prostatic hypertrophy; BUN = blood urea nitrogen; CHF = congestive heart failure; FENa = fractional excretion of sodium [(urine Na × SCr) ÷ (serum Na × urine Cr) × 100%]; GFR = glomerular filtration rate; NSAID = nonsteroidal anti-inflammatory drug; RBC = red blood cell count; SCr = serum creatinine; WBC = white blood cell count.

e. Calculation of fractional excretion of sodium (FENa – percentage of Na filtered at the glomerulus that is excreted in the urine).

$$FENa\ (\%) = \frac{(urine\ Na)/(urine\ Cr)}{(serum\ Na/SCr)} \times 100$$

D. Prevention of AKI
   1. Avoid nephrotoxic drugs when possible
   2. Ensure adequate hydration
   3. Patient education
   4. Drug therapies to decrease the incidence of contrast-induced nephropathy: See "Drug-Induced Kidney Damage" section

E. Treatment and Management of Established AKI
   1. Prerenal azotemia: Correct primary hemodynamics.
      a. Normal saline if volume depleted
      b. Pressure management if needed
      c. Blood products if needed
   2. Intrinsic: No specific therapy universally effective
      a. Eliminate the causative hemodynamic abnormality or toxin.
      b. Avoid additional insults.
      c. Fluid and electrolyte management to prevent volume depletion or overload and electrolyte imbalances
      d. Nutrition support is important, but no specific recommendations are widely accepted.
      e. Medical therapy
         i. Loop diuretics: Recommend not using to prevent AKI (Kidney Disease: Improving Global Outcomes [KDIGO], Grade 1B) and suggest not using to treat AKI, except to manage hypervolemia (KDIGO, Grade 2C)
         ii. Fenoldopam: Suggest not using to prevent or treat AKI (KDIGO, Grade 2C)
         iii. Dopamine: Recommend not using low-dose dopamine to prevent or treat AKI (KDIGO, Grade 1A)
         iv. Atrial natriuretic peptide: Suggest not using to prevent (KDIGO, Grade 2C) or treat (KDIGO, Grade 2B) AKI
         v. Recombinant human (rh)IGF-1 (insulin-like growth factor-1): Recommend not using to prevent or treat AKI (KDIGO, Grade 1B)
   3. Postrenal AKI: Relieve obstruction. Early identification is important. Consult urology and/or radiology.
   4. Indications for renal replacement therapy (RRT) in AKI:
      a. Blood urea nitrogen (BUN) greater than 100 mg/dL
      b. Volume overload unresponsive to diuretics
      c. Uremia or encephalopathy
      d. Life-threatening electrolyte imbalance: hyperkalemia, hypermagnesemia
      e. Refractory metabolic acidosis

Patient Cases

5. A 67-year-old man is referred for intermittent chest pain. His medical history is significant for KDIGO Category G3a CKD, type 2 diabetes mellitus, and hypertension. Medications include enalapril, hydrochlorothiazide, and pioglitazone. Laboratory values include SCr 1.8 mg/dL, glucose 189 mg/dL, hemoglobin 12 g/dL, and hematocrit 36%. His physical examination is normal. The plan is to undergo elective cardiac catheterization. Which approach is the best choice for hydration?

    A. 0.45% NaCl.

    B. 0.9% NaCl.

    C. 5% dextrose/0.45% NaCl.

    D. Oral hydration with water.

6. After the administration of radiocontrast, which is the optimal time to reevaluate renal function to assess for possible contrast-associated nephropathy?

    A. 6 hours.

    B. 24 hours.

    C. 4 days.

    D. 7 days.

II. DRUG-INDUCED KIDNEY DAMAGE

  A. Introduction: Drugs can cause kidney damage through many mechanisms. Evaluate potential drug-induced nephropathy on the basis of the period of ingestion, patient risk factors, and the propensity of the suspected agent to cause kidney damage.

    1. Risk factors

      a. History of CKD

      b. Advanced age

    2. Epidemiology

      a. 7% of all drug toxicities

      b. 18%–27% of AKI in hospitals

      c. 1%–5% of NSAID users in community

      d. Most implicated medications: aminoglycosides, NSAIDs, ACEIs, intravenous contrast dye, amphotericin

    3. The kidneys are at elevated risk of toxic injury because:

      a. High exposure to toxin: Kidney receives 20%–25% cardiac output.

      b. Autoregulation and specialized blood flow through glomerulus

      c. High intrarenal drug metabolism

      d. Tubular transport processes

      e. Concentration of solutes (i.e., toxins) in tubules

      f. High energy requirements of tubule epithelial cells

      g. Urine acidification

    4. Pseudonephrotoxicity

      a. Drugs that inhibit the tubular secretion of Cr: trimethoprim, cimetidine

      b. Drugs that increase BUN: corticosteroids, tetracycline

      c. Drugs that interfere with Cr assay: cefoxitin and other cephalosporins

B. Acute Tubular Necrosis
   1. Most common drug-induced kidney disease in the inpatient setting
   2. Aminoglycoside nephrotoxicity
      a. Incidence: 1.7%–58% of patients
      b. Pathogenesis
         i. Caused by proximal tubular damage leading to obstruction of the lumen
         ii. Cationic charge of drug leads to binding to tubular epithelial cells and uptake into those cells.
         iii. Accumulation of phospholipids and toxicity
      c. Presentation
         i. Gradual rise in SCr concentrations and decrease in GFR after 6–10 days of therapy
         ii. Patients usually have nonoliguric kidney failure.
         iii. Wasting of electrolytes (i.e., hypokalemia and hypomagnesemia) may occur.
      d. Risk factors
         i. Related to dosing: large total cumulative dose, prolonged therapy, trough concentration exceeding 2 mg/L, recent previous aminoglycoside therapy
         ii. Concurrent use of other nephrotoxins (cyclosporine, amphotericin B, diuretics, vancomycin)
         iii. Patient related: preexisting kidney disease or damage, advanced age, poor nutrition, shock, gram-negative bacteremia, liver disease, hypoalbuminemia, obstructive jaundice, dehydration, and K and Mg deficiencies
      e. Prevention
         i. Avoid use in high-risk patients.
         ii. Maintain adequate hydration.
         iii. Limit the total cumulative aminoglycoside dose.
         iv. Avoid use of other nephrotoxins.
         v. Use extended-interval (once-daily) dosing; need to monitor these and other high-risk patients closely
   3. Radiographic contrast media nephrotoxicity related to intravenous contrast use
      a. Incidence
         i. Third leading cause of inpatient AKI
         ii. Less than 2% and up to 50% of patients, depending on risk
         iii. Associated with a high (34%) in-hospital mortality rate
      b. Pathogenesis
         i. Renal ischemia caused by alteration in intrarenal hemodynamics
            (a) Osmotic diuresis and dehydration. Contrast media based on osmolality: high-osmolar contrast media around 2000 mOsm/kg, low-osmolar contrast media 600–800 mOsm/kg, iso-osmolar contrast media 290 mOsm/kg
            (b) Some contrast agents also cause systemic hypotension on injection and renal vasoconstriction caused by the release of adenosine, endothelin, and other vasoconstrictors.
         ii. Direct tubular toxicity caused by reactive oxygen species; directly influenced by tubular flow rates and duration of exposure of tubules
      c. Presentation
         i. Initial transient osmotic diuresis, followed by tubular proteinuria
         ii. SCr rises and peaks about 2–5 days after the procedure.
         iii. 50% of patients develop oliguria, and some will require dialysis.
      d. Risk factors for toxicity
         i. Preexisting kidney disease (SCr more than 1.5 mg/dL or CrCl less than 60 mL/minute)
         ii. Diabetes mellitus
         iii. Volume depletion

      iv. Age older than 75 years

      v. Anemia

      vi. Conditions with decreased blood flow to the kidney (e.g., CHF)

      vii. Hypotension

      viii. Other nephrotoxins

      ix. Large doses of contrast (more than 140 mL) or hyperosmolar contrast agents

   e. Prevention

      i. Volume expansion with either intravenous isotonic saline or sodium bicarbonate (KDIGO recommendation, Grade 1A) beginning 6–12 hours before procedure; maintain urine output greater than 150 mL/hour.

      ii. Use an alternative imaging study, if possible.

      iii. Discontinue nephrotoxic agents and avoid diuretics.

      iv. Use low-osmolar or iso-osmolar contrast agents in patients at risk (KDIGO recommendation, Grade 1B).

      v. Medications used to prevent contrast-induced nephropathy

         (a) *N*-Acetylcysteine (NAC): Antioxidant and vasodilatory mechanism. Accumulation of glutathione takes time, so it may not be as effective in emergency cases. Various dosing recommendations. Widely used. Conflicting evidence. Considered safe. May use oral NAC in combination with intravenous hydration (KDIGO suggestion, Grade 2D)

         (b) Ascorbic acid: Antioxidant. One large study showed benefit when used immediately before. Not confirmed. Give oral ascorbic acid 3 g before procedure and 2 g twice daily for two doses after procedure. May have role in emergency cases

         (c) Theophylline: Do not use (KDIGO suggestion, Grade 2C).

         (d) Fenoldopam: Do not use (KDIGO recommendation, Grade 1B).

         (e) Prophylactic hemodialysis (HD) and hemofiltration: Do not use (KDIGO suggestion, Grade 2C).

   f. The Joint National Committee (JNC) standards on medication management regarding radiologic contrast media

      i. Treated as a drug

      ii. Subject to all the standards for medication management in a health system

   g. Nephrogenic systemic fibrosis (also known as nephrogenic fibrosing dermopathy)

      i. Rare but associated with gadolinium-based agents used in high doses for magnetic resonance angiogram

      ii. Occurs in patients with moderate CKD to end-stage kidney disease (ESKD) given intravenous contrast, and systemic acidosis seems to be a risk factor (Magnevist, Omniscan, and OptiMARK considered inappropriate for use in patients with AKI or CKD).

      iii. Onset 2–18 days after exposure

      iv. Presents as burning; itching; swelling, hardening, or tightening of skin; skin patches; spots on eyes; joint stiffness; and muscle weakness

      v. Can cause organ damage, and deaths have occurred

      vi. In 2010, the U.S. Food and Drug Administration (FDA) required the addition of a warning to prescribing information.

4. Cisplatin and carboplatin nephrotoxicity

   a. Incidence: 6%–13% with appropriate dosing and administration

   b. Pathogenesis: Complex; direct tubular toxins

   c. Presentation

      i. SCr peaks 10–12 days after therapy starts but may continue to rise with subsequent cycles of therapy.

          ii.   Renal Mg wasting is common (may be severe with central nervous system symptoms) and may be accompanied by hypokalemia and hypocalcemia.

          iii.   May result in irreversible kidney damage

      d.   Risk factors for toxicity: Many courses of cisplatin, advanced patient age, dehydration, concurrent nephrotoxins, kidney irradiation, alcohol abuse

      e.   Prevention

          i.   Avoid concurrent use of nephrotoxins.

          ii.   Use smallest dose possible and decrease frequency of administration.

          iii.   Aggressive intravenous hydration: 1–4 L within 24 hours of high-dose cisplatin or carboplatin

          iv.   Amifostine: Cisplatin-chelating agent that should be considered in patients at risk of nephrotoxicity

  5.   Amphotericin B nephrotoxicity

      a.   Incidence

          i.   Increases as cumulative dose increases

          ii.   Approaches 80% with cumulative doses of 4 g or more

      b.   Pathogenesis

          i.   Direct proximal and distal tubular toxicity

          ii.   Arterial vasoconstriction

      c.   Presentation

          i.   Manifests after administration of 2–3 g

          ii.   Loss of tubular function leads to electrolyte wasting (especially K^+, Na^+, and Mg^{2+}) and distal tubular acidosis.

          iii.   Patients may require substantial K^+ and Mg^{2+} replacement.

          iv.   SCr increases and GFR decreases because of a decrease in kidney blood flow from vasoconstriction caused by amphotericin.

      d.   Risk factors for toxicity: Existing kidney dysfunction, high average daily doses, diuretic use, volume depletion, concomitant nephrotoxins, rapid infusion

      e.   Prevention

          i.   Avoid other nephrotoxins (especially cyclosporine) and limit the total cumulative dose.

          ii.   Intravenous hydration with 0.9% NaCl at least 1 L/day before each dose

          iii.   Use a liposomal product in high-risk patients.

C. Functional (Hemodynamically Mediated) AKI

  1.   Caused by a decrease in intraglomerular pressure through the vasoconstriction of afferent arterioles or the vasodilation of efferent arterioles

  2.   ACEIs and ARBs

      a.   Pathogenesis

          i.   Vasodilation of the efferent arteriole

          ii.   Leads to a decrease in glomerular hydrostatic pressure and a resultant decrease in GFR

      b.   Presentation

          i.   Exerts a predictable dose-related reduction in GFR

          ii.   SCr is usually expected to rise by up to 30%.

             (a) Usually occurs within 2–5 days

             (b) Usually stabilizes in 2–3 weeks

             (c) Increases greater than 30% may be detrimental.

             (d) Usually reversible on drug discontinuation

      c.   Risk factors for toxicity: Patients with bilateral (or unilateral with a solitary kidney) renal artery stenosis, decreased effective kidney blood flow (CHF, cirrhosis), preexisting kidney disease, and volume depletion

d. Prevention
  i. Initiate therapy with low doses and gradually titrate upward.
  ii. Switch to long-acting agents once tolerance is established.
  iii. Initially, monitor kidney function and SCr concentrations daily for inpatients, weekly for outpatients.
  iv. Avoid use of concomitant diuretics, if possible, during therapy initiation.
  v. Avoid use of concomitant NSAIDs.

3. Nonsteroidal anti-inflammatory drugs (NSAIDs)
  a. Incidence: Estimates indicate that 500,000–2.5 million people develop NSAID-induced nephrotoxicity annually in the United States.
  b. Pathogenesis
    i. Vasodilatory prostaglandins help maintain glomerular hydrostatic pressure by afferent arteriolar dilation, especially in times of decreased kidney blood flow.
    ii. Administration of an NSAID in the setting of decreased kidney perfusion reduces this compensatory mechanism by decreasing the production of prostaglandins, resulting in afferent vasoconstriction and reduced glomerular blood flow.
  c. Presentation
    i. Can occur within days of starting therapy
    ii. Patients generally have low urine volume and Na; may also observe an increase in BUN, SCr, K+, edema, and weight
  d. Risk factors for toxicity: Preexisting kidney disease, systemic lupus erythematosus, high plasma renin activity (e.g., CHF, hepatic disease), diuretic therapy, atherosclerotic disease, and advanced age
  e. Prevention
    i. Use therapies other than NSAIDs when appropriate (e.g., acetaminophen for osteoarthritis).
    ii. Question the utility of COX-2–specific inhibitors because they have not been found to prevent kidney dysfunction, and they increase cardiovascular complications.
  f. Treatment
    i. If NSAID-induced AKI is suspected, discontinue drug and give supportive care.
    ii. Avoid use of concomitant medications affecting the renin-angiotensin-aldosterone system.
    iii. Recovery is usually rapid.

4. Cyclosporine and tacrolimus
  a. Incidence
    i. The 5-year risk of developing CKD after transplantation of a nonrenal organ ranges from 7% to 21%.
    ii. The occurrence of kidney failure in the transplant recipient population increases the risk of death fourfold.
  b. Pathogenesis
    i. Caused by a dose-related hemodynamic mechanism; calcineurin inhibitors may also cause chronic interstitial nephritis through a separate mechanism that is not dose related.
    ii. Causes vasoconstriction of afferent arterioles through possible increased activity of various vasoconstrictors (thromboxane A_2, endothelin, sympathetic nervous system) or decreased activity of vasodilators (nitric oxide, prostacyclin)
    iii. Increased vasoconstriction from angiotensin II may also contribute.
    iv. Effects usually resolve with a dose reduction.
  c. Presentation
    i. Can occur within days of starting therapy
    ii. SCr rises and eGFR decreases.
    iii. Patients often have hypertension, hyperkalemia, and hypomagnesemia.

      iv. A biopsy is often needed for kidney transplant recipients to distinguish drug-induced injury from acute allograft rejection.

   d. Risk factors for toxicity include advanced age, high initial cyclosporine dose, kidney graft rejection, hypotension, infection, and concomitant nephrotoxins.

   e. Prevention

      i. Monitor serum cyclosporine and tacrolimus concentrations closely.

      ii. Use lower doses in combination with other nonnephrotoxic immunosuppressants (e.g., steroids, mycophenolate mofetil).

      iii. Calcium channel blockers *may* help antagonize the vasoconstrictor effects of cyclosporine by dilating afferent arterioles.

D. Tubulointerstitial Disease

  1. Involves the renal tubules and the surrounding interstitium

  2. Onset can be acute or chronic.

    a. Acute onset generally involves interstitial inflammatory cell infiltrates, rapid loss of kidney function, and systemic symptoms (i.e., fever and rash).

    b. Chronic onset shows interstitial fibrosis, slow decline in kidney function, and no systemic symptoms.

  3. Acute allergic interstitial nephritis

    a. Cause of up to 3% of all AKI cases; caused by an allergic hypersensitivity reaction that affects the interstitium of the kidney

    b. Many medications and medication classes can cause this type of kidney failure, including β-lactams and the NSAIDs (although the presentations are different).

      i. Penicillins: Classic presentation of acute allergic interstitial nephritis. Signs and symptoms occur about 1–2 weeks after therapy initiation and include fever, maculopapular rash, eosinophilia, pyuria, hematuria, and proteinuria. Eosinophiluria may also be present.

      ii. NSAIDs: Onset much more delayed; typically begins about 6 months into therapy. Usually occurs in older adults on chronic NSAID therapy. Patients usually do not have systemic symptoms.

    c. Kidney biopsy may be needed to confirm diagnosis.

    d. Treatment includes discontinuing the offending agent and possibly initiating steroid therapy.

  4. Chronic interstitial nephritis

    a. Often progressive and irreversible

    b. Lithium

      i. Toxicity results from a duration-related decrease in response to antidiuretic hormone after long-term use (more than 10 years of therapy).

      ii. Clinical presentation

        (a) Often asymptomatic, with slow progression over years

        (b) May be recognized by slow increases in blood pressure (BP) or BUN and SCr

      iii. Risks include long duration of use, elevated serum concentrations, and repeated episodes of AKI from lithium toxicity.

      iv. Prevention is accomplished by maintaining the lowest serum lithium concentrations possible, avoiding dehydration, and monitoring kidney function closely.

    c. Cyclosporine and tacrolimus: Presents later in therapy (about 6–12 months) than hemodynamically mediated toxicity

  5. Papillary necrosis

    a. Form of chronic interstitial nephritis affecting the papillae, causing necrosis of the collecting ducts

       b.   Results from the long-term use of analgesics
- i. "Classic" example was with products that contained phenacetin.
- ii. Occurs more often with combination products
- iii. Products containing caffeine may also increase risk.

       c.   Evolves slowly as time progresses

       d.   Affects women more often than men

       e.   Difficult to diagnose, and much controversy remains about risk, prevention, and cause

E. Postrenal (Obstructive) Nephropathy
1. Results from obstruction of the flow of urine after glomerular filtration
2. Renal tubular obstruction
   - a. Caused by intratubular precipitation of tissue degradation products or precipitation of drugs or their metabolites
     - i. Tissue degradation products
       - (a) Uric acid intratubular precipitation after tumor lysis after chemotherapy
       - (b) Drug-induced rhabdomyolysis leading to intratubular precipitation of myoglobin
       - (c) Results in rapid decline in kidney function, with resultant oliguric or anuric kidney failure
     - ii. Drug precipitation: Sulfonamides, methotrexate, acyclovir, ascorbic acid; needlelike crystals observed in leukocytes found on urinalysis can prompt diagnosis.
   - b. Prevention includes pretreatment hydration, maintenance of high urinary volume, and alkalinization of the urine.
3. Extrarenal urinary tract obstruction
   - a. Benign prostatic hypertrophy can be worsened by anticholinergics.
   - b. Bladder outlet or ureteral obstruction from fibrosis after cyclophosphamide for hemorrhagic cystitis
4. Nephrolithiasis
   - a. Usually does not affect GFR, so does not have the classic signs and symptoms of nephrotoxicity
   - b. Some medications contribute to the formation of kidney stones: triamterene, sulfadiazine, indinavir, and ephedrine derivatives.

F. Glomerular Disease
1. Proteinuria is the hallmark of glomerular disease and may occur with or without a decrease in GFR.
2. A few distinct drugs can cause glomerular disease:
   - a. NSAIDs: Associated with acute allergic interstitial nephritis
   - b. Heroin: Can be caused by direct toxicity or toxicity from additives or infection from injection, and ESKD develops in most cases
   - c. Parenteral gold: Results from immune complex formation along glomerular capillary loops

III. CHRONIC KIDNEY DISEASE

A. Background
1. Prevalence: Difficult to assess. According to the 2013 U.S. Renal Data System Annual Report, 14.0% of adults (20 years or older) in the National Health and Nutrition Examination Survey population (2005–2010) have CKD. There were 430,273 patients on dialysis in 2011 and 185,626 transplant recipients. Incidence rate is flat, so growth in the number of patients with ESKD results mainly from the longer life span of these patients.

2. Definition of CKD
   a. According to the National Kidney Foundation Kidney Disease Outcome Quality Initiative (KDOQI): Kidney damage for more than 3 months, as defined by structural or functional abnormality of the kidney, with or without decreased GFR. Manifested by either pathologic abnormalities or markers of kidney damage—including abnormalities in the composition of blood or urine or abnormalities in imaging tests—*or* GFR less than 60 mL/minute/1.73 m^2 for 3 months, with or without kidney damage (Table 3).

Table 3. KDOQI Stages in CKD

Stage of Renal Disease	Damage	GFR (mL/minute/1.73 m^2)
Increased risk of developing kidney disease	Risk factors for CKD (diabetes, HTN, family history)	Greater than or equal to 90
Stage 1	Kidney damage with normal GFR	Greater than or equal to 90
Stage 2	Kidney damage with mild decrease in GFR	60–89
Stage 3	Moderate decrease in GFR	30–59
Stage 4	Severe decrease in GFR	15–29
Stage 5	Kidney failure	Less than 15

CKD = chronic kidney disease; GFR = glomerular filtration rate; HTN = hypertension; KDOQI = Kidney Disease Outcomes Quality Initiative.

   b. According to the KDIGO clinical practice guideline for the evaluation and management of CKD, CKD is defined as abnormalities of kidney structure or function for more than 3 months. These abnormalities may be seen as persistent markers of kidney damage or GFR less than 60 mL/minute/1.73 m^2 (Table 4).

Table 4. KDIGO Categories in CKD

GFR Category	Terms	GFR (mL/minute/1.73 m^2)
G1	Kidney damage with normal or high GFR	Greater than or equal to 90
G2	Kidney damage with mildly decreased GFR	60–89
G3a	Mildly to moderately decreased GFR	45–59
G3b	Moderately to severely decreased GFR	30–44
G4	Severely decreased GFR	15–29
G5	Kidney failure	Less than 15

CKD = chronic kidney disease; GFR = glomerular filtration rate.

B. Etiology
   1. Diabetes (40% of new cases of ESKD in the United States)
   2. Hypertension (25% of new cases)
   3. Glomerulonephritis (10%)
   4. Others: urinary tract disease, polycystic kidney disease, lupus, analgesic nephropathy, unknown

C. Risk Factors
   1. Susceptibility (associated with an increased risk but not proved to cause CKD): Advanced age, reduced kidney mass, low birth weight, racial or ethnic minority, family history, low income or education, systemic inflammation, and dyslipidemia; mostly not modifiable

2. Initiation (directly cause CKD): Diabetes, hypertension, autoimmune disease, polycystic kidney diseases, and drug toxicity; may be modifiable by drug therapy

3. Progression (result in faster decline in kidney function): Hyperglycemia, elevated BP, proteinuria, and smoking

---

Patient Cases

7. A 55-year-old man has a history of hypertension and newly diagnosed type 2 diabetes mellitus. He denies alcohol use but does smoke cigarettes (1 pack/day). His medications include atenolol 50 mg/day and a multivitamin. At your pharmacy, his BP is 149/92 mm Hg. His albumin/creatinine ratio (ACR) is 400 mg/g. A recent SCr is 1.9 mg/dL, which is consistent with a value measured 3 months earlier. His eGFR is 50 mL/minute. Which is the best assessment of his kidney disease based on KDIGO criteria?

    A. Category G2.

    B. Category G3a.

    C. Category G3b.

    D. Category G4.

8. Assuming that nonpharmacologic approaches have been optimized, which action is best to limit the progression of his kidney disease?

    A. Add nifedipine.

    B. Add diltiazem.

    C. Add enalapril.

    D. Increase atenolol.

9. Enalapril was added to this patient's regimen. Two weeks later, he presents back to his physician. His BP is 139/89 mm Hg. A repeat SCr is 2.3 mg/dL, and serum potassium is 5.2 mEq/L. Which is the best recommendation for this patient?

    A. Change enalapril to diltiazem ER. Monitor BP, SCr, and K in 2 weeks.

    B. Add chlorthalidone 50 mg/day. Monitor BP, SCr, and K in 2 weeks.

    C. Change enalapril to valsartan.

    D. Increase atenolol.

10. A study compared the use of an angiotensin receptor blocker alone or in combination with an ACEI in patients with chronic kidney disease. AKI occurred in 80 of 724 (11%) patients in receiving monotherapy and in 130 of 724 patients (18%) receiving combination therapy. Based on this information, what is the number of patients needed to harm?

    A. 7.

    B. 15.

    C. 50.

    D. 105.

D. Albuminuria or Proteinuria
  1. Marker of kidney damage, progression factor, and cardiovascular risk factor. Can be classified as in Table 5

Table 5. KDIGO Categories of Albuminuria

Category	Classification	ACR (mg/g)	Daily Excretion (mg/24 hours)
A1	Normal to mildly increased	Less than 30	Less than 30
A2	Moderately increased	30–300	30–300
A3	Severely increased albuminuria	Greater than 300	Greater than 300
	Nephrotic-range proteinuria		Greater than 3000

ACR = albumin/creatinine ratio.

Note: Classified as "normal" or "increased urinary albumin excretion" in 2014 American Diabetes Association clinical practice guidelines. Diabetes Care 2014;37(suppl 1):S14-S80.

  2. Assessment for proteinuria: Usually assessed by measuring urinary ACR. Spot urine: Untimed sample is adequate for adults and children (screening test).

E. Assessment of Kidney Function
  1. Serum creatinine (SCr)
    a. Avoid use as the sole assessment of kidney function.
    b. Depends on age, sex, weight, and muscle mass
    c. All laboratories now use "standardized" SCr traceable to isotope dilution mass spectrometry, which decreases variability in results between laboratories.
  2. Measurement of GFR: Inulin, iothalamate, and others are very rarely used in clinical practice.
  3. Measurement of CrCl through urine collection
    a. Reserve for vegetarians, patients needing dietary assessment, or those with abnormal muscle mass (e.g., patients with low muscle mass, patients with amputations) or when documenting need to start or continue dialysis.
    b. Urine collection yields a better estimate in patients with very low muscle mass.
    c. In most cases, equations overestimate kidney function because SCr concentrations are low in patients with very low muscle mass.
  4. Estimated CrCl using **Cockcroft-Gault equation** (mL/minute): Overestimates GFR

$$CrCl = \frac{[(140 - age) \times body\ weight]}{[SCr \times 72]} \times (0.85\ if\ female)$$

Although controversial, ideal body weight is often used in place of actual body weight for obese patients.
  5. Estimated GFR with **MDRD** study data equation
    a. Estimated GFR (mL/minute/1.73 m^2) in patients with known CKD (GFR less than 90 mL/minute)
    b. Isotope dilution mass spectrometry–traceable four-variable MDRD formula correlates well with the original MDRD formula; simpler to use:

$$eGFR\ (mL/minute/1.73\ m^2) = 175 \times SCr^{-1.154} \times age^{-0.203} \times (0.742\ if\ female) \times (1.212\ if\ African\ American)$$

    c. This equation is available at http://nkdep.nih.gov/lab-evaluation/gfr-calculators.shtml (accessed December 15, 2014) or www.kidney.org.

6. CKD-EPI equation: Alternative equation based on race, sex, SCr range, and age. More accurate at GFRs greater than 60 mL/minute/1.73 m². Available at http://www.kidney.org/professionals/KDOQI/gfr_calculator (accessed October 3, 2014)

7. For children, use Schwartz and Counahan-Barratt formulas.

F. Diabetic Nephropathy
   1. Pathogenesis
      a. Hypertension (systemic and intraglomerular)
      b. Glycosylation of glomerular proteins
      c. Genetic links
   2. Diagnosis
      a. Long history of diabetes
      b. Proteinuria
      c. Retinopathy (suggests microvascular disease)
   3. Monitoring
      a. Type 1 diabetes mellitus: Begin annual monitoring for albuminuria 5 years after diagnosis.
      b. Type 2 diabetes mellitus: Begin annual monitoring for albuminuria immediately (do not know how long patient has had diabetes mellitus).
   4. Management and slowing progression
      a. Aggressive BP management
         i. Goal BP readings in patients with diabetes

Group	Severity of Albuminuria	Goal Blood Pressure (maximum)	Level of Evidence
ADA 2014	Any	140/80 mm Hg[a]	B
KDIGO	Normal to mild albuminuria	140/90 mm Hg	1B
KDIGO	Moderate to severe albuminuria	130/80 mm Hg	2D
JNC 8	Any	140/90 mm Hg	E

[a]Systolic BP less than 130 mm Hg may be appropriate in some patients.

ADA = American Diabetes Association; JNC =Joint National Committee; KDIGO = Kidney Disease: Improving Global Outcomes.

        ii. ACEIs or ARBs are preferred and should be used with any degree of proteinuria, even if the patient is not hypertensive.
          (a) Use moderate to high doses with proteinuria.
          (b) Hold ACEI or ARB if serum potassium is greater than 5.6 mEq/L or if there is a rise in SCr greater than 30% after initiation.
          (c) Increased risk of hyperkalemia if combined with direct renin inhibitor
        iii. Most patients will require diuretic in combination (thiazide with stages 1–3 and loop diuretics in stages 4 and 5). If BP is greater than 160/100 mm Hg, start with a two-drug regimen.
        iv. Calcium channel blockers (nondihydropyridine) are second line to ACEIs and ARBs. Data are emerging for combined therapy.
        v. Dietary Na consumption should be less than 2.4 g/day. Modify Dietary Approaches to Stop Hypertension (DASH) diet to limit K intake as well.
      b. Intensive blood glucose control. Glycosylated hemoglobin (A1C) less than 7%. Less aggressive with more advanced CKD
      c. Protein restriction: Data are insufficient in diabetes, but 0.8 g/kg/day might slightly reduce progression and decrease the risk of ESKD. Patients should avoid high-protein diets.

G. Nondiabetic Nephropathy
1. Management of hypertension
   a. BP goals
      i. KDIGO guidelines

Target Group	Severity of Albuminuria	Goal Blood Pressure (maximum)	Level of Evidence
Nondiabetic CKD	Normal to mild albuminuria	140/90 mm Hg	1B
Nondiabetic CKD	Moderate to severe albuminuria	130/80 mm Hg	2D moderate 2C severe

      ii. JNC 8 guidelines: Patients 18 years and older with CKD: Goal BP less than 140/90 mm Hg (Grade E, Expert Opinion)
   b. If proteinuric and hypertensive, use ACEI *or* ARB. Often, need to add (or start with) combination. Diuretic is usual second drug. Monitor serum potassium.
2. Minimize protein in diet. Controversial. May slow progression according to MDRD study but may also impair nutrition. Very low-protein diet may increase mortality.

H. Other Guidelines to Slow Progression
1. Hyperlipidemia
   a. Assessment
      i. Newly identified CKD: Recommend evaluation of lipid profile (KDIGO, Grade 1C).
      ii. Follow-up measurement of lipid levels not necessary for most patients (not graded)
   b. Treatment recommendations (KDIGO)

Target Group	Treatment Recommendation	Grade
Adults more than 50 years old, GFR category G1–G2	Statin	1B
Adults more than 50 years old, GFR category G3a–G5	Statin or statin/ezetimibe	1A
Adults 18–49 years old with CKD before dialysis or transplant with CAD, diabetes, stroke, or estimated risk of coronary death or MI greater than 10%	Statin	2A
Adults on therapy when dialysis initiated	Continue statin or statin/ezetimibe	2C
Adults with dialysis-dependent CKD	Do *not* start therapy	2A
Adult kidney transplant recipients	Statin	2A

CAD, coronary artery disease.
KDIGO guideline for lipid management in CKD. Kidney Int 2014;85:1303-9.

2. Smoking cessation.

Patient Cases

11. A 70-year-old man is being assessed for HD access. He has a history of diabetes mellitus and hypertension but is otherwise healthy. Which dialysis access has the lowest rate of complications and the longest life span and is thus the best access to use?

    A. Subclavian catheter.

    B. Tenckhoff catheter.

    C. Arteriovenous graft.

    D. Arteriovenous fistula.

12. A patient undergoing long-term HD experiences intradialytic hypotension. After nonpharmacologic approaches have been optimized, which medication is best to manage his low BP?

    A. Levocarnitine.

    B. NaCl tablets.

    C. Fludrocortisone.

    D. Midodrine.

13. A patient with CKD on peritoneal dialysis presents with fever and abdominal pain. She also notes that her peritoneal dialysate has become cloudy. Laboratory evaluation of dialysate reveals many white blood cells, primarily neutrophils. Gram stain and culture of the fluid are ordered. According to the 2010 recommendations for peritoneal dialysis–related peritonitis, which is the best empiric therapy for this patient?

    A. Intravenous metronidazole plus gentamicin.

    B. Cefazolin plus ceftazidime instilled intraperitoneally.

    C. Intravenous clindamycin plus vancomycin.

    D. Vancomycin instilled intraperitoneally.

IV. RENAL REPLACEMENT THERAPY

A. Indications for RRT
   1. A: acidosis (not responsive to bicarbonate)
   2. E: electrolyte abnormality (hyperkalemia, hyperphosphatemia)
   3. I: intoxication (boric acid, ethylene glycol, lithium, methanol, phenobarbital, salicylate, theophylline)
   4. O: fluid overload (symptomatic [pulmonary edema])
   5. U: uremia (pericarditis and weight loss)

B. Two Primary Modes of Dialysis
   1. Hemodialysis: Most common modality in United States
   2. Peritoneal dialysis

C. Hemodialysis (intermittent for ESKD)
   1. Access
      a. Arteriovenous fistula: Preferred access
         i. Natural, formed by anastomosis of artery and vein
         ii. Lowest incidence of infection and thrombosis, lowest cost, longest survival
         iii. Takes weeks or months to "mature"

      b.   Arteriovenous graft
         i.   Usually synthetic (polytetrafluoroethylene)
         ii. Often used in patients with vascular disease
      c.   Catheters
         i.   Commonly used if permanent access unavailable
         ii. Problems include high infection and thrombosis rates. Low blood flow leads to inadequate dialysis.
  2. Dialysis membranes
      a.   Conventional: Not often used anymore. Small pores. Made of cuprophane
      b.   High flux (large pores) and high efficiency (large surface area). Can remove drugs that were impermeable to standard membranes (vancomycin). Large amounts of fluid removal (ultrafiltrate)
  3. Adequacy
      a. Kt/V: Unitless parameter. K = clearance, t = time on dialysis, and V = volume of distribution of urea. KDOQI set a minimum of 1.2 or more (target Kt/V of 1.4).
      b.   URR: Urea reduction ratio. URR = [(preBUN − postBUN)/preBUN] * 100%. Goal URR is greater than 65% (target URR of 70%).
  4. Common complications of HD
      a.   Intradialytic
         i.   Hypotension: Related primarily to fluid removal. Common in older adults and in people with diabetes mellitus
            (a) Acute treatment: Trendelenburg position, decrease ultrafiltration rate; administer saline boluses
            (b) Prevention: Accurately set "dry weight"; limit fluid gains between sessions; midodrine 2.5–10 mg orally before dialysis
            (c) Less well-studied agents include fludrocortisone, selective serotonin reuptake inhibitors
         ii. Cramps: Vitamin E 400 international units at bedtime
         iii. Nausea and vomiting
         iv. Headache, chest pain, or back pain
      b.   Vascular access complications: Most common with catheters
         i.   Infection: *S. aureus.* Need to treat aggressively. May need to remove catheter
         ii. Thrombosis: Suspected with low blood flow. Oral antiplatelet agents for prevention not used because of lack of efficacy. Can treat with alteplase 2 mg or reteplase 0.4 unit per lumen; try to aspirate after 30 minutes; may repeat dose after 120 minutes
  5. Factors that affect the efficiency of HD
      a.   Type of dialyzer used (changes in membrane surface area and pore size)
      b.   Length of therapy
      c.   Dialysis flow rate
      d.   Blood flow rate

D. Continuous RRT for AKI
  1. Continuous venovenous hemofiltration: Removes fluid and solutes by convection rather than by diffusion
      a.   Drug removal depends on ultrafiltrate production rate and protein binding of drug. Predict drug removal by the sieving coefficient (SC):

$$SC = \frac{\text{concentration of drug in ultrafiltrate}}{\text{concentration of drug in blood}}$$

      b.   Requires replacement fluid because of high ultrafiltrate rate
  2. Continuous venovenous hemodialysis: Dialysate flows countercurrent to blood flow, and solute is removed by diffusion.

E. Peritoneal Dialysis
1. Peritoneal dialysis membrane is 1–2 m² (approximates the body surface area) and consists of the vascular wall, the interstitium, the mesothelium, and the adjacent fluid films. From 1.5 to 3 L of peritoneal dialysate fluid may be instilled in the peritoneum (fill), allowed to dwell for a specified time, and then drained.
2. Solutes and fluid diffuse across the peritoneal membrane.
3. Peritoneal dialysis is usually *not* used to treat AKI in adults.
4. Peritonitis
   a. Infection of the peritoneal cavity. Patient technique and population variables influence the infection rate. Older adults or those with diabetes have a higher infection rate. Peritonitis is a main cause of failure of peritoneal dialysis.
   b. Treatment
      i. Most common gram-positive organisms include *Staphylococcus epidermis, S. aureus,* and streptococci. Most common gram-negative organisms include *Escherichia coli* and *Pseudomonas aeruginosa.*
      ii. Empiric treatment should cover gram-positive and gram-negative bacteria.
         (a) Intraperitoneal administration of vancomycin or first-generation cephalosporin *and* intraperitoneal third-generation cephalosporin or aminoglycoside
         (b) Adjust as needed.
5. Types of peritoneal dialysis
   a. Continuous ambulatory peritoneal dialysis: Classic. Requires mechanical process, which requires many manual changes throughout the day. Can disrupt daytime routine
   b. Automated peritoneal dialysis: Many variants exist, but continuous cycling peritoneal dialysis is the most common. Patient undergoes many exchanges during sleep by a cycling machine. May have one or two dwells during day. Minimizes potential contamination. Lowest incidence of peritonitis

---

Patient Cases

14. A 60-year-old patient on HD has had ESKD for 10 years. His HD access is a left arteriovenous fistula. He has a history of hypertension, coronary artery disease (CAD), mild CHF, type 2 diabetes mellitus, and a seizure disorder. Medications are as follows: epoetin alfa 14,000 units intravenously three times/week at dialysis, a renal multivitamin once daily, atorvastatin 20 mg/day, insulin, calcium acetate 2 tablets three times/day with meals, phenytoin 300 mg/day, and intravenous iron 100 mg/month. Laboratory values are as follows: hemoglobin 10.2 g/dL, immunoassay for PTH 800 pg/mL, Na 140 mEq/L, K 4.9 mEq/L, Cr 7.0 mg/dL, calcium 9.5 mg/dL, albumin 2.5 g/dL, and phosphorus 7.8 mg/dL. Serum ferritin is 550 ng/mL, and transferrin saturation (TSAT) is 32%. The red blood cell count (RBC) indices are normal. His white blood cell count (WBC) is normal, and he is afebrile. Which is most likely to be contributing to relative epoetin resistance in this patient?

   A. Iron deficiency.

   B. Hyperparathyroidism.

   C. Phenytoin therapy.

   D. Infection.

15. In addition to diet modification and emphasizing adherence, which is the best approach to managing this patient's hyperparathyroidism and renal osteodystrophy?

   A. Increase calcium acetate.

   B. Change calcium acetate to sevelamer and add cinacalcet.

   C. Hold calcium acetate and add intravenous vitamin D analog.

   D. Add intravenous vitamin D analog.

V. MANAGING THE COMPLICATIONS OF CHRONIC KIDNEY DISEASE

A. Anemia
1. Several factors are responsible for anemia in CKD: Decreased erythropoietin production (most important), shorter life span of red blood cells, blood loss during dialysis, iron deficiency, anemia of chronic disease, and renal osteodystrophy.
2. Prevalence: 26% of patients with a GFR greater than 60 mL/minute have anemia, compared with 75% of patients with a GFR less than 15 mL/minute.
3. Signs and symptoms: Similar to those of anemia associated with other causes
4. Treatment: Treatment of anemia in CKD can decrease morbidity and mortality, reduce left ventricular hypertrophy, increase exercise tolerance, and increase quality of life.
5. Recent studies suggest that treatment with erythropoiesis-stimulating agents (ESAs) to high hemoglobin concentrations (greater than 13 g/dL) increases cardiovascular events. Most recently, the Trial to Reduce Cardiovascular Events with Aranesp Therapy failed to show a benefit in outcomes, but treatment with ESAs was associated with increased stroke (N Engl J Med 2009;361:2019-32).
   a. Anemia workup: Initiate evaluation when CrCl is less than 60 mL/minute *or* when hemoglobin is less than 13 g/dL (men) or less than 12 g/dL (women)
      i. Hemoglobin and hematocrit monitoring recommendations
         (a) Stage 3 CKD: At least annually
         (b) Stage 4 and 5 (nondialysis): At least twice per year
         (c) Stage 5 (dialysis): At least every 3 months
      ii. Mean corpuscular volume
      iii. Reticulocyte count
      iv. Iron studies
         (a) TSAT (serum iron/total iron-binding capacity): Assesses available iron
         (b) Ferritin: Measures stored iron
      v. Serum vitamin B_{12} and folate levels
      vi. Stool guaiac

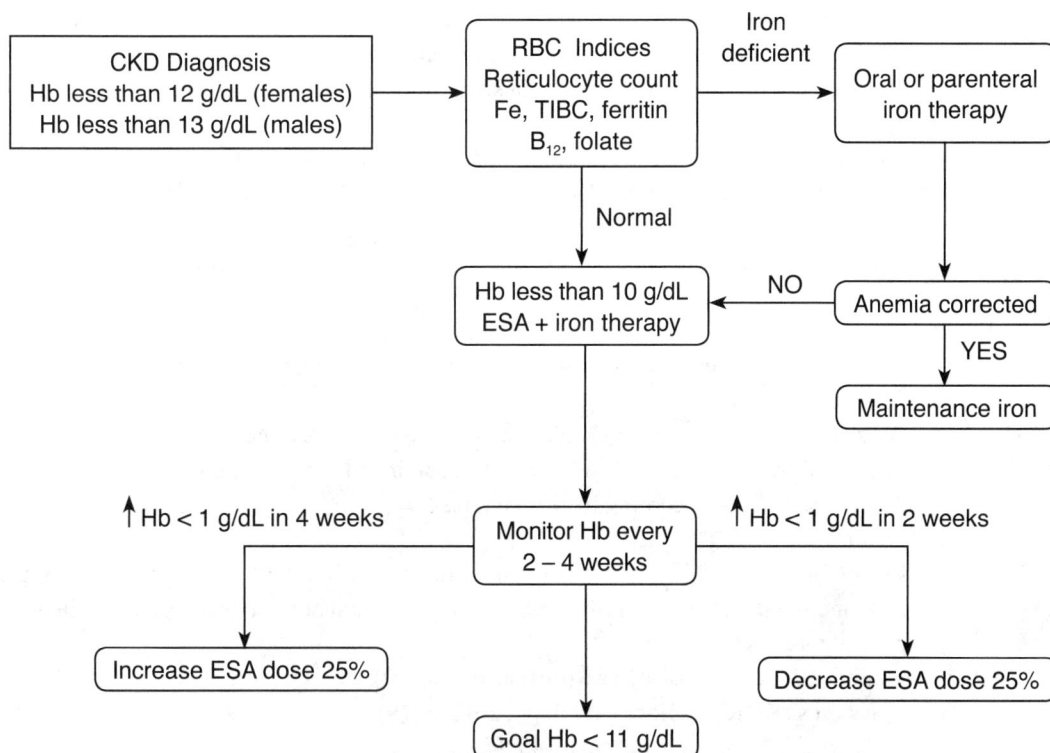

Figure 1. Management of anemia of CKD based on KDIGO and KDOQI guidelines. TIBC = total iron-binding capacity.

b. Erythropoiesis-stimulating agents (ESAs) (*Note: ESAs are under the FDA's Risk Evaluation and Mitigation Strategies program.*)

   i. Initiation of ESAs
      (a) Patients with CKD (nondialysis): Not to be initiated if hemoglobin is greater than 10 g/dL. If hemoglobin is less than 10 g/dL, consider the rate of decline in hemoglobin and the need to reduce the likelihood of transfusion (particularly in patients who may receive a renal transplant).
      (b) Patients with CKD (dialysis): Initiate therapy for hemoglobin less than 10 g/dL (KDIGO guidelines recommend avoiding until hemoglobin is less than 9 g/dL).
      (c) Use with caution, if at all, in patients with a history of stroke or cancer (evidence is stronger in nondialysis patients than in dialysis patients with CKD).

   ii. Maintenance of ESAs: Individualize dosing and use the lowest dose of ESA sufficient to reduce the need for red blood cell transfusions; adjust dosing as appropriate.

   iii. Epoetin alfa
      (a) Same molecular structure as human erythropoietin (recombinant DNA technology)
      (b) Binds to and activates erythropoietin receptor
      (c) Administered subcutaneously or intravenously
      (d) Subcutaneous dosage requirement is typically 30% less than intravenous dosage requirement.

   iv. Darbepoetin alfa
      (a) Molecular structure of human erythropoietin has been modified from 3 *N*-linked carbohydrate chains to 5 *N*-linked carbohydrate chains; increased duration of activity

(b) The advantage is less-frequent dosing (e.g., once weekly, once every 2–3 weeks).

(c) Binds to and activates erythropoietin receptor

(d) May be administered subcutaneously or intravenously

c. Therapy goals

    i. Use the lowest possible dose of ESA to prevent blood transfusion.

    ii. In nondialysis patients with CKD, hold or reduce dose when hemoglobin is greater than 10 g/dL.

    iii. In dialysis patients, hold or reduce dose when hemoglobin is greater than 11 g/dL (KDIGO suggests an upper limit of 11.5 g/dL).

d. ESA dose adjustment is based on hemoglobin response.

    i. Adjustment parameters are similar for epoetin alfa and darbepoetin alfa.

    ii. Maximal increase in hemoglobin is about 1 g/dL every 2–4 weeks.

    iii. Dosage adjustments upward should not be made more often than every 4 weeks.

    iv. In general, dose adjustments are made in 25% increments (i.e., dosages adjusted upward or downward by 25% according to current dose).

e. ESA monitoring

    i. Hemoglobin every 2–4 weeks during initiation phase. In maintenance phase of therapy, monitor hemoglobin at least monthly in dialysis patients and at least every 3 months in nondialysis patient with CKD.

    ii. Monitor BP because it may rise (treat as necessary).

    iii. Iron stores (KDIGO, Kidney Int Suppl 2012;2:279)

        (a) Ferritin: Goal is greater than 500 ng/mL.

        (b) TSAT target is greater than 30%.

f. Common causes of inadequate response to ESA therapy

    i. Iron deficiency is the most common cause of erythropoietin resistance; however, increased use of intravenous iron products has reduced this problem.

    ii. Infection and inflammation

    iii. Other causes include chronic blood loss, hyperparathyroidism, aluminum toxicity, folate or vitamin B_{12} deficiency, malignancies, malnutrition, hemolysis, and vitamin C deficiency.

g. Iron therapy

    i. Most patients with CKD who are receiving ESAs require parenteral iron therapy to meet needs (increased requirements, decreased oral absorption).

    ii. For adult patients who undergo dialysis, an empiric cumulative or total dose of 1000 mg is usually given, and equations are rarely used.

    iii. Follow TSAT and ferritin as noted during erythropoietic therapy.

    iv. Adverse effects

        (a) Anaphylactic-type reactions with iron dextran require test dose. Hypersensitivity reaction may occur with all parenteral iron products.

        (b) Hypotension with administration of sodium ferric gluconate, iron sucrose, and ferumoxytol. Monitor during and up to 30 minutes after administration.

        (c) Hypertension. Transient increases in BP with ferric carboxymaltose

    v. Seven commercial iron preparations are approved in the United States (Table 6).

    vi. Oral iron not recommended in patients with CKD on dialysis

Table 6. Iron Therapy

Iron Product	Replacement Therapy (TSAT less than 30% and ferritin less than 500 ng/mL)	Maintenance Therapy (iron stores in goal)	Initial Test Dose
Iron dextran (high-molecular-weight iron dextran: Dexferrum) (low-molecular-weight iron dextran: INFeD)	IVP: 100 mg IV 3 times/week during HD for 10 doses (1 g) IVPB: 500–1000 mg in 250 mL of NS infused for at least 1 hour (option for non-HD patients)	25–100 mg/week IV × 10 weeks	Yes; 25-mg 1-time test dose
Sodium ferric gluconate complex (Ferrlecit and generic)	125 mg IV 3 times/week during HD for 8 doses (1 g)	31.25–125 mg/week IV × 10 weeks	None needed
Iron sucrose (Venofer)	100 mg IV 3 times/week during HD for 10 doses (1 g) For non-HD CKD, 200 mg IV × 5 doses	25–100 mg/week IV × 10 weeks	None needed
Ferumoxytol (Feraheme)	510 mg at up to 30 mg/second, followed by a second 510-mg IV dose 3–8 days later (all CKD)	N/A	None needed
Ferric carboxymaltose (Injectafer)	15 mg/kg IV up to 750 mg; may repeat after at least 7 days (maximum 1500 mg elemental iron per 2-dose course)	N/A	None needed

CKD = chronic kidney disease; HD = hemodialysis; IV = intravenous(ly); IVP = IV push; IVPB = IV piggyback; N/A = not applicable; NS = normal saline solution; TSAT = transferrin saturation.

B. CKD-Mineral Bone Disorder (CKD-MBD) and Renal Osteodystrophy
   1. Pathophysiology: Calcium and phosphorus homeostasis is complex, involving the interplay of hormones affecting the bone, gastrointestinal (GI) tract, kidneys, and PTH. Process may begin as early as GFR 60 mL/minute. Factors contributing to CKD-MBD and renal osteodystrophy include:
      a. Hyperphosphatemia
      b. Decreased production of 1,25-dihydroxyvitamin D_3
      c. Reduced absorption of calcium in the gut
      d. Decreased ionized (free) calcium concentrations
      e. Direct stimulation of PTH secretion
      f. Elevated PTH concentrations cause decreased reabsorption of phosphorus and increased reabsorption of calcium in the proximal tube. This adaptive mechanism is lost as GFR falls below 30 mL/minute. Important: Calcium is not well absorbed through the gut at this point, and calcium concentrations are maintained by increased bone resorption through elevated PTH. Unabated calcium loss from the bone results in renal osteodystrophy.
   2. Prevalence
      a. Main cause of morbidity and mortality in patients undergoing dialysis
      b. Very common

3. Signs and symptoms
   a. Insidious onset: Patients may experience fatigue and musculoskeletal and GI pain; calcification may be visible on radiography; bone pain and fractures can occur if progression is left untreated.
   b. Laboratory abnormalities (Table 7)
      i. Phosphorus
      ii. Corrected calcium
      iii. Intact PTH
      iv. Alkaline phosphatase
      v. 25-OH vitamin D

Table 7. KDIGO Guidelines for Frequency of Laboratory Monitoring in CKD Stages 3–5

	Stage 3 CKD	Stage 4 CKD	Stage 5 CKD
Calcium	Every 6–12 months	Every 3–6 months	Every 1–3 months
Phosphorus	Every 6–12 months	Every 3–6 months	Every 1–3 months
Intact PTH	Baseline	Every 6–12 months	Every 3–6 months
Alkaline phosphatase	Baseline	Every 12 months	Every 12 months
25-OH vitamin D	Baseline	Baseline	Baseline

CKD = chronic kidney disease; KDIGO = Kidney Disease: Improving Global Outcomes; PTH = parathyroid hormone.

4. Treatment
   a. Therapy goals (Table 8)

Table 8. KDIGO Guidelines for Calcium, Phosphorus, and Intact PTH in CKD Stages 3–5

	CKD Stage 3	CKD Stage 4	CKD Stage 5	CKD Stage 5 on Dialysis
Calcium	Normal	Normal	Normal	Normal
Phosphorus	Normal	Normal	Normal	Near normal
Intact PTH	Normal	Normal	Normal	2–9 times upper normal

CKD = chronic kidney disease; KDIGO = Kidney Disease: Improving Global Outcomes; PTH = parathyroid hormone.

   b. Nondrug therapy
      i. Dietary phosphorus restriction 800–1000 mg/day in stage 3 CKD or higher
      ii. Dialysis removes various amounts of phosphorus, depending on treatment modalities; however, by itself it is insufficient to maintain phosphorus balances in most patients.
      iii. Parathyroidectomy: Reserved for patients with unresponsive hyperparathyroidism
   c. Drug therapy
      i. Phosphate binders: Take with meals to bind phosphorus in the gut; products from different groups may be used together for additive effect.

Table 9. Phosphate Binders

Product	Dosage Form	Typical Dose
Calcium carbonate	500, 1000, 1250 mg (40% elemental Ca)	1250 mg TID with meals
Calcium acetate (PhosLo, Phoslyra)	667-mg capsule, tablet 667-mg/5 mL solution (25% elemental Ca)	2001 mg TID with meals
Sevelamer hydrochloride (Renagel)	400-, 800-mg tablet	800–2400 mg TID with meals
Sevelamer carbonate (Renvela)	800-mg tablet 0.8-g, 2.4-g packet	800–2400 mg TID with meals
Lanthanum carbonate (Fosrenol)	500-, 750-, 1000-mg chewable tablet	250–500 mg TID with meals
Sucroferric oxyhydroxide (Velphoro)	500-mg chewable tablet	500 mg TID with meals
Aluminum hydroxide	320-mg/5 mL suspension	300–600 mg TID with meals
Ferric citrate	210 mg tablet	420 mg TID with meals

TID = three times/day.

(a) Aluminum-containing phosphate binders (aluminum hydroxide, aluminum carbonate, and sucralfate). Effectively lower phosphorus concentrations. In general, avoid. Not used as often because of aluminum toxicity (adynamic bone disease, encephalopathy, and erythropoietin resistance). Use should be limited to a single short-term (4-week) course.

(b) Calcium-containing phosphate binders (calcium carbonate and calcium acetate)

    (1) Widely used phosphate binder. Calcium binders are often the initial binder of choice for stage 3 and 4 CKD. Calcium or nonionic binders are considered initial binder of choice in stage 5 CKD. Carbonate salt is inexpensive.

    (2) Carbonate is also used to treat hypocalcemia, which sometimes occurs in patients with CKD, and can decrease metabolic acidosis.

    (3) Calcium acetate is a better binder than carbonate and contains less elemental calcium. Less calcium absorption

    (4) Use may be limited by development of hypercalcemia; reduce dose or discontinue.

    (5) Total elemental calcium is 2000 mg/day (1500-mg binder; 500-mg diet).

(c) Sevelamer: A nonabsorbable phosphate binder

    (1) Effectively binds dietary phosphorus

    (2) As with calcium, considered primary therapy in stage 5 CKD. In particular, consider whether the patient has hypercalcemia or whether calcium intake exceeds the recommended dose with calcium-containing binders.

    (3) Decreases low-density lipoprotein cholesterol and increases high-density lipoprotein cholesterol

    (4) Metabolic acidosis may worsen with sevelamer hydrogen chloride (HCl).

(d) Lanthanum carbonate

    (1) As effective as aluminum in phosphate-binding capability. Not widely used, but indications similar to sevelamer

    (2) Flavorless, chewable tablet

    (3) Consider using if patient has hypercalcemia

(e) There are no data indicating that any phosphate binder is superior to another in clinical outcomes (mortality or hospitalization). However, sevelamer and lanthanum do cause less hypercalcemia and reduce calcium burden.

ii. Vitamin D and vitamin D analogs: Suppress PTH synthesis and reduce PTH concentrations; therapy is limited by resultant hypercalcemia. Products include calcitriol, doxercalciferol, and paricalcitol.

   (a) Ergocalciferol (vitamin D_2): May be used in stage 3–5 CKD for patients with low serum 25-hydroxyvitamin D concentrations; repeat vitamin D levels after 6 months of therapy.

   (b) Cholecalciferol (vitamin D_3): May be used as alternative to ergocalciferol.

Table 10. Vitamin D Repletion

Serum 25-OH Vitamin D (ng/mL)	Assessment	Dosing Regimen
Less than 5	Severe deficiency	Weekly PO doses × 12 weeks; then monthly *or* Single IM dose
5–15	Mild deficiency	Weekly PO doses × 4 weeks, then monthly
16–30	Insufficiency	Monthly PO doses

IM = intramuscular; PO = oral.

   (c) Calcitriol, the pharmacologically active form of 1,25-dihydroxyvitamin D_3, is FDA label approved for the management of hypocalcemia and the prevention and treatment of secondary hyperparathyroidism.
      (1) Oral and parenteral formulations
      (2) Does not require hepatic or renal activation
      (3) Low-dose daily oral therapy reduces hypocalcemia but does not reduce PTH concentrations significantly.
      (4) High incidence of hypercalcemia, limiting PTH suppression
      (5) Dose adjustment at 4-week intervals

   (d) Paricalcitol: Vitamin D analog; FDA label approved for the treatment and prevention of secondary hyperparathyroidism
      (1) Parenteral and oral formulations
      (2) Does not require hepatic or renal activation
      (3) Lower incidence of hypercalcemia compared with calcitriol (decreased mobilization of calcium from the bone and decreased absorption of calcium from the gut)

   (e) Doxercalciferol: Vitamin D analog; FDA label approved for the treatment and prevention of secondary hyperparathyroidism
      (1) Parenteral and oral formulations
      (2) Prodrug; requires hepatic activation; may have more physiologic levels
      (3) Lower incidence of hypercalcemia compared with calcitriol (decreased mobilization of calcium from the bone and decreased absorption of calcium from the gut)

iii. Cinacalcet HCl: A calcimimetic that attaches to the calcium receptor on the parathyroid gland and increases the sensitivity of receptors to serum calcium concentrations, thus reducing PTH. Especially useful in patients with high calcium and phosphate concentrations and high PTH concentrations when vitamin D analogs cannot be used or cannot be increased

   (a) The initial dose is 30 mg, irrespective of PTH concentration.

   (b) Monitor serum calcium every 1–2 weeks (risk of hypocalcemia is about 5%); do not initiate therapy if corrected serum calcium is less than 8.4 mg/dL.

(c) Can be used in patients irrespective of phosphate binder or vitamin D analog use

(d) Caution in patients with seizure disorder (hypocalcemia may exacerbate)

(e) Adverse effects are nausea (30%) and diarrhea (20%).

(f) Cinacalcet inhibits cytochrome P450 (CYP) 2D6 metabolism, thereby inhibiting the metabolism of CYP2D6 substrates such that dose reductions in drugs with narrow therapeutic indices may be required (e.g., flecainide, tricyclic antidepressants, thioridazine).

(g) Cinacalcet is metabolized primarily by CYP3A, so drugs that are potent inhibitors of CYP3A (ketoconazole) may increase cinacalcet concentrations up to twofold.

Patient Case

16. A 40-year-old patient on dialysis with a history of grand mal seizures takes phenytoin 300 mg/day. His albumin concentration is 3.0 g/dL. His total phenytoin concentration is 5.0 mcg/mL. Which is the best interpretation of the phenytoin concentrations?

   A. The concentration is subtherapeutic, and a dose increase is warranted.

   B. The concentration is therapeutic, and no dosage adjustment is needed.

   C. The concentration is toxic, and a dose reduction is needed.

   D. The level is not interpretable.

VI. DOSAGE ADJUSTMENTS IN KIDNEY DISEASE

A. Dosages of Many Drugs Will Require Adjustment to Prevent Toxicity in Patients with CKD. Adjustment strategies vary depending on whether the patient is receiving RRT and, if so, the type of RRT. The National Kidney Disease Education Program of the National Institutes of Health/National Institute of Diabetes and Digestive and Kidney Diseases suggests that either eGFR or eCrCl be used for drug dosing. If eGFR is used in very large or small patients, the eGFR should be multiplied by the actual body surface area to obtain eGFR in milliliters per minute.

B. Pharmacokinetic Principles Guiding Therapy Adjustments
   1. Absorption: Oral absorption can be decreased.
      a. Nausea and vomiting
      b. Increased gastric pH (uremia)
      c. Edema
      d. Physical binding of drugs to phosphate binders
   2. Distribution
      a. Changes in concentrations in highly water-soluble drugs occur as extracellular fluid status changes.
      b. Acidic and neutral protein-bound drugs are displaced by toxin buildup. Other mechanisms include conformational changes of the plasma protein–binding site. Phenytoin is a classic example. The "normal" free fraction of phenytoin is 10%. Free fraction can be as high as 30% in patients with ESKD and hypoalbuminemia.
         i. Hypoalbuminemia correction:
            Concentration adjusted = Concentration measured/[(0.2 × measured albumin) + 0.1]
         ii. Renal failure adjustment:
            Concentration adjusted = Concentration measured/[(0.1 × measured albumin) + 0.1]

       iii. Patients have lower total concentrations, despite having adequate free concentrations (increased free fraction).

       iv. Dosage adjustment of phenytoin not needed, just a different approach to evaluating concentrations.

   3. Metabolism: Variable changes can occur with uremia; metabolites can accumulate.

   4. Excretion: Decreased

C. Pharmacodynamic changes can also occur (e.g., patients with CKD can be more sensitive to benzodiazepines).

D. General Recommendations
   1. Patient history and clinical data
   2. Estimate CrCl (Jeliffe or Brater equation in AKI; Cockcroft-Gault or MDRD study equations in stable kidney function).
   3. Identify medications that require modification (Table 11).

Table 11. Dose Adjustments in Decreased Kidney Function

Drug Class	Agents Requiring Dose Adjustment
Antibiotics	Almost all antibiotics require dosage adjustment (exceptions: cloxacillin, clindamycin, linezolid, metronidazole, and macrolides)
Cardiac medications	Atenolol, ACEIs, digoxin, nadolol, sotalol; avoid potassium-sparing diuretics if CrCl less than 30 mL/minute
Lipid-lowering therapy	Clofibrate, fenofibrate, statins (particularly rosuvastatin)
Narcotics	Codeine, avoid meperidine; other agents may also accumulate
Antipsychotic and antiepileptic agents	Chloral hydrate, gabapentin, lithium, paroxetine, primidone, topiramate, trazodone, vigabatrin
Hypoglycemic agents	Acarbose, chlorpropamide, glyburide, glipizide, insulins, and metformin
Antiretrovirals	Individualize therapy: Monitor CD4 counts, viral load, and adverse effects (agents requiring dose adjustment: lamivudine, adefovir, didanosine, stavudine, tenofovir, zalcitabine, and zidovudine)
Miscellaneous	Allopurinol, colchicine, H_2-receptor antagonists, diclofenac, ketorolac, acyclovir, valacyclovir, and terbutaline

ACEIs = angiotensin-converting enzyme inhibitors; CrCl = creatinine clearance; H_2 = histamine-2.

   4. Calculate drug doses individualized for the patient.
     a. Published data
     b. Rowland-Tozer estimate
       i. $Q = 1 - [Fe(1 - KF)]$
       ii. Q = kinetic parameter or drug dose adjustment factor
       iii. Fe = fraction of drug excreted unchanged in the urine
       iv. KF = ratio of patient's CrCl to normal (120 mL/minute)
   5. Monitor patient (e.g., kidney function, clinical parameters) and drug concentration (if applicable).
   6. Revise regimen as appropriate.

E. Drug Dosing in HD
   1. Dosing changes in patients with HD may be necessary because of accumulation caused by kidney failure *or* because the procedure may remove the drug from the circulation *or* because of pharmacodynamic effects (e.g., BP medication reduction because of intradialytic hypotension).

2. Drug-related factors affecting drug removal during dialysis
   a. Molecular weight: With high-flux membranes, larger molecules (e.g., vancomycin) can be removed compared with conventional filters.
   b. Water soluble: Nonsoluble drugs are not likely to be removed.
   c. Protein binding: Because albumin cannot pass through membranes, protein-bound drugs cannot either.
   d. Volume of distribution: Drugs with a small Vd (less than 1 L/kg) available in central circulation for removal. Large Vds cannot be removed (digoxin and tricyclic antidepressants), even if the protein binding is very low.
3. Procedure-related factors affecting drug removal
   a. Type of dialyzer: High flux, widely used now
   b. Blood flow rate: Elevated rates increase delivery and maintain gradient across membrane.
   c. Duration of dialysis session
   d. Dialysate flow rate. High rates of flow increase removal by maintaining the gradient across membranes.

REFERENCES

Kidney Disease

1. National Kidney Foundation's Kidney Disease Outcome Quality Initiative (NKF KDOQI). Available at www.kidney.org/professionals/kdoqi/index.cfm.

2. National Kidney Disease Education Program (NKDEP). www.nkdep.nih.gov/.

3. Kidney Disease: Improving Global Outcomes (KDIGO). http://kdigo.org/home/guidelines/.

Acute Kidney Injury

1. Bellomo R, Ronco C, Kellum JA, et al.; the ADQI Workgroup. Acute renal failure—definition, outcome measures, animal models, and information technology needs: the Second International Consensus Conference of the Acute Dialysis Quality Initiative (ADQI) Group. Crit Care 2004;8:R204-R212.

2. Dager W, Halilovic J. Acute kidney injury. In: DiPiro JT, Talbert RL, Yee GC, et al., eds. Pharmacotherapy: A Pathophysiologic Approach, 9th ed. New York: McGraw-Hill, 2014:611-32.

3. Kellum JA. Acute kidney injury. Crit Care Med 2008;36:S141-5.

4. Kidney Disease: Improving Global Outcomes (KDIGO) Acute Kidney Injury Work Group. KDIGO practice guideline for acute kidney injury. Kidney Int Suppl 2012;2:1-138.

5. Mehta RL, Kellum JA, Shah SV, et al. Acute Kidney Injury Network: report of an initiative to improve outcomes in acute kidney injury. Crit Care 2007;11:R31.

6. Palevsky PM, Liu KD, Brophy PD, et al. KDOQI U.S. commentary on the 2012 KDIGO clinical practice guidelines for acute kidney injury. Am J Kidney Dis 2013;61:649-72.

7. Stamatakis MK. Acute kidney injury. In: Chisholm-Burns MA, Wells BG, Schwinghammer TL, et al., eds. Pharmacotherapy: Principles and Practice, 2nd ed. New York: McGraw-Hill, 2010:431-44.

8. Ympa YP, Sakr Y, Reinhart K, et al. Has mortality from acute kidney injury decreased? A systematic review of the literature. Am J Med. 2005;118:827-32.

Glomerulonephritis

1. Beck L, Bomback AS, Choi MJ, et al. KDOQI U.S. commentary on the 2012 clinical practice guideline for glomerulonephritis. Am J Kidney Dis 2013;62:403-41.

2. Kidney Disease: Improving Global Outcomes (KDIGO). Glomerulonephritis Work Group. KDIGO clinical practice guideline for glomerulonephritis. Kidney Int Suppl 2012;2:139-274.

3. Lau AH. Glomerulonephritis. In: DiPiro JT, Talbert RL, Yee GC, et al., eds. Pharmacotherapy: A Pathophysiologic Approach, 9th ed. New York: McGraw-Hill, 2014:705-28.

Drug-Induced Kidney Damage

1. Nolin TD, Himmelfarb J. Drug-induced kidney disease. In: DiPiro JT, Talbert RL, Yee GC, et al., eds. Pharmacotherapy: A Pathophysiologic Approach, 9th ed. New York: McGraw-Hill, 2014:687-704.

2. Schweiger MJ, Chambers CE, Davidson CJ, et al. Prevention of contrast induced nephropathy: recommendations for the high risk patient undergoing cardiovascular procedures. Catheter Cardiovasc Interv 2007;69:135-40.

Chronic Kidney Disease and Complications

1. Inker LA, Astor BC, Fox CH, et al. KDOQI commentary on the 2012 Clinical Practice Guideline for the evaluation and management of CKD. Am J Kidney Dis 2014;63:713-35.

2. American Diabetes Association. Standards of medical care in diabetes: 2014. Diabetes Care 2014;37(suppl 1):S14-80.

3. Hudson JQ, Wazny LD. Chronic kidney disease: management of complications. In: DiPiro JT, Talbert RL, Yee GC, et al., eds. Pharmacotherapy: A Pathophysiologic Approach, 9th ed. New York: McGraw-Hill, 2014:633-63.

4. Kidney Disease: Improving Global Outcomes (KDIGO) CKD Work Group. KDIGO 2012 clinical practice guideline for the evaluation and management of chronic kidney disease. Kidney Int Suppl 2013;3:1-150.

5. Levey AS, Coresh J. Chronic kidney disease. Lancet 2012;379:165-80.

6. National Kidney Foundation. KDOQI. Clinical practice guidelines and clinical practice recommendations for diabetes and chronic kidney disease. Am J Kidney Dis 2007;49(suppl 2):S1-180.

7. National Kidney Foundation. K/DOQI clinical practice guidelines for chronic kidney disease: evaluation: classification, and stratification. Am J Kidney Dis 2002;39(suppl 1):S1-266.

8. National Kidney Foundation. KDOQI clinical practice guideline for diabetes and CKD: 2012 update. Am J Kidney Dis 2012;60:850-86.

9. National Kidney Foundation. KDOQI clinical practice guidelines on hypertension and antihypertensive agents in chronic kidney disease. Am J Kidney Dis 2004;43(suppl 5):S1.

10. Schonder KS. Chronic and end-stage renal disease. In: Chisholm-Burns MA, Wells BG, Schwinghammer TL, et al., eds. Pharmacotherapy: Principles and Practice, 2nd ed. New York: McGraw-Hill, 2010:445-78.

11. Taler SJ, Agarwal R, Bakris GL, et al. KDOQI U.S. commentary on the 2012 KDIGO clinical practice guideline for management of blood pressure in CKD. Am J Kidney Dis 2013;62:201-13.

12. Wanner C, Tonelli M; KDIGO Lipid Guideline Development Work Group Members. KDIGO clinical practice guideline for lipid management in CKD: summary of recommendation statements and clinical approach to the patient. Kidney Int 2014;85:1303-9.

Anemia of Chronic Kidney Disease

1. Kidney Disease: Improving Global Outcomes (KDIGO) Anemia Work Group. KDIGO clinical practice guideline for anemia in chronic kidney disease. Kidney Int Suppl 2012;2:279-335.

2. Kliger AS, Foley RN, Goldfarb DS, et al. KDOQI U.S. commentary on the 2012 KDIGO clinical practice guideline for anemia in CKD. Am J Kidney Dis 2013;62:849-59. Available at http://www.kidney.org/sites/default/files/docs/kdoqi_commentary_on_kdigo_anemia.pdf. Accessed October 3, 2014.

3. National Kidney Foundation. KDOQI clinical practice guidelines and recommendations for anemia of chronic kidney disease. Am J Kidney Dis 2006;47(suppl 3):S1-146. Available at http://www2.kidney.org/professionals/KDOQI/guidelines_anemia/. Accessed October 3, 2014.

Mineral and Bone Disorder

1. Kidney Disease: Improving Global Outcomes (KDIGO) CKD-MBD Work Group. KDIGO clinical practice guideline for the diagnosis, evaluation, prevention, and treatment of chronic kidney disease–mineral and bone disorder (CKD-MBD). Kidney Int 2009;76(suppl 113):S1-130.

2. Uhlig K, Berns JS, Kestenbaum B, et al. KDOQI U.S. commentary on the 2009 KDIGO clinical practice guideline for the diagnosis, evaluation, and treatment of CKD–mineral and bone disorder (CKD-MBD). Am J Kidney Dis 2010;55:773-99.

Renal Replacement Therapy

1. Li PK, Szeto CC, Piraino B, et al. Peritoneal dialysis-related infections recommendations: 2010 update. Perit Dial Int 2010;30:393-423.

2. Ballinger AE, Palmer SC, Wiggins KJ, et al. Treatment for peritoneal dialysis-associated peritonitis. Cochrane Database of Systematic Reviews 2014;4:CD005284. doi:10.1002/14651858. CD005284.pub3.

3. Sowinski KM, Churchwell MD, Decker BS. Hemodialysis and peritoneal dialysis. In: DiPiro JT, Talbert RL, Yee GC, et al., eds. Pharmacotherapy: A Pathophysiologic Approach, 9th ed. New York: McGraw-Hill, 2014:665-85.

4. O'Mara NB. Management of patients on dialysis. In: Murphy JE, Lee MW, eds. Pharmacotherapy Self-Assessment Program, 2014 Book 2. Chronic Illnesses. Lenexa, KS: American College of Clinical Pharmacy, 2014:203-207.

Drug Therapy Adjustment in CKD

1. National Kidney Disease Education Program. Chronic kidney disease and drug dosing: information for providers. Revised January 2010. Available at http://nkdep.nih.gov/resources/ckd-drug-dosing-508.pdf. Accessed October 3, 2014.

2. Kappel J, Calissi P. Nephrology: 3. Safe drug prescribing for patients with renal insufficiency. Can Med Assoc J 2002;166:473-7.

3. Mohammad RS, Matzke GR. Drug therapy individualization for patients with chronic kidney disease. In: DiPiro JT, Talbert RL, Yee GC, et al., eds. Pharmacotherapy: A Pathophysiologic Approach, 9th ed. New York: McGraw-Hill, 2014:729-43.

ANSWERS AND EXPLANATIONS TO PATIENT CASES

1. Answer: D

Estimating CrCl in a patient with unstable kidney function is difficult. The Jeliffe or Brater equation has been recommended as preferable to other equations. In this case, the patient is anuric; therefore, a CrCl (GFR) of less than 10 mL/minute (Answer D) should be assumed. Answer A (Cockcroft-Gault) is inappropriate because Cockcroft-Gault should be used only with stable kidney function. The use of MDRD (Answer B) in unstable kidney function is also inappropriate. Although Answer C, the Brater equation, may be used, it would still overestimate kidney function in this patient because the patient is anuric.

2. Answer: B

This patient probably has ATN, which is a type of intrinsic renal failure (Answer B). The rapid rise in SCr, the BUN/Cr ratio of about 10, and the muddy casts all point to ATN. There is no evidence of prerenal causes (hypotension, volume depletion) (Answer A). Naproxen is associated with functional AKI (Answer D), but the urine in these patients is bland without casts. Answer C is incorrect because there is no evidence of obstruction in this patient.

3. Answer: A

One of the strategies in managing AKI is to remove potentially nephrotoxic drugs, either direct toxins or medications that alter intrarenal hemodynamics. It is common to see the following orders for patients in AKI: no ACEIs, ARBs, NSAIDs, or intravenous contrast. However, low-dose aspirin can be continued without adversely affecting kidney function. It is also important to remove (or reduce the dose of) agents that are cleared renally. Metformin, which accumulates in decreased kidney function, should be temporarily discontinued at this time because of an increased risk of lactic acidosis, not because of an adverse effect on kidney function. In this case, lisinopril is most likely to affect kidney function so it should be discontinued.

4. Answer: C

This patient presents with ATN, anuria, and volume overload. Although loop diuretics have not been shown to improve clinical outcomes in patients with AKI, they may increase urine output, which will help with fluid and electrolyte balance. In addition, this patient is hypervolemic, so a trial of intravenous loop diuretics would be appropriate (Answer C). Adding 0.9% NaCl (Answer A) would worsen fluid overload. Hydrochlorothiazide (Answer B) would not be appropriate because thiazide diuretics are unlikely to be effective with such poor kidney function. Fluid restriction (Answer D) may be necessary if furosemide fails to increase urine output, but it would not be the first-line approach.

5. Answer: B

Intravenous 0.9% NaCl is considered the most effective hydration for the prevention of contrast-induced nephropathy (Answer B). The other solutions, particularly oral, would not be appropriate. Although not listed as a choice, intravenous sodium bicarbonate solutions have also been used in this setting.

6. Answer: B

Contrast-associated nephropathy is associated with an acute rise in BUN and SCr within 24–48 hours, with a peak at 3–5 days. Monitoring of SCr at 24 hours will help identify the development of contrast-associated nephropathy. In contrast, 6 hours is too early to detect a significant change, and waiting more than 48 hours would delay the detection of renal damage.

7. Answer: B

The patient is currently at category 3a CKD (GFR 45–59 mL/minute/1.73 m^2), which can be calculated by the MDRD formula or Cockcroft-Gault. The five categories range from mild kidney damage (G1) to kidney failure (G5).

8. Answer: C

Given the diagnosis of diabetes mellitus and the presence of overt proteinuria, this patient probably has diabetic nephropathy. Progression will be accelerated by smoking, poor diabetes control, and poor BP control. In patients with diabetes, a target A1C of less than 7% is associated with a decrease in the rate of disease progression. Blood pressure control of less than 130/80 mm Hg in patients also decreases the progression of kidney disease. The standard of care in patients with diabetic nephropathy is ACEIs (evidence for a reduction in mortality and reduced progression of CKD) or ARBs (evidence for a reduction in progression but no mortality data), so enalapril (Answer C) is the best choice. A nondihydropyridine (Answer B) might be initiated in patients who cannot tolerate ACEI or ARB therapy but would not be a choice yet. Dihydropyridine therapy (Answer A) is not recommended in diabetic nephropathy because of conflicting literature on its efficacy. An increase in atenolol (Answer D) might control BP, but inhibition of the renin-angiotensin system is still the best answer. In addition, a recent meta-analysis evaluating atenolol in hypertensive patients with diabetes mellitus found either no difference or worse outcomes.

9. Answer: B

The BP is not at goal (should be less than 130/80 mm Hg). To improve BP control and increase the effect of the ACEI, chlorthalidone should be added to the regimen (Answer B). Monitoring of SCr and serum potassium is appropriate in this patient. There is less than a 30% increase in SCr, so enalapril should be continued, making Answer A and Answer C inappropriate. Adding chlorthalidone will also counter the tendency for hyperkalemia. Answer D would probably lower BP but would not be the preferred route because renal protection probably would not be improved.

10. Answer: B

Calculation of the number needed to harm (NNH) is similar to the calculation of the number needed to treat but is focused on a negative outcome. In this study, the risk of acute kidney injury was 11% in the monotherapy group and 18% in the combination therapy group, a difference of 7%. The NNH is calculated as 1/(absolute risk increase) = 1/(0.07) = 14.3. So the best estimate is that 1 additional patient would develop AKI for approximately every 15 patients treated with combination therapy compared with angiotensin receptor blocker therapy alone.

11. Answer: D

A native arteriovenous fistula is the preferred access for chronic HD. If an arteriovenous fistula cannot be constructed, a synthetic arteriovenous graft (Answer C) is considered second line. A subclavian catheter (Answer A) is a poor choice because of the greater risk of infection and thrombosis and because of the poor blood flow obtained through a catheter. A Tenckhoff catheter (Answer B) is incorrect because this is a catheter for peritoneal dialysis.

12. Answer: D

The best-studied agent is midodrine, an α_1-agonist. Levocarnitine (Answer A) has been tried, but data are limited on its benefit. Fludrocortisone (Answer C) is a synthetic mineralocorticoid that is used for hypotension in other situations; however, the primary mechanism is caused by Na and water restriction in the kidney; therefore, this drug is less likely to work. Sodium chloride tablets (Answer B) would not work acutely, and they should generally be avoided.

13. Answer: B

Empiric coverage for the treatment of peritoneal dialysis–related peritonitis should include activity against both gram-positive and gram-negative organisms. Intraperitoneal administration is preferred to intravenous administration. The use of cefazolin will provide activity against *Staphylococcus* unless an area has a high rate of methicillin-resistant organisms. The choice of antibiotic for gram-negative coverage can include a third-generation cephalosporin with activity against *Pseudomonas* (e.g., ceftazidime or cefepime or an aminoglycoside). Short-term use of an aminoglycoside should not adversely affect residual renal function. For patients with dialysis-related peritonitis, empiric anaerobic coverage is not necessary.

14. Answer: B

Hyperparathyroidism is associated with epoetin resistance in patients on HD (Answer B). Although iron deficiency is the most common cause of epoetin deficiency, the laboratory results in this patient do not indicate iron deficiency (Answer A). Phenytoin therapy (Answer C) has been associated with anemia in other patient populations but not in patients on HD. Infection (Answer D) and inflammation are very common causes of epoetin deficiency in patients on HD, but nothing in this patient's presentation suggests an infectious or inflammatory process.

15. Answer: B

This patient requires treatment for his elevated intact PTH (800 pg/mL), which puts him at high risk of renal osteodystrophy. He has high serum phosphorus, and although the measured serum calcium concentration is normal, his corrected calcium concentration is elevated according to the presence of hypoalbuminemia (corrected calcium is 10.7 mg/dL). Current phosphate binder therapy is contributing to calcium exposure; therefore, calcium acetate should be discontinued and sevelamer initiated. Cinacalcet will lower intact PTH and potentially serum calcium. Answer A is incorrect because increasing the calcium acetate may worsen the hypercalcemia. Answer C is incorrect for two reasons. First, the patient needs some type of phosphate binder; second, intravenous vitamin D analogs can worsen hypercalcemia and are not very effective at reducing elevated intact PTH in the presence of hyperphosphatemia. Answer D is incorrect because intravenous vitamin D analogs can worsen hypercalcemia and are not very effective in reducing elevated intact PTH in the presence of hyperphosphatemia. Because this patient also has a seizure disorder, close monitoring of serum calcium concentrations is recommended with the introduction of cinacalcet and discontinuation of calcium acetate. Significant reductions in serum calcium can lower the seizure threshold and potentially worsen seizures.

16. Answer: B
The presence of kidney failure and low albumin results in an increased free fraction of phenytoin. Using the correction equation gives a corrected level of 12.5, which is therapeutic. A free phenytoin concentration can also be drawn.

ANSWERS AND EXPLANATIONS TO SELF-ASSESSMENT QUESTIONS

1. Answer: C

Initial treatment of AKI requires the identification and reversal (if possible) of the insult to the kidney. This patient's symptoms and presentation are consistent with prerenal azotemia because of volume depletion, so fluid administration is the best choice in this case. There is no suggestion of obstruction (distended abdomen, history of benign prostatic hypertrophy). Diuretic administration would be inappropriate because it would worsen his volume depletion and probably further impair his kidney function. Fluid management is critical to managing AKI, necessitating a careful assessment of the patient. Although his glucose concentration is elevated, insulin is not necessary at this time.

2. Answer: C

The patient has intrinsic azotemia, resulting in damage to the kidneys. Aminoglycosides can cause direct damage to the tubules. The BUN/SCr ratio is normal (an increased BUN/SCr ratio reflecting hypovolemia is common in prerenal azotemia). Decreased urinary sodium of less than 20 mOsm/L is also a marker of hypovolemia. Fractional excretion of sodium additionally distinguishes prerenal and intrinsic renal damage. A low FENa (less than 1%) in an oliguric patient suggests that tubular function is still intact. A FENa greater than 2% is commonly seen in intrinsic renal failure. The specific gravity is normal in intrinsic renal failure. Elevated specific gravity greater than 1.018 is seen in prerenal failure, reflecting concentrated urine caused by hypovolemia. Cellular debris is often present in intrinsic renal failure because of renal tubular cell death or damage.

3. Answer: B

Application of the Rowland-Tozer equation yields the following calculation:

$Q = 1 - [Fe(1 - KF)]$

$Q = 1 - [0.4(1 - 25/120)]$

$Q = 1 - [0.4(0.79)]$

$Q = 1 - 0.32$

$Q = 0.68$ or 68% of usual dose

Drug X usual dose = 600 mg

Formulation = 100 mg/mL in a 6-mL vial

Adjusted dose = (usual dose) × (Q)

= (600 mg)(0.68) = 410 mg

Volume drug = (dose)/(concentration)

= (410 mg)/(100 mg/mL) = 4.1 mL

4. Answer: C

In most cases, either the Cockcroft-Gault or the MDRD equation is appropriate (and best) to assess kidney function. However, this patient is significantly below his ideal body weight and has malnutrition, so equations will overestimate. An iothalamate study will measure GFR, but it is not used clinically.

5. Answer: C

This patient is not at goal for hemoglobin. Iron studies show the patient is iron deficient, with TSAT less than 30% and ferritin less than 500 ng/mL. Although a trial of oral iron might be indicated in nondialysis patients with CKD, patients on HD should be given intravenous iron as first line.

6. Answer: B

The BUN/SCr ratio, urine osmolality, and presence of urinary casts all point to ATN. Prerenal and functional AKI look similar in urinalysis. Classically, AIN has eosinophils in the urine.

7. Answer: B

Hemoglobin represents continuous data. Because each treatment is administered to a separate group of patients, the data are not paired (i.e., they are unpaired). Assuming the data are normally distributed, continuous unpaired data should be evaluated using a t-test. Analysis of variance can be used for continuous data, but only when three groups of data are compared. However, chi-square is used for nominal data.

8. Answer: D

A cost-utility analysis is an extension of the cost-effectiveness analysis in which outcomes measured are lives saved, adjusted for changes in quality of life, measured as quality-adjusted life-years. A cost minimization study compares the costs and consequences of two or more interventions that have equivalent outcomes, so the primary focus is on cost. A cost-effectiveness analysis compares costs and consequences to determine which treatment can achieve the best outcomes at the lowest cost. A cost-benefit analysis measures costs and consequences in monetary terms. It may be useful to compare costs with unrelated outcomes.

Infectious Diseases

Curtis L. Smith, Pharm.D., BCPS

Ferris State University
Lansing, Michigan

INFECTIOUS DISEASES

CURTIS L. SMITH, PHARM.D., BCPS

FERRIS STATE UNIVERSITY
LANSING, MICHIGAN

Learning Objectives

1. Describe appropriate treatment of patients with respiratory tract infections, urinary tract infections, central nervous system (CNS) infections, skin and soft tissue infections, osteomyelitis, intra-abdominal infections, and endocarditis.
2. Identify appropriate preventive therapy for respiratory tract infections, CNS infections, endocarditis, and surgical wound infections.

Self-Assessment Questions

Answers and explanations to these questions can be found at the end of this chapter.

1. P.E. is a 56-year-old man who comes to the clinic with a 3-day history of fever, chills, pleuritic chest pain, malaise, and cough productive of sputum. In the clinic, his temperature is 102.1°F (38.9°C) (all other vital signs are normal). His chest radiograph shows consolidation in the right lower lobe. His white blood cell count (WBC) is 14,400 cells/mm³, but all other laboratory values are normal. He is given a diagnosis of community-acquired pneumonia (CAP). He has not received any antibiotics in 5 years and has no chronic disease states. Which is the best empiric therapy for P.E.?

   A. Doxycycline 100 mg orally twice daily.
   B. Cefuroxime axetil 250 mg orally twice daily.
   C. Levofloxacin 750 mg/day orally.
   D. Trimethoprim/sulfamethoxazole double strength orally twice daily.

2. H.W. is a 38-year-old woman who presents with high temperature, malaise, dry cough, nasal congestion, and severe headaches. Her symptoms began suddenly 3 days ago, and she has been in bed since then. She reports no other illness in her family, but several people have recently called in sick at work. Which is best for H.W.?

   A. Azithromycin 500 mg, followed by 250 mg/day orally for 4 more days.
   B. Amoxicillin/clavulanic acid 875 mg orally twice daily.
   C. Oseltamivir 75 mg twice daily orally for 5 days.
   D. Symptomatic treatment only.

3. A study is designed to assess the risk of pneumococcal pneumonia in older adults 10 years or more after their pneumococcal vaccination, compared with older adults who have never received the vaccination. Which study design is best?

   A. Case series.
   B. Case-control study.
   C. Prospective cohort study.
   D. Randomized controlled trial.

4. S.C. is a 46-year-old woman who presents to the clinic with purulent nasal discharge, nasal and facial congestion, headaches, fever, and dental pain. Her symptoms began about 10 days ago, improved after about 4 days, and then worsened again a few days later. Which is the best empiric therapy for S.C.?

   A. Cefpodoxime 200 mg twice daily.
   B. Clindamycin 300 mg orally four times daily.
   C. Amoxicillin/clavulanate 875 mg/125 mg every 12 hours.
   D. No antibiotic therapy needed because this is a typical viral infection.

5. N.R. is a 28-year-old woman who presents to the clinic with a 2-day history of dysuria, frequency, and urgency. She has no significant medical history, and the only drug she takes is oral contraceptives. Which is the best empiric therapy for N.R.?

   A. Oral nitrofurantoin extended release (ER) 100 mg twice daily for 3 days.
   B. Oral ciprofloxacin 500 mg twice daily for 7 days.
   C. Oral trimethoprim/sulfamethoxazole double strength twice daily for 3 days.
   D. Oral cephalexin 500 mg four times daily for 3 days.

6. B.Y. is an 85-year-old woman who is bedridden and lives in a nursing home. She is chronically catheterized, and her urinary catheter was last changed 3 weeks ago. Today, her urine is cloudy, and a urinalysis shows many bacteria. B.Y. is not noticing any symptoms. A urine culture is obtained. Which option is best for B.Y.?

A. No therapy because she is chronically catheterized and has no symptoms.

B. No antibiotic therapy, but the catheter should be changed.

C. Oral ciprofloxacin 500 mg twice daily for 7 days and a new catheter.

D. Oral ciprofloxacin 500 mg twice daily for 14–21 days without a change in catheter.

7. V.E. is a 44-year-old man who presents to the emergency department with a warm, erythematous, and painful right lower extremity. There is no raised border at the edge of the infection. Three days ago, he scratched his leg on a barbed wire fence on his property. His temperature has been as high as 101.8°F (38°C) with chills. Doppler studies of his lower extremity are negative. Blood cultures were drawn, and they are negative to date. Which is the best empiric therapy for V.E.?

A. Nafcillin 2 g intravenously every 6 hours. The infection may worsen, and necrotizing fasciitis must be ruled out.

B. Penicillin G, 2 million units intravenously every 4 hours. This is probably erysipelas.

C. Piperacillin/tazobactam 3.375 g intravenously every 6 hours. Surgical debridement is vitally important.

D. Enoxaparin 80 mg subcutaneously twice daily and warfarin 5 mg/day orally.

8. R.K. is a 36-year-old woman who presents to the emergency department with a severe headache and neck stiffness. Her temperature is 99.5°F (37.5°C). After a negative computed tomographic scan of the head, a lumbar puncture is performed, showing the following: glucose 54 mg/dL (peripheral, 104), protein 88 mg/dL, and WBC 220 cells/mm³ (100% lymphocytes). The Gram stain shows no organisms. Which option describes the best therapy for R.K.?

A. This is aseptic (probably viral) meningitis, and no antibiotics are necessary.

B. Administer ceftriaxone 2 g intravenously every 12 hours until the cerebrospinal fluid (CSF) cultures are negative for bacteria.

C. Administer ceftriaxone 2 g intravenously every 12 hours and vancomycin 1000 mg intravenously every 12 hours until the CSF cultures are negative for bacteria.

D. Administer acyclovir 500 mg intravenously every 8 hours until the CSF culture results are complete.

9. L.G. is a 49-year-old woman with a history of mitral valve prolapse. She presents to her physician's office with malaise and a low-grade fever. Her physician notes that her murmur is louder than normal and orders blood cultures and an echocardiogram. A large vegetation is observed on L.G.'s mitral valve, and her blood cultures are growing *Enterococcus faecalis* (susceptible to all antibiotics). Which is the best therapy for L.G.?

A. Penicillin G plus gentamicin for 2 weeks.

B. Vancomycin plus gentamicin for 2 weeks.

C. Ampicillin plus gentamicin for 4–6 weeks.

D. Cefazolin plus gentamicin for 4–6 weeks.

10. N.L. is a 28-year-old woman with no significant medical history. She reports to the emergency department with fever and severe right lower quadrant pain. She has had a dull pain for the past few days, but it suddenly became severe during the past 8 hours. Her temperature is 103.5°F (39.7°C), and she has rebound tenderness on abdominal examination. She is taken to surgery immediately, where a perforated appendix is diagnosed and repaired. Which is the best follow-up antibiotic regimen?

A. Vancomycin 1000 mg intravenously every 12 hours plus metronidazole 500 mg intravenously every 8 hours.

B. Ceftriaxone 1 g/day intravenously plus ciprofloxacin 400 mg intravenously every 12 hours.

C. Ertapenem 1 g/day intravenously.

D. No antibiotics needed after surgical repair of a perforated appendix.

I. RESPIRATORY TRACT INFECTIONS

A. Pneumonia
   1. Pneumonia is the most common cause of death attributable to infectious diseases (very high rates in older adults) and in the top 10 causes of death in the United States.
   2. Hospital-acquired pneumonia is the second most common nosocomial infection (0.6%–1.1% of all hospitalized patients). There is a higher incidence in patients in the intensive care unit recovering from thoracic or upper abdominal surgery and in older adults.
   3. Mortality rates
       a. Community-acquired pneumonia (CAP) without hospitalization: less than 1%
       b. CAP with hospitalization: about 14%
       c. Nosocomial: about 33%–50%

B. Community-Acquired Pneumonia
   1. Definition: Acute infection of the pulmonary parenchyma, accompanied by an acute infiltrate consistent with pneumonia on chest radiograph or auscultatory findings. Patients must also *not* have any of the following characteristics: hospitalization 2 days or more in the past 90 days; residence in a long-term care facility; receipt of intravenous antibiotic therapy, chemotherapy, or wound care in the past 30 days; or attendance at a hospital or hemodialysis clinic.
   2. Symptoms of CAP are listed below. Older adults often have fewer and less severe findings (mental status changes are common).
       a. Fever or hypothermia
       b. Rigors
       c. Sweats
       d. New cough with or without sputum (90%)
       e. Chest discomfort (50%)
       f. Onset of dyspnea (66%)
       g. Fatigue, myalgias, abdominal pain, anorexia, and headache
   3. Predictors of a complicated course of CAP are listed below. Hospitalization should be based on the severity-of-illness scores (e.g., CURB-65, pneumonia severity index).
       a. Age greater than 65 years
       b. Comorbid illness (diabetes mellitus, congestive heart failure, lung disease, renal failure, liver disease)
       c. High temperature: more than 101°F (38°C)
       d. Bacteremia
       e. Altered mental status
       f. Immunosuppression (e.g., steroid use, cancer)
       g. High-risk etiology (*Staphylococcus aureus, Legionella,* gram-negative bacilli, anaerobic aspiration)
       h. Multilobe involvement or pleural effusions
   4. Severity-of-illness scoring systems in CAP
       a. CURB-65

Table 1. CURB-65 Scoring

CURB-65[a]	
Symptom	**Points**
Confusion	1
Urea >19 mg/dL	1
Respiratory rate ≥30 breaths/minute	1
SBP <90 mm Hg, DBP ≤60 mm Hg	1
Age ≥65 years	1

[a]CRB-65 (without a blood urea nitrogen level) is useful in a primary practice setting.

DBP = diastolic blood pressure; SBP = systolic blood pressure.

Table 2. CURB-65 Location of Therapy

CURB-65		
Score	**Risk of Death at 30 Days (%)**	**Location of Therapy**
0	0.7	Treat as outpatient
1	2.1	Treat as outpatient
2	9.2	Outpatient or inpatient
3	14.5	Inpatient (±ICU)
4	40.0	Inpatient (±ICU)
5	57.0	Inpatient (±ICU)

ICU = intensive care unit.

    b. Pneumonia severity index (or Pneumonia Patient Outcomes Research Team score)
       i. Evaluates 20 patient characteristics
       ii. Assesses risk of mortality, similar to CURB-65
       iii. Has predictive ability similar to that of CURB-65 but better in patients with lower mortality risk

C. Nosocomial Pneumonia
    1. Hospital-acquired pneumonia: Pneumonia that occurs 48 hours or more after admission and was not incubating at the time of admission
    2. Ventilator-associated pneumonia: Pneumonia that arises more than 48–72 hours after endotracheal intubation
    3. Health care–associated pneumonia: Pneumonia developing in a patient who was hospitalized 2 days or more in the past 90 days; who resided in a nursing home or long-term care facility; who received intravenous antibiotic therapy, intravenous chemotherapy, or wound care in the past 30 days; or who attended a hospital or hemodialysis clinic
    4. Risk factors for nosocomial pneumonia
       a. Intubation and mechanical ventilation
       b. Supine patient position
       c. Enteral feeding
       d. Oropharyngeal colonization
       e. Stress bleeding prophylaxis
       f. Blood transfusion
       g. Hyperglycemia

h. Immunosuppression or corticosteroids
i. Surgical procedures: thoracoabdominal, upper abdominal, thoracic
j. Immobilization
k. Nasogastric tubes
l. Previous antibiotic therapy
m. Admission to the intensive care unit
n. Advanced age
o. Underlying chronic lung disease

D. Microbiology (Table 3)

Table 3. Incidence of Pneumonia by Organism

Community Acquired (%)		Hospital Acquired (%)	
Unidentifiable	40–60	Unidentifiable	50
Mycoplasma pneumoniae	13–37	S. aureus	10
Streptococcus pneumoniae	9–20	Pseudomonas aeruginosa	8
Haemophilus influenzae	3–10	*Enterobacter* spp.	5
Chlamydia pneumoniae	1–17	*K. pneumoniae*	4
Legionella pneumophila	0.7–13	*Candida* spp.	3
Viruses	Common	*Acinetobacter* spp.	2
Others:	Uncommon	*Serratia marcescens*	2
Staphylococcus aureus		*Escherichia coli*	2
Moraxella catarrhalis		*S. pneumoniae*	1
Pneumocystis pneumonia			
Anaerobes			
Gram-negative bacilli			
(e.g., *Klebsiella pneumoniae*)			
Specific populations in community-acquired pneumonia:		Issues in hospital-acquired pneumonia:	
Alcoholics: *S. pneumoniae*, oral anaerobes, gram-negative bacilli (e.g., *Klebsiella*)		*P. aeruginosa* is transmitted by health care workers' hands or respiratory equipment	
Nursing home: *S. pneumoniae, H. influenzae*, gram-negative bacilli, *S. aureus*		*S. aureus* is transmitted by health care workers' hands	
COPD: *S. pneumoniae, H. influenzae, M. catarrhalis*		Enterobacteriaceae endogenously colonize hospitalized patients' airways (healthy people seldom have gram-negative upper airway colonization)	
Postinfluenza: *H. influenzae, S. aureus, S. pneumoniae*		Stress changes respiratory epithelial cells so that gram-negative organisms can adhere	
Exposure to water: *Legionella*		Up to 70% of patients in the intensive care unit have gram-negative upper airway colonization, and 25% of them will become infected through aspiration	
Poor oral hygiene: oral anaerobes			
HIV infection: *Pneumocystis jirovecii, S. pneumoniae, M. pneumoniae, Mycobacterium*			

COPD = chronic obstructive pulmonary disease; HIV = human immunodeficiency virus.

Patient Case

1. R.L. is a 68-year-old man who presents to the emergency department with coughing and shortness of breath. His symptoms, which began 4 days ago, have worsened during the past 24 hours. He is coughing up yellow-green sputum, and he has chills, with a temperature of 102.4°F (39°C). His medical history includes coronary artery disease with a myocardial infarction 5 years ago, congestive heart failure, hypertension, and osteoarthritis. He rarely drinks alcohol and has not smoked since his myocardial infarction. His medications on admission include lisinopril 10 mg/day, hydrochlorothiazide 25 mg/day, and acetaminophen 650 mg four times/day. On physical examination, he is alert and oriented, with the following vital signs: temperature 101.8°F (38°C), heart rate 100 beats/minute, respiratory rate 24 breaths/minute, and blood pressure 142/94 mm Hg. His laboratory results are normal except for blood urea nitrogen (BUN) 32 mg/dL (serum creatinine 1.23 mg/dL). A sputum specimen is not available. If R.L. were hospitalized, which would be the best empiric therapy for him?

   A. Ampicillin/sulbactam 1.5 g intravenously every 6 hours.

   B. Piperacillin/tazobactam 4.5 g intravenously every 6 hours plus gentamicin 180 mg intravenously every 12 hours.

   C. Ceftriaxone 1 g intravenously every 24 hours plus azithromycin 500 mg/day intravenously.

   D. Doxycycline 100 mg intravenously every 12 hours.

E. Therapy: Pneumonia
   1. CAP
      a. Empiric treatment of nonhospitalized patients
         i. Previously healthy and no antibiotic therapy in the past 3 months
            (a) Macrolide (clarithromycin or azithromycin if *Haemophilus influenzae* is suspected)
            (b) Doxycycline
         ii. Comorbidities (chronic obstructive pulmonary disease [COPD], diabetes mellitus, chronic renal or liver failure, congestive heart failure, malignancy, asplenia, or immunosuppression) *or* recent antibiotic therapy (within the past 3 months)
            (a) Respiratory fluoroquinolone (moxifloxacin, gemifloxacin, or levofloxacin [750 mg])
            (b) Macrolide (or doxycycline) with high-dose amoxicillin (1 g three times/day) or amoxicillin/clavulanate (2 g twice daily) or a cephalosporin (ceftriaxone, cefuroxime, or cefpodoxime)
      b. Empiric treatment of hospitalized patients with moderately severe pneumonia
         i. Respiratory fluoroquinolone (moxifloxacin, gemifloxacin [oral only], or levofloxacin [750 mg])
         ii. Ampicillin, ceftriaxone, or cefotaxime (ertapenem in select patients) plus a macrolide (or doxycycline)
      c. Empiric treatment of hospitalized patients with severe pneumonia necessitating intensive care unit treatment (may need to add other antibiotics if *P. aeruginosa* or methicillin-resistant *S. aureus* [MRSA] is suspected)
         i. Ampicillin/sulbactam plus either a respiratory fluoroquinolone or azithromycin
         ii. Ceftriaxone plus either a respiratory fluoroquinolone or azithromycin
         iii. Cefotaxime plus either a respiratory fluoroquinolone or azithromycin
      d. Treatment duration: At least 5 days, with 48–72 hours afebrile and no more than one sign of clinical instability (elevated temperature, heart rate, or respiratory rate; decreased systolic blood pressure; or arterial oxygen saturation) before therapy discontinuation

---

Patient Case

2. B.P. is a 66-year-old woman who underwent a two-vessel coronary artery bypass graft 8 days ago and has been on a ventilator in the surgical intensive care unit since then. Her temperature is now rising, and a tracheal aspirate shows many white blood cells and gram-negative rods. Her medical history includes coronary artery disease with a myocardial infarction 2 years ago, COPD, and hypertension. Which is the best empiric therapy for B.P.?

   A. Ceftriaxone 1 g/day intravenously plus gentamicin 480 mg intravenously every 24 hours plus linezolid 600 mg intravenously every 12 hours.

   B. Piperacillin/tazobactam 4.5 g intravenously every 6 hours.

   C. Levofloxacin 750 mg/day intravenously plus linezolid 600 mg intravenously every 12 hours.

   D. Cefepime 2 g intravenously every 12 hours plus tobramycin 480 mg intravenously every 24 hours plus vancomycin 15 mg/kg intravenously every 12 hours.

---

2. Hospital-acquired pneumonia
   a. Early onset (less than 5 days) and no risk factors for multidrug-resistant (MDR) organisms. Common organisms include *Streptococcus pneumoniae, H. influenzae,* methicillin-sensitive *S. aureus* (MSSA), *Escherichia coli, Klebsiella pneumoniae, Enterobacter* spp., and *Proteus* spp.
      i. Third-generation cephalosporin (ceftriaxone)
      ii. Fluoroquinolone (levofloxacin, moxifloxacin, ciprofloxacin)
      iii. Ampicillin/sulbactam
      iv. Ertapenem
   b. Late onset (5 days or longer) or risk factors for MDR organisms. Common organisms include those listed above for early onset plus *Pseudomonas aeruginosa, K. pneumoniae* (extended-spectrum β-lactamase positive), *Acinetobacter* spp., MRSA, and *Legionella pneumophila.*
      i. Ceftazidime or cefepime plus aminoglycoside or fluoroquinolone (ciprofloxacin, levofloxacin)
      ii. Imipenem, meropenem, or doripenem plus aminoglycoside or fluoroquinolone (ciprofloxacin, levofloxacin)
      iii. Piperacillin/tazobactam plus aminoglycoside or fluoroquinolone (ciprofloxacin, levofloxacin)
      iv. Vancomycin or linezolid should be added to the above regimens only if MRSA risk factors (e.g., history of MRSA infection or colonization, recent hospitalization or antibiotic use, presence of invasive health care devices) are present or there is a high incidence locally (greater than 10%–15%).
   c. Treatment duration: Efforts should be made to decrease therapy duration to as short as 7 or 8 days (14 days for pneumonia secondary to *P. aeruginosa* or *Acinetobacter*).
   d. Risk factors for MDR organisms
      i. Antibiotic therapy within the past 90 days
      ii. Hospitalization of 5 days or more
      iii. High resistance in community or hospital unit
      iv. Risk factors for health care–associated pneumonia
         (a) Hospitalization for 2 or more days in the preceding 90 days
         (b) Residence in a nursing home or extended care facility
         (c) Intravenous therapy (including antibiotics) or intravenous chemotherapy within 30 days
         (d) Attendance at a hospital or hemodialysis clinic
         (e) Home wound care within 30 days
      v. Family member with MDR pathogen
      vi. Immunosuppressive disease or therapy

Patient Case

3. B.P., who eventually improves, is transferred to a regular floor. She cannot remember receiving any recent vaccinations. Which is the best vaccination recommendation for this patient?

    A. B.P. needs no vaccinations.

    B. B.P. should receive the pneumococcal vaccine now and the influenza vaccine in the fall.

    C. B.P. should receive the influenza vaccine in the fall, but because of her current infection, the pneumococcal vaccine is unnecessary.

    D. B.P. should receive the pneumococcal vaccine now, but she is not in a group in which the influenza vaccine is recommended.

    F. Influenza
        1. Characteristics of influenza infection
            a. Epidemic with significant mortality
            b. Epidemics begin abruptly → peak in 2–3 weeks → resolve in 5–6 weeks
            c. Occurs almost exclusively in the winter
            d. Average overall attack rates of 10%–20%
            e. Mortality greatest in those older than 65 years (especially with heart and lung disease): More than 80% of deaths caused by influenza are from this age group (20,000 deaths a year in the United States).
        2. Is it a cold or the flu? (Table 4)

Table 4. Differentiating the Symptoms of Cold and Influenza

Signs and Symptoms	Influenza	Cold
Onset	Sudden	Gradual
Temperature	Characteristic, high (>101°F [38°C]) of 3–4 days' duration	Occasional
Cough	Dry; can become severe	Hacking
Headache	Prominent	Occasional
Myalgia (muscle aches and pains)	Usual; often severe	Slight
Tiredness and weakness	Can last 2–3 weeks	Very mild
Extreme exhaustion	Early and prominent	Never
Chest discomfort	Common	Mild to moderate
Stuffy nose	Sometimes	Common
Sneezing	Sometimes	Usual
Sore throat	Sometimes	Common

        3. Pathophysiology
            a. Type A
                i. Influenza further grouped by variations in hemagglutinin and neuraminidase (e.g., H1N1, H3N2)
                ii. Changes through antigenic drift or shift
                    (a) Drift: Annual, gradual change caused by mutations, substitutions, and deletions
                    (b) Shift: Less common dramatic change leading to pandemics
                iii. Causes epidemics every 1–3 years

---

b. Type B

    i. Type B influenza carries one form of hemagglutinin and one form of neuraminidase, both of which are less likely to mutate than the hemagglutinin and neuraminidase of type A influenza.

    ii. Changes through antigenic drift (minor mutations from year to year); when enough drifts occur, an epidemic is likely.

    iii. Causes epidemics every 5 years

4. Therapy

  a. Treatment indicated in patients with confirmed or suspected influenza and the following conditions (use only the neuraminidase inhibitors):

    i. Hospitalized patients

    ii. Severe, complicated, or progressive illness

    iii. High risk of influenza complications:

      (a) Patients younger than 2 years or 65 years and older

      (b) Patients with chronic disease states: Pulmonary (including asthma), cardiovascular (except hypertension alone), renal, hepatic, hematologic (including sickle cell disease), metabolic disorders (including diabetes mellitus), or neurologic and neurodevelopment conditions

      (c) Immunosuppressed patients

      (d) Pregnant women

      (e) Patients younger than 19 years who are receiving long-term aspirin therapy

      (f) American Indians and Alaska Natives

      (g) Patients who are morbidly obese

      (h) Residents of nursing homes and other long-term care facilities

    iv. Treatment may be considered for those without risk factors according to clinical judgment (must initiate within 48 hours).

  b. Adamantanes

    i. Amantadine (Symmetrel), rimantadine (Flumadine)

    ii. Inhibit viral uncoating and release of viral nucleic acid by inhibiting M2 protein

      (a) Never effective against influenza B virus

      (b) Not recommended for treatment because of current universal resistance in influenza A

  c. Neuraminidase inhibitors

    i. Oseltamivir (Tamiflu), Zanamivir (Relenza)

    ii. Inhibit neuraminidase; symptoms resolve 1–1.5 days sooner.

    iii. Adverse effects

      (a) Oseltamivir: Gastrointestinal (nausea and vomiting)

      (b) Zanamivir: Bronchospasm, cough (not recommended in patients with asthma or COPD)

    iv. Dose

      (a) Oseltamivir: 75 mg orally twice daily for 5 days; decrease dose to 75 mg/day orally in patients with creatinine clearance less than 30 mL/minute.

      (b) Zanamivir: Two inhalations (5 mg/inhalation) twice daily for 5 days

      (c) Initiate within 48 hours of symptom onset.

5. Prevention

  a. Chemoprophylaxis only for influenza-related complications in patients at very high risk (e.g., severely immunosuppressed patients) who cannot be protected by the vaccine when a high risk of exposure exists

  b. Amantadine, rimantadine: Not recommended for prevention because of current universal resistance

c. Neuraminidase inhibitors
    i. Oseltamivir (Tamiflu)
       (a) Oseltamivir administered 75 mg/day orally for 6 weeks during peak influenza season showed 74% protective efficacy (as prophylaxis in unvaccinated people).
       (b) Begin oseltamivir 75 mg/day orally within 2 days of close contact with an infected person and continue for no more than 10 days.
    ii. Zanamivir (Relenza)
       (a) Zanamivir 10 mg/day through inhalation for 4 weeks during peak influenza season showed 67% protective efficacy (as prophylaxis in unvaccinated people).
       (b) Begin zanamivir 10 mg/day within 5 days of community outbreak and continue for 4 weeks during peak influenza season.

G. Immunizations Related to the Respiratory Tract
  1. Pneumococcal vaccines
    a. Characteristics: Pneumococcal polysaccharide vaccine (PPSV23)
      i. PPSV contains 23 purified capsular polysaccharide antigens of *S. pneumoniae*.
      ii. The 23 capsular types account for 85%–90% of invasive *S. pneumoniae* infection.
      iii. Antibody levels remain elevated for at least 5 years.
    b. Characteristics: Pneumococcal conjugate vaccine (PCV13)
      i. PCV contains 13 purified capsular polysaccharide antigens of *S. pneumoniae* conjugated to a carrier protein.
      ii. The 13 capsular types are all in PPSV23 except for one.
      iii. If both PCV13 and PPSV23 are required, PCV13 should be given first, followed by PPSV23 at least 8 weeks later. If PPSV23 is given first, PCV13 should be given at least 6–12 months later.
    c. Recommendations (Table 5)

Table 5. Pneumococcal Vaccine Recommendations (all recommendations are for PPSV23 except where noted)

Vaccination-Recommended Group	Revaccination
Immunocompetent People	
People ≥65 years of age These people should receive PCV13 and PPSV23	Ideally give PCV13 first followed by PPSV23 in 8 weeks Second dose of PPSV23 if patient received vaccine ≥5 years previously and was <65 years old at the time of vaccination
People 2–64 years of age with chronic cardiovascular disease, chronic pulmonary disease, diabetes mellitus, alcoholism, chronic liver disease, cochlear implants or CSF leaks; adult asthmatics or adult smokers People with cochlear implants or CSF leaks should also receive PCV13	Not recommended
People 2–64 years of age living in nursing homes or long-term care facilities	Not recommended

Table 5. Pneumococcal Vaccine Recommendations *(continued)*

Vaccination-Recommended Group	Revaccination
Immunocompromised People	
Immunocompromised people ≥2 years old, including those with HIV infection, leukemia, lymphoma, Hodgkin disease, multiple myeloma, generalized malignancy, chronic renal failure, or nephrotic syndrome; those receiving immunosuppressive chemotherapy (including corticosteroids); and those who have received an organ or bone marrow transplant These people should also receive PCV13	Single revaccination recommended after 5 years (for anyone ≥2 years)
People 2–64 years of age with functional or anatomic asplenia These people should also receive PCV13	Single revaccination recommended after 5 years (for anyone ≥2 years old)

CSF = cerebrospinal fluid; HIV = human immunodeficiency virus; PCV = pneumococcal conjugate vaccine; PPSV = pneumococcal polysaccharide vaccine.

2. Influenza vaccine
   a. Characteristics
      i. Each year's vaccine contains two strains of type A and one strain of type B, selected by worldwide surveillance and antigenic characterization.
      ii. Prevents illness in 70%–90% of healthy people younger than 65 years
      iii. Prevents illness in 53%, hospitalization in 50%, and death in 68% of older adults
      iv. Administer yearly in September or October.
   b. Recommendations
      i. Everyone older than 6 months should receive the vaccine annually.
      ii. Children younger than 9 years should receive two doses, at least 1 month apart, the first season they receive the vaccine. Intranasal live attenuated influenza vaccine recommended in children 2–8 years old.
      iii. In adults the Centers for Disease Control and Prevention (CDC) currently does not recommend one vaccine over any other.
      iv. Patients with egg allergies:
         (a) Only hives after egg exposure: Administer recombinant inactivated influenza vaccine (Flublok) or administer inactivated influenza vaccine but only by a health care provider familiar with egg allergies.
         (b) More severe symptoms after egg exposure: Administer recombinant inactivated influenza vaccine (Flublok) or refer to an allergist for risk assessment.
   c. Influenza vaccine products (Table 6)

Table 6. Influenza Vaccine Products

Influenza Vaccine	Indications	Notes
Inactivated influenza vaccine trivalent (IIV3, multiple brands)	6 months and older	Primary influenza vaccine; at this time, the CDC has no preference for using any other vaccine over this IIV3 vaccine
Intranasal live attenuated influenza vaccine quadrivalent (LAIV4, FluMist)	2–49 years without underlying illnesses (including health care workers)	Pregnant women should receive the inactivated vaccine Use of inactivated vaccine is preferred for vaccinating household members, health care workers, and others who have close contact with severely immunosuppressed people
High-dose trivalent influenza vaccine (high-dose Fluzone)	65 years and older	The CDC has no preference for using this vaccine over the regular influenza vaccine
Inactivated influenza vaccine quadrivalent (IIV4, Fluzone, and Fluarix)	6 months and older	The CDC has no preference for using this vaccine over the regular influenza vaccine
Intradermal inactivated influenza vaccine trivalent (IIV3, Fluzone intradermal)	18–64 years	Much smaller needle, but local reactions are significantly greater than with the IM vaccines
Inactivated influenza vaccine trivalent – cell culture based (IIV3, Flucelvax)	18 years and older	Grown in mammalian cell lines, but still exposed to eggs early in production Same cautions for patients with egg allergies
Recombinant inactivated influenza vaccine trivalent (RIV3, Flublok)	18 years and older	Produced by recombinant technology; safe for patients with egg allergies

CDC = Centers for Disease Control and Prevention; IM = intramuscular.

H. Sinusitis
   1. Definition and etiology
      a. Inflammation of the mucosal lining of the nasal passage and paranasal sinuses lasting up to 4 weeks
      b. Many different causes, including viruses, bacteria, and fungi
      c. Viruses account for more than 90% of cases, whereas bacteria account for less than 10%.
   2. Diagnosis
      a. Presence of at least two major symptoms or one major and two or more minor symptoms (Table 7)

Table 7. Symptoms Associated with Diagnosis of Sinusitis

Major Symptoms	Minor Symptoms
Purulent anterior nasal discharge	Headache
Purulent or discolored posterior nasal discharge	Ear pain, pressure, or fullness
Nasal congestion or obstruction	Halitosis
Facial congestion or fullness	Dental pain
Facial pain or pressure	Cough
Hyposmia or anosmia	Fever (for subacute or chronic sinusitis)
Fever (for acute sinusitis only)	Fatigue

b. Viral or bacterial? (Table 8)

Table 8. Differentiating Viral from Bacterial Sinusitis

	Viral	**Bacterial**
Symptoms	Nasal discharge, congestion, and scratchy throat	Nasal discharge, congestion, and scratchy throat
Nasal discharge	Clear to purulent to clear; purulence not present until days 4–5	Persistent purulent discharge (>10 days) *or* early and severe (first 3–4 days) *or* increased on days 5–6 after typical viral infection ("double-sickening")
Fever	None (or early in course, resolving in 48 hours)	High temperature (≥39°C) and early (first 3–4 days)
Other symptoms	Headache, facial pain, and myalgia (resolving in 48 hours)	Headache, facial pain, myalgia, daytime cough
Peak symptoms	Days 3–6	Persistent >10 days *or* early and severe (first 3–4 days) *or* improved symptoms that worsen on days 5–6
Duration	5–10 days	In general, >10 days

3. Treatment
   a. Begin antibiotics as soon as *bacterial* sinusitis is diagnosed (see criteria in Table 8).
   b. First-line therapy
      i. Amoxicillin/clavulanate
      ii. High-dose amoxicillin/clavulanate (2 g twice daily in adults or 90 mg/kg/day divided twice daily) in:
         (a) Geographic regions with high endemic rates (greater than 10%) of invasive penicillin-nonsusceptible *S. pneumoniae*
         (b) Those with a severe infection (e.g., evidence of systemic toxicity with a temperature of 39°C or higher and a threat of suppurative complications)
         (c) Attendance at day care
         (d) Age younger than 2 years or older than 65 years
         (e) Recent hospitalization
         (f) Antibiotic use within the past month
         (g) Those who are immunocompromised
   c. Second-line therapy
      i. Respiratory fluoroquinolone (including children with type I hypersensitivity to penicillin)
      ii. Doxycycline
      iii. Cefixime or cefpodoxime with clindamycin (for children with non–type I hypersensitivity to penicillin)
      iv. Intranasal saline irrigation as adjunctive therapy
      v. Intranasal corticosteroids as adjunctive therapy in patients with allergic rhinitis
   d. Therapy duration
      i. Adults: 5–7 days
      ii. Children: 10–14 days

II. URINARY TRACT INFECTIONS

A. Introduction
1. Most common bacterial infection in humans: 7 million office visits per year; 1 million hospitalizations
2. Many women (15%–20%) will have a urinary tract infection (UTI) during their lifetime.
3. From 1–50 years of age, UTIs occur predominantly in women; after 50, men are affected because of prostate problems.

B. Microbiology (Table 9)

Table 9. Incidence of Urinary Tract Infections by Organism

Community Acquired (%)		Nosocomial (%)	
Escherichia coli	73	E. coli	31
Staphylococcus saprophyticus	13	*Pseudomonas aeruginosa*	10
Proteus mirabilis	5	Other gram-negative bacilli	10
Klebsiella pneumoniae	4	*K. pneumoniae*	9
Enterococcus	2	*Staphylococcus aureus*	6
		P. mirabilis	5
		Enterococcus	2
		Fungal	14

C. Predisposing Factors
1. Age
2. Female sex
3. Diabetes mellitus
4. Pregnancy
5. Immunosuppression
6. Urinary tract instrumentation
7. Urinary tract obstruction
8. Renal disease; renal transplantation
9. Neurologic dysfunction

Patient Case

4. G.N. is a 62-year-old woman who presents to the clinic with a 3-day history of urinary frequency and dysuria. During the past 24 hours, she has had nausea, vomiting, and flank pain. G.N. has a history of type 2 diabetes mellitus, which is poorly controlled, with some diabetes-related complications. G.N. also has hypertension and a history of several episodes of deep venous thrombosis. Her medications include glyburide 5 mg/day orally, enalapril 10 mg orally twice daily, warfarin 3 mg/day orally, and metoclopramide 10 mg four times/day. On physical examination, she is alert and oriented, with the following vital signs: temperature 102.8°F (39°C), heart rate 120 beats/minute, respiratory rate 16 breaths/minute, supine blood pressure 140/75 mm Hg, and standing blood pressure 110/60 mm Hg. Her laboratory values are within normal limits except for elevated international normalized ratio 2.7, BUN 26 mg/dL, serum creatinine 1.88 mg/dL, and white blood cell count (WBC) 12,000 cells/mm³ (78 polymorphonuclear leukocytes, 7 band neutrophils, 10 lymphocytes, and 5 monocytes). Her urinalysis shows turbidity, 2+ glucose, pH 7.0, protein 100 mg/dL, 50–100 WBC, positive nitrites, 3–5 red blood cells, and many bacteria and positive casts. Which is the best empiric therapy for G.N.?

A. Trimethoprim/sulfamethoxazole double strength orally twice daily; duration of antibiotics 7 days.

B. Ciprofloxacin 400 mg intravenously twice daily and then 500 mg orally twice daily; duration of antibiotics 10 days.

C. Gentamicin 140 mg intravenously every 24 hours; duration of antibiotics 3 days.

D. Tigecycline 100 mg once, then 50 mg every 12 hours and then doxycycline 100 mg twice daily; duration of antibiotics 10 days.

D. Clinical Presentation
1. Lower UTI: Cystitis (older adults may have only nonspecific symptoms, such as mental status changes, abdominal pain, and decreased eating or drinking)
   a. Dysuria
   b. Frequent urination
   c. Urgency
   d. Occasionally, gross hematuria
   e. Occasionally, foul-smelling urine
2. Upper UTI: Pyelonephritis (older adults may have only nonspecific symptoms, such as mental status changes, abdominal pain, and decreased eating or drinking)
   a. Frequency, dysuria, hematuria
   b. Suprapubic pain
   c. Costovertebral angle tenderness; flank pain
   d. Fever, chills
   e. Elevated WBC
   f. Nausea, vomiting
3. Factors associated with or used to define complicated UTI
   a. Male sex
   b. Hospital acquired
   c. Pregnancy
   d. Anatomic abnormality of the urinary tract
   e. Childhood UTIs
   f. Recent antimicrobial use
   g. Indwelling urinary catheter
   h. Recent urinary tract instrumentation
   i. Immunosuppression

4. Recurrent cystitis
   a. Relapse: Infection with the same organism within 14 days of discontinuing antibiotics for the preceding UTI
   b. Reinfection: Infection with a completely different organism; most common cause of recurrent cystitis

E. Diagnosis: Urinalysis (blood cultures will be positive in 20% of patients with upper UTIs)
   1. Pyuria (WBC greater than 5–10 cells/mm^3)
   2. Bacteriuria (more than 10^2 colony-forming units per milliliter is diagnostic)
   3. Red blood cells
   4. Cloudiness
   5. Nitrite positive
   6. Leukocyte esterase positive
   7. Casts (if pyelonephritis)

F. Therapy
   1. Uncomplicated cystitis
      a. Recommended therapy
         i. Trimethoprim/sulfamethoxazole 160 mg/800 mg twice daily for 3 days.
            Avoid if resistance prevalence is known to exceed 20% or if used for UTI in previous 3 months.
         ii. Nitrofurantoin 100 mg twice daily for 5 days
         iii. Fosfomycin 3 g, one dose
      b. Alternatives
         i. Fluoroquinolones for 3 days
         ii. β-Lactams for 3–7 days
   2. Uncomplicated pyelonephritis
      a. Outpatient therapy (if patient is not immunocompromised or does not have nausea and vomiting)
         i. Trimethoprim/sulfamethoxazole for 14 days
         ii. Fluoroquinolone for 5–7 days
         iii. β-Lactam for 10–14 days (less effective than first two options)
      b. Uropathogen resistance greater than 10%: Use initial dose of an intravenous, long-acting β-lactam (e.g., ceftriaxone) or once-daily aminoglycoside.
   3. Complicated UTIs
      a. Inpatient therapy
         i. Fluoroquinolone
         ii. Aminoglycoside
         iii. Extended-spectrum β-lactam
      b. Therapy duration: 5–14 days (5 days with levofloxacin)
   4. Pregnancy (pregnant women should be screened for bacteriuria and treated, even if asymptomatic)
      a. 7-day treatment regimen
         i. Amoxicillin
         ii. Nitrofurantoin (avoid after 38 weeks' gestation and during labor and delivery)
         iii. Cephalexin
      b. Antibiotics to avoid
         i. Fluoroquinolones
         ii. Tetracyclines
         iii. Aminoglycosides
         iv. Trimethoprim/sulfamethoxazole (used frequently but avoidance recommended, especially during the late third trimester)

5. Recurrent cystitis
   a. Relapse
      i. Assess for pharmacologic reason for treatment failure.
      ii. Longer treatment (for 2–6 weeks, depending on length of initial course)
   b. Reinfection (reassess need for continuous prophylactic antibiotics every 6–12 months)
      i. If patient has two or fewer UTIs in 1 year, use patient-initiated therapy for symptomatic episodes (3-day treatment regimens).
      ii. If patient has three or more UTIs in 1 year and they are temporally related to sexual activity, use postintercourse prophylaxis with trimethoprim/sulfamethoxazole single strength, cephalexin 250 mg, or nitrofurantoin 50–100 mg.
      iii. If patient has three or more UTIs in 1 year that are not related to sexual activity, use daily or three times per week prophylaxis with trimethoprim 100 mg, trimethoprim/sulfamethoxazole single strength, cephalexin 250 mg, or nitrofurantoin 50–100 mg.
6. Catheter-related UTIs
   a. Short-term indwelling catheters
      i. About 5% of patients develop a UTI per each day of catheterization; by 30 days, 75%–95% of patients with an indwelling catheter will have bacteriuria.
      ii. Preventive antimicrobial therapy is not recommended; it only increases the chance of selecting out resistant organisms.
      iii. Asymptomatic patients with bacteriuria should not be treated.
      iv. Symptomatic patients with bacteriuria should be treated with 7 days of antibiotics if symptoms resolve promptly and with 10–14 days of antibiotics if there is a delayed response (both durations whether or not catheter removed). Treat for 5 days with levofloxacin if the patient is not severely ill; treat for 3 days in women 65 years and younger who have their catheters removed and who do not have upper urinary tract symptoms.
      v. The most common organisms are *E. coli* (21.4%), *Candida* spp. (21.0%), *Enterococcus* spp. (14.9%), *P. aeruginosa* (10.0%), *K. pneumoniae* (7.7%), and *Enterobacter* spp. (4.1%).
   b. Long-term indwelling catheters
      i. Almost all patients will be bacteriuric with two to five organisms.
      ii. Asymptomatic patients should not be treated.
      iii. Symptomatic patients should be treated for a short period (7 days) to prevent resistance, and catheter replacement may be indicated.
7. Prostatitis and epididymitis
   a. Acute bacterial prostatitis
      i. Primarily gram-negative organisms
      ii. Therapy duration, 4 weeks
         (a) Trimethoprim/sulfamethoxazole
         (b) Fluoroquinolones
   b. Chronic bacterial prostatitis
      i. Difficult to treat
      ii. Therapy duration, 1–4 months
         (a) Trimethoprim/sulfamethoxazole
         (b) Fluoroquinolones
8. Epididymitis
   a. Older than 35 years, probably caused by enteric organisms
      i. Therapy duration: 10 days to 4 weeks
      ii. Antibiotics: trimethoprim/sulfamethoxazole or fluoroquinolones

      b.   Younger than 35 years, probably gonococcal or chlamydial infection
          i.   Therapy duration: 10 days
          ii. Antibiotics: ceftriaxone 250 mg intramuscularly once plus doxycycline 100 mg twice daily

III. SKIN AND SKIN STRUCTURE INFECTIONS

A. Cellulitis
  1. Description
     a. Acute spreading skin infection that involves primarily the deep dermis and subcutaneous fat
     b. Nonelevated, poorly defined margins
     c. Warmth, pain, erythema and edema, and tender lymphadenopathy
     d. Malaise, fever, and chills
     e. Usually, patient has had previous minor trauma, abrasions, ulcers, or surgery (could be tinea infections, psoriasis, or eczema).
     f. Often, patients have impaired lymphatic drainage.
  2. Microorganism: usually *S. pyogenes* and occasionally *S. aureus* (rarely other organisms)
  3. Treatment: 5–10 days (may extend therapy if infection has not improved)
     a. Antistaphylococcal penicillin (nafcillin, oxacillin, or dicloxacillin)
     b. Penicillin G if definitively streptococcal
     c. Alternatives
        i. Clindamycin
        ii. β-Lactamase inhibitor combinations
        iii. First-generation cephalosporin
     d. Treat empirically for MRSA if associated with penetrating trauma, especially from illicit drug use, purulent drainage, or with concurrent evidence of MRSA infection elsewhere
        i. Outpatient: clindamycin, trimethoprim/sulfamethoxazole (add β-lactam for *Streptococcus*), doxycycline (add β-lactam for *Streptococcus*),
        ii. Inpatient: vancomycin, linezolid, daptomycin, or telavancin

B. Erysipelas
  1. Description
     a. Acute spreading skin infection that involves primarily the superficial dermis
     b. Spreads rapidly through the lymphatic system in the skin (patients may have impaired lymphatic drainage)
     c. Usually occurs in infants and older adults
     d. Usually occurs on the legs and feet (facial erysipelas can occur, but this is less common)
     e. Warmth, erythema, and pain
     f. Edge of infection is elevated and sharply demarcated from the surrounding tissue.
     g. Systemic signs of infection are common, but blood cultures are positive only 5% of the time.
  2. Microorganism: group A *Streptococcus* (*S. pyogenes*), but occasionally groups G, C, and B are seen
  3. Treatment: 5 days (may extend therapy if infection has not improved)
     a. Penicillin G
     b. Clindamycin

C. Necrotizing Fasciitis
  1. Description
     a. Acute, necrotizing cellulites that involve the subcutaneous fat and superficial fascia
     b. Infection extensively alters surrounding tissue, leading to cutaneous anesthesia or gangrene.

  c. Very painful (pain out of proportion to appearance)

  d. Streptococcal infection: Either spontaneous or attributable to varicella, minor trauma (cuts, burns, and splinters), surgical procedures, or muscle strain; mixed infection generally secondary to abdominal surgery or trauma

  e. Significant systemic symptoms, including shock and organ failure

 2. Microorganisms

  a. *S. pyogenes*

  b. Mixed infection with facultative and anaerobic bacteria

 3. Treatment

  a. Surgical debridement: Most important therapy and often repeated debridement is necessary

  b. Antibiotics are not curative; given in addition to surgery (if used early, may be effective alone)

  c. Empiric therapy: Vancomycin or linezolid plus piperacillin/tazobactam or a carbapenem or ceftriaxone with metronidazole

  d. Streptococcal necrotizing fasciitis: High-dose intravenous penicillin plus clindamycin

D. Varicella-Zoster Virus Immunization: Shingles Vaccine (Zostavax)

 1. Characteristics

  a. Zoster vaccine is a live attenuated vaccine, identical to the chicken pox vaccine (Varivax) but with significantly more plaque-forming units of virus per vaccination.

  b. Significantly decreases the number of cases and the burden of illness in vaccinated patients (50% effective, but decreases with age). In addition, significantly decreases the incidence and persistence of post-herpetic neuralgia (40% effective)

 2. Recommendations

  a. One dose: Recommended for all adults 60 years and older (regardless of chickenpox or zoster history); indicated in adults 50 years and older

  b. Not indicated for treatment of active herpes zoster infections or post-herpetic neuralgia

---

Patient Case

5. G.N. returns to the clinic in 6 months with no urinary symptoms, but her chief concern is now an ulcer on her right foot. She recently returned from a vacation in Florida and thinks she might have stepped on something while walking barefoot on the beach. Her foot is not sore but is red and swollen around the ulcer. The ulcer is deep, and the infection may involve the underlying bone. Her medications are the same as before. Vital signs are stable, and there is nothing significant on physical examination except for the right foot ulcer. Laboratory values are within normal limits (serum creatinine 0.86 mg/dL). Which best describes the organisms likely to be responsible for G.N.'s foot ulcer?

A. Multiple anaerobic organisms.

B. *P. aeruginosa.*

C. *S. aureus.*

D. Polymicrobial with gram-positive, gram-negative, and anaerobic organisms.

IV. DIABETIC FOOT INFECTIONS

A. Epidemiology
   1. 25% of people with diabetes develop foot infections.
   2. 1 in 15 requires amputation.

B. Etiology
   1. Neuropathy: Motor and autonomic
      a. Mechanical or thermal injuries lead to ulcerations without patient knowledge.
      b. Gait disturbances and foot deformities; maldistribution of weight on the foot
      c. Diminished sweating, causing dry, cracked skin
   2. Vasculopathy: Decreased lower limb perfusion
   3. Immunologic defects: Cellular and humoral

C. Causative Organisms: In general, polymicrobial (average, 2.1–5.8 microorganisms)
   1. *S. aureus*
   2. *Streptococcus*
   3. *Enterococcus*
   4. *Proteus*
   5. *E. coli*
   6. *Klebsiella*
   7. *Enterobacter*
   8. *P. aeruginosa*
   9. *Bacteroides fragilis*
   10. *Peptococcus*

D. Therapy
   1. Preventive therapy
      a. Examine feet daily for calluses, blisters, trauma, and so forth.
      b. Wear properly fitting shoes.
      c. No barefoot walking
      d. Keep feet clean and dry.
      e. Have toenails cut properly.

Patient Case

6. Which is the best empiric therapy for G.N.?

   A. Nafcillin 2 g intravenously every 6 hours; duration of antibiotics 6–12 weeks.

   B. Tobramycin 120 mg intravenously every 12 hours plus levofloxacin 750 mg/day intravenously; duration of antibiotics 1–2 weeks.

   C. Ampicillin/sulbactam 3 g intravenously every 6 hours; duration of antibiotics 2–3 weeks.

   D. Below-the-knee amputation followed by ceftriaxone 1 g intravenously every 24 hours; duration of antibiotics 1 week.

---

2. Antimicrobial therapy
   a. Mild infections (and no antibiotics in the past month)
      i. No MRSA risk factors: penicillinase-resistant penicillin, first-generation cephalosporin, fluoroquinolone, or clindamycin
      ii. MRSA risk factors: doxycycline or trimethoprim/sulfamethoxazole
   b. Moderate to severe infections
      i. Ampicillin/sulbactam
      ii. Ertapenem
      iii. Cefoxitin
      iv. Third-generation cephalosporin
      v. Moxifloxacin alone or ciprofloxacin/levofloxacin plus clindamycin
      vi. Tigecycline
      vii. If risk of *P. aeruginosa* (uncommon in diabetic foot infections and frequently a nonpathogenic colonizer), use piperacillin/tazobactam, ceftazidime, cefepime, or carbapenem. Risk factors for *Pseudomonas* include patients soaking their feet, lack of response to nonpseudomonal therapy, or a severe infection.
      viii. If risk of MRSA, use vancomycin, linezolid, or daptomycin. Risk factors for MRSA include history of MRSA infection or colonization, high local prevalence of MRSA, or a severe infection.
   c. Treatment duration: 1–2 weeks for mild to moderate infections and 2–3 weeks for severe infections. Four weeks or more is necessary for osteomyelitis; after amputation treatment, duration is 2–5 days if there is no remaining infected tissue or 4 weeks or more if infected tissue remains.

E. Surgical Therapy
   1. Drainage and debridement (appropriate wound care) are very important.
   2. Amputation is often necessary; if infection is discovered early, can maintain structural integrity of the foot.

Patient Case

7. W.A. is a 55-year-old man who presents with weight loss, malaise, and severe back pain and spasms that have progressed during the past 2 months. He has also experienced loss of sensation in his lower extremities. Four months before this admission, he had surgery for a fractured tibia, followed by an infection treated with unknown antibiotics. W.A. has hypertension and diverticulitis. On physical examination, he is alert and oriented, with the following vital signs: temperature 99.4°F (37.4°C), heart rate 88 beats/minute, respiratory rate 14 breaths/minute, and blood pressure 130/85 mm Hg. His laboratory values are within normal limits, except for WBC 14,300 cells/mm^3, erythrocyte sedimentation rate 89 mm/hour, and C-reactive protein 12 mg/dL. Magnetic resonance imaging shows bony destruction of lumbar vertebrae 1 and 2, which is confirmed by a bone scan. A computed tomography–guided bone biopsy shows gram-positive cocci in clusters. Which is the best initial therapy for W.A.?

A. Vancomycin 15 mg/kg intravenously every 12 hours; duration of antibiotics 6 weeks.

B. Nafcillin 2 g intravenously every 6 hours; duration of antibiotics 2 weeks.

C. Levofloxacin 750 mg/day orally; duration of antibiotics 6 weeks.

D. Ampicillin/sulbactam 3 g intravenously every 6 hours; duration of antibiotics 2 weeks.

V. OSTEOMYELITIS

A. Introduction
   1. Infection of the bone with subsequent bone destruction
   2. Around 20 cases per 100,000 people

B. Characteristics (Table 10)

Table 10. Characteristics of Osteomyelitis

	Hematogenous Spread	**Contiguous Spread**	**Vascular Insufficiency**
Definition	Spread of bacteria through the blood-stream from a distant site	Spread of bacteria from an adjacent tissue infection or by direct inoculation	Infection results from insufficient blood supply to fight the bacteria
Patient population	Children (<16 years): femur, tibia, humerus Adult: vertebrae	Adults (25–50 years): femur, tibia, skull	Adults (>50 years)
Predisposing factors	Bacteremia (e.g., IV catheters, IVDU, skin infections, URI) Sickle cell anemia	Open reduction of fractures Gunshot wound Dental or sinus infections Soft tissue infections	Diabetes PVD Post-CABG (sternum)
Common pathogens	Usually monomicrobial Children: *Staphylococcus aureus* (60%–90%), *Staphylococcus epidermidis, Streptococcus pyogenes, Streptococcus pneumoniae, Haemophilus influenzae, Pseudomonas aeruginosa, Enterobacter, Escherichia coli* (all <5%) Adults: *S. aureus* and gram-negative bacilli Sickle cell anemia: *Salmonella* (67%), *S. aureus, S. pneumoniae* IV drug users: *P. aeruginosa*	Usually mixed infection: *S. aureus* (60%), *S. epidermidis, Streptococcus* Gram-negative bacilli: *P. aeruginosa* (foot punctures), *Proteus, Klebsiella, E. coli* Anaerobic (human bites, decubitus ulcers)	Usually polymicrobial: *S. aureus, S. epidermidis, Streptococcus* Gram-negative bacilli Anaerobic (*Bacteroides fragilis* group) Infected prosthesis: *S. aureus, S. epidermidis*

CABG = coronary artery bypass graft; IV = intravenous; IVDU = intravenous drug use; PVD = pulmonary vascular disease; URI = upper respiratory infection.

C. Clinical Presentation
   1. Signs and symptoms
      a. Fever and chills
      b. Localized pain, tenderness, and swelling
      c. Neurologic symptoms if spinal cord compression
   2. Laboratory tests
      a. Elevated WBC
      b. Elevated erythrocyte sedimentation rate
      c. Elevated C-reactive protein

3. Diagnostic tests
   a. Radiographic tests: Positive results lag behind infectious process.
   b. Computed tomography and magnetic resonance imaging scans
   c. Radionuclide imaging: Positive as soon as 24–48 hours after infectious process begins.

D. Empiric Therapy
   1. Neonates younger than 1 month
      a. Nafcillin plus cefotaxime *or*
      b. Nafcillin plus an aminoglycoside
   2. Infants (1–36 months)
      a. Cefuroxime
      b. Ceftriaxone
      c. Nafcillin plus cefotaxime
   3. Pediatrics (older than 3 years)
      a. Nafcillin
      b. Cefazolin
      c. Clindamycin
   4. Adults
      a. Nafcillin, cefazolin, or vancomycin
      b. Choose additional antibiotics according to patient-specific characteristics.
   5. Patients with sickle cell anemia: Ceftriaxone/cefotaxime or ciprofloxacin/levofloxacin (no studies assessing best empiric therapy)
   6. Prosthetic joint infections
      a. Debridement and retention of prosthesis or one-stage exchange of prosthesis
         i. Staphylococcal: Pathogen-specific intravenous therapy plus rifampin 350–400 mg twice daily for 2–6 weeks, followed by rifampin plus ciprofloxacin or levofloxacin for 3 months (hip, elbow, shoulder, ankle prosthesis) or 6 months (knee prosthesis)
         ii. Nonstaphylococcal: Pathogen-specific intravenous (or highly bioavailable oral) therapy for 4–6 weeks, followed by indefinite oral suppression therapy
      b. Resection of prosthesis with or without planned reimplantation or amputation
         i. Pathogen-specific intravenous (or highly bioavailable oral) therapy for 4–6 weeks
         ii. Only 24–48 hours of antibiotic therapy after amputation if all infected tissue is removed

E. Therapy Length
   1. Acute osteomyelitis: 4–6 weeks
   2. Chronic osteomyelitis: 6–8 weeks of parenteral therapy and 3–12 months of oral therapy

F. Criteria for Effective Oral Therapy for Osteomyelitis
   1. Adherence
   2. Identified organism that is highly susceptible to the oral antibiotic used
   3. C-reactive protein less than 2.0 mg/dL
   4. Adequate surgical debridement
   5. Resolving clinical course

VI. CENTRAL NERVOUS SYSTEM (CNS) INFECTIONS

A. Meningitis: Introduction
 1. Incidence: About 8.6 cases per 100,000 people
 2. Occurs more often in male than in female patients
 3. More common in children

B. Microbiology (Table 11)
 1. Bacterial (septic meningitis)

Table 11. Bacterial Etiology of Meningitis, Based on Age

Age	Most Likely Organisms	Less Common Organisms
<1 month (newborns)	*Streptococcus agalactiae* *Listeria monocytogenes* *Streptococcus pneumoniae* *Neisseria meningitidis*	*Escherichia coli* *Klebsiella* spp. Herpes simplex type 2
1–23 months	*S. pneumoniae* *N. meningitidis* *Haemophilus influenzae* *Streptococcus agalactiae*	Viruses *E. coli*
2–50 years	*N. meningitidis* *S. pneumoniae*	*H. influenzae* Viruses
>50 years	*S. pneumoniae* *N. meningitidis* *H. influenzae*	*L. monocytogenes, Streptococcus agalactiae,* aerobic gram-negative bacilli, viruses

 2. Other causes (aseptic meningitis)
  a. Viral
  b. Fungal
  c. Parasitic
  d. Tubercular
  e. Syphilis
  f. Drugs (e.g., trimethoprim/sulfamethoxazole, ibuprofen)

C. Predisposing Factors
 1. Head trauma
 2. Immunosuppression
 3. CNS shunts
 4. Cerebrospinal fluid (CSF) fistula or leak
 5. Neurosurgical patients
 6. Alcoholism
 7. Local infections
  a. Sinusitis
  b. Otitis media
  c. Pharyngitis
  d. Bacterial pneumonia

8. Splenectomized patients
9. Sickle cell disease
10. Congenital defects

D. Clinical Presentation
   1. Symptoms
      a. Fever, chills
      b. Headache, backache, nuchal rigidity, mental status changes, photophobia
      c. Nausea, vomiting, anorexia, poor feeding habits (infants)
      d. Petechiae or purpura (*Neisseria meningitidis* meningitis)
   2. Physical signs
      a. Brudzinski sign
      b. Kernig sign
      c. Bulging fontanel

E. Diagnosis
   1. History and physical examination
   2. Lumbar puncture
      a. Elevated opening pressure
      b. Composition in bacterial meningitis (Table 12)

Table 12. CSF Changes in Bacterial Meningitis

Component	Normal CSF	Bacterial Meningitis
Glucose	30–70 mg/dL (2/3 peripheral)	<50 mg/dL (≤0.4 CSF/blood)
Protein	<50 mg/dL	>150 mg/dL
WBC	<5 cells/mm^3	>1200 cells/mm^3
pH	7.3	7.1
Lactic acid	<14 mg/dL	>35 mg/dL

CSF = cerebrospinal fluid; WBC = white blood cell count.

      c. CSF stains and studies
         i. Gram stain (microorganisms): Helps identify organism in 60%–90% of cases
         ii. Latex agglutination: High sensitivity, 50%–100%, for common organisms
            (a) Not recommended routinely
            (b) Most useful in patients pretreated with antibiotics with subsequent negative CSF Gram stains and cultures
         iii. Acid-fast staining (tubercular meningitis)
         iv. India ink test (*Cryptococcus*)
         v. Cryptococcal antigen
         vi. Herpes simplex virus polymerase chain reaction
   3. Laboratory findings
      a. Elevated WBC with a left shift
      b. CSF Gram stain
      c. CSF cultures (positive in 75%–80% of bacterial meningitis cases)
      d. Blood cultures (±)
      e. C-reactive protein concentrations: High negative predictive value

Patient Case

8. D.M. is a 21-year-old university student who presents to the emergency department with the worst headache of his life. During the past few days, he has felt slightly ill but has been able to go to class regularly and eat and drink adequately. This morning, he awoke with a terrible headache and pain whenever he moved his neck. He has no significant medical history and takes no medications. He cannot remember the last time he received a vaccination. On physical examination, he is in extreme pain (10/10) with the following vital signs: temperature 102.4°F (39.1°C), heart rate 110 beats/minute, respiratory rate 18 breaths/minute, and blood pressure 130/75 mm Hg. His laboratory values are within normal limits, except for WBC 22,500 cells/mm^3 (82 polymorphonuclear leukocytes, 11 band neutrophils, 5 lymphocytes, and 2 monocytes). A computed tomography scan of the head is normal, so a lumbar puncture is performed with the following results: glucose 44 mg/dL (peripheral, 110), protein 220 mg/dL, and WBC 800 cells/mm^3 (85% neutrophils, 15% lymphocytes). Gram staining shows abundant gram-negative cocci. Which is the best empiric therapy for D.M.?

    A. Penicillin G 4 million units intravenously every 4 hours plus dexamethasone 4 mg intravenously every 6 hours.

    B. Ceftriaxone 2 g intravenously every 12 hours.

    C. Ceftriaxone 2 g intravenously every 12 hours plus dexamethasone 4 mg intravenously every 6 hours.

    D. Ceftriaxone 2 g intravenously every 12 hours plus vancomycin 1000 mg intravenously every 12 hours.

F. Empiric Therapy
    1. Neonates younger than 1 month
        a. Ampicillin plus aminoglycoside *or*
        b. Ampicillin plus cefotaxime
    2. Infants (1–23 months): Third-generation cephalosporin (cefotaxime or ceftriaxone) plus vancomycin
    3. Children and adults (2–50 years): Third-generation cephalosporin (cefotaxime or ceftriaxone) plus vancomycin
    4. Older adults (50 years and older): Third-generation cephalosporin (cefotaxime or ceftriaxone) plus vancomycin plus ampicillin
    5. Penetrating head trauma, neurosurgery, or CSF shunt: Vancomycin plus cefepime, ceftazidime, or meropenem

G. Therapy for Common Pathogens
    1. *S. pneumoniae*
        a. A minimum inhibitory concentration (MIC) of 0.1 mcg/mL or less
            i.   Penicillin G 4 million units intravenously every 4 hours
            ii. Ampicillin 2 g intravenously every 4 hours
            iii. Alternative: Third-generation cephalosporin or chloramphenicol
        b. An MIC 0.1–1.0 mcg/mL
            i.   Third-generation cephalosporin
            ii. Alternative: cefepime or meropenem
        c. An MIC 2.0 mcg/mL or greater
            i.   Vancomycin plus a third-generation cephalosporin
            ii. Alternative: moxifloxacin
    2. *N. meningitidis*
        a. An MIC less than 0.1 mcg/mL
            i.   Penicillin G 4 million units intravenously every 4 hours
            ii. Ampicillin 2 g intravenously every 4 hours
            iii. Alternative: third-generation cephalosporin or chloramphenicol

        b.   An MIC 0.1–1.0 mcg/mL

           i.   Third-generation cephalosporin

           ii.   Alternative: chloramphenicol, fluoroquinolone, or meropenem

  3.   *H. influenzae*

        a.   β-Lactamase negative

           i.   Ampicillin 2 g intravenously every 4 hours

           ii.   Alternative: third-generation cephalosporin, cefepime, chloramphenicol, or fluoroquinolone

        b.   β-Lactamase positive

           i.   Third-generation cephalosporin

           ii.   Alternative: cefepime, chloramphenicol, or fluoroquinolone

  4.   *Streptococcus agalactiae*

        a.   Penicillin G 4 million units intravenously every 4 hours

        b.   Ampicillin 2 g intravenously every 4 hours

        c.   Alternative: third-generation cephalosporin

  5.   *Listeria monocytogenes*

        a.   Penicillin G 4 million units intravenously every 4 hours

        b.   Ampicillin 2 g intravenously every 4 hours

        c.   Alternative: trimethoprim/sulfamethoxazole or meropenem

H. Therapy Length: Based on clinical experience, not on clinical data

  1.   *N. meningitidis:* 7 days

  2.   *H. influenzae:* 7 days

  3.   *S. pneumoniae:* 10–14 days

I. Adjunctive Corticosteroid Therapy

  1.   Risks and benefits

        a.   Significantly less hearing loss and other neurologic sequelae in children receiving dexamethasone for *H. influenzae* meningitis

        b.   Significantly improved outcomes, including decreased mortality, in adults receiving dexamethasone for *S. pneumoniae* meningitis

        c.   May decrease antibiotic penetration (decreased penetration of vancomycin in animals after dexamethasone)

  2.   Dose and administration

        a.   Give corticosteroids 10–20 minutes before or at same time as antibiotics.

        b.   Dexamethasone 0.15 mg/kg every 6 hours for 2–4 days

        c.   Use in children with *H. influenzae* meningitis or in adults with pneumococcal meningitis; however, may need to initiate before knowing specific causative bacteria

Patient Case

9. After D.M.'s diagnosis, there is concern about prophylaxis. Which is the best recommendation for meningitis prophylaxis?

   A. The health care providers in close contact with D.M. should receive rifampin 600 mg every 12 hours for four doses.

   B. Everyone in D.M.'s dormitory and in all of his classes should receive rifampin 600 mg/day for 4 days.

   C. Everyone in the emergency department at the time of D.M.'s presentation should receive the meningococcal conjugate vaccine.

   D. Everyone in the emergency department at the time of D.M.'s presentation should receive rifampin 600 mg every 12 hours for four doses.

J. Prophylaxis
   1. *S. pneumoniae*
      a. PCV: 13 valent
         i. All children younger than 23 months
         ii. Children 24–59 months with high-risk status
            (a) Certain chronic diseases
            (b) Alaska Native or American Indian
            (c) African American
            (d) Day care attendees
         iii. Adults 65 years or older
         iv. Adults with asplenia or who are immunocompromised
      b. PPSV23 valent: Give to those at risk (see patient groups in Pneumonia section above).
   2. *N. meningitidis*
      a. Chemoprophylaxis: For close contacts (household or day care) and exposure to oral secretions of index case
         i. Rifampin
            (a) Adults: 600 mg every 12 hours × 4 doses
            (b) Children: 10 mg/kg every 12 hours × 4 doses
            (c) Infants (younger than 1 month): 5 mg/kg every 12 hours × 4 doses
         ii. Ciprofloxacin 500 mg orally × 1 (adults only)
         iii. Ceftriaxone 125–250 mg intramuscularly × 1
      b. Meningococcal polysaccharide vaccine (Menomune) and meningococcal conjugate vaccine (Menactra, Menveo) (both lack serogroup B)
         i. Indications (use Menactra or Menveo unless patient is older than 55 years)
            (a) Young adolescents (11–12 years)
            (b) College freshmen living in dormitories (4 cases per 100,000 per year, especially freshmen living in dormitories)
            (c) Military recruits
            (d) Travel to "meningitis belt" of Africa and Asia, Saudi Arabia for Islamic Hajj pilgrimage
            (e) People with asplenia (anatomic or functional)
            (f) People with terminal complement component deficiencies
            (g) Outbreaks of meningococcal disease

        ii.   Booster dose

           (a) Adolescents: Recommended at 16 years of age if they received a first dose at age 11–12 years or at 5 years after the first dose, up to age 21 years, to those who first received the vaccine at age 13–15 years

           (b) Asplenic or immunocompromised patients: Recommended in 2 months and then every 5 years

3.   *H. influenzae*

    a.   Chemoprophylaxis: For everyone in households with unvaccinated children

        i.   Adults: Rifampin 600 mg/day for 4 days

        ii.   Children (1 month to 12 years): Rifampin 20 mg/kg/day for 4 days

        iii.   Infants younger than 1 month: Rifampin 10 mg/kg/day for 4 days

    b.   *H. influenzae* type B polysaccharide vaccine

        i.   All children

        ii.   Indications regardless of age

           (a) Asplenia (anatomic or functional)

           (b) Sickle cell disease

           (c) Hodgkin disease

           (d) Hematologic neoplasms

           (e) Solid organ transplantation

           (f) Severely immunocompromised (non–HIV related)

        iii.   Consider for people with HIV infection.

K. Brain Abscess

   1.   Pathophysiology

      a.   Direct extension or retrograde septic phlebitis from otitis media, mastoiditis, sinusitis, and facial cellulitis

      b.   Hematogenous: Particularly lung abscess or infective endocarditis: 3%–20% have no detectable focus.

   2.   Signs and symptoms

      a.   Expanding intracranial mass lesion: Focal neurologic deficits

      b.   Headache

      c.   Fever

      d.   Seizures

      e.   Mortality is about 50%.

   3.   Microbiology

      a.   Usually polymicrobial

      b.   *Streptococcus* spp. in 50%–60%

      c.   Anaerobes in about 40%

   4.   Therapy

      a.   Incision and drainage: By craniotomy or stereotaxic needle aspiration

      b.   Suggested empiric regimens based on source of infection

         i.   Otitis media or mastoiditis: metronidazole plus third-generation cephalosporin

         ii.   Sinusitis: metronidazole plus third-generation cephalosporin

         iii.   Dental sepsis: penicillin plus metronidazole

         iv.   Trauma or neurosurgery: vancomycin plus third-generation cephalosporin

         v.   Lung abscess, empyema: penicillin plus metronidazole plus sulfonamide

         vi.   Unknown: vancomycin plus metronidazole plus third-generation cephalosporin

      c.   Corticosteroids if elevated intracranial pressure

Patient Case

10. T.S. is a 48-year-old man who presents to the emergency department with fever, chills, nausea and vomiting, anorexia, lymphangitis in his right hand, and lower back pain. He has no significant medical history except for kidney stones 4 years ago. He has no known drug allergies. He is homeless and was an intravenous drug abuser (heroin) for the past year but quit 2 weeks ago. On physical examination, he is alert and oriented, with the following vital signs: temperature 100.8°F (38°C), heart rate 114 beats/minute, respiratory rate 12 breaths/minute, and blood pressure 127/78 mm Hg. He has a faint systolic ejection murmur, and his right hand is erythematous and swollen. His laboratory values are all within normal limits. He had an HIV test 1 year ago, which was negative. One blood culture was obtained that later grew MSSA. Two more cultures were obtained that are now growing gram-positive cocci in clusters. A transesophageal echocardiogram shows vegetation on the mitral valve. Which is the best therapeutic regimen for T.S.?

   A. Nafcillin intravenous therapy; antibiotic duration 2 weeks.

   B. Nafcillin intravenously plus rifampin therapy; antibiotic duration 6 weeks or longer.

   C. Nafcillin intravenously plus gentamicin intravenous therapy; antibiotic duration 2 weeks of both antibiotics.

   D. Nafcillin intravenously plus gentamicin; antibiotic duration 6 weeks (nafcillin) with gentamicin for the first 3–5 days.

VII. ENDOCARDITIS

  A. Introduction
     1. Infection of the heart valves or other endocardial tissue
     2. Platelet-fibrin complex becomes infected with microorganisms: vegetation
     3. Main risk factors include mitral valve prolapse, prosthetic valves, and intravenous drug abuse.
     4. Three or four cases per 100,000 people per year

  B. Presentation and Clinical Findings
     1. Signs and symptoms
        a. Fever: Low grade and remittent
        b. Cutaneous manifestations (50% of patients): petechiae (including conjunctival), Janeway lesions, splinter hemorrhage
        c. Cardiac murmur (90% of patients)
        d. Arthralgias, myalgias, low back pain, arthritis
        e. Fatigue, anorexia, weight loss, night sweats
     2. Laboratory findings
        a. Anemia: normochromic, normocytic
        b. Leukocytosis
        c. Elevated erythrocyte sedimentation rate and C-reactive protein
        d. Positive blood culture in 78%–95% of patients
     3. Complications
        a. Congestive heart failure: 38%–60% of patients
        b. Emboli: 22%–43% of patients
        c. Mycotic aneurysm: 5%–10% of patients

C. Microbiology (Table 13)
1. Three to five blood cultures of at least 10 mL each should be drawn during the first 24–48 hours.
2. Empiric therapy should be initiated only in acutely ill patients. In these patients, three blood samples should be drawn during a 15- to 20-minute period before antibiotics are initiated.

Table 13. Incidence of Microorganisms in Endocarditis

Organism	Incidence (%)
Streptococcus	50
Staphylococcus aureus	25
Enterococcus	8
Coagulase-negative *Staphylococcus*	7
Gram-negative bacilli	6
Candida albicans	2

D. Treatment (Table 14)

Table 14. Treatment Recommendation for Endocarditis

Organism	Recommended Therapy	Length of Therapy (weeks)	
		Native Valve	Prosthetic Valve
Viridans streptococci (with PCN MIC ≤0.12 mcg/mL)	PCN G	4	—
	PCN G + gentamicin	2	6[a]
	Ceftriaxone	4	—
	Ceftriaxone + gentamicin	2	6[a]
	Vancomycin	4	6
Viridans streptococci (with PCN MIC >0.12 mcg/mL)	PCN G + gentamicin	4[b]	6
	Ceftriaxone + gentamicin	4[b]	6
	Vancomycin	4	6
Staphylococcus, methicillin sensitive	Oxacillin or nafcillin ± Gentamicin for 3–5 days Plus rifampin in prosthetic valves	6	≥6[b]
	Cefazolin ± Gentamicin for 3–5 days Plus rifampin in prosthetic valves	6	≥6[b]
	Vancomycin (only if severe PCN allergy) Plus rifampin in prosthetic valves	6	≥6[b]
Staphylococcus, methicillin resistant	Vancomycin Plus rifampin and gentamicin in prosthetic valves Daptomycin (not for prosthetic valves)	6	≥6[b]
Enterococcus	PCN G or ampicillin + gentamicin or streptomycin	4–6	6
	Vancomycin + gentamicin or streptomycin	6	6

Table 14. Treatment Recommendation for Endocarditis *(continued)*

Organism	Recommended Therapy	Length of Therapy (weeks)	
		Native Valve	Prosthetic Valve
Enterococcus, PCN resistant	Ampicillin/sulbactam or vancomycin + gentamicin	6	6
Enterococcus faecium, PCN, aminoglycoside, and vancomycin resistant	Linezolid	≥8	≥8
	Quinupristin/dalfopristin	≥8	≥8
Enterococcus faecalis, PCN, aminoglycoside, and vancomycin resistant	Imipenem/cilastatin + ampicillin	≥8	≥8
	Ceftriaxone + ampicillin	≥8	≥8
HACEK group	Ceftriaxone	4	6
	Ampicillin/sulbactam	4	6
	Fluoroquinolone (ciprofloxacin, levofloxacin, moxifloxacin)	4	6

[a]Gentamicin can be added for 2 weeks if creatinine clearance is greater than 30 mL/minute.
[b]Gentamicin for 2 weeks.
HACEK = *Haemophilus, Actinobacillus Cardiobacterium, Eikenella, Kingella*; MIC = minimum inhibitory concentration; PCN = penicillin.

E. Prophylaxis (Table 15)

Table 15. Endocarditis Prophylaxis

Conditions in Which Prophylaxis Is Necessary	Dental Procedures That Require Prophylaxis
Prosthetic cardiac valves including bioprosthetic and homograft valves	Any dental procedure that involves the gingival tissues or periapical region of a tooth and for procedures that perforate the oral mucosa
Previous bacterial endocarditis	
Congenital heart disease	
Unrepaired cyanotic congenital heart disease	**Other Procedures That Require Prophylaxis**
Completely repaired congenital heart defect with prosthetic material or device, during the first 6 months after the procedure	Respiratory tract
	Tonsillectomy or adenoidectomy
Repaired congenital heart disease with residual defects adjacent to or at the site of a prosthetic patch or device	Surgical operations that involve an incision or biopsy of the respiratory mucosa
Cardiac transplant recipients who develop cardiac valvulopathy	

F. Recommended Prophylaxis for Dental or Respiratory Tract Procedures (Table 16)

Table 16. Prophylaxis for Dental or Respiratory Tract Procedures

Situation	Agent	Regimen
Standard general prophylaxis	Amoxicillin	Adults: 2 g; children: 50 mg/kg 1 hour before procedure
Unable to take oral medications	Ampicillin	Adults: 2 g IM/IV; children: 50 mg/kg IM/IV within 30 minutes before procedure
	Cefazolin or ceftriaxone	Adults: 1 g IM/IV; children: 50 mg/kg IM/IV within 30 minutes before procedure
Allergic to penicillin	Clindamycin	Adults: 600 mg; children: 20 mg/kg 1 hour before procedure
	Cephalexin	Adults: 2 g; children: 50 mg/kg 1 hour before procedure
	Azithromycin or clarithromycin	Adults: 500 mg; children: 15 mg/kg 1 hour before procedure
Allergic to penicillin and unable to take oral medications	Clindamycin	Adults: 600 mg; children: 20 mg/kg IV within 30 minutes before procedure
	Cefazolin or ceftriaxone	Adults: 1 g IM/IV; children: 50 mg/kg IM/IV within 30 minutes before procedure

IM = intramuscularly; IV = intravenously.

Patient Case

11. Six months after treatment of his endocarditis, T.S. is visiting his dentist for a tooth extraction. Which antibiotic is best for prophylaxis?

    A. Tooth extractions do not require endocarditis prophylaxis.

    B. Administer amoxicillin 2 g 1 hour before the extraction.

    C. Administer amoxicillin 3 g 1 hour before the extraction and 1.5 g 6 hours for four doses after the extraction.

    D. T.S. is not at increased risk of endocarditis and does not need prophylactic antibiotics.

VIII. PERITONITIS AND INTRA-ABDOMINAL INFECTIONS

A. Introduction
    1. Definition: Inflammation of the peritoneum (serous membrane lining the abdominal cavity)
    2. Types
        a. Primary: Spontaneous or idiopathic, no primary focus of infection
        b. Secondary: Occurs secondary to an abdominal process

B. Primary Peritonitis
    1. Etiology
        a. Alcoholic cirrhosis and ascites (peritonitis occurs in 10% of these patients)
        b. Other: postnecrotic cirrhosis, chronic active hepatitis, acute viral hepatitis, congestive heart failure, systemic lupus erythematous, metastatic malignancy (common underlying problem is ascites)

2. Microbiology
   a. *E. coli*
   b. *K. pneumoniae*
   c. *S. pneumoniae*
   d. Group A *Streptococcus*
3. Pathogenesis
   a. Hematogenous: Portosystemic shunting increases bacteria in the blood, infecting ascitic collection.
   b. Lymphogenous
   c. Transmural through the intact gut wall from the lumen
   d. Vaginally through the fallopian tubes
4. Clinical manifestations and diagnosis
   a. Fever
   b. Abdominal pain
   c. Nausea, vomiting, diarrhea
   d. Diffuse abdominal tenderness, rebound tenderness, hypoactive or no bowel sounds
   e. Ascitic fluid
      i. Protein: Low because of hypoalbuminemia or dilution with transudate fluid from the portal system
      ii. WBC more than 300 cells/mm^3 (85% have more than 1000 cells/mm^3), primarily granulocytes
      iii. pH: Less than 7.35
      iv. Lactic dehydrogenase: More than 25 mg/dL
      v. Gram stain: 60%–80% are negative, but diagnostic if it is positive

C. Secondary Peritonitis
   1. Etiology
      a. Injuries to the gastrointestinal tract, including
         i. Peptic ulcer perforation
         ii. Perforation of a gastrointestinal organ
         iii. Appendicitis
         iv. Endometritis secondary to intrauterine device
         v. Bile peritonitis
         vi. Pancreatitis
         vii. Operative contamination
         viii. Diverticulitis
         ix. Intestinal neoplasms
         x. Secondary to peritoneal dialysis
   2. Microbiology of intra-abdominal infections
      a. Stomach and proximal small intestine: aerobic and facultative gram-positive and gram-negative organisms
      b. Ileum: *E. coli, Enterococcus,* anaerobes
      c. Large intestine: obligate anaerobes (i.e., *Bacteroides, Clostridium perfringens*), aerobic and facultative gram-positive and gram-negative organisms (i.e., *E. coli, Streptococcus, Enterococcus, Klebsiella, Proteus, Enterobacter*)
   3. Clinical manifestations and diagnosis
      a. Fever, tachycardia
      b. Elevated WBC
      c. Abdominal pain aggravated by motion, rebound tenderness
      d. Bowel paralysis

e. Pain with breathing

f. Decreased renal perfusion

g. Ascitic fluid

   i. Protein: High (more than 3 g/dL); exudate fluid

   ii. WBCs: Many, primarily granulocytes

D. Therapy

1. Therapy or prophylaxis should be limited in:

  a. Bowel injuries caused by trauma that are repaired within 12 hours (treat for less than 24 hours)

  b. Intraoperative contamination by enteric contents (treat for less than 24 hours)

  c. Perforations of the stomach, duodenum, and proximal jejunum (unless patient is on antacid therapy or has malignancy) (prophylactic antibiotics for less than 24 hours)

  d. Acute appendicitis without evidence of perforation, abscess, or peritonitis (treat for less than 24 hours)

2. Mild to moderate community-acquired infection

  a. Cefoxitin

  b. Cefazolin, cefuroxime, ceftriaxone, or cefotaxime plus metronidazole

  c. Ticarcillin/clavulanate

  d. Ertapenem

  e. Moxifloxacin

  f. Ciprofloxacin or levofloxacin plus metronidazole

  g. Tigecycline

3. High-risk or severe community-acquired or health care–acquired infection

  a. Piperacillin/tazobactam

  b. Ceftazidime or cefepime plus metronidazole

  c. Imipenem/cilastatin, meropenem, or doripenem

  d. Ciprofloxacin or levofloxacin plus metronidazole (not for health care–acquired infections)

  e. Aminoglycoside when extended-spectrum β-lactamase–producing Enterobacteriaceae or *P. aeruginosa* is of concern (health care–acquired infections only)

  f. Vancomycin for MRSA (health care–acquired infections only)

4. Therapy duration: 4–7 days (unless source control is difficult)

IX. *CLOSTRIDIUM DIFFICILE* INFECTION

A. Introduction

1. *Clostridium difficile* is transmitted by the fecal-oral route.

2. Overgrowth in the gastrointestinal tract occurs after antibiotic therapy.

3. Risk factors: hospital stays, medical comorbidities, extremes of age, immunodeficiency states, advancing age, use of broad-spectrum antibiotics for extended periods

4. Production of endotoxins A and B causes pathogenesis.

5. Symptoms: watery diarrhea, abdominal pain, leukocytosis, gastrointestinal tract complications

6. New strain (BI/NAP1) produces more enterotoxin, produces binary toxin, has increased sporulation capacity, and is resistant to fluoroquinolones. Increased risk of metronidazole failure, morbidity, and mortality

B. Therapy
1. Initial episode and first recurrence
   a. Metronidazole 500 mg orally (or intravenously) three times a day for 10–14 days
      i. For mild to moderate episodes
      ii. Oral is the preferred route.
   b. Vancomycin 125 mg orally four times a day for 10–14 days, for severe episodes.
   c. Fidaxomicin 200 mg orally twice daily for 10 days: No difference in clinical cure rates compared with vancomycin but lower incidence of recurrence
2. Second and third recurrences
   a. Consider fidaxomicin if not already given.
   b. Can consider higher doses of vancomycin (500 mg orally four times a day)
   c. Taper therapy: Vancomycin 125 mg orally four times a day for 14 days, twice daily for 7 days, and daily for 7 days
   d. Pulse therapy: Recommended vancomycin course of therapy for initial episode (for 10–14 days), followed by vancomycin every other day for 8 days, and then every 3 days for 15 days
   e. Consider rifaximin 400 mg twice daily for 14 days or nitazoxanide 500 mg twice daily for 10 days.

Patient Case

12. You are a pharmacist who works closely with the surgery department to optimize therapy for patients undergoing surgical procedures at your institution. The surgeons provide you with principles of surgical prophylaxis that they believe are appropriate. Which is the best practice for optimizing surgical prophylaxis?

   A. Antibiotics should be redosed for extended surgical procedures; redose if the surgery lasts longer than 4 hours or involves considerable blood loss.

   B. All patients should be given antibiotics for 24 hours after the procedure; this will optimize prophylaxis.

   C. Preoperative antibiotics can be given up to 4 hours before the incision; this will make giving the antibiotics logistically easier.

   D. Vancomycin should be the antibiotic of choice for surgical wound prophylaxis because of its long half-life and activity against MRSA.

X. MEDICAL AND SURGICAL PROPHYLAXIS

A. Introduction
1. Prophylaxis: Administering the putative agent before bacterial contamination occurs
2. Early therapy: Immediate or prompt institution of therapy as soon as the patient presents; usually, contamination or infection will have preceded the initiation of therapy (e.g., dirty wounds).

B. Classification of Surgical Procedures (Table 17)

Table 17. Classification of Surgical Procedures

Surgical Procedure	Infection Rate (%)
Clean: No entry is made in the respiratory, gastrointestinal, or genitourinary tracts or in the oropharyngeal cavity In general, it is elective with no break in technique and no inflammation encountered	1–4
Clean contaminated: Entry in the respiratory, gastrointestinal, genitourinary, or biliary tracts or oropharyngeal cavity without unusual contamination Includes clean procedures with a minor break in technique	5–15
Contaminated: Includes fresh traumatic wounds, gross spillage from the gastrointestinal tract (without a mechanical bowel preparation), a major break in technique, or incisions encountering acute, nonpurulent inflammation	16–25
Dirty: Includes procedures involving old traumatic wounds, perforated viscera, or clinically evident infection	30–100

C. Risk Factors for Postoperative Wound Infections
  1. Bacterial contamination
    a. Exogenous sources: Flaw in aseptic technique
    b. Endogenous sources
      i. Most important except in clean procedures
      ii. Patient flora causes infection.
  2. Host resistance
    a. Extremes of age
    b. Nutrition (i.e., malnourished patients)
    c. Obesity
    d. Diabetes mellitus (decreased wound healing and increased risk of infection)
    e. Immunocompromised
    f. Hypoxemia
    g. Remote infection
    h. Presence of foreign body
      i. Healthy person tolerates inoculum of 10^5.
      ii. In presence of foreign body, need only 10^2

D. Indications for Surgical Prophylaxis
  1. Common postoperative infection with low morbidity
  2. Uncommon postoperative infection with significant morbidity and mortality

E. Principles of Prophylaxis (Figure 1; Tables 18 and 19)
  1. Timing: Antibiotics must be present in the tissues at the time of bacterial contamination (incision) and throughout the operative period; "on-call" dosing is not acceptable.
    a. Administering antibiotics earlier than immediately preoperatively (within 60 minutes before incision or 60–120 minutes if using vancomycin or a fluoroquinolone) is unnecessary.
    b. Initiating antibiotics postoperatively is no more effective than administering no prophylaxis.
    c. Antibiotics should be redosed for extended surgical procedures.
    d. Redose if the surgery lasts longer than 4 hours (or more than 2 half-lives of the antibiotic) or involves considerable blood loss.

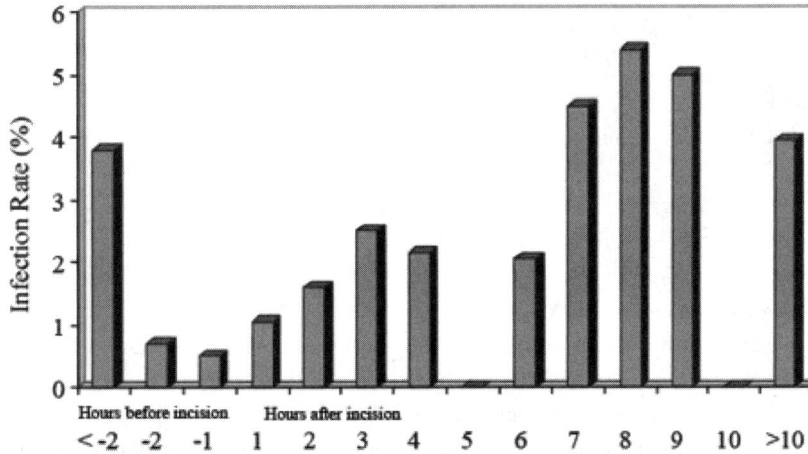

Figure 1. Principles of prophylaxis.

Information from Classen DC, Evans RS, Pestotnik SL, et al. The timing of prophylactic administration of antibiotics and the risk of surgical-wound infection. N Engl J Med 1992;326:281-6.

Table 18. Temporal Relation Between the Administration of Prophylactic Antibiotics and Rates of Surgical Wound Infection

Time of Administration[a]	No. of Patients	No. (%) of Infections	Relative Risk (95% CI)	Odds Ratio (95% CI)
Early	369	14 (3.8)	6.7 (2.9–14.7)	4.3 (1.8–10.4)
Preoperative	1708	10 (0.59)	1.0	
Perioperative	282	4 (1.4)	2.4 (0.9–7.9)	2.1 (0.6–7.4)
Postoperative	488	16 (3.3)	5.8 (2.6–12.3)	5.8 (2.4–13.8)
All	2847	44 (1.5)	—	—

[a]For administering antibiotics; "early" denotes 2–24 hours before the incision, "preoperative" 0–2 hours before the incision, "perioperative" within 3 hours after the incision, and "postoperative" more than 3 hours after the incision.

CI = confidence interval.

Table 19. Duration of Surgical Procedure and Risk of Infection

Duration of Surgical Procedure	Infections/Total Patients (%)	Infections/Standard Regimen Patients (%)	Infections/Cefoxitin Regimen Patients (%)
<3 hours	0/46	0/29	0/17
≥3 hours to ≤4 hours	4/46 (8.7)	2/21 (9.5)	2/25 (8.0)
>4 hours	5/27 (18.5)	0/13	5/14 (35.7)

Information from Kaiser AB, Herrington JL Jr, Jacobs JK, et al. Cefoxitin versus erythromycin, neomycin, and cefazolin in colorectal operations. Importance of the duration of the surgical procedure. Ann Surg 1983;98:525-30.

2. Duration
   a. Most procedures, including gastrointestinal, orthopedic, and gynecologic procedures, require antibiotics only as long as the patient is in the operating room; administration beyond surgical closure is not necessary.
   b. Cardiac procedures may require 24 hours of antibiotics after surgery.

3. Spectrum
   a. Need only activity against skin flora unless the operation violates a hollow viscus mucosa
   b. Gastrointestinal, genitourinary, hepatobiliary, and some pulmonary operations require additional antibiotics.
   c. Colorectal surgery is one procedure in which broad-spectrum aerobic and anaerobic coverage is most effective.
   d. Attempt to avoid a drug that may be needed for therapy if infection occurs.
4. Adverse reactions and bacterial resistance
   a. Antibiotic prophylaxis should not cause greater morbidity than the infection it prevents.
   b. Overuse may lead to resistance, which could prevent further use of the antibiotic for surgical prophylaxis or other infections (duration of administration is an important factor).
5. Cost
   a. Prophylaxis can account for a substantial portion of the antibiotic budget.
   b. Must be weighed against the cost of treating one person with a postoperative infection

F. Antibiotic Prophylaxis in Specific Surgical Procedures
   1. Gastrointestinal
      a. Gastric or duodenal
         i. Because of acidity, little normal flora
         ii. Rates of intragastric organisms and postoperative infections increase with increasing pH.
         iii. Indicated for morbid obesity, esophageal obstruction, decreased gastric acidity, or decreased gastrointestinal motility
         iv. Recommendation: Cefazolin 2 g before induction
      b. Biliary
         i. Biliary tract normally has no organisms.
         ii. Indicated for high-risk patients. (Often, intraoperative cholangiography shows unexpected common duct stones, so some studies recommend using antibiotics in all biliary surgery. In addition, studies have shown an increase in infection rates without risk factors.)
            (a) Acute cholecystitis
            (b) Obstructive jaundice
            (c) Common duct stones
            (d) Age older than 70 years
         iii. Recommendation: Cefazolin, cefoxitin, cefotetan, or ceftriaxone 2 g or ampicillin/sulbactam 3 g before induction
      c. Appendectomy
         i. Acutely inflamed or normal appendix: Less than 10% risk
         ii. Evidence of perforation: More than 50% risk (treatment necessary)
         iii. If perforated appendix, treat for 3–7 days
         iv. Recommendation: Cefoxitin or cefotetan 2 g (or cefazolin plus metronidazole) before induction
      d. Colorectal
         i. A 30%–77% infection rate without antibiotics
         ii. One of the few surgical procedures in which coverage for aerobes *and* anaerobes has proved most effective
         iii. Preoperative antibiotics
            (a) Combined oral and parenteral regimens may be better than parenteral regimens alone.
            (b) Oral regimens are inexpensive; however, some data suggest they are less effective when used alone (without parenteral agents), have greater toxicity, and may increase the risk of *C. difficile* infections.

        (c) Recommendation: Cefoxitin or cefotetan 2 g (or cefazolin or ceftriaxone plus metronidazole or ampicillin/sulbactam or ertapenem) before induction *or* gentamicin/tobramycin 5 mg/kg and clindamycin 900 mg–metronidazole 500 mg preinduction with or without neomycin 1 g and erythromycin 1 g at 19, 18, and 9 hours before surgery or neomycin 2 g and metronidazole 2 g at 13 and 9 hours before surgery

        (d) Mechanical bowel preparation is not recommended and may be harmful.

2. Obstetrics and gynecology
    a. Vaginal or abdominal hysterectomy
        i. Antibiotics are most effective in vaginal hysterectomies but generally are given for both procedures.
        ii. Recommendation: Cefazolin or cefoxitin or cefotetan 2 g (or ampicillin/sulbactam) before induction
    b. Cesarean section. Recommendation: Cefazolin 2 g after the cord is clamped

3. Cardiothoracic
    a. Cardiac surgery
        i. Antibiotics decrease the risk of mediastinitis.
        ii. Recommendation: Cefazolin or cefuroxime 2 g preinduction (plus intraoperative doses), if MRSA is probable or patient has been hospitalized, and then vancomycin
    b. Pulmonary resection (i.e., lobectomy and pneumonectomy). Recommendation: Cefazolin 2 g before induction (or ampicillin/sulbactam or vancomycin)
    c. Vascular surgery
        i. High mortality with infected grafts
        ii. Recommendation: Cefazolin 2 g before induction and every 8 hours for three doses; if MRSA is probable, then use vancomycin

4. Orthopedic
    a. Prophylaxis is indicated when surgery involves prosthetic materials (i.e., total hip or knee, nail, or plate).
    b. Recommendation: Cefazolin 2 g before induction (or vancomycin)

5. Head and neck
    a. Indicated for major surgical procedures when an incision is made through the oral or pharyngeal mucosa
    b. Recommendation: Cefazolin or cefuroxime 2 g plus metronidazole or ampicillin/sulbactam 3 g or clindamycin 900 mg before induction

6. Urologic
    a. In general, not recommended
    b. Indicated if patient has a positive urine culture before surgery (should treat and then operate)
    c. If therapy is unsuccessful, cover for the infecting organism and operate.

REFERENCES

Respiratory Tract Infections

1. Mandell LA, Wunderink RG, Anzueto A, et al. Infectious Diseases Society of America/American Thoracic Society consensus guidelines on the management of community-acquired pneumonia in adults. Clin Infect Dis 2007;44(suppl 2):S27-S72.

2. American Thoracic Society; Infectious Diseases Society of America. Guidelines for the management of adults with hospital-acquired, ventilator-associated, and healthcare-associated pneumonia. Am J Respir Crit Care Med 2005;171:388-416.

3. Centers for Disease Control and Prevention (CDC). Antiviral agents for the treatment and chemoprophylaxis of influenza: Recommendations of the Advisory Committee on Immunization Practices (ACIP). MMWR 2011;60:1-28.

4. Grohskopf LA, Olsen SJ, Sokolow LZ, et al.; Influenza Division, National Center for Immunization and Respiratory Diseases, CDC. Prevention and control of seasonal influenza with vaccines: recommendations of the Advisory Committee on Immunization Practices (ACIP)—United States, 2014–15 influenza season. MMWR Morb Mortal Wkly Rep 2014;63(32):691-7.

5. Chow AW, Benninger MS, Brook I, et al.; Infectious Diseases Society of America. IDSA clinical practice guideline for acute bacterial rhinosinusitis in children and adults. Clin Infect Dis 2012;54:e72-e112.

Urinary Tract Infections

1. Gupta K, Hooton TM, Naber KG, et al.; Infectious Diseases Society of America; European Society for Microbiology and Infectious Diseases. International clinical practice guidelines for the treatment of acute uncomplicated cystitis and pyelonephritis in women: a 2010 update by the Infectious Diseases Society of America and the European Society for Microbiology and Infectious Diseases. Clin Infect Dis 2011;52:e103-20.

Skin and Soft Tissue Infections

1. Stevens DL, Bisno AL, Chambers HF, et al. Practice guidelines for the diagnosis and management of skin and soft tissue infections: 2014 update by the Infectious Diseases Society of America. Clin Infect Dis 2014;XX:1-43.

2. Lipsky BA, Berendt AR, Cornia PB, et al.; Infectious Diseases Society of America. 2012 Infectious Diseases Society of America clinical practice guideline for the diagnosis and treatment of diabetic foot infections. Clin Infect Dis 2012;54:e132-73.

3. Liu C, Bayer A, Cosgrove SE, et al.; Infectious Diseases Society of America. Clinical practice guidelines by the Infectious Diseases Society of America for the treatment of methicillin-resistant *Staphylococcus aureus* infections in adults and children. Clin Infect Dis 2011;52:e18-55.

4. Stevens DL, Bisno AL, Chambers HF, et al. Practice guidelines for the diagnosis and management of skin and soft-tissue infections. Clin Infect Dis 2005;41:1373-406.

Osteomyelitis

1. Osmon DR, Berbari EF, Berendt AR, et al.; Infectious Diseases Society of America. Diagnosis and management of prosthetic joint infection: clinical practice guidelines by the Infectious Diseases Society of America. Clin Infect Dis 2013;56:e1-e25.

Central Nervous System Infections

1. Tunkel AR, Hartman BJ, Kaplan SL, et al. Practice guidelines for the management of bacterial meningitis. Clin Infect Dis 2004;39:1267-84.

Endocarditis

1. Baddour LM, Wilson WR, Bayer AS, et al. Infective endocarditis: diagnosis, antimicrobial therapy, and management of complications. Circulation 2005;111:3167-84.

2. Wilson W, Taubert KA, Gewitz M, et al. Prevention of infective endocarditis. Guidelines from the American Heart Association. Circulation 2007;115:1656-8.

Intra-abdominal Infections

1. Solomkin JS, Mazuski JE, Bradley JS, et al.; Infectious Diseases Society of America. Diagnosis and management of complicated intra-abdominal infection in adults and children: guidelines by the Surgical Infection Society and the Infectious Diseases Society of America. Clin Infect Dis 2010;50:133-64.

Clostridium difficile Infections

1. Cohen SH, Gerding DN, Johnson S, et al.; Society for Healthcare Epidemiology of America; Infectious Diseases Society of America. Clinical practice guidelines for *Clostridium difficile* infection in adults: 2010 update by the Society for Healthcare Epidemiology of America (SHEA) and the Infectious Diseases Society of America (IDSA). Infect Control Hosp Epidemiol 2010;31:431-55.

2. Surawicz CM, Brandt LJ, Binion DG, et al. Guidelines for diagnosis, treatment, and prevention of *Clostridium difficile* infections. Am J Gastroenterol 2013;108(4):478-98.

Medical and Surgical Prophylaxis

1. Bratzler DW, Dellinger EP, Olsen KM, et al. Surgical Infection Prevention Guidelines Writers Workgroup. Clinical practice guidelines for antimicrobial prophylaxis in surgery. Am J Health Syst Pharm 2013;70:195-283.

ANSWERS AND EXPLANATIONS TO PATIENT CASES

1. Answer: C

Although ampicillin/sulbactam has good activity against *H. influenzae, Moraxella catarrhalis,* and *S. pneumoniae* (but not drug-resistant *S. pneumoniae* [DRSP]), it has no activity against atypical organisms (*L. pneumophila, Mycoplasma pneumoniae, Chlamydia pneumoniae*). Current recommendations are to include a macrolide with a β-lactam antibiotic for hospitalized patients with community-acquired pneumonia (CAP). Piperacillin/tazobactam has good activity against *H. influenzae, M. catarrhalis,* and *S. pneumoniae* (but not DRSP) and, with gentamicin, is excellent for pneumonia caused by most gram-negative organisms. However, this increased activity is not necessary for CAP, and the combination has no activity against atypical organisms. Ceftriaxone plus azithromycin is the best initial choice. It has excellent activity against atypical organisms (because of azithromycin), *H. influenzae, M. catarrhalis,* and *S. pneumoniae* (even intermediate DRSP). Although doxycycline has activity against atypical organisms and most of the typical organisms that cause CAP, it is not recommended as monotherapy in hospitalized patients. In addition, its activity against *S. pneumoniae* may be limited (if the patient lives in an area with extensive DRSP). Doxycycline would not be the best initial choice.

2. Answer: D

Ceftriaxone plus gentamicin plus linezolid is not good empiric therapy because ceftriaxone has limited activity against *P. aeruginosa,* and gentamicin has variable activity against *P. aeruginosa,* depending on the institution. Because the patient has been on a ventilator and in an intensive care unit for 8 days, she is at increased risk of nosocomial pneumonia, specifically caused by *P. aeruginosa* (and possibly MRSA, depending on the institution). Although piperacillin/tazobactam has good activity against most common causes of nosocomial pneumonia (including *P. aeruginosa*), the most recent guidelines recommend two antibiotics with activity against *P. aeruginosa* for patients with severe nosocomial pneumonia, and she may require an antibiotic with MRSA activity. Levofloxacin has only moderate activity against *P. aeruginosa,* and two drugs should be used. Cefepime plus tobramycin plus vancomycin is the best empiric therapy because it includes two antibiotics with excellent activity against *P. aeruginosa* and another agent for MRSA.

3. Answer: B

This patient should receive vaccinations now. There are no contraindications to receiving either pneumococcal or influenza vaccine immediately after an episode of pneumonia. It is best to vaccinate whenever patients are available. This patient's age and medical history put her at risk of both pneumococcal disease and influenza. Therefore, administration of pneumococcal and influenza vaccines is indicated (if it is during the middle of influenza season and she was not vaccinated in the fall, she can receive the influenza vaccine now). The patient's age places her in a group needing the pneumococcal vaccine, and everyone should receive the influenza vaccine. The causative agent for her current infection does not affect the recommendation for vaccination.

4. Answer: B

Although the treatment duration is correct for this patient's diagnosis (7 days), oral trimethoprim/sulfamethoxazole is inappropriate for complicated pyelonephritis. It will also interact with warfarin, increasing the risk of bleeding. Ciprofloxacin 400 mg intravenously twice daily and then 500 mg orally twice daily for 10 days is an appropriate choice and duration (7–14 days) for this complicated pyelonephritis (it may also interact with warfarin but to a lesser extent than trimethoprim/sulfamethoxazole). It would be expected to have activity against the common organisms causing complicated pyelonephritis. Gentamicin for 3 days is too short a treatment duration, and tigecycline, followed by doxycycline, is not recommended for complicated pyelonephritis (although tigecycline is found unchanged in the urine).

5. Answer: D

Diabetic foot infections are generally polymicrobial (average organisms, 2.5–5.8).

6. Answer: C

Nafcillin has excellent activity against gram-positive organisms, but it would miss the gram-negative organisms and anaerobes often involved in moderate to severe diabetic foot infections. Tobramycin and levofloxacin would be good against aerobic organisms, but levofloxacin has only limited activity against anaerobes. Tobramycin may also not be a good choice for a patient with diabetes mellitus with long-term complications (because of the increased risk of nephrotoxicity). β-Lactamase inhibitor combinations are good agents because they have activity against the organisms that are often involved. At this time, a regimen active against *P. aeruginosa* is probably not necessary. Treatment duration may need to be extended if the bone is involved. Aggressive antibiotic treatment often prevents the need for an amputation.

7. Answer: A

Because sensitivities of the gram-positive organism are still unknown, vancomycin is the best choice. In addition, the therapy duration for osteomyelitis is 4–6 weeks. Therefore, the 2-week duration with nafcillin is too short. Although levofloxacin is advantageous because it can be given orally, it will probably not achieve adequate bone concentrations to eradicate *S. aureus* (the most likely organism). Ampicillin/sulbactam is effective against *S. aureus* (except for MRSA); its broad spectrum of activity is not necessary in this situation, and the duration is too short.

8. Answer: B

From his presentation and laboratory values, this patient has bacterial meningitis. The gram-negative cocci on Gram stain are probably *N. meningitidis*. Penicillin is effective against *N. meningitidis;* however, some strains are resistant, and until culture results are received, it is unwise to use this agent alone. Ceftriaxone alone is effective for meningococcal meningitis, and this is the best answer (although some may continue to use vancomycin until the cultures actually grow *N. meningitidis*). Dexamethasone is beneficial only in adults with pneumococcal meningitis (not meningococcal meningitis). Ceftriaxone is the appropriate empiric antibiotic therapy in this situation. Vancomycin is generally used empirically because of its activity against highly penicillin-resistant *S. pneumoniae*. Because this is probably not pneumococcal meningitis, vancomycin can be discontinued.

9. Answer: A

Only people in close contact to a patient with meningococcal meningitis require prophylaxis (primarily those who live closely with the patient and those who are exposed to oral secretions). The correct regimen is rifampin 600 mg every 12 hours for four doses. Although the vaccine is a good idea for those at future risk of acquiring this infection (e.g., college students living in dormitories), its use during an outbreak is very limited.

10. Answer: D

The treatment duration in Answer A is too short (nafcillin intravenously × 2 weeks) for *S. aureus* endocarditis. Only streptococcal endocarditis can be treated for 2 weeks. Although nafcillin intravenously plus rifampin therapy for 6 weeks or longer is an appropriate duration for MSSA, the rifampin does not need to be added in patients with native valve endocarditis. Nafcillin intravenously plus gentamicin intravenously × 2 weeks is too short for *S. aureus* endocarditis. Nafcillin intravenously × 6 weeks with gentamicin for the first 3–5 days is the recommended treatment for MSSA endocarditis. Gentamicin should be added for 3–5 days to decrease the duration of bacteremia.

11. Answer: B

This patient is at increased risk of endocarditis because of his history of the disease. Tooth extractions require prophylaxis for those at risk. Amoxicillin 2 g, 1 hour before the tooth extraction, is the current recommended dose. The 2-g dose is adequate for protection, and a follow-up dose is not needed. Amoxicillin 3 g, 1 hour before the extraction, and 1.5 g, 6 hours for four doses after the extraction, is the older recommended dose. A follow-up dose is not needed.

12. Answer: A

Redosing antibiotics for surgical prophylaxis is very important, especially for antibiotics with short half-lives, for extended surgical procedures, or for when there is extensive blood loss. Antibiotics given beyond the surgical procedure are generally unnecessary and only increase the potential for adverse drug reactions and resistant bacteria. Although preoperative antibiotics given up to 4 hours before the incision may improve the logistics of administering surgical prophylaxis, study results show that antibiotics must be given as close to the time of the incision as possible (definitely within 2 hours). Vancomycin should not be used routinely for surgical prophylaxis. The Centers for Disease Control and Prevention does not recommend the use of vancomycin for "routine surgical prophylaxis other than in a patient with life-threatening allergy to β-lactam antibiotics."

ANSWERS AND EXPLANATIONS TO SELF-ASSESSMENT QUESTIONS

1. Answer: A

The patient has CAP that does not require hospitalization (CURB-65 score is 1 at most [no mention of mental status]). Because he has not received any antibiotics in the past 3 months and has no comorbidities, he is at low risk of DRSP. Therefore, the drug of choice is either a macrolide or doxycycline. Cefuroxime is not recommended for treatment of CAP. Fluoroquinolones are recommended only if the patient has had recent antibiotics or has comorbidities. Trimethoprim/sulfamethoxazole is not used for CAP.

2. Answer: D

The symptoms of this patient (high temperature, malaise, dry cough, nasal congestion, and severe headaches) are most consistent with influenza; therefore, an antibacterial agent would not affect recovery. Oseltamivir should be initiated within 48 hours of symptom onset, so because this patient is more than 3 days out from symptom onset, oseltamivir will not affect recovery. Because of the viral etiology and time since symptom onset, symptomatic treatment is all that is indicated.

3. Answer: B

A case-control study would be the most appropriate study design because it is the most ethical, cost-effective, timely method. A stronger study design—for instance, a prospective cohort study or a randomized controlled trial—has many disadvantages if used to answer this question. In a prospective cohort study, too many patients would need to be observed because of the low incidence of confirmed pneumococcal pneumonia. This study would therefore be too costly and take too long to complete. Randomized controlled trials also have many disadvantages in this situation. First, patients would need to be vaccinated and then observed for at least 10 years. Second, too many patients would need to be observed because of the low incidence of confirmed pneumococcal pneumonia. Third, it would be unethical to randomly assign half the patients to no vaccination. This study would therefore be too costly, unethical, and time-consuming. A case series would evaluate only a few patients given a diagnosis of pneumococcal pneumonia 10 or more years after vaccination. It would not provide comparative data, nor would it provide a strong study design.

4. Answer: C

This patient has symptoms suggestive of bacterial sinusitis, including two major symptoms and a few minor symptoms. The fact that the symptoms improved and then worsened suggests a bacterial sinusitis that followed a viral infection. Although the combination of cefpodoxime and clindamycin is an option for sinusitis in penicillin-allergic patients, it is not recommended to give either of these alone for treatment. The best option is amoxicillin/clavulanate, which has activity against organisms commonly seen in bacterial sinusitis and is considered a first-line agent.

5. Answer: C

Although nitrofurantoin is a recommended first-line agent, the therapy duration is too short for its use. Because this patient has no contraindications to the use of trimethoprim/sulfamethoxazole or nitrofurantoin, and trimethoprim/sulfamethoxazole resistance rates are not mentioned as being high, fluoroquinolones would not be considered appropriate as first-line therapy in this particular case. In addition, 7 days of therapy is not necessary. The best choice for this patient is trimethoprim/sulfamethoxazole double strength twice daily orally for 3 days. The patient should be counseled about the potential interaction between antibiotics and oral contraceptives. β-Lactams are not as effective as trimethoprim/sulfamethoxazole, and data are limited on their use for 3 days.

6. Answer: A

For the asymptomatic patient who is bedridden and chronically catheterized, with cloudy urine and bacteria shown by urinalysis, no therapy is indicated. All patients with chronic urinary catheters will be bacteriuric. Because this patient is asymptomatic, the catheter does not need to be replaced. If she were symptomatic, catheter replacement might be indicated. Antibiotics are not indicated; however, a 7-day course would be appropriate if treatment were instituted. A long course of treatment only increases the risk of acquiring resistant organisms.

7. Answer: A

Because cellulitis (which the patient appears to have) is usually caused by *Streptococcus* or *Staphylococcus*, nafcillin is the drug of choice (vancomycin could be initiated empirically if MRSA were a concern in this patient). Necrotizing fasciitis must be ruled out because other organisms may be involved, and surgery would be crucial. Although penicillin is the treatment of choice for erysipelas, the patient probably has acute cellulitis (there is no raised border at the edge of the infection, which is indicative of erysipelas). Although piperacillin/tazobactam has activity against both *Streptococcus* and *Staphylococcus,* this treatment is too broad spectrum for an acute cellulitis. Because Doppler studies are negative, the likelihood of a deep venous thrombosis is low.

8. Answer: C

Even if a patient is believed to have aseptic meningitis after analysis of the CSF, antibiotics must be given until CSF cultures are negative. In empiric therapy for bacterial meningitis in adults (i.e., when the CSF Gram stain is negative), ceftriaxone should be used in combination with vancomycin. The vancomycin is necessary for activity against resistant *S. pneumoniae.* Although the symptoms and CSF results are similar to what is expected for herpes simplex encephalitis, the use of acyclovir alone in this patient is inappropriate. Antibacterials must be used as well. Viral meningitis is generally caused by coxsackie virus, echovirus, and enterovirus, which are not treated with acyclovir.

9. Answer: C

Enterococcal endocarditis should be treated for 4–6 weeks. The 2-week treatment regimen is indicated only for streptococcal endocarditis. There is also no indication that the patient is penicillin allergic; thus, vancomycin should not be used as first-line treatment. Ampicillin plus gentamicin for 4–6 weeks is the regimen of choice for penicillin-susceptible enterococcal endocarditis. Cephalosporins have no activity against *Enterococcus;* therefore, the regimen with cefazolin is inappropriate.

10. Answer: C

A perforated appendix requires antibiotics after surgery for an intra-abdominal infection. The combination of vancomycin and metronidazole does not have adequate activity against aerobic, gram-negative organisms (e.g., *E. coli*). The combination of ceftriaxone and ciprofloxacin does not have adequate activity against anaerobic organisms (e.g., *B. fragilis* group). Ertapenem is a good choice for intra-abdominal infections, although it has limited activity against *Enterococcus.*

HIV/Infectious Diseases

Curtis L. Smith, Pharm.D., BCPS

Ferris State University
Lansing, Michigan

HIV/Infectious Diseases

Curtis L. Smith, Pharm.D., BCPS

Ferris State University
Lansing, Michigan

Learning Objectives

1. Formulate an appropriate regimen to prevent or treat human immunodeficiency virus infections, including initiation and monitoring therapy.
2. Discuss appropriate treatment of the various acquired immunodeficiency syndrome opportunistic infections, including primary and secondary prophylaxis.
3. Describe appropriate treatment and preventive therapy for tuberculosis, including infections with drug-resistant organisms.
4. Classify the various antifungal agents and explain their role in common fungal infections.

Self-Assessment Questions

Answers and explanations to these questions can be found at the end of this chapter.

1. K.E. is a 29-year-old asymptomatic patient who is human immunodeficiency virus (HIV) positive. She recently found out she is pregnant and is estimated to be early in her first trimester. Her most recent CD4 count was 170 cells/mm^3, and her viral load was 100,000 copies/mL by reverse transcriptase polymerase chain reaction. Which is the best therapy for K.E. to prevent HIV transmission to her child?

   A. No drug therapy is needed; the risks to the fetus outweigh any benefits.

   B. Administer zidovudine 300 mg twice daily orally throughout the pregnancy, followed by zidovudine during labor and consequently to the baby for 6 weeks.

   C. No drug therapy is required now, but administer a single dose of nevirapine at the onset of labor.

   D. Administer a potent combination antiretroviral therapy (ART) regimen that includes zidovudine throughout the pregnancy.

2. R.E. is a 33-year-old man who has been HIV positive since 2005. Recently, his CD4 counts started to decrease significantly, and his viral load started to increase. He is initiated on tenofovir, emtricitabine, and atazanavir/ritonavir. Which is the best counseling for R.E.?

   A. Watch for yellowing of the skin and eyes because atazanavir can cause hyperbilirubinemia.

   B. If you think you are having a drug-related adverse effect, cut the dose of all of your drugs in half.

   C. Talk to your pharmacist about drug interactions because both atazanavir and tenofovir inhibit cytochrome P450 (CYP) 3A4.

   D. Tenofovir and emtricitabine cause additive peripheral neuropathy, so let your pharmacist know if you experience tingling in your extremities.

3. One year later, R.E. is concerned that his ART is not working and asks whether he should make some changes. Which statement best represents what to tell him?

   A. His therapy should be changed only if he is deteriorating clinically (e.g., having more opportunistic infections).

   B. His therapy should be changed if his viral load increases significantly after initial suppression to undetectable concentrations.

   C. If he is concerned about his regimen not being effective, then atazanavir/ritonavir should be changed to fosamprenavir/ritonavir.

   D. Resistance usually occurs with emtricitabine, so this should be changed to lamivudine.

4. F.V. is a 46-year-old man who has been HIV positive for 15 years. He has been receiving potent combination ART for the past 5 years, including zidovudine, lamivudine, and lopinavir/ritonavir. He is now experiencing hyperglycemia, fat redistribution, and lipid abnormalities. Which is the best management strategy for F.V.'s drug-related symptoms?

   A. Change regimen to tenofovir, emtricitabine, and rilpivirine.

   B. Change regimen to abacavir, lamivudine, and raltegravir.

   C. Add simvastatin for the lipid abnormalities and treat according to the recommendations from the National Cholesterol Education Program.

D. Add pioglitazone for the glucose abnormalities and treat according to the recommendations from the American Diabetes Association.

5. P.P., a 43-year-old man who is HIV positive, presents to the clinic with a headache that has gradually worsened during the past 2 weeks. He does not feel very sick and has not experienced any focal seizures. His most recent CD4 count was 35 cells/mm^3. His laboratory profile is performed with the following results: Gram stain negative, white blood cell count 2 cells/mm^3, protein 35 mg/dL, glucose 75 mg/dL (peripheral 110 mg/dL), India ink positive, and cryptococcal antigen 1:1024. Which is the best therapy for P.P.?

A. Fluconazole 200 mg/day orally for 8 weeks.

B. Amphotericin B deoxycholate 0.3 mg/kg/day alone for 2 weeks.

C. Amphotericin B deoxycholate 0.3 mg/kg/day plus flucytosine 37.5 mg/kg every 6 hours for 4 weeks.

D. Amphotericin B deoxycholate 0.7 mg/kg/day plus flucytosine 25 mg/kg every 6 hours for 2 weeks, followed by fluconazole 400 mg/day for 8 weeks.

6. A study is performed to compare the incidence of active tuberculosis (TB) infection in patients receiving isoniazid versus rifampin for latent TB infection. After completing therapy (6 months for isoniazid and 4 months for rifampin), 0.3% in the isoniazid group and 0.8% in the rifampin group progress to active disease. Which best represents how many patients would need to be treated with isoniazid over rifampin to prevent one progression to active disease?

A. 5.

B. 50.

C. 200.

D. Insufficient information to calculate this number.

7. G.T. is a 34-year-old woman positive for HIV who is brought to the emergency department by her boyfriend after experiencing headaches, a change in mental status, and loss of feeling on her right side. A computed tomographic scan shows two large ring-enhancing lesions in her brain. Her most recent CD4 count was 85 cells/mm^3, but that was 4 months ago. She currently takes no antiretroviral agents but does take dapsone for *Pneumocystis jiroveci* pneumonia (PCP) prophylaxis. Which is the best therapy for G.T.?

A. Atovaquone for 4–6 weeks.

B. High-dose trimethoprim/sulfamethoxazole plus clindamycin for 6 weeks.

C. Pyrimethamine plus sulfadiazine for 6 weeks.

D. Pyrimethamine plus clindamycin and leucovorin for 6 weeks.

8. H.Y., a 49-year-old man with acute myeloid leukemia is given a diagnosis of TB and initiated on empiric therapy with rifampin, isoniazid, ethambutol, and pyrazinamide. Three months into his TB therapy, he is hospitalized and given a diagnosis of aspergillosis; treatment is needed in addition to his TB treatment. Which is the best antifungal to use in H.Y.?

A. Fluconazole.

B. Voriconazole.

C. Flucytosine.

D. Micafungin.

9. P.I. is a 35-year-old woman who presents to the clinic with a 2-week history of night sweats, fatigue, weight loss, and a persistent cough. A purified protein derivative (PPD) is placed, and a sputum sample is taken; then, P.I. is sent home with a prescription for levofloxacin 750 mg/day orally. Two days later, her PPD is measured at 20-mm induration, and her sputum sample is positive for acid-fast bacilli. P.I., who has no pertinent medical history, has never been outside the United States. She lives in an area with an extremely low incidence of multidrug-resistant TB. Which regimen is the best therapy for P.I.?

A. Isoniazid 300 mg/day orally for 6 months.

B. Isoniazid, rifampin, pyrazinamide, and ethambutol for 2 months, followed by isoniazid and rifampin for 4 more months.

C. Isoniazid and rifampin for 6 months.

D. Levofloxacin 750 mg/day orally for both TB and other bacterial causes of pneumonia.

10. A prospective, double-blind study compared the effects of two therapies—a potent combination ART with a ritonavir-boosted protease inhibitor (PI) and a potent combination ART with efavirenz—in 350 patients with HIV. Which is the best statistical test to use to compare end points such as the mean change in viral load or mean change in CD4 counts?

    A. Analysis of variance.

    B. Chi-square test.

    C. Student t-test.

    D. Wilcoxon rank sum test.

I. HUMAN IMMUNODEFICIENCY VIRUS

A. Transmission of HIV
  1. Sexual transmission
     a. Homosexual or heterosexual
     b. Increases with increased number of sexual partners
     c. Prevention
        i. Latex condom
        ii. Circumcision (males)
        iii. Preexposure prophylaxis
            (a) Use in those who are at substantial risk of acquiring HIV, including anyone in an ongoing relationship with an HIV-positive partner; anyone who is not in a mutually monogamous relationship with an HIV-negative partner and is either a gay or bisexual man who has had anal sex without a condom or been diagnosed with an STD in the past 6 months or a heterosexual man or woman who does not regularly use condoms during sex with partners of unknown HIV status who are at substantial risk of HIV infection; anyone who injects illicit drugs in the past 6 months and who have shared injection equipment or been in drug treatment in the past 6 months.
            (b) Document negative HIV antibody.
            (c) Use tenofovir 300 mg plus emtricitabine 200 mg (Truvada) daily.
            (d) Test every 90 days for HIV antibody (and if prophylaxis is discontinued).
  2. Parenteral exposure to blood or blood products
     a. Intravenous drug abuser: Increased with increased needle sharing
     b. Hemophiliacs and blood transfusion recipients: Decreased since 1985
  3. Universal precautions (Table 1)
     a. Purpose is prevention of parenteral, mucous membrane, and nonintact skin exposures to blood-borne pathogens
     b. Bodily fluids

Table 1. Universal Precautions

Universal Precautions Apply to:	Universal Precautions Do Not Apply to:
Blood	Feces
Bodily fluids containing visible blood	Nasal secretions
Semen and vaginal secretions	Sputum
Tissue	Sweat
Cerebrospinal fluid	Tears
Synovial fluid	Urine
Pleural fluid	Vomitus
Peritoneal fluid	Breast milk
Pericardial fluid	Saliva (precautions recommended for dentistry)
Amniotic fluid	

     c. General guidelines
        i. Take care when using and disposing of needles, scalpels, and other sharp instruments.
        ii. Use protective barriers (i.e., gloves, masks, and protective eyewear).
        iii. Wash hands and skin immediately if they are contaminated with body fluids to which universal precautions apply.

4. Perinatal transmission
    a. Antepartum: Through maternal circulation
    b. During delivery
    c. Postpartum: Breastfeeding
    d. Zidovudine therapy decreases risk of transmission from 23% to 3%–4% (less than 2% with combination therapy).

B. Diagnosis
    1. Step 1
        a. Fourth-generation HIV test
        b. Positive: 2–3 weeks after the infection
        c. Negative tests require no further testing; positive tests proceed to step 2.
        d. Sensitivity and specificity: Greater than 99%
        e. Fourth-generation tests: Abbott Architect HIV Ag/Ab Combo Assay; Bio-Rad GS HIV Combo Ag/Ab EIA
    2. Step 2
        a. HIV test that differentiates HIV-1 from HIV-2
        b. If positive: Diagnosis made
        c. If negative or indeterminate: Proceed to step 3
        d. Sensitivity and specificity: Greater than 99%
        e. Multispot HIV-1/HIV-0 Rapid Test
    3. Step 3
        a. HIV-1 nucleic acid amplification test (screening for HIV-1 RNA)
        b. If positive: Diagnosis made
        c. If negative: Negative for HIV-1
        d. HIV-1 NAT tests: APTIMA HIV-1 RNA Qualitative Assay; Procleix Ultrio
    4. Test for HIV RNA
        a. Detects HIV RNA in serum (tests for the virus, not for antibodies)
        b. Branched-chain DNA, Versant (Siemens)
            i. Signal amplification
            ii. Sensitive to 75 copies/mL of HIV RNA
        c. Reverse transcriptase polymerase chain reaction, Amplicor HIV-1 Monitor (Roche) or Abbott RealTime HIV-1 (Abbott): Sensitive to 50 copies/mL of HIV RNA
        d. Nucleic acid sequence–based amplification, NucliSens (bioMérieux): Sensitive to 40 copies/mL of HIV RNA
        e. Values expressed as copies of HIV RNA per milliliter or the log of copies of HIV RNA per milliliter
        f. For all tests, less than 200 copies/mL is considered undetectable.
        g. Changes greater than threefold (about 0.5 log) are clinically significant.
    5. Use of HIV RNA testing (viral load)
        a. Most important use of the viral load is to monitor the effectiveness of therapy after initiation of antiretroviral therapy (ART).
        b. Newly diagnosed HIV infection (for baseline value to follow)
        c. Every 3–6 months without therapy (also check CD4 count)
        d. From 2 to 4 (no more than 8) weeks after starting or changing therapy (should detect a significant decrease)
        e. Every 3–6 months while on therapy (checking for increase—therapy failure); (also check CD4 count)
        f. Whenever there is a clinical event or decrease in CD4 count

6. Who should be screened for HIV?
   a. All patients 13–64 years of age (in all health care settings)
   b. Adults and adolescents at high risk of HIV infection should be checked annually (intravenous drug users, those who have unprotected sex with several partners, men who have sex with men, men or women who have sex for money or drugs, people being treated for sexually transmitted diseases, recipients of several blood transfusions 1975–1985)
   c. Pregnant women
7. CD4 T-cell count
   a. Measure of immune function, used to determine the timing of ART, opportunistic infection prophylaxis, disease progression, and survival
   b. Normal values: 500–1300 cells/mm^3
   c. Changes greater than 30% in CD4 counts are considered clinically significant.
   d. CD4 counts decrease, on average, 50–80 cells/mm^3 per year in untreated HIV-infected patients.
   e. With potent combination ART, CD4 counts increase, on average, 50–100 cells/mm^3 per year.
   f. Monitor at diagnosis (baseline), after ART is started to guide discontinuation of opportunistic infection prophylaxis, every 12 months for those consistently on therapy and with CD4 counts between 300 and 500 cells/mm^3 for at least 2 years, and optional if CD4 is greater than 500 cells/mm^3 in those virologically suppressed for at least 2 years. More frequent monitoring (every 3 to 6 months) may be needed based on clinical symptoms and viral load testing.
8. Case definition for HIV, 2008 (Table 2)

Table 2. Case Definition for HIV, 2008

Stage	Laboratory Evidence[a]	Clinical Evidence
Stage 1	Laboratory confirmation of HIV infection *and* CD4 count of ≥500/μL *or* CD4 percentage of ≥29	None required (but no AIDS-defining condition)
Stage 2	Laboratory confirmation of HIV infection *and* CD4 count of 200–499/μL *or* CD4 percentage of ≥14–28	None required (but no AIDS-defining condition)
Stage 3 (AIDS)	Laboratory confirmation of HIV infection *and* CD4 count of <200/μL *or* CD4 percentage of <14	*Or* documentation of an AIDS-defining condition (with laboratory confirmation of HIV infection)
Stage unknown	Laboratory confirmation of HIV infection *and* No information on CD4 count or percentage	*And* no information on presence of AIDS-defining conditions

[a]Laboratory confirmation: Positive result from an HIV antibody screening test (e.g., reactive enzyme immunoassay) confirmed by a positive result from a supplemental HIV antibody test (e.g., Western blot or indirect immunofluorescence assay test) *or* positive result or report of a detectable quantity (i.e., within the established limits of the laboratory test) from any of the following HIV virologic (i.e., nonantibody) tests.

9. Acquired immunodeficiency syndrome (AIDS)-defining conditions (Table 3)

Table 3. AIDS-Defining Conditions

Bacterial infections, multiple or recurrent (<13 years)	Lymphoid interstitial pneumonia or pulmonary
Candidiasis: bronchi, trachea, or lungs	lymphoid hyperplasia complex (<13 years)
Candidiasis: esophageal	Lymphoma: Burkitt (or equivalent term)
Cervical cancer: invasive	Lymphoma: immunoblastic (or equivalent term)
Coccidioidomycosis: disseminated or extrapulmonary	Lymphoma: primary or brain
Cryptococcosis: extrapulmonary	*Mycobacterium avium* complex or *M. kansasii:*
Cryptosporidiosis: chronic intestinal (>1 month in duration)	disseminated or extrapulmonary
Cytomegalovirus disease (other than liver, spleen, or nodes)	*M. tuberculosis:* any site (pulmonary or
Cytomegalovirus retinitis (with loss of vision)	extrapulmonary)
Encephalopathy: HIV related	*Mycobacterium:* other species or unidentified
Herpes simplex: chronic ulcer(s) (>1 month in duration);	species; disseminated or extrapulmonary
bronchitis, pneumonitis, or esophagitis	*Pneumocystis jirovecii* pneumonia
Histoplasmosis: disseminated or extrapulmonary	Pneumonia: recurrent
Isosporiasis: chronic intestinal (>1 month in duration)	Progressive multifocal leukoencephalopathy
Kaposi sarcoma	*Salmonella septicemia* (recurrent)
	Toxoplasmosis of brain
	Wasting syndrome caused by HIV

C. Primary HIV Infection
1. Characteristics of the primary HIV infection
   a. About 40%–60% develop symptoms from the primary infection.
   b. Abrupt onset: Duration 3–14 days
   c. Occurs 5 days to 3 months after HIV exposure (generally within 2–4 weeks)
   d. Fevers, sweats, lethargy, malaise, myalgias, arthralgias, headache, photophobia, diarrhea, sore throat, lymphadenopathy
   e. Treatment of an acute HIV infection is generally not recommended.
2. Progression of HIV
   a. HIV replicates actively at all stages of the infection.
   b. 10^9 to 10^{10} virions are produced every day.
   c. Half-life of virions is about 6 hours.
3. Immunization of patients with HIV (no live virus vaccines if CD4 count is less than 200 cells/mm^3)
   a. Influenza virus vaccine: Annually before the influenza season
   b. Pneumococcal vaccine: Once (ideally, before CD4 count is less than 200 cells/mm^3)
   c. Hepatitis B vaccine: For all susceptible patients
   d. Hepatitis A vaccine: For all at-risk patients

D. Treatment of HIV
1. Reverse transcriptase inhibitors (RTIs) (nucleoside [NRTIs], nucleotide, and nonnucleoside [NNRTIs])
   a. Reverse transcriptase: Enzyme required to copy viral RNA to DNA
   b. See Tables 4 and 5 for RTI characteristics.
2. Protease inhibitors (PIs)
   a. Protease: Enzyme required to cleave polyproteins into mature viral protein components
   b. See Table 6 for PI characteristics.
3. Entry inhibitors (Table 7)
   a. Block binding and entry of the virus into human cells
   b. See Table 7 for entry inhibitor characteristics.
4. Integrase inhibitors (INSTIs) (Table 7)
   a. Integrase: Enzyme required for integration of viral DNA into the host cellular genome
   b. See Table 7 for INSTI characteristics.
5. Prevention of maternal-fetal transmission
   a. Pregnant women with HIV receiving no ART
      i. Women who meet the criteria for beginning HIV therapy in adults should receive a potent three-drug combination ART (to prevent resistance); initiate therapy as soon as possible, even in the first trimester.
      ii. Women who do not meet the criteria for beginning HIV therapy should still receive potent combination ART (to prevent transmission); delay therapy until after first trimester, but no later than 28 weeks' gestation, though earlier therapy can be considered.
      iii. Use zidovudine as a component of therapy unless there is severe toxicity or resistance, or unless the woman is already on a fully suppressive regimen.
      iv. Avoid efavirenz in women of childbearing age to prevent first-trimester exposure.
      v. Women who have received ART in the past but who are currently on no therapy should have HIV antiretroviral resistance testing completed before starting therapy.
      vi. Continue combination regimen through the intrapartum period (with zidovudine infusion added) and treat baby for 6 weeks.
   b. Pregnant women with HIV receiving potent combination ART
      i. Continue current combination regimens (preferably with zidovudine) if already receiving therapy. Avoid efavirenz in the first trimester.
      ii. Continue combination regimen through intrapartum period (with zidovudine infusion added) and treat baby for 6 weeks.
   c. Pregnant women with HIV in labor (with or without therapy during pregnancy)
      i. At labor, zidovudine 2 mg/kg intravenously for 1 hour, followed by a 1-mg/kg/hour infusion until cord is clamped. Discontinue oral zidovudine but continue any other oral antiretrovirals (except for stavudine).
      ii. Continue ART as much as possible during labor.
   d. Infants born to mothers who are HIV positive
      i. Zidovudine 4-mg/kg/dose every 12 hours for 6 weeks
      ii. Infants born to mothers who did not receive antiretrovirals during pregnancy: Zidovudine for 6 weeks (see dose above) plus nevirapine 8–12 mg/dose (based on weight) at birth, 48 hours later, and 96 hours after second dose

6. Prevention of postexposure infection
    a. Use universal precautions.
    b. Nonoccupational exposures: Treat if exposure of vagina, rectum, eye, mouth, mucous membrane, or nonintact skin with blood, semen, vaginal secretions, or breast milk of a person with a known HIV infection
    c. Occupational exposures: Needlesticks or cuts (1 in 300 risk) and mucous membrane exposure (1 in 1000 risk)
    d. Postexposure prophylaxis can reduce HIV infection by about 80%.
    e. Nonoccupational exposures: Begin within 72 hours.
    f. Occupational exposures: Begin treatment within hours; if HIV status of source patient is unknown, start treatment while status is being evaluated.
    g. Treatment should be administered for 4 weeks.
    h. Recommended therapy for nonoccupational exposure is potent combination ART.
    i. Regimens for occupational postexposure prophylaxis
        i. Preferred regimen: raltegravir *plus* tenofovir/emtricitabine
        ii. Alternative regimens
            (a) One of the following agents: raltegravir, darunavir/ritonavir, etravirine, rilpivirine, atazanavir/ritonavir, or lopinavir/ritonavir *plus* one of the following combinations: tenofovir/emtricitabine, tenofovir/lamivudine, zidovudine/lamivudine, or zidovudine/emtricitabine *or*
            (b) Elvitegravir, cobicistat, tenofovir, emtricitabine (Stribild)

Table 4. Nucleoside RTIs

	Abacavir (ABC) (Ziagen, Epzicom, Trizivir, Triumeq)	Didanosine (ddI) (Videx)	Emtricitabine (FTC) (Emtriva, Truvada, Atripla, Complera, Stribild)	Lamivudine (3TC) (Epivir, Combivir, Epzicom, Trizivir, Triumeq)	Stavudine (d4T) (Zerit)	Zidovudine (ZDV) (AZT, Retrovir, Combivir, Trizivir)
Form	300-mg tablets 20 mg/mL liquid Trizivir: 300 mg of ABC/ 150 mg of 3TC/300 mg of ZDV Triumeq: 600 mg of ABC, 50 mg of DTG, 300 mg of 3TC Epzicom (see Lamivudine)	125-, 200-, 250-, 400-mg enteric-coated capsules 10-mg/mL solution	200-mg capsules 10 mg/mL liquid Truvada: 200 mg of FTC/300 mg of TDF Atripla (see Efavirenz) Complera (see Rilpivirine) Stribild (see Elvitegravir)	150-, 300-mg tablets 10 mg/mL liquid Combivir: 150 mg of 3TC/300 mg of ZDV Epzicom: 300 mg of 3TC/600 mg of ABC Trizivir (see Abacavir)	15-, 20-, 30-, 40-mg capsules 1 mg/mL solution	100-mg capsules, 300-mg tablets 50 mg/5 mL liquid 10 mg/mL injection
Dosing	300 mg BID or 600 mg/day[a]	>60 kg: 200 mg BID or 400 mg/day[b] ≤60 kg: 125 mg BID or 250 mg/day[b]	200 mg/day or 240 mg liquid/day[b]	150 mg BID or 300 mg/day[b] <50 kg: 4 mg/kg BID[b]	>60 kg: 40 mg BID[b] ≤60 kg: 30 mg BID[b]	200 mg TID or 300 mg BID[b]
Oral bioavailability	82%	40% Empty stomach	93%	86%	86%	60%
Serum half-life	1½ hours	1½ hours	10 hours	5–7 hours	1 hour	1.1 hours
Intracellular half-life	12–26 hours	>20 hours	>20 hours	18–22 hours	7½ hours	7 hours
Elimination	Metabolized by alcohol dehydrogenase and glucuronyl transferase Metabolites; renal	Renal excretion 50%	Renal excretion (86%)	Renally excreted unchanged (70%)	Renal excretion 50%	Metabolized to ZDV glucuronide (GZDV) Renal excretion of GZDV
Major toxicity (Note: All may cause lactic acidosis with hepatic steatosis)	Hypersensitivity, fever, rash, GI symptoms, malaise, fatigue, anorexia, and myocardial infarction	Pancreatitis (5%) Peripheral neuropathy (35%) Nausea, diarrhea	Diarrhea, nausea, headache, rash, and hyperpigmentation	Diarrhea, nausea, abdominal pain, insomnia, and headaches (minimal toxicity)	Peripheral neuropathy (20%–30%) Elevated liver enzymes Pancreatitis	Bone marrow suppression, GI intolerance, headache, insomnia, asthenia, nail pigmentation, and myalgia
Drug interactions	Ethanol may increase ABC concentrations	Fluoroquinolones, tetracycline; ketoconazole, dapsone; tenofovir		TMP/SMZ may increase 3TC concentrations		Myelosuppressive agents Rifampin
Miscellaneous information	Hypersensitivity reaction may be fatal; discontinue drug immediately Screen for *HLA-B*5701* before initiation; cross-resistance with ddI and 3TC		Activity in resting macrophages Avoid combination products (Atripla, Complera, and Stribild) in renal dysfunction, and use appropriately adjusted individual agents instead	Resistance develops quickly with monotherapy Activity in resting macrophages	Activity in activated lymphocytes	Activity in activated lymphocytes

[a]Dosage adjustment in hepatic insufficiency.

[b]Dosage adjustment in renal insufficiency.

AZT = azidothymidine; BID = twice daily; DTG = dolutegravir; GI = gastrointestinal; TDF = tenofovir disoproxil fumarate; TID = three times daily; TMP/SMZ = trimethoprim/sulfamethoxazole.

Table 5. Nonnucleoside and Nucleotide RTIs

	Delavirdine (DLV) (Rescriptor)	Efavirenz (EFV) (Sustiva, Atripla)	Etravirine (ETR) (Intelence)	Nevirapine (NVP) (Viramune, Viramune XR)	Rilpivirine (RPV) (Edurant, Complera)	Tenofovir disoproxil fumarate (TDF) (Viread, Truvada, Atripla, Complera, Stribild)
RTI type	Nonnucleoside	Nonnucleoside	Nonnucleoside	Nonnucleoside	Nonnucleoside	Nucleotide
Form	100-, 200-mg tablets	50-, 200-mg capsules 600-mg tablets Atripla: 200 mg of FTC/300 mg of TDF/efavirenz 600 mg	100-, 200-mg tablets	200-mg tablets 400-mg XR tablets 50 mg/5 mL suspension	25-mg tablets Complera: 200 mg FTC/300 mg TDF/rilpivirine 25 mg	300-mg tablets Truvada: 200 mg FTC/300 mg TDF Atripla (see Efavirenz)
Dosing	400 mg PO TID	400–600 mg PO qHS	200 mg PO BID	200 mg/day for 14 days, then 200 mg PO BID or 400 mg PO daily (XR)[a]	25 mg PO daily	300 mg PO daily[b]
Oral bioavailability	85% Avoid antacids	42% Avoid with high-fat meal	Take with food	>90%	Take with food	40% Take with food
Serum half-life	5.8 hours	40–55 hours	41 hours	25–30 hours	50 hours	10–14 hours
Elimination	Metabolized by CYP3A4, 51% excreted in urine (<5% unchanged), 44% in feces	Metabolized by CYP3A4, 14%–34% excreted in urine, 16%–61% in feces	Metabolized by CYP3A4, CYP2C9, CYP2C19	Metabolized by CYP3A4; 80% excreted in urine (<5% unchanged), 10% in feces	Metabolized by CYP3A4	Eliminated by renal filtration and active secretion
Major toxicity	Rash (less than nevirapine) Headache Elevated LFTs	Rash (less than delavirdine) CNS symptoms (insomnia, impaired concentration, nightmares, mania) Elevated LFTs	Rash Nausea Hypersensitivity reaction	Rash GI toxicity Elevated LFTs; hepatotoxicity	Rash Depression Insomnia Headache	GI toxicity Headache May cause lactic acidosis with hepatic steatosis (mitochondrial toxicity may be less)
Drug interactions	Inhibits CYP3A4 Separate administration with antacids and ddI	Induces CYP3A4	Induces CYP3A4 Inhibits CYP2C9 and CYP2C19	Induces CYP3A4 Watch rifampin, rifabutin, OCs, protease inhibitors, triazolam, midazolam	PPIs (contra-indicated), H₂-blockers, antacids	Increases ddI concentration; separate administration
Miscellaneous information	Extensive cross-resistance in class	Extensive cross-resistance in class Avoid in first trimester of pregnancy (teratogenic) Do not use Atripla if CrCl < 50 mL/minute	Can dissolve in water for patients who cannot swallow May be effective against HIV strains resistant to efavirenz or nevirapine	Extensive cross-resistance in class Do not initiate in women with CD4⁺ counts >250 cells/mm³ or in men with CD4⁺ counts >400 cells/mm³ (liver toxicity)	Use with caution if viral load > 100,000 copies/mL	May be effective against HIV strains resistant to other RTIs

[a]Dosage adjustment in hepatic insufficiency.
[b]Dosage adjustment in renal insufficiency.

BID = twice daily; CNS = central nervous system; CrCl = creatinine clearance; CYP = cytochrome P450; ddI = didanosine; FTC = emtricitabine; GI = gastrointestinal; LFT = liver function test; OC = oral contraceptive; PO = orally; PPI = proton pump inhibitor; qHS = every night; RTI = reverse transcriptase inhibitor; TID = three times daily; XR = extended release.

Table 6. Protease Inhibitors

	Atazanavir (ATV) (Reyataz)	Darunavir (DRV) (Prezista)	Fosamprenavir (FPV) (Lexiva)	Indinavir (IDV) (Crixivan)	Lopinavir/ Ritonavir (LPV/r) (Kaletra)	Nelfinavir (NFV) (Viracept)	Ritonavir (RTV) (Norvir)	Saquinavir (SQV) (Invirase)	Tipranavir (TPV) (Aptivus)
Form	100-, 150-, 200-, 300-mg capsules	75-, 150-, 300-, 400-, 600-mg tablets	700-mg tablets; 50-mg/mL liquid; prodrug of amprenavir	100-, 200-, 400-mg capsules	100/25-, 200/50-mg tablets; 80/20-mg/mL solution	250-, 625-mg tablets; 50-mg/g oral powder	100-mg tablets or capsules; 80-mg/mL liquid Refrigerate capsules	200-mg capsules, 500-mg tablets	250-mg capsules; 100-mg/mL solution Refrigerate capsules
Dosing	400 mg/day[a,b] If taken with efavirenz: RTV 100 mg + ATV 400 mg daily If taken without efavirenz: RTV 100 mg + ATV 300 mg daily	800 mg/day with RTV 100 mg daily or 600 mg BID with RTV 100 mg BID[a]	1400 mg bid (or 1400 mg + RTV 100–200 mg/day; or 700 mg + RTV 100 mg BID) With efavirenz: 700 mg + RTV 100 mg BID[a]	800 mg q8h 800 mg + RTV 100–200 mg q12h[a]	400/100 mg BID or 800/200 mg/day with food If taking efavirenz or nevirapine: 500 mg/125 mg BID	750 mg TID or 1250 mg BID[a]	"Boosting dose" = 100–400 mg divided once or twice daily	1000 mg BID with ritonavir 100 mg; take within 2 hours of a meal[a]	500 mg BID with RTV 200 mg BID[a]
Oral bioavailability	Food increases absorption and bioavailability; take with food	Food increases absorption and bioavailability; take with food	Take without respect to food (take with food if given with ritonavir)	65%; 1 hour before or 2 hours after meals (may take with low-fat meal)	Take solution with food; take tablets without respect to food	20%–80%; take with meal or snack	65%–75%; take with food	Take with food	Take without respect to food (take with food if given with ritonavir)
Serum half-life	7 hours	15 hours	7 hours	1.52 hours	56 hours	3.55 hours	35 hours	12 hours	6 hours
Elimination	CYP3A4	CYP3A4	CYP3A4	CYP3A4; renal, 20%	CYP3A4	CYP3A4	CYP3A4 > CYP2D6 > CYP2C9/10	CYP3A4	CYP3A4
Major toxicity	Indirect hyperbilirubinemia rash, elevated transaminases, prolonged PR interval and heart block, endocrine disturbances[c]	Rash (sulfa); hepatotoxicity; endocrine disturbances[c]	Rash; GI intolerance; oral paresthesias; elevated LFTs; endocrine disturbances[c]	Nephrolithiasis; GI intolerance; alopecia, dry skin and lips; endocrine disturbances[c]	GI intolerance; fatigue; asthenia; pancreatitis; PR and QTc prolongation; endocrine disturbances[c]	Diarrhea (mild); endocrine disturbances[c]	GI intolerance; paresthesias (circumoral and extremities); taste disturbances; asthenia; endocrine disturbances[c]	GI intolerance (mild); PR and QT prolongation; endocrine disturbances[c]	Hepatotoxicity; rash (sulfa); intracranial hemorrhage; endocrine disturbances[c]
Drug interactions	Inhibits CYP3A4, PPIs, H$_2$-blockers, antacids	Inhibits CYP3A4	Inhibits CYP3A4 (<RTV)	Inhibits CYP3A4 (<RTV); ddI decreases absorption	Inhibits CYP3A4, CYP2D6	Inhibits CYP3A4 (<RTV)	Inhibits CYP3A4, CYP2D6 (potent) ddI decreases absorption Induces glucuronyl transferases	Inhibits CYP3A4 (<RTV)	Inhibits CYP3A4, CYP2D6
Miscellaneous information	Less lipid effects	Good for PI-resistant virus		Fluid intake of at least 1.5 L/day			Cross-resistance with IDV	Do not use with IDV	Good for PI-resistant virus; must give with RTV

[a]Dosage adjustment in hepatic insufficiency.
[b]Dosage adjustment in renal insufficiency.
[c]Endocrine disturbances include insulin resistance (type 2 diabetes mellitus in 8%–10%), peripheral fat loss and central fat accumulation (in 50%), and lipid abnormalities (in 70%).

BID = twice daily; CYP = cytochrome P450; ddI = didanosine; GI = gastrointestinal; LFT = liver function test; PI = protease inhibitor; PPI = proton pump inhibitor; q8h = every 8 hours; q12h = every 12 hours; TID = three times daily.

Table 7. Entry Inhibitors and Integrase Inhibitors

	Enfuvirtide (Fuzeon)	Maraviroc (MVC) (Selzentry)	Dolutegravir (DTG) (Tivicay, Triumeq)	Elvitegravir (EVG) (Stribild, Vitekta)	Raltegravir (RAL) (Isentress)
Class	Entry inhibitor	Entry inhibitor	Integrase inhibitor	Integrase inhibitor	Integrase inhibitor
Form	90-mg vials	150-, 300-mg tablets	50-mg tablets Triumeq: 600 mg of ABC, 50 mg of DTG, 300 mg of 3TC	Tablets with elvitegravir 150 mg/cobicistat 150 mg/tenofovir 300 mg emtricitabine 200 mg[a] Vitekta: 85-mg or 150-mg tabs	25-, 100-, 400-mg tablets
Dosing	90 mg SC BID	150–600 mg PO BID (depending on concomitant drug interactions)[a]	50 mg PO once daily	Stribild: once daily Vitekta: once daily; dose depends on combination	400 mg PO BID
Oral bioavailability	N/A	23%–33%	Take with or without food	Food increases absorption and bioavailability Take with food	
Serum half-life	3.8 hours	14–18 hours	14 hours	13 hours	9 hours
Elimination	Metabolized by hydrolysis	Metabolized by CYP3A	Metabolized by glucuronidation by UGT1A1/3 enzymes and by CYP3A	Metabolized by CYP3A and glucuronidation by UGT1A1/3 enzymes Cobicistat is metabolized by CYP3A and CYP2D6	Metabolized by hepatic glucuronidation by uridine 5'-diphospho--glucuronosyltransferase
Major toxicity	Hypersensitivity reactions; local injection-site reactions (98%); pneumonia	Abdominal pain, cough, dizziness, musculoskeletal symptoms, pyrexia, rash, upper respiratory tract infections, hepatotoxicity, orthostatic hypotension	Insomnia and diarrhea Benign increases in creatinine (inhibits creatinine secretion) and bilirubin (blocks bilirubin clearance)	Renal toxicity (avoid concomitant nephrotoxic agents); discontinue if CrCl is less than 50 mL/minute	Nausea, headache, diarrhea, pyrexia, creatine kinase elevation
Drug interactions	None	CYP3A substrate (watch CYP3A inducers and inhibitors)	Inhibitors and inducers of UGT1A3, UGT1A9, BCRP, and P-glycoprotein	Monitor closely if used with CYP3A inducers or inhibitors	Inducers of UGT1A1: rifampin, efavirenz, tipranavir/ritonavir, and rifabutin
Mechanism of action	Attachment of gp120 to CD4 receptor and coreceptors CCR5 or CXCR4 results in exposure of the specific peptide sequence of gp41; enfuvirtide binds to this gp41 peptide sequence, preventing fusion	Binds to the CCR5 receptor of the CD4 T cell, preventing fusion and HIV entry	Inhibits strand transfer of viral DNA to host cell DNA by the integrase enzyme	Inhibits strand transfer of viral DNA to host cell DNA by the integrase enzyme Cobicistat is a potent CYP3A inhibitor used for pharmacokinetic enhancement; also inhibits tubular secretion of creatinine	Inhibits strand transfer of viral DNA to host cell DNA by the integrase enzyme

[a]Dosage adjustment in renal insufficiency.

3TC = lamivudine; ABC = abacavir; BID = twice daily; CrCl = creatinine clearance; CYP = cytochrome P450; N/A = not applicable; PO = orally; qHS = every night; SC = subcutaneously; TID = three times daily.

Patient Case

1. F.G. is a 27-year-old man who is HIV positive but asymptomatic. One year ago, his CD4 count was 815 cells/mm^3, and his viral load was 1500 copies/mL (by reverse transcriptase polymerase chain reaction). F.G. continues to be monitored; his CD4 count has decreased (most recent was 240 cells/mm^3), and his viral load has increased (most recent was 60,000 copies/mL by reverse transcriptase polymerase chain reaction). Which is the best treatment for F.G.?

    A. ART should not be given because F.G.'s CD4 count is still above 200 cells/mm^3.

    B. Initiate F.G. on zidovudine alone because his CD4 count is still above 200 cells/mm^3.

    C. Initiate F.G. on combination therapy of zidovudine, lamivudine, and nevirapine.

    D. Initiate F.G. on combination therapy of tenofovir, emtricitabine, and atazanavir/ritonavir.

---

7. Treatment of the patient who is HIV positive
    a. Initiating potent combination ART in an antiretroviral-naive patient
        i.   Any patient who is HIV positive (regardless of viral load or CD4 count) with the following conditions
            (a) Pregnancy
            (b) History of AIDS-defining illness
            (c) HIV-associated nephropathy
            (d) HIV/hepatitis B coinfection
        ii. Any HIV-positive patient with the following CD4 counts
            (a) Less than 350 cells/mm^3 (strongest recommendation)
            (b) CD4 350–500 cells/mm^3 (lower strength of recommendation)
            (c) More than 500 cells/mm^3 (lowest strength of recommendation)
        iii. Any HIV-positive patient at risk of transmitting HIV to sexual partners
    b. Recommended therapy regardless of baseline viral load or CD4 count: The optimal ART for a treatment-naive patient consists of two NRTIs in combination with a third active drug from one of three drug classes: an NNRTI, a PI boosted with ritonavir, or an INSTI
        i.   NNRTI-based regimen: efavirenz/tenofovir/emtricitabine (EFV/TDF/FTC)
        ii. PI-based regimens
            (a) Atazanavir/ritonavir plus tenofovir/emtricitabine (ATV/r plus TDF/FTC)
            (b) Darunavir/ritonavir plus tenofovir/emtricitabine (DRV/r plus TDF/FTC)
        iii. INSTI-based regimens
            (a) Dolutegravir/abacavir/lamivudine (DTG plus ABC/3TC); only for patients who are HLA-B* 5701 negative
            (b) Dolutegravir/tenofovir/emtricitabine (DTG plus TDF/FTC)
            (c) Elvitegravir/cobicistat plus tenofovir/emtricitabine (EVG/cobi/TDF/FTC); only for patients with pre-ART CrCl >70 mL/min
            (d) Raltegravir/Tenofovir/Emtricitabine (RAL plus TDF/FTC)
    c. Recommended therapy only for patients with viral load <100,000 copies/mL
        i.   NNRTI-based regimens
            (a) Efavirenz/abacavir/lamivudine (EFV plus ABC/3TC); only for patients who are HLA-B* 5701 negative
            (b) Rilpivirine/tenofovir/emtricitabine (RPV/TDF/FTC); only for patients with CD4 count >200 cells/mm^3
        ii. PI-based regimen: Atazanavir/ritonavir plus abacavir/lamivudine (ATV/r plus ABC/3TC); only for patients who are HLA-B*5701 negative

---

      iii. Recommended therapy only for patients with viral load <100,000 copies/mL: Efavirenz *or* atazanavir/ritonavir *plus* abacavir/lamivudine; rilpivirine *plus* tenofovir/emtricitabine (only if CD4 count > 200 cells/mm^3)

  d. Alternative therapy: Based on individual patient characteristics and needs, an "alternative regimen" may be the optimal regimen for a given patient.

    i. PI-based regimens

      (a) Darunavir/ritonavir *plus* abacavir/lamivudine (DRV/r plus ABC/3TC); only for patients who are HLA-B*5701 negative

      (b) Lopinavir/ritonavir *plus* abacavir/lamivudine or tenofovir/emtricitabine (LPV/r [once or twice daily] plus ABC/3TC); only for patients who are HLA-B*5701 negative

      (c) Lopinavir/ritonavir *plus* abacavir/lamivudine or tenofovir/lamivudine (LPV/r [once or twice daily] plus TDF/FTC)

    ii. INSTI-based regimen: Raltegravir *plus* abacavir/lamivudine (RAL plus ABC/3TC); only for patients who are HLA-B*5701 negative

---

Patient Cases

2. Six months after he starts appropriate therapy, F.G.'s CD4 count is 620 cells/mm^3, and his viral load is undetectable. Two years later, his CD4 count decreases to 310 cells/mm^3, and his viral load is 15,000 copies/mL. Resistance testing is performed, and resistance is detected to atazanavir but not the other PIs. Which change is best for F.G.'s therapy?

  A. Stress adherence and continue the same regimen.

  B. Change atazanavir/ritonavir to efavirenz.

  C. Change tenofovir and emtricitabine to abacavir and lamivudine.

  D. Change the entire regimen to abacavir, lamivudine, and darunavir/ritonavir.

3. Which is the best parameter to monitor if F.G. is to receive darunavir/ritonavir?

  A. Peripheral neuropathy.

  B. Drug interactions with drugs metabolized by CYP1A2.

  C. Endocrine disturbances such as hyperglycemia, fat redistribution, and lipid abnormalities.

  D. Nephrolithiasis.

---

  f. Change therapy for the following reasons:

    i. Practical reasons

      (a) Reduce pill burden

      (b) Decrease adverse events

      (c) Change food or fluid requirements

      (d) Minimize drug interactions

      (e) Optimize therapy during or before pregnancy

      (f) Reduce costs

    ii. Virologic failure

      (a) Not achieving HIV RNA less than 200 copies/mL

      (b) Two consecutive HIV RNA levels more than 200 copies/mL after 24 weeks of therapy

      (c) HIV RNA levels more than 200 copies/mL after initial suppression to undetectable levels

   iii. Immunologic failure

    (a) No specific definition

    (b) Some studies have used the following:

     (1) Failure to increase 50–100 cells/mm^3 above the baseline CD4 cell count during the first year of therapy

     (2) Failure to increase the CD4 count above 350 cells/mm^3 in 4–7 years

 g. Regimen switching for practical reasons

   i. Review past treatment history and resistance testing. Consider consulting an HIV specialist.

   ii. Do not switch without assurance that the new regimen will be as active as the current one.

   iii. Within-class switches due to adverse events usually maintain suppression.

   iv. If there is no drug resistance, switches to lower-toxicity, lower–pill burden regimens generally results in similar if not better outcomes.

   v. Monitor the patient closely during the first 3 months after a switch.

 h. Options for treatment failure

   i. Perform resistance testing (while patient is on failing regimen or within 4 weeks of discontinuing).

    (a) More accurate result if HIV RNA levels are >1,000 copies/mL

    (b) If HIV RNA levels are >500 but <1,000 copies/mL, testing may be unsuccessful but should still be considered.

   ii. Prior therapy with no resistance

    (a) Check adherence and address underlying causes. Consider reinitiating the same regimen.

    (b) Initiate a new regimen.

    (c) Intensify one therapy or boost one therapy based on pharmacokinetic parameters.

   iii. Prior therapy with resistance: Start a new regimen with at least two and preferably three fully active agents.

   iv. Extensive therapy with resistance: Resuppress viral load maximally or at least adequately to prevent clinical progression.

   v. New regimen with at least two fully active agents is not possible: Continue current regimen.

 i. Resistance testing

   i. Types of testing

    (a) Genotypic

     (1) Testing for the presence of mutations known to cause drug resistance

     (2) Comparing the HIV-1 pol gene with a wild-type gene

     (3) Recommended to guide therapy in patients with virologic failure while on their first or second regimen

    (b) Phenotypic

     (1) Test for inhibitory concentration needed to decrease HIV replication by 50% (IC_{50})

     (2) Values are reported as fold changes in sensitivity.

     (3) An increase of less than fourfold in IC_{50} is defined as sensitive.

     (4) A four- to tenfold increase in IC_{50} is defined as intermediate.

     (5) An increase of more than tenfold in IC_{50} is defined as resistant.

     (6) Added to genotypic testing in patients with complex drug resistance mutation patterns

   ii. Indications

    (a) Recommended: Upon entrance into care

    (b) Recommended: Virologic failure during potent combination ART

    (c) Recommended: All pregnant women with HIV

    (d) Recommended: Suboptimal suppression of viral load after initiation of potent combination ART

(e) Recommended: Acute HIV infection before initiating therapy to determine whether a drug-resistant virus was transmitted

(f) Genotypic testing recommended for treatment-naive patients

(g) Phenotypic testing recommended for treatment-experienced patients with complex resistance patterns

iii. Benefits

(a) Resistance testing is an independent indicator of virologic outcome (better short-term viral load response in those who had testing completed).

(b) May also benefit patients by limiting drug exposures, toxicities, and expense

iv. Limitations

(a) The effect of resistance testing is limited in heavily treated patients.

(b) The HIV RNA value must be greater than 1000 copies/mL (500–1000 copies/mL acceptable).

(c) Current need for expert interpretation

(d) Difficult-to-detect small mutant populations (less than 20%)

(e) Cost: About $400–$500 per test

II. OPPORTUNISTIC INFECTIONS: PATIENTS WITH HIV

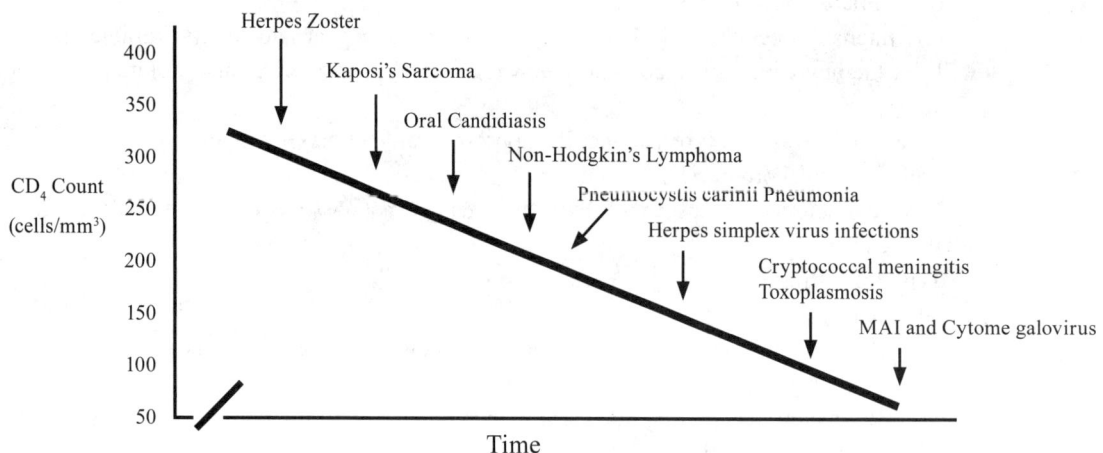

Figure 1. Relationship between CD4 count and risk of HIV-related opportunistic infections.
MAI = *Mycobacterium avium-intracellulare.*

A. Overview of HIV-Associated Opportunistic Infections

1. Principle 1: The fungal, parasitic, and viral infections acquired by people who are infected with HIV are rarely curable. At best, the infection is controllable during an acute episode but usually requires long-term suppressive therapy.

2. Principle 2: Most HIV-associated infections represent endogenous reactivation of previously acquired organisms and do not represent a threat to others.

3. Principle 3: Concurrent or consecutive infections with different organisms are a common clinical occurrence in severely immunosuppressed people with HIV infection.

4. Principle 4: The observed frequency of certain parasitic and fungal infections depends on the prevalence of asymptomatic infection with these pathogens in the local population.

5. Principle 5: Infections associated with HIV are severe, often disseminated and atypical, and characterized by a high density of organisms.

6. Principle 6: Certain B-cell–associated infections are seen with greater frequency in people with HIV infections (e.g., pneumococcal infection).

Patient Cases

4. Three years later, F.G. (from Patient Case questions 1–3) has not responded to any of his ART regimens because of resistance or intolerance. His CD4 count has decreased to 135 cells/mm^3. For which infection is it most important that F.G. receive primary prophylaxis?

   A. *Pneumocystis jirovecii* pneumonia (PCP).

   B. Cryptococcal meningitis.

   C. Cytomegalovirus (CMV).

   D. *Mycobacterium avium* complex (MAC).

5. B.L. is a 44-year-old man positive for HIV who arrives at the emergency department severely short of breath. He is an extremely nonadherent patient and has not seen a health care provider in more than 3 years. A chest radiograph shows pulmonary infiltrates in both lung fields. The results of the laboratory tests are as follows: sodium 147 mEq/L, potassium 4.2 mEq/L, chloride 104 mEq/L, bicarbonate 25.2 mEq/L, glucose 107 mg/dL, blood urea nitrogen 38 mg/dL, serum creatinine 1.1 mg/dL, aspartate aminotransferase 28 IU/L, alanine aminotransferase 32 IU/L, lactate dehydrogenase 386 IU/L, alkaline phosphate 75 IU/L, pH 7.45, P_{O_2} 63 mm Hg, P_{CO_2} 32 mm Hg, and oxygen saturation 85%. Sputum Gram stain is negative; silver stain is also negative. Which is the best therapy for B.L.?

   A. Pentamidine intravenously with adjuvant prednisone therapy for 21 days.

   B. Trimethoprim/sulfamethoxazole for 21 days.

   C. Trimethoprim/sulfamethoxazole intravenously with adjuvant prednisone therapy for 21 days.

   D. Atovaquone for 21 days.

B. Initiating Potent Combination ART in the Setting of Acute Opportunistic Infections
   1. Opportunistic infections with no effective therapy require prompt initiation of ART: cryptosporidiosis, microsporidiosis, promyelocytic leukemia, and Kaposi sarcoma.
   2. ART should begin within 2 weeks of acute opportunistic infections, except for tuberculosis (TB), in which therapy should begin within 2 weeks when the CD4 count is less than 50 cells/mm^3 and by 8–12 weeks for all others.

C. *Pneumocystis jirovecii* pneumonia (PCP)
   1. Clinical presentation
      a. Fever, shortness of breath, and nonproductive cough
      b. Elevated lactate dehydrogenase
      c. Diffuse pulmonary infiltrates
      d. In general, with CD4 counts less than 200 cells/mm^3
      e. Hypoxemia with elevated alveolar-arterial (A-a) gradient and decreased P_{O_2}; A-a gradient = 150 – P_{O_2} – P_{CO_2}

2. Diagnosis
   a. Induced sputum or bronchoalveolar lavage or transbronchial biopsy
   b. Methenamine silver stain of sputum sample
3. Therapy
   a. Trimethoprim/sulfamethoxazole (preferred)
      i. Dose: 15–20 mg/kg/day of trimethoprim divided every 6–8 hours for 21 days (intravenously for moderate to severe PCP); trimethoprim/sulfamethoxazole double strength 2 tablets three times daily (for mild to moderate PCP)
      ii. Adverse effects (80% of patients, with 20%–60% requiring discontinuation)
         (a) Nausea and vomiting
         (b) Rash
         (c) Anemia, thrombocytopenia, leucopenia
         (d) Renal impairment or hyperkalemia (also, small increases in serum creatinine occur because of competition between trimethoprim and creatinine for renal secretion)
      iii. Prophylaxis dose
         (a) Preferred: Trimethoprim/sulfamethoxazole double strength or single strength once daily (pediatric dose, 150 mg/m^2 per dose of trimethoprim and 750 mg/m^2 per dose of sulfamethoxazole)
         (b) Alternative: Trimethoprim/sulfamethoxazole double strength three times/week
   b. Clindamycin and primaquine
      i. Dose: Clindamycin 600 mg every 6 hours or 900 mg every 8 hours intravenously or 300 mg every 6 hours or 450 mg every 8 hours orally and primaquine base 30 mg/day for 21 days
      ii. Adverse effects
         (a) Rash
         (b) Anemia, methemoglobinemia
         (c) Diarrhea
   c. Pentamidine
      i. Dose: 4 mg/kg/day intravenously for 21 days
      ii. Adverse effects
         (a) Hypotension
         (b) Rash
         (c) Electrolyte disturbances
         (d) Hypoglycemia or hyperglycemia
         (e) Pancreatitis
      iii. Prophylaxis dose: 300 mg by nebulization (Respirgard) once monthly (can predose with β-agonist to diminish respiratory irritation)
   d. Trimethoprim and dapsone
      i. Dose: 15 mg/kg/day of trimethoprim divided every 8 hours and dapsone 100 mg/day for 21 days (only for mild to moderate PCP)
      ii. Adverse effects
         (a) Nausea and vomiting
         (b) Anemia
      iii. Prophylactic dose: Dapsone 100 mg/day (pediatric dose, 1 mg/kg/day) alone or 50 mg/week with 50–75 mg of pyrimethamine and 25 mg of leucovorin
   e. Atovaquone (Mepron)
      i. Dose: 750 mg twice daily for 21 days given with a high-fat meal (only for mild to moderate PCP)
      ii. Pediatric dose (less than 40 kg [88 lb]) = 40 mg/kg/day divided twice daily

        iii. Equal to trimethoprim/sulfamethoxazole for PCP but not an antibacterial

        iv. Potential for decreased efficacy in patients with diarrhea (because of poor absorption)

        v. Adverse effects

           (a) Nausea and vomiting

           (b) Rash

           (c) Transient increase in liver function tests

           (d) Insomnia, headache, fever

        vi. Prophylactic dose = 1500 mg once daily (alternative to trimethoprim/sulfamethoxazole)

    f. Adjuvant therapy: corticosteroids

        i. Used in patients with severe PCP (A-a gradient of 35 or more or Po_2 of 70 or less); start within 72 hours.

        ii. Decreases mortality

        iii. Dose: 40 mg twice daily of prednisone for 5 days, followed by 40 mg/day for 5 days, and then 20 mg/day for remainder of PCP therapy (use cautiously in patients with TB)

4. Prophylaxis

    a. Secondary prophylaxis in patients after PCP (may be discontinued if CD4 count is more than 200 cells/mm³ for 3 months or longer because of potent combination ART)

    b. Primary prophylaxis in patients with CD4 count less than 200 cells/mm³ (may be discontinued if CD4 count is more than 200 cells/mm³ for 3 months or longer because of potent combination ART)

D. *Candida* Infections

    1. Oral *Candida* infections (thrush)

        a. More than 90% of patients with AIDS sometime during their illness

        b. Signs and symptoms

            i. Creamy white, curdlike patches on the tongue and other oral mucosal surfaces

            ii. Pain; decreased food and fluid intake

    2. *Candida* esophagitis

        a. Not always an extension of oral thrush (30% do not have oral thrush)

        b. Signs and symptoms: painful swallowing, obstructed swallowing, substernal pain

    3. Diagnosis

        a. Signs and symptoms of infection

        b. Fungal cultures, potassium hydroxide smear

        c. Endoscopic evaluation

    4. Therapy (oral candidiasis is easy to treat [3–14 days' duration], but it relapses within 30 days)

        a. Nystatin

            i. Indicated for mucous membrane and cutaneous *Candida* infections

            ii. Use for initial episodes in patients with CD4 count more than 50 cells/mm³.

            iii. 5 mL (100,000 units/mL); swish and swallow four times daily.

            iv. Poor adherence

        b. Clotrimazole (alternative to nystatin)

            i. Use for initial episodes in patients with CD4 count more than 50 cells/mm³.

            ii. Clotrimazole (Mycelex) troches 10 mg five times daily

            iii. Poor adherence (generally better tolerated than nystatin)

        c. Fluconazole

            i. Indicated for oropharyngeal and esophageal candidiasis

            ii. 2% relapse on fluconazole versus 28% on placebo

            iii. 10% of patients develop fluconazole-resistant infections.

            iv. 100–400 mg/day

    d. Itraconazole
       i. Indicated for oropharyngeal and esophageal candidiasis
       ii. Oral solution: 200 mg/day
       iii. Significant drug-drug interactions

Patient Case

6. G.H. is a 33-year-old man positive for HIV who presents to the clinic with a severe headache that has gradually worsened during the past 3 weeks. He also has memory problems and is always tired. He has refused ART in the past, and his most recent CD4 count was 75 cells/mm³. He is given a diagnosis of cryptococcal meningitis and is successfully treated. Which is the best follow-up therapy for G.H.?

    A. No maintenance treatment is necessary.

    B. Administer fluconazole 200 mg/day orally.

    C. Administer amphotericin B 1 mg/kg/week intravenously.

    D. He is protected as long as he is also receiving PCP prophylaxis.

  E. Cryptococcosis
    1. *Cryptococcus neoformans*
    2. Occurs in 6%–10% of patients with AIDS
    3. In general, occurs in patients with CD4 counts less than 50 cells/mm³
    4. Acute mortality is 10%–25%, and 12-month mortality is 30%–60%.
    5. Worldwide distribution
      a. Found in aged pigeon droppings and nesting places (e.g., barns, window ledges)
      b. Organism must be aerosolized and inhaled; it then disseminates hematogenously.
    6. Signs and symptoms
      a. Almost always meningitis (66%–84%)
      b. Usually present for weeks or months (1 day to 4 months; average, 31 days)
      c. Insidious onset
        i. Low-grade fever (80%–90%)
        ii. Headaches (80%–90%)
        iii. Altered sensorium (20%): irritability, somnolence, clumsiness, impaired memory and judgment, behavioral changes
        iv. Seizures may occur late in the course (less than 10%).
        v. Minimal nuchal rigidity, meningismus, photophobia
    7. Diagnosis
      a. Cerebrospinal fluid (CSF) changes including:
        i. Positive CSF cultures
        ii. CSF India ink
        iii. CSF cryptococcal antigen titer (91%)
        iv. Elevated opening pressure greater than 20 cm H_2O
      b. Serum cryptococcal antigen more than 1:8
    8. Therapy
      a. Preferred: Lipid amphotericin 3–4 mg/kg/day *plus* flucytosine 25 mg/kg every 6 hours for at least 2 weeks, followed by fluconazole 400 mg/day for at least 8 weeks
      b. Alternative
        i. Lipid amphotericin 5 mg/kg/day *plus* flucytosine 25 mg/kg every 6 hours for at least 2 weeks, followed by fluconazole 400 mg/day for at least 8 weeks

      ii. Amphotericin B deoxycholate 0.7–1 mg/kg/day *plus* flucytosine 25 mg/kg every 6 hours for at least 2 weeks, followed by fluconazole 400 mg/day for at least 8 weeks

      iii. Lipid amphotericin 3–4 mg/kg/day *plus* fluconazole 800 mg/day for at least 2 weeks, followed by fluconazole 400 mg/day for at least 8 weeks

      iv. Lipid amphotericin 3–4 mg/kg/day alone for at least 2 weeks, followed by fluconazole 400 mg/day for at least 8 weeks

      v. Amphotericin B deoxycholate 0.7–1 mg/kg/day *plus* fluconazole 800 mg/day for 2 weeks, followed by fluconazole 800 mg/day for at least 8 weeks

      vi. Fluconazole 400–800 mg/day *plus* flucytosine 25 mg/kg every 6 hours for 6 weeks

      vii. Fluconazole 800–2000 mg/day for 10–12 weeks

9. Outcome
   a. Therapeutic response: 42%–75%
   b. Length of therapy is controversial, but antifungals should probably be continued as long as CSF and other body fluid cultures are positive and for 1 month after negative cultures.
   c. Relapse: 50%–90% (with about 100% mortality)

10. Prophylaxis
    a. Relapses usually occur within first year after therapy (less often with potent combination ART).
    b. Secondary prophylaxis: Fluconazole 200 mg/day (may consider discontinuing after a minimum of 1 year of chronic maintenance therapy if CD4 count is more than 100 cells/mm^3 for 3 months or longer after potent combination ART; reinitiate if CD4 count decreases to less than 100 cells/mm^3)
    c. Primary prophylaxis: Not indicated (decreases the incidence of cryptococcosis but does not decrease mortality and may lead to resistance)

Patient Cases

7. After being treated for cryptococcal meningitis, G.H. is initiated on potent combination ART. For 2, 6, and 8 months after starting the therapy, his CD4 counts are 212, 344, and 484 cells/mm^3, respectively. Which is the best follow-up therapy for G.H. now?

    A. Continue fluconazole maintenance therapy.

    B. Maintenance therapy with fluconazole should be given for at least 1 year; then, it can be discontinued because the CD4 counts have increased.

    C. Maintenance therapy with fluconazole should be continued until CD4 counts are greater than 500 cells/mm^3.

    D. Maintenance therapy with fluconazole can be discontinued.

8. J.C., a 36-year-old woman positive for HIV, has severe anemia. She has been tested for iron deficiency and has been taken off zidovudine and trimethoprim/sulfamethoxazole. She has also started to lose weight and to have severe diarrhea. A blood culture is positive for MAC. Which treatment is best for J.C.?

    A. Clarithromycin plus ethambutol for 2 weeks, followed by maintenance with clarithromycin alone.

    B. Azithromycin ethambutol for at least 12 months.

    C. Clarithromycin plus isoniazid for 2 weeks, followed by maintenance with clarithromycin alone.

    D. Ethambutol plus rifabutin indefinitely.

F. *M. avium* Complex
1. Organism characteristics
   a. Complex is similar (main species are *M. avium* and *Mycobacterium intracellulare,* which are not differentiated microbiologically).
   b. Ubiquitous in soil and water
      i. Organisms gain access through the gastrointestinal tract.
      ii. After access, the organism spreads hematogenously.
   c. Usually occurs in patients with HIV having a CD4 count less than 50 cells/mm^3
2. Signs and symptoms (nonspecific)
   a. Weight loss, intermittent fevers, chills, night sweats, abdominal pain, diarrhea, chronic malabsorption, and progressive weakness
   b. Anemia
   c. Elevated alkaline phosphatase
3. Diagnosis
   a. Blood culture
   b. Bone marrow biopsy
   c. Stool cultures (do not treat if cultured only in the stool)
4. Therapy
   a. MAC is independently associated with risk of death, and treatment prolongs survival.
   b. Preferred therapeutic regimen is macrolide plus ethambutol: Clarithromycin 500 mg (7.5–15 mg/kg) twice daily (*or* azithromycin 500–600 mg/day 10–20 mg/kg if drug interactions or intolerance to clarithromycin) *plus* ethambutol 15 mg/kg/day for 12 months
   c. Other agents: Consider adding to preferred therapy if advanced immunosuppression (CD4 count <50 cells/mm^3), high mycobacterial loads (>2 log colony-forming units/mL of blood), or in the absence of effective ART.
      i. Rifabutin (Mycobutin) 150–600 mg/day (rifabutin dose chosen on the basis of other antiretrovirals because of drug-drug interactions)
      ii. A fluoroquinolone such as levofloxacin 500 mg oral daily or moxifloxacin 400 mg oral daily
      iii. An aminoglycoside such as amikacin 10–15 mg/kg intravenously daily or streptomycin 1 g intravenously or intramuscularly daily
   d. Chronic maintenance therapy or secondary prophylaxis may be discontinued after 12 months of therapy if CD4 count is more than 100 cells/mm^3 for 6 months or longer because of potent combination ART and if patient is asymptomatic. Restart if CD4 count drops below 100 cells/mm^3.
5. Primary prophylaxis in patients with CD4 counts less than 50 cells/mm^3 (may be discontinued if CD4 count is more than 100 cells/mm^3 for 3 months or longer because of potent combination antiretroviral therapy)
   a. Clarithromycin 500 mg orally twice daily: Lower incidence of MAC bacteremia (vs. placebo)
   b. Azithromycin 1200 mg orally once weekly
   c. Azithromycin 600 mg orally twice weekly
   d. Rifabutin 300 mg/day (150 mg orally twice daily with food if there are gastrointestinal adverse effects)
      i. Two times longer until a positive MAC culture (vs. placebo)
      ii. Decreased incidence of symptoms related to MAC
      iii. Adverse effects: rash, gastrointestinal disturbances, neutropenia, body fluid discoloration
      iv. *Do not* give alone to patients with active TB.

G. Cytomegalovirus (CMV)
   1. Characteristics of CMV infection
      a. Fifty-three percent of Americans between 18 and 25 years of age are CMV positive.
      b. Eighty-one percent of Americans older than 35 years are CMV positive.
      c. More than 95% of homosexual men are CMV positive.
      d. About 90% of CMV infections are asymptomatic (if illness occurs, it resembles mononucleosis).
      e. Virus remains latent in the host after initial infection but may reactivate if patient becomes immunocompromised (especially cell-mediated immunity).
      f. Before highly active antiretroviral therapy, 90% of patients with AIDS developed CMV infections, and 25% experienced life- or sight-threatening disease.
   2. Diagnosis of CMV infection
      a. Serology (detects exposure to CMV)
      b. Virus isolation
         i. Tissue culture: Takes up to 6 weeks
         ii. Shell vial technique: Takes only 16 hours; organism is incubated overnight and then detected by immunofluorescence microscopy with monoclonal antibodies.
      c. Cytology and histology
         i. Large (cytomegalic) cell with a large, central, basophilic, intranuclear inclusion ("owl's eye")
         ii. Low yield
   3. Manifestations of CMV
      a. Gastrointestinal
         i. Colitis: 5%–10% of patients with AIDS
         ii. Esophagitis and gastritis uncommon
         iii. Hepatitis: 33%–50% with histologic evidence but minimal clinical importance
         iv. Maintenance drugs not needed
      b. Pneumonia
         i. CMV is commonly in bronchial secretions; of questionable importance
         ii. Chest radiography results are similar to those seen with PCP.
         iii. Symptoms: Shortness of breath; dyspnea on exertion; dry, nonproductive cough
         iv. Treat if:
            (a) Documented tissue infection
            (b) CMV is only pathogen
            (c) Deteriorating illness
         v. About 50%–60% of patients will respond; no need for maintenance
      c. Retinitis
         i. Occurs in 10%–15% of patients with AIDS; is clinically most important CMV infection
         ii. In general, patients have CD4 counts less than 100 cells/mm^3.
         iii. Begins unilaterally and spreads bilaterally
         iv. Early complaints: "floaters," pain behind the eye
         v. In general, progressive; no spontaneous resolution (blindness in weeks to months)
         vi. Twenty-six percent progression, even with treatment; retinal detachment very common
   4. Therapy for CMV infections
      a. Ganciclovir (Cytovene-IV, Cytovene), valganciclovir (Valcyte)
         i. Competes with deoxynucleosides, inhibiting viral DNA synthesis
         ii. Must be triphosphorylated; the rate-limiting step in this process is the first phosphorylation. CMV induces the production of the enzymes necessary for the monophosphorylation of ganciclovir but not acyclovir.

    iii. Valganciclovir is a prodrug rapidly converted to ganciclovir in the intestinal wall and liver (bioavailability about 60%).

    iv. Adverse effects

        (a) 65% have adverse effects, and 76% have moderate to severe neutropenia (25% less than 1000 cells/mm^3, 16% less than 500 cells/mm^3).

           (1) In general, after 10 days

           (2) Ganciclovir plus zidovudine: 82% will have severe hematologic toxicity.

           (3) Patients receiving ganciclovir can tolerate no more than 300 mg/day of zidovudine.

        (b) Thrombocytopenia (9% less than 20,000 cells/mm^3)

        (c) Confusion, convulsions, dizziness, headache, thought disorders

        (d) Nausea, vomiting, diarrhea, abnormal liver function tests

        (e) Possible reproductive toxicity

    v. Dose

        (a) Induction: Valganciclovir 900 mg orally twice daily for 14–21 days (alternative: ganciclovir 5 mg/kg intravenously every 12 hours for 14–21 days)

        (b) Maintenance: Valganciclovir 900 mg/day orally (alternative: ganciclovir 5 mg/kg/day intravenously)

        (c) All (100%) patients will relapse in 1–8 weeks without maintenance.

        (d) Intravenous maintenance therapy requires establishment of central venous access.

b. Foscarnet

    i. Inhibits viral-induced DNA polymerase; no effect on human DNA polymerase

    ii. Effective against all herpes viruses (especially CMV), HBV (±), and HIV

    iii. Foscarnet and ganciclovir are equally effective against CMV, but foscarnet decreases (by about 4 months) mortality because of its anti-HIV effects.

    iv. Foscarnet is active against ganciclovir resistant CMV with mutations in the UL97 region of the viral genome.

    v. Adverse effects

        (a) Renal impairment

           (1) Especially occurs if the patient is dehydrated or taking other renal toxic drugs

           (2) A two- to threefold elevation in serum creatinine (more than 50% had to discontinue)

           (3) Usually reversible

           (4) Prevented by administering 2.5 L/day of normal saline

        (b) Decrease in hemoglobin and hematocrit

        (c) Altered serum electrolytes (calcium, phosphorus, magnesium)

        (d) Penile ulcerations

    vi. Preparation and dose

        (a) Commercial preparation is available in 500-mL glass bottles at 24 mg/mL; 24 mg/mL should be administered centrally. For peripheral administration, use 12 mg/mL.

        (b) One gram of foscarnet contains about 600 mg of sodium chloride.

        (c) Induction: 60 mg/kg every 8 hours or 90 mg/kg every 12 hours for 14–21 days (administer for 1 hour)

        (d) Maintenance: 90–120 mg/kg/day (administer for 2 hours)

        (e) Decrease dose by 3.5 mg/kg for each 0.1 mL/minute/kg of CrCl below 1.6 mL/minute/kg.

        (f) Maintenance therapy requires establishment of central venous access.

c. Cidofovir (Vistide)

    i. Acts as a nucleoside monophosphate, inhibiting viral DNA polymerase

    ii. Intracellular activation required

iii. Cidofovir is active against ganciclovir-resistant CMV with mutations in the UL97 region of the viral genome

iv. Adverse effects

    (a) Renal impairment

    (b) Manifested as proteinuria and elevated creatinine concentrations

    (c) Decreased with concurrent probenecid (2 g, 3 hours before infusion and 1 g, 2 and 8 hours after infusion, to decrease renal secretion) and saline hydration

    (d) Probenecid may cause nausea, vomiting, headache, fever, and flushing.

v. Neutropenia (15% of patients)

vi. Dose

    (a) Induction: 5 mg/kg/week for 2 weeks

    (b) Maintenance: 5 mg/kg every other week

    (c) Maintenance therapy does not require the establishment of central venous access.

    (d) Adequate saline hydration plus probenecid (2 g, 3 hours before infusion and 1 g, 2 and 8 hours after infusion) must be administered with drug.

    (e) Avoid regimen in patients with sulfa allergy because of cross-hypersensitivity with probenecid.

5. Prophylaxis

    a. Secondary prophylaxis is required for all patients (see individual drugs for specific doses); it may be discontinued if the CD4 count is more than 100 cells/mm^3 for 3–6 months or longer because of potent combination ART. Reinitiate secondary prophylaxis if the CD4 count decreases to less than 100 cells/mm^3.

    b. Primary prophylaxis not recommended. In patients with CD4 counts less than 50 cells/mm^3, regular funduscopic examinations are recommended.

H. Toxoplasmosis

1. Description

    a. *Toxoplasma gondii* (protozoan)

    b. Felines are the hosts for sporozoite production (change litter box daily, wash hands after changing litter box or have someone else change the litter box, and, ideally, keep the cat indoors).

    c. From 15% to 68% of adults in the United States are seropositive for *T. gondii*.

    d. Secondary to undercooked beef, lamb, or pork (stress avoidance in patients with HIV)

    e. Case-defining illness in 2.1% of patients with AIDS

2. Signs and symptoms

    a. Fever, headache, altered mental status

    b. Focal neurologic deficits (60%): hemiparesis, aphasia, ataxia, visual field loss, nerve palsies

    c. Seizures (33%)

    d. CSF: mild pleocytosis, increased protein, normal glucose

3. Diagnosis

    a. Brain biopsy: Only definitive diagnosis but generally not done

    b. Antibodies or *T. gondii* isolation in serum or CSF

    c. Magnetic resonance imaging scan or computed tomographic scan: Multiple, bilateral, hypodense, ring-enhancing mass lesions (magnetic resonance imaging scan more sensitive than computed tomographic scan)

4. Therapy

    a. Standard therapy

      i. Pyrimethamine 50–75 mg/day (loading dose, 200 mg in two doses) *plus*

      ii. Sulfadiazine 1000–1500 mg every 6 hours (watch crystalluria)
- (a) Bone marrow suppression: thrombocytopenia, granulocytopenia, anemia
- (b) Add folinic acid (leucovorin) 10–25 mg/day to reduce bone marrow effects of pyrimethamine.
- (c) Duration: 6 weeks or after signs and symptoms resolve

  b. Alternative therapy
- i. Clindamycin
   - (a) Dosage: 600–1200 mg intravenously every 6 hours for 6 weeks; after 3 weeks, can change to oral 600 mg every 8 hours
   - (b) Used in combination with pyrimethamine/leucovorin for sulfa intolerance or by itself when bone marrow suppression occurs
- ii. Atovaquone
   - (a) Dosage: 1500 mg orally twice daily
   - (b) Used in combination with pyrimethamine/leucovorin or in combination with sulfadiazine or alone
- iii. Azithromycin
   - (a) Dosage: 900–1200 mg/day orally
   - (b) Used in combination with pyrimethamine (do not use alone for acute therapy)

5. Prophylaxis
   a. Relapse rates approach 80% without maintenance therapy.
   b. Toxoplasma-seropositive patients with a CD4 count of 100 cells/mm^3 or less should receive primary prophylaxis.
   c. For primary prophylaxis, use trimethoprim/sulfamethoxazole double strength once daily or dapsone/pyrimethamine/leucovorin or atovaquone with or without pyrimethamine at doses used for PCP prophylaxis (may be discontinued if the CD4 count is more than 200 cells/mm^3 for 3 months or longer because of potent combination ART).
   d. For secondary prophylaxis, use the following (may be discontinued if the CD4 count is more than 200 cells/mm^3 for 6 months or longer because of potent combination ART):
      i. Pyrimethamine 25–50 mg/day plus leucovorin 10–25 mg/day with sulfadiazine 2–4 g/day
      ii. Clindamycin 600 mg every 8 hours can be substituted if sulfa intolerance occurs.
      iii. Atovaquone 750 mg orally every 6–12 hours with or without pyrimethamine/leucovorin or sulfadiazine

III. TUBERCULOSIS

A. *M. tuberculosis*
   1. Factors associated with acquiring TB
      a. Exposure to people with active pulmonary TB
      b. Geographic location
      c. Low socioeconomic status
      d. Nonwhite race
      e. Male sex
      f. AIDS
      g. Foreign birth
   2. Epidemiology (Figure 2)

**Number of persons with reported cases of
tuberculosis, 1986-2012**

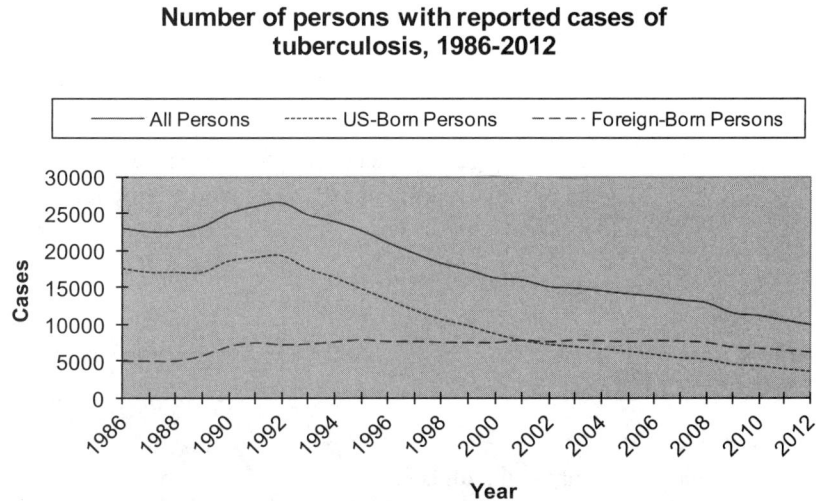

Figure 2. Epidemiology of tuberculosis.

B. Pathophysiology (Figure 3)
   1. Person-to-person transmission: Airborne droplets carrying *M. tuberculosis* are inhaled.
   2. Infection primarily pulmonary, although can occur in other organ systems

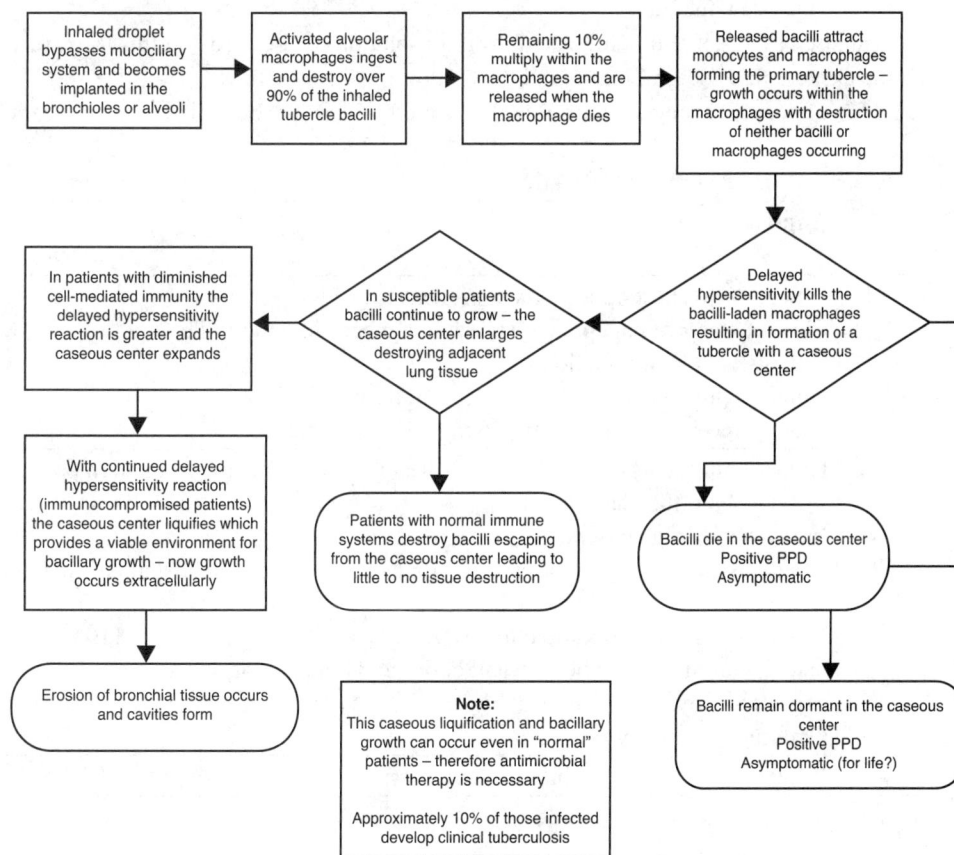

Figure 3. Pathophysiology of tuberculosis.

PPD = purified protein derivative.

C. Diagnosis (Table 8)

Table 8. Diagnosis of Tuberculosis

Nonspecific Signs and Symptoms	Radiology	Microbiology
Cough Malaise Weight loss Fever, chills Night sweats Pleuritic pain	Chest radiograph: patchy or nodular infiltrates in upper lobes; cavitary lesions	Sputum smear for AFB Sputum culture for *Mycobacterium tuberculosis*

AFB = acid-fast bacillus.

1. Skin test for PPD (Table 9)
   a. Recommended dose is 5 tuberculin units/0.1 mL.
   b. Mantoux method
      i. Intradermal injection of tuberculin into forearm
      ii. Measure diameter of induration after 48–72 hours.
      iii. Use two-step PPD for initial testing of people who will be tested periodically (e.g., health care workers).
   c. False-negative tests occur in 15%–20% of people infected with *M. tuberculosis,* primarily in those recently infected or anergic.
   d. Two hundred fifty tuberculin units per 0.1 mL of solution can be used, but this is not recommended by the Centers for Disease Control and Prevention.
   e. Only 8% of people vaccinated with Bacille Calmette-Guérin at birth will react 15 years later.

Table 9. Recommendation for Purified Protein Derivative Skin Test

Criterion for Positive Skin Test (mm)	Applicable Group
5	Patients with chest radiograph consistent with TB Close contacts of patients with newly diagnosed infectious TB Patients with HIV infection Patients with documented defects in cellular immunity Patients receiving prednisone ≥15 mg/day for ≥1 month
10	Recent immigrants (within the past 5 years) from countries with a high prevalence of TB (even if they had BCG) Intravenous drug abusers Residents and employees of prisons or jails, nursing homes, hospitals, and homeless shelters Patients with diseases known to be associated with a higher risk of TB (diabetes mellitus, silicosis, leukemias and lymphomas, chronic renal failure), gastrectomy, and jejunoileal bypass Children <4 years old
15	Patients with no identifiable risk factors

BCG = Bacille Calmette-Guérin; TB = tuberculosis.

2. Interferon gamma release assays and targeted blood tests
   a. QuantiFERON-TB Gold and T-SPOT.TB
   b. Blood test that detects the release of interferon gamma in response to *M. tuberculosis* infection
   c. Less sensitivity, but greater specificity than the PPD test for predicting future active infection
   d. Can be used interchangeably with PPD: Most beneficial to verify a positive PPD in patients with a history of Bacille Calmette-Guérin vaccine or for patients who will not or cannot return for a PPD reading
3. Booster effect
   a. The TB test can restimulate hypersensitivity in those exposed in the past.
   b. Occurs within 1 week of the test and persists for more than 1 year
   c. Those with small TB test reactions can be retested in 1 week; if positive, result should be attributed to boosting of a subclinical hypersensitivity; chemoprophylaxis is not necessary.

Patient Case

9. J.M. is a 42-year-old man who has a yearly PPD skin test because he works at a long-term care facility. Forty-eight hours after the PPD is placed, he has an 18-mm induration. This is the first time he has reacted to this test. His chest radiograph is negative. Which is best in view of J.M.'s positive PPD?

   A. No treatment is necessary, and J.M. should have another PPD skin test in 1 year.

   B. Another PPD skin test should be performed in 1 week to see whether this is a booster effect.

   C. J.M. should be monitored closely, but no treatment is necessary because he is older than 35 years.

   D. J.M. should be initiated on isoniazid 300 mg/day orally for 9 months.

D. Therapy
   1. Treatment of latent TB infection
      a. The goal is to prevent latent (asymptomatic) infection from progressing to clinical disease.
      b. The treatment of latent TB infection should be instituted in the following groups with a positive PPD skin test:
         i. Close contacts of people with newly diagnosed infectious TB
         ii. Health care workers at facilities treating patients with TB
         iii. Foreign-born people from high-prevalence countries (immigration within 5 years)
         iv. Homeless people
         v. People working at or living in long-term care facilities
         vi. Patients with HIV infection
         vii. Recent converters (within a 2-year period)
         viii. People with abnormal chest radiographs that show fibrotic lesions, likely to represent old, healed TB
         ix. People with medical conditions that have been reported to increase the risk of TB: intravenous drug use, diabetes mellitus, silicosis, Hodgkin disease, leukemia, immunosuppressive therapy, corticosteroids, end-stage renal disease
      c. Dosing regimens
         i. Patients who are not infected with HIV
            (a) Isoniazid 300 mg/day or 900 mg twice weekly for 6–9 months (9 months preferred)
            (b) Rifampin 600 mg/day for 4 months
            (c) Rifapentine 900 mg plus isoniazid 900 mg/week for 12 weeks (with directly observed therapy)

       (d) Rifampin 600 mg/day plus isoniazid 300 mg/day for 3 months (not recommended by the Centers for Disease Control and Prevention)

    ii. Patients who are coinfected with HIV

       (a) Administer isoniazid 300 mg/day for 9 months.

       (b) Alternative: Isoniazid 900 mg two times/week for 9 months with directly observed therapy (lower strength of evidence)

    iii. Areas with multidrug-resistant isolates: Two drugs with activity against the isolate for 6–12 months

---

Patient Case

10. R.J. is a 32-year-old man positive for HIV infection who presents to the clinic with increased weight loss, night sweats, and a cough productive of sputum. He is currently receiving fosamprenavir/ritonavir 700 mg/100 mg twice daily, zidovudine 300 mg twice daily, lamivudine 150 mg twice daily, fluconazole 200 mg/day orally, and trimethoprim/sulfamethoxazole double strength daily. A sputum sample is obtained, which is positive for acid-fast bacillus. R.J. lives in an area with a low incidence of multidrug-resistant TB. Which is the best initial treatment?

    A. Initiate isoniazid, rifampin, and pyrazinamide with no change in HIV medications.

    B. Initiate isoniazid, rifampin, and pyrazinamide; increase the dosage of fosamprenavir/ritonavir; and use a higher dosage of rifamycin.

    C. Initiate isoniazid, rifabutin, pyrazinamide, and ethambutol, with a lower dosage of rifabutin.

    D. Initiate isoniazid, rifabutin, pyrazinamide, and ethambutol, and decrease the dosage of fosamprenavir/ritonavir.

---

    2. Treatment of active TB infection (Table 10)

      a. Principles of treatment

        i. Regimens must contain many drugs to which the organisms are susceptible.

        ii. Drug therapy must continue for a sufficient period.

Table 10. Pharmacotherapeutic Agents in the Treatment of Tuberculosis

First-Line Agents	Second-Line Agents
Isoniazid	Bedaquiline
Rifampin	Para-aminosalicylic acid
Pyrazinamide	Ethionamide
Ethambutol	Cycloserine
Streptomycin	Kanamycin/amikacin
	Capreomycin
	Fluoroquinolones
	Rifabutin
	Rifapentine

      b. Therapeutic options for patients without HIV infection. (Note: Any regimen administered two, three, or five times/week should be done by directly observed therapy.)

        i. Option 1: Isoniazid, rifampin, pyrazinamide, and ethambutol for 2 months (daily, five times weekly, three times weekly, or twice weekly), followed by isoniazid and rifampin for 4 months (daily, five times weekly, three times weekly, or twice weekly)

      ii.   Option 2: Isoniazid, rifampin, and ethambutol for 2 months (daily or five times/week), followed by isoniazid and rifampin for 7 months (daily, five times/week, or two times/week)

  c. Therapeutic options for patients with HIV

      i.   Option 1: Isoniazid, rifampin, pyrazinamide, and ethambutol for 2 months (daily or five times/week), followed by isoniazid and rifampin for 4 months (daily or five times/week or three times/week)

      ii.   Option 2: Isoniazid, rifampin, and ethambutol for 2 months (daily or five times/week), followed by isoniazid and rifampin for 7 months (daily or five times/week)

  d. Concurrent therapy in patients with HIV

      i.   For ART-naive patients, ART should be initiated within 2 weeks when the CD4 count is less than 50 cells/mm^3 and by 8–12 weeks for all others.

      ii.   PIs and NNRTIs (except for efavirenz or nevirapine) should not be administered concurrently with rifampin; NRTIs can be administered with rifampin.

      iii.   A washout period of 1–2 weeks may be necessary once rifampin is discontinued before PIs or NNRTIs are initiated.

      iv.   Rifabutin can be substituted for rifampin; patients may take NNRTIs with rifabutin, but doses may need to be increased to 450–600 mg/day (see HIV guidelines).

      v.   Patients may take PIs with rifabutin, but the rifabutin dose should be decreased to 150 mg every day or every other day (300 mg three times weekly may be an option).

      vi.   Patients taking rifabutin and PIs or NNRTIs should have HIV RNA concentrations performed periodically.

  e. Known drug resistance to isoniazid: Administer rifampin, pyrazinamide, ethambutol, and moxifloxacin or levofloxacin for 2 months; rifabutin may be substituted for rifampin in patients with HIV. Continuation phase should be completed with rifampin (or rifabutin) plus ethambutol plus moxifloxacin (or levofloxacin) for 7 months.

  f. Known drug resistance to rifampin: Administer isoniazid, pyrazinamide, and ethambutol for 9–12 months; streptomycin may be added for the first 2 months to shorten the total treatment time to 9 months.

  g. Total duration of therapy should be based on number of doses received, not on calendar time.

      i.   Pulmonary TB: 6 months

      ii.   Pulmonary TB and culture positive after 2 months of TB treatment: 9 months

      iii.   Extrapulmonary TB with central nervous system (CNS) infection: 9–12 months

      iv.   Extrapulmonary TB with bone or joint involvement: 6 to 9 months

      v.   Extrapulmonary TB in other sites: 6 months

Patient Case

11. Which represents the best follow-up for R.J.?

   A. Treatment with the initial drugs should continue for 6 months.

   B. Treatment can be decreased to just isoniazid and a rifamycin after 2 months for a total treatment of 18–24 months.

   C. Treatment can be decreased to just isoniazid and a rifamycin after 2 months for a total treatment of 6 months; HIV RNA concentrations should be observed closely during therapy.

   D. Treatment can be decreased to isoniazid, a rifamycin, and either pyrazinamide or ethambutol after 2 months for a total treatment of 6 months; HIV RNA concentrations should be observed closely during therapy.

IV. ANTIFUNGAL THERAPY

Patient Case

12. C.A. is a 66-year-old man with a history of advanced non–small cell lung cancer. After his most recent chemotherapy, he became severely neutropenic, and he was given a diagnosis of *Aspergillus* pneumonia. C.A.
has acute renal failure related to his chemotherapy and is receiving warfarin, diltiazem, dronedarone, atorvastatin, pantoprazole, and carbamazepine. Which of the following antifungals would be the best therapy for
C.A.?

   A. Lipid amphotericin.

   B. Micafungin.

   C. Fluconazole.

   D. Voriconazole.

A. Amphotericin B (Fungizone, Abelcet, Amphotec, AmBisome)
   1. Mechanism of action: Binds to ergosterol in the fungal cell membrane, altering membrane permeability
      and causing cell lysis
   2. Spectrum of activity
      a. *Candida, Blastomyces dermatitidis, Coccidioides immitis, C. neoformans, Paracoccidioides,
         Histoplasma capsulatum, Sporothrix, Aspergillus,* mucormycoses
      b. Clinical use
         i. Cryptococcal meningitis
         ii. Systemic fungal infections caused by sensitive fungi
         iii. Limited use clinically with newer antifungals
   3. Adverse effects
      a. Renal toxicity (glomerular and tubular)
         i. Glomerular filtration rate decreases by about 40% within 2 weeks and usually stabilizes at
            20%–60% of normal.
         ii. In general, reversible unless total dose is more than 4–5 g
         iii. Manifestations: renal tubular acidosis, urine casts, azotemia, oliguria, magnesium, and potas-
            sium wasting
         iv. Prevention
            (a) Correct salt depletion: 3 L normal saline for 24 hours or 500 mL normal saline before and
               after amphotericin dose
            (b) Avoid diuretics and liberalize salt intake; risk-benefit with other disease states
      b. Thrombophlebitis prevention
         i. Dilute to 0.1 mg/mL and infuse for at least 4 hours; a faster infusion (i.e., 45 minutes to
            2 hours) may be tolerated.
         ii. Use a central site.
         iii. Adding heparin may decrease phlebitis.
      c. Anemia
      d. Fever and chills
         i. Mechanism: Amphotericin B induces prostaglandin synthesis.
         ii. Premedications
            (a) Hydrocortisone: 25 mg intravenously before the dose or in the bottle decreases fever and
               chills (higher doses are not significantly better)

       (b) Ibuprofen (10 mg/kg up to 600 mg 30 minutes before infusion): Significantly more fever and chills in placebo (87%) than in ibuprofen group (48%)

       (c) Acetylsalicylic acid, acetaminophen, diphenhydramine: Never shown to be effective (but not specifically studied)

  e. Rigors treatment

     i. Meperidine 50 mg: Stops reaction within 30 minutes (mean, 10.8 minutes)

     ii. If the patient consistently needs meperidine, then prophylactic doses may be appropriate.

4. Dosing

  a. Start therapy with 0.25 mg/kg (some suggest 5–10 mg) administered for 4–6 hours.

  b. Increase gradually to desired milligram per kilogram concentration (i.e., 5- to 10-mg increments).

  c. May increase rapidly in fulminant infections or immunocompromised patients

  d. Amphotericin can be given on alternate days by doubling the daily dose to a maximum of 1.5 mg/kg.

5. Lipid amphotericin formulations (liposome, lipid complex, and colloidal dispersion)

  a. Lipid formulations are designed to maintain therapeutic efficacy, but they diminish renal- and infusion-related toxicity.

Table 11. Amphotericin Formulations

	Amphotericin B Deoxycholate	Abelcet	Amphotec	AmBisome
Lipid type		Multilamellar vesicle with ribbonlike structure (lipid complex)	Colloidal dispersion in aqueous solution (disk-shaped bilayer)	Unilamellar liposome
Dose	0.7–1 mg/kg/day	5 mg/kg/day for 2 hours	3–4 mg/kg/day for 3–4 hours	3–5 mg/kg/day
Test dose	Yes	None	Yes	None
Chills or rigors (%)	54–56	18	77	18
Fever (%)	44–47	14	55	17
Nephrotoxicity (%)	34–47	28	8	19
Hypokalemia (%)	12–29	5	26	7
Hypomagnesemia (%)	11–26	NA	6	20

  b. Mostly taken up by macrophages in the lung, liver, spleen, bone marrow, and circulating monocytes

  c. Liposomes target fungal cell membranes much more than human cell membranes.

  d. Amphotericin dissociates from the liposome over time, decreasing its toxicity (only free drug is toxic).

  e. Primary use in patients with aspergillosis and cryptococcal meningitis who cannot tolerate amphotericin B deoxycholate

  f. Potential use for invasive candidiasis

B. Azole Antifungals

1. Mechanism of action: Inhibits the synthesis of ergosterol, a component of the fungal cell membrane, vital for normal growth

2. Ketoconazole (Nizoral): Use only if no option for using alternative antifungals.
   a. Spectrum of activity
      i. *Candida* spp., *Blastomyces,* histoplasmosis, *Coccidioides, Sporothrix,* dermatophytes
      ii. Clinical use: Histoplasmosis, superficial *Candida* and other infections, blastomycosis, coccidioidomycosis
   b. Adverse effects
      i. Nausea, abdominal pain, headache, rash
      ii. Adrenal insufficiency, decreased libido, impotence, gynecomastia, menstrual irregularities (inhibits steroidogenesis)
      iii. Elevated liver function tests, potential fulminate hepatitis
   c. Drug interactions (CYP3A4 substrate and inhibitor)
      i. Antacids, histamine-2 (H_2)-blockers, proton pump inhibitors, didanosine (gastrointestinal absorption)
      ii. Rifampin (decreases ketoconazole concentrations)
      iii. Cyclosporine
      iv. Phenytoin
      v. Warfarin
      vi. Methylprednisolone, midazolam, alprazolam, simvastatin, lovastatin
      vii. Protease inhibitors
   d. Dosing: 200–400 mg/day
3. Fluconazole (Diflucan)
   a. Spectrum of activity
      i. *Candida* spp. (poor activity against *C. glabrata* and no activity against *C. krusei*), *Cryptococcus, Blastomyces, Histoplasma,* dermatophytes
      ii. Clinical use
         (a) *Candida* infections (primarily *C. albicans* and *C. parapsilosis*)
         (b) Cryptococcal meningitis
   b. Pharmacokinetics
      i. Well absorbed orally (bioavailability 100%); also available intravenously
      ii. Half-life is about 30 hours; primarily eliminated unchanged in the urine
   c. Adverse effects
      i. Nausea, abdominal pain, headache, reversible alopecia
      ii. Elevated liver function tests
   d. Drug interactions (CYP3A4 inhibitor at more than 400 mg/day and CYP2C9 inhibitor at lower doses)
      i. Cyclosporine
      ii. Phenytoin
      iii. Warfarin
   e. Dosing
      i. Oral candidiasis: 100–200 mg/day
      ii. Esophageal candidiasis: 200–400 mg/day
      iii. Invasive candidiasis: 400–800 mg/day
      iv. Acute cryptococcal meningitis: 400–800 mg/day
      v. Cryptococcal meningitis prophylaxis: 200 mg/day
4. Itraconazole (Sporanox)
   a. Spectrum of activity
      i. *Candida* spp. (usually just *C. albicans*), *Cryptococcus, Aspergillus, Blastomyces, Histoplasma,* dermatophytes

      ii. Clinical use

        (a) Onychomycosis

        (b) Histoplasmosis

        (c) Aspergillosis

        (d) Blastomycosis

  b. Pharmacokinetics

      i. Oral absorption about 55% when given with food

      ii. Half-life is about 20 hours; extensively metabolized; hydroxy itraconazole is active.

  c. Adverse effects

      i. Nausea, abdominal pain, headache, rash

      ii. Elevated liver function tests, potential fulminate hepatitis

      iii. Caution in heart failure (avoid doses ≥400 mg/day; do not use for treatment of onychomycosis if heart failure)

  d. Drug interactions (CYP3A4 inhibitor at more than 400 mg/day and CYP2C9 inhibitor at lower doses)

      i. Antacids, H_2-blockers, proton pump inhibitors, didanosine (gastrointestinal absorption)

      ii. Cyclosporine

      iii. Digoxin (decreases digoxin volume of distribution)

      iv. Phenytoin

      v. Warfarin

      vi. Protease inhibitors

      vii. HMG-CoA (3-hydroxy-3-methylglutaryl coenzyme A) reductase inhibitors

  e. Dosing: 100–200 mg/day. Oral capsules with food; oral solution without food

5. Voriconazole (Vfend)

  a. Spectrum of activity

      i. *Candida* spp., *Aspergillus, Fusarium, Scedosporium, Histoplasma, Cryptococcus*

      ii. Clinical use

        (a) Resistant *Candida* infections (especially *C. glabrata* and *C. krusei*)

        (b) Aspergillosis

        (c) Histoplasmosis

  b. Pharmacokinetics

      i. Oral absorption about 95%; also available intravenously

      ii. Half-life is about 6 hours; extensively metabolized; CYP2C9, CYP3A4, CYP2C19

  c. Adverse effects

      i. Abnormal vision 30% (abnormal vision, color changes, photophobia). Short-term (20–30 minutes) effects on retina. Dose related. Not studied for more than 28 days of therapy

      ii. Elevated liver function tests, rash, nausea

  d. Drug interactions (CYP3A4 and CYP2C9 inhibitor and substrate; see Table 12)

  e. Dosing

      i. Aspergillosis: Loading dose, 6 mg/kg two times intravenously (infuse for 2 hours); maintenance dose, 4 mg/kg every 12 hours intravenously (infuse for 2 hours)

      ii. Candidiasis and candidemia: 400 mg orally or intravenously every 12 hours for two doses, then 200 mg every 12 hours

        (a) For patients who are receiving phenytoin, increase dose to 5 mg/kg every 12 hours intravenously or 200–400 mg every 12 hours orally.

        (b) Dose reduction for moderate or severe cirrhosis: After loading dose, decrease dose by 50% in Child-Pugh class A/B. No information for patients in Child-Pugh class C

(c) No adjustment of the oral dose for renal insufficiency; patients with CrCl less than 50 mL/minute should not receive the intravenous product because of accumulation of the intravenous vehicle sulfobutyl ether-β-cyclodextrin.

(d) Therapeutic drug monitoring indicated because of polymorphism in CYP2C19 metabolism

Table 12. Drug Interactions Reported with Voriconazole

Drug	Effect	Recommendation
Rifampin (CYP inducer)	↓ Voriconazole	Coadministration contraindicated
Rifabutin (CYP inducer)	↓ Voriconazole ↑ Rifabutin	Coadministration contraindicated
Carbamazepine (CYP inducer)	↓ Voriconazole	Coadministration contraindicated
Barbiturates, long acting (CYP inducers)	↓ Voriconazole	Coadministration contraindicated
Pimozide (CYP3A4 substrate)	↑ Pimozide ↑ Risk QT prolongation	Coadministration contraindicated
Quinidine (CYP3A4 substrate)	↑ Quinidine ↑ Risk QT prolongation	Coadministration contraindicated
Ergot alkaloids	↑ Ergot alkaloids ↑ Risk ergotism	Coadministration contraindicated
Sirolimus (CYP3A4 substrate)	↑ Sirolimus	Coadministration contraindicated
Cyclosporine (CYP3A4 substrate)	↑ Cyclosporine	Reduce cyclosporine dose by half when initiating voriconazole Monitor levels closely Increase cyclosporine dose as necessary when voriconazole is discontinued
Tacrolimus (CYP3A4 substrate)	↑ Tacrolimus	Reduce tacrolimus dose to one-third of initial dose when initiating voriconazole Monitor levels closely Increase tacrolimus dose as necessary when voriconazole is discontinued
Omeprazole (CYP2C19 inhibitor, CYP2C19 and CYP3A4 substrate)	↑ Voriconazole ↑ Omeprazole	In patients receiving omeprazole doses ≥40 mg, reduce omeprazole dose by half
Warfarin (CYP2C9 substrate)	↑ Warfarin ↑ PT	Closely monitor PT/INR and adjust warfarin dose as needed

CYP = cytochrome P450; INR = international normalized ratio; PT = prothrombin time.

6. Posaconazole (Noxafil)
   a. Spectrum of activity
      i. *Candida* spp., *Cryptococcus, Trichosporon, Aspergillus, Fusarium, Zygomycetes*
      ii. Clinical use
         (a) *Candida* infections
         (b) Aspergillosis
         (c) Zygomycoses
         (d) Fusariosis

    b. Pharmacokinetics
       i. Oral absorption of suspension increased by a high-fat meal
       ii. New oral tablet formulation: Food has less impact on absorption.
       iii. Half-life is about 24–30 hours; primarily eliminated unchanged in the feces
    c. Adverse effects
       i. Nausea, vomiting, diarrhea
       ii. Elevated liver function tests, rash, hypokalemia, thrombocytopenia
       iii. Corrected QT (QTc) interval prolongation
    d. Drug interactions: CYP3A4 inhibitor; decreased posaconazole absorption with proton pump inhibitors and H_2-blockers
    e. Dosing: Oropharyngeal candidiasis, 100 mg/day; refractory oropharyngeal candidiasis, 400 mg twice daily; prophylaxis of invasive fungal infections in neutropenic and patients with graft-versus-host disease, 200 mg three times daily (suspension), 300 mg daily (tablet or intravenous)

C. Echinocandins
  1. Mechanism of action: Inhibits synthesis of 1,3-β-D-glucan, an essential component of the fungal cell wall
  2. Caspofungin (Cancidas), micafungin (Mycamine), anidulafungin (Eraxis)
    a. Spectrum of activity
       i. *Candida* spp. (weak against *C. parapsilosis*), *Aspergillus*
       ii. Clinical use
         (a) *Candida:* Invasive candidiasis, candidemia, intra-abdominal abscesses, peritonitis, and pleural space infections
         (b) Esophageal candidiasis
         (c) Invasive aspergillosis (refractory to or intolerant of other therapies)
    b. Pharmacokinetics
       i. Only available intravenously
       ii. Half-life of about 1–2 days; caspofungin and micafungin hepatically metabolized; anidulafungin chemically degraded in the blood
    c. Adverse effects: Infusion site–related reactions, headache, gastrointestinal symptoms
    d. Drug interactions
       i. Caspofungin: Avoid concomitant use with cyclosporine or tacrolimus.
       ii. Micafungin: Avoid concomitant sirolimus or nifedipine.
       iii. Anidulafungin: None
    e. Dosing
       i. Caspofungin: 70 mg once intravenously, followed by 50 mg/day intravenously (lower dose for Child-Pugh class B: 70 mg loading, then 35–50 mg daily)
       ii. Micafungin: Candidemia 100 mg/day; esophageal candidiasis or aspergillosis 150 mg/day
       iii. Anidulafungin: 200 mg once intravenously, followed by 100 mg/day intravenously

REFERENCES

Human Immunodeficiency Virus

1. Kuhar DT, Henderson DK, Struble KA, et al.; U.S. Public Health Service Working Group. Updated U.S. Public Health Service guidelines for the management of occupational exposures to human immunodeficiency virus and recommendations for postexposure prophylaxis. Infect Control Hosp Epidemiol 2013;34:875-92.

2. Panel on Antiretroviral Guidelines for Adults and Adolescents. Guidelines for the Use of Antiretroviral Agents in HIV-1-Infected Adults and Adolescents. Department of Health and Human Services. May 1, 2014:1-267. Available at www.aidsinfo.nih.gov/ContentFiles/AdultandAdolescentGL.pdf. Accessed August 26, 2014.

3. Panel on Treatment of HIV-Infected Pregnant Women and Prevention of Perinatal Transmission. Recommendations for Use of Antiretroviral Drugs in Pregnant HIV-1-Infected Women for Maternal Health and Interventions to Reduce Perinatal HIV Transmission in the United States. September 14, 2011:1-207. Available at http://aidsinfo.nih.gov/ContentFiles/PerinatalGL.pdf. Accessed October 10, 2012.

4. Günthard HF, Aberg JA, Eron JJ, et al.; International Antiviral Society–USA Panel. Antiretroviral treatment of adult HIV infection: 2014 recommendations of the International Antiviral Society–USA Panel. JAMA. 2014;312(4):410-25.

Opportunistic Infections in Patients with HIV

1. Panel on Opportunistic Infections in HIV-Infected Adults and Adolescents. Guidelines for the Prevention and Treatment of Opportunistic Infections in HIV-Infected Adults and Adolescents: Recommendations from the Centers for Disease Control and Prevention, the National Institutes of Health, and the HIV Medicine Association of the Infectious Diseases Society of America. Available at http://aidsinfo.nih.gov/contentfiles/lvguidelines/adult_oi.pdf. Accessed September 27, 2013.

Tuberculosis

1. American Thoracic Society/Centers for Disease Control and Prevention/Infectious Diseases Society of America. Treatment of tuberculosis. Am J Respir Crit Care Med 2003;167:603-62.

2. Horsburgh CR Jr, Rubin EJ. Clinical practice. Latent tuberculosis infection in the United States. N Engl J Med 2011;364:1441-8.

3. Targeted tuberculin testing and treatment of latent tuberculosis infection. Am J Respir Crit Care Med 2000;161:S221-47.

4. Zumla A, Raviglione M, Hafner R, et al. Tuberculosis. N Engl J Med 2013;368:745-55.

Antifungal Therapy

1. Limper AH, Knox KS, Sarosi GA, et al.; American Thoracic Society Fungal Working Group. An official American Thoracic Society statement: treatment of fungal infections in adult pulmonary and critical care patients. Am J Respir Crit Care Med 2011;183:96-128.

2. Pappas PG, Kauffman CA, Andes D, et al. Infectious Diseases Society of America. Clinical practice guidelines for the management of candidiasis: 2009 update by the Infectious Diseases Society of America. Clin Infect Dis 2009;48:503-35.

3. Perfect JR, Dismukes WE, Dromer F, et al. Clinical practice guidelines for the management of cryptococcal disease: 2010 update by the Infectious Diseases Society of America. Clin Infect Dis 2010;50:291-322.

ANSWERS AND EXPLANATIONS TO PATIENT CASES

1. Answer: D

The patient should be treated at this time; a potent combination ART definitely should be initiated when CD4 counts fall below 350 cells/mm³ and can be initiated in patients with CD4 counts greater than 350 cells/mm³ (although this is a lower strength of recommendation). The combination therapy of tenofovir, emtricitabine, and atazanavir/ritonavir is a preferred initial therapeutic regimen. Monotherapy is not indicated for HIV. Although treatment with zidovudine, lamivudine, and nevirapine is an acceptable alternative, it should not be first-line therapy.

2. Answer: D

A change in potent combination ART should be made when the viral load becomes detectable after a period of levels below detection. Some clinicians would wait and monitor the patient closely if the viral load increased to 10,000 copies/mL. However, these patients generally will require changes in therapy in the future. Testing is showing resistance to atazanavir. Because of that, changes in ART must be made. Simply stressing adherence and continuing the same regimen is inappropriate. Ideally, a new regimen should contain at least two, preferably three fully active drugs. In general, changing a single antiretroviral in a failing regimen is not recommended because of the risk of rapid development of resistance. Changing only one drug in a regimen should be done only for intolerance. Therefore, initiating an entirely new regimen of abacavir, lamivudine, and darunavir/ritonavir is best because changing all three agents simultaneously limits the possibility of resistance to the new regimen occurring quickly.

3. Answer: C

A patient taking darunavir/ritonavir should be monitored for endocrine disturbances (e.g., hyperglycemia, fat redistribution, lipid abnormalities) because all PIs can cause endocrine disturbances. Because darunavir/ritonavir does not cause peripheral neuropathy (although didanosine, zalcitabine, and stavudine do), this does not need to be monitored. Drug interaction with drugs metabolized by CYP1A2 is not of concern because darunavir is an inhibitor of CYP3A4, and ritonavir is an inhibitor of CYP2D6 and CYP3A4.

Darunavir does not cause nephrolithiasis; thus, the patient does not need to be monitored for this (although a patient taking indinavir does).

4. Answer: A

When the CD4 count decreases to 135 cells/mm³, the patient should receive primary prophylactic treatment against PCP (CD4 count less than 200 cells/mm³). Primary prophylaxis is necessary for MAC when the CD4 count is less than 50 cells/mm³. For CMV, patients with CD4 counts less than 50 cells/mm³ should receive regular funduscopic examinations. In general, primary prophylaxis is not used for cryptococcal meningitis.

5. Answer: C

Although pentamidine would be an appropriate therapeutic option for a patient who is HIV positive with PCP, the optimal empiric therapy is trimethoprim/sulfamethoxazole intravenously with adjuvant prednisone therapy for 21 days. Although trimethoprim/sulfamethoxazole is the drug of choice for PCP, adjuvant prednisone therapy is indicated because the patient's A-a gradient is 55, and the patient's Po_2 is less than 70. Atovaquone is indicated only for patients with mild to moderate PCP who cannot tolerate trimethoprim/sulfamethoxazole. This patient does not meet this criterion.

6. Answer: B

Patients with cryptococcal meningitis should always receive secondary prophylaxis. One of the principles of treating AIDS-related illnesses is that the infections are seldom curable, and generally, long-term preventable therapy is required. Weekly amphotericin B has been studied for secondary prophylaxis, but fluconazole is the best agent for secondary prophylaxis. The agents that are effective for PCP prophylaxis have no activity against *Cryptococcus*.

7. Answer: B

Maintenance therapy for cryptococcal meningitis with fluconazole can be discontinued after a minimum of 1 year of long-term maintenance therapy if the CD4 count increases to more than 100 cells/mm³ for 3 months or longer after potent combination ART. Because this patient's CD4 counts have been greater than 100 cells/

mm³ for at least 3 months, maintenance therapy can be discontinued after he has been treated for 1 year.

8. Answer: B

For the treatment of MAC, azithromycin plus ethambutol for at least 12 months is the best therapeutic combination; this combination includes one of the newer macrolides and a second agent (ethambutol is usually the preferred second agent). Therapy may be discontinued after 12 months if CD4 counts increase with potent combination ART and if the patient is asymptomatic. Clarithromycin plus ethambutol for 2 weeks, followed by maintenance with clarithromycin alone, is incorrect because there is no induction therapy followed by maintenance monotherapy for MAC. A therapeutic regimen of clarithromycin plus isoniazid is not the best because isoniazid has no activity against MAC. Although ethambutol plus rifabutin has activity against MAC, the current recommendations are that all therapeutic regimens include either azithromycin or clarithromycin; therefore, the ethambutol plus rifabutin regimen is not the treatment of choice.

9. Answer: D

A patient with an induration of greater than 15 mm after a PPD skin test for TB needs to be assessed for treatment. Because this patient's PPD skin test was negative last year, he is considered a recent converter and needs to be treated. He would also need to be treated if there were patients with TB at the long-term care facility. The booster effect is a phenomenon associated with an initial small reaction causing immunologic stimulation, followed by a larger reaction with a subsequent test. This patient had an initial large reaction (18-mm induration). Age is not a factor to consider in treating latent TB. Initiating isoniazid 300 mg/day orally for 9 months is the best recommendation for managing this patient's positive PPD.

10. Answer: C

This patient's HIV medications should be changed (rifampin will induce the metabolism of fosamprenavir and ritonavir). He should not receive a PI (except for full-dose ritonavir) or an NNRTI (except for efavirenz) with rifampin. Patients who are HIV positive should be initiated on four drugs for TB, and fosamprenavir should not be used with rifampin. The best recommendation is isoniazid, rifabutin, pyrazinamide, and ethambutol,

with a lower dose of rifabutin; it includes the four drugs for TB and a lower dose of rifabutin (because of fosamprenavir/ritonavir inhibition). The fosamprenavir/ritonavir dose does not need to be changed when adding rifabutin.

11. Answer: C

For this patient, only rifamycin and isoniazid need to be continued after 2 months of therapy with the four drugs for TB. The regimen can be simplified to a rifamycin and isoniazid after 2 months, but the recommended treatment duration is 6 months. The concentrations of HIV RNA should be monitored closely because of potential alterations in drug concentrations of the PI.

12. Answer: B

Micafungin has activity against *Aspergillus* and is the best option for this patient because it does not require dosage adjustment for renal dysfunction and has limited drug interactions. Lipid amphotericin has activity against *Aspergillus* and could be used for this infection, but because of its renal toxicity, Lipid amphotericin is not the best choice in this patient with acute renal failure. Fluconazole has no activity against *Aspergillus* and also may potentially interact with the some of the drugs the patient is receiving. Voriconazole has activity against *Aspergillus,* but it significantly interacts with a number of the drugs the patient is receiving (atorvastatin, dronedarone, warfarin, carbamazepine), making it a less than ideal choice in this patient.

ANSWERS AND EXPLANATIONS TO SELF-ASSESSMENT QUESTIONS

1. Answer: D
Transmission of HIV to a child is decreased if the mother's viral load is decreased. The benefits of therapy far outweigh the risk. A potent combination ART that includes zidovudine throughout the pregnancy is the most appropriate therapeutic regimen for an asymptomatic patient with HIV who is pregnant (even in the first trimester) and has a low CD4 count and high viral load (although if the woman is on a fully suppressed regimen without zidovudine, that regimen should be continued without changes). Although zidovudine 300 mg twice daily orally throughout the pregnancy, followed by zidovudine during labor and to the baby for 6 weeks, was the regimen originally studied to decrease HIV transmission, potent combination ART is indicated because of the patient's low CD4 count and high viral load; therefore, single-drug therapy is inappropriate. A single dose of nevirapine at the onset of labor will not affect viral load or lower the risk of HIV transmission as much as potent combination ART throughout the pregnancy. Single-dose nevirapine is indicated in women in labor who were not treated during their pregnancy.

2. Answer: A
The patient should be told that atazanavir can cause hyperbilirubinemia. This patient should be told to talk to a pharmacist about the current combination therapy because there are many drug interactions with antiretroviral agents. However, although atazanavir inhibits CYP3A4, tenofovir does not (it is an NRTI, not a PI). In addition, informing the patient to cut the dose in half if there are adverse effects is incorrect because antiretroviral drugs, especially PIs, should never be used below the recommended dose. Informing the patient that tenofovir and emtricitabine cause additive peripheral neuropathy is incorrect because neither of these drugs is associated with that adverse effect.

3. Answer: B
There are many other reasons to change ART in addition to clinical deterioration. These include an inability to decrease viral load to undetectable levels, the detection of virus after initial suppression to undetectable levels, a failure to increase the CD4 count by 50–100 cells/mm³ during the first year of therapy, and a failure

to increase the CD4 count above 350 cells/mm³ while on therapy. If there is a question of ineffective ART, single drugs should be changed only with caution (consider changing the entire regimen). Resistance does not occur more commonly with emtricitabine than with other antiretroviral agents.

4. Answer: A
A change in therapy is indicated for the patient taking potent combination ART and experiencing hyperglycemia, fat redistribution, and lipid abnormalities. Although adding lipid-lowering agents may be indicated to lower cardiovascular risks, simvastatin should not be used with lopinavir or ritonavir because of the drug interaction (increased simvastatin concentrations lead to an increased risk of myalgias). Pravastatin is a better choice (even though it may decrease ritonavir concentrations). Although adding an insulin-sensitizing agent may be indicated, pioglitazone should not be used with lopinavir or ritonavir because of the drug interaction (increased pioglitazone concentrations and potential induction of PI metabolism by pioglitazone). At this time, changing agents (if possible) to an effective regimen that does not cause endocrine disturbances is the best option. The NRTIs that can increase lipid levels include stavudine, zidovudine, and abacavir; therefore, these agents should be avoided. Abacavir is also associated with an increased incidence of myocardial infarction. All of the ritonavir-boosted PIs can increase lipid concentrations, as can efavirenz; therefore, these agents should be avoided. The best option is therefore tenofovir, emtricitabine, and rilpivirine.

5. Answer: D
The current recommended regimen for treating cryptococcal meningitis in patients positive for HIV is amphotericin B 0.7 mg/kg/day plus flucytosine 25 mg/kg every 6 hours for 2 weeks, followed by fluconazole 400 mg/day. Fluconazole alone is recommended only for mild to moderate cryptococcal meningitis, and the dose should be 400 mg/day. Studies have shown that early mortality is greater with fluconazole alone than with amphotericin B alone. When amphotericin B is used alone for cryptococcal meningitis, the dose should be 0.7 mg/kg per day, not 0.3 mg/kg per day. The flucytosine dose of 37.5 mg/kg every 6 hours is high and is

especially likely to cause bone marrow suppression in patients who are HIV positive.

6. Answer: C
The number of patients needed to treat with isoniazid over rifampin to prevent one progression to active disease is $200 = 1/(0.008 - 0.003)$. The only information needed is the absolute risk in both groups, which is provided.

7. Answer: D
Pyrimethamine plus clindamycin and leucovorin for 6 weeks is the correct choice for treating toxoplasmosis in a patient who is HIV positive, not taking antiretrovirals, and taking dapsone for PCP prophylaxis. Atovaquone is not first-line therapy, although data support its effectiveness in combination with sulfadiazine or pyrimethamine; trimethoprim/sulfamethoxazole is not effective for treatment or secondary prophylaxis of toxoplasmosis. Pyrimethamine and sulfadiazine are the first-line agents for toxoplasmosis; however, leucovorin should always be used with pyrimethamine to prevent myelosuppression.

8. Answer: D
Fluconazole does not have activity against aspergillus, so it would not be an option for therapy. Although voriconazole has activity against aspergillus, there is a significant interaction with rifampin, resulting in lower voriconazole concentrations. Flucytosine does not have activity against aspergillus. Micafungin would be the best option because of its activity against aspergillus and lack of drug interaction with any of the TB medications.

9. Answer: B
Because the patient is symptomatic and her sputum is acid-fast bacillus positive, she should be treated for an active TB infection. The recommended therapy for active TB is isoniazid, rifampin, pyrazinamide, and ethambutol for 2 months, followed by isoniazid and rifampin for 4 more months. Patients should be initiated on at least three antibiotics for the first 2 months. Although fluoroquinolones have some activity against TB, their use as first-line monotherapy is inappropriate.

10. Answer: C
Data are continuous and probably normally distributed (given the large population of 350 patients in the study); therefore, a parametric test is indicated. The t-test is the best parametric test for comparing two groups. Although an analysis of variance is a parametric test, it is used to compare more than two groups. A chi-square test is used to compare nominal or categorical data between two groups. The end points in this study are continuous and should therefore not be compared using this statistical test. The Wilcoxon rank sum test is a nonparametric analog to the t-test.

Pharmacokinetics: A Refresher

Curtis L. Smith, Pharm.D., BCPS

Ferris State University
Lansing, Michigan

PHARMACOKINETICS: A REFRESHER

CURTIS L. SMITH, PHARM.D., BCPS

FERRIS STATE UNIVERSITY
LANSING, MICHIGAN

Learning Objectives

1. Identify and provide examples using basic pharmacokinetic concepts commonly used in clinical practice, including elimination rate constant, volume of distribution, clearance, and bioavailability.
2. Describe specific pharmacokinetic characteristics of commonly used therapeutic agents, including aminoglycosides, vancomycin, phenytoin, and digoxin, as well as pharmacokinetic alterations in patients with renal and hepatic disease.
3. Define important issues as they pertain to drug concentration sampling and interpretation.

Self-Assessment Questions

Answers and explanations to these questions can be found at the end of this chapter.

1. J.H., a 65-year-old woman (65 kg), was recently initiated on tobramycin and piperacillin/tazobactam for the treatment of hospital-acquired pneumonia. After the first tobramycin dose of 120 mg (infused from noon to 1:00 p.m.), serum tobramycin concentrations are drawn. They are 4.4 mg/L at 3:00 p.m. and 1.2 mg/L at 7:00 p.m. Which is the best assessment regarding the calculation of tobramycin pharmacokinetic parameters in this patient?

    A. Data are sufficient to determine the half-life but not the volume of distribution (Vd).

    B. Data are sufficient to determine both the half-life and the Vd.

    C. Data are insufficient to determine either the half-life or the Vd.

    D. Data are sufficient to determine the Vd but not the half-life.

2. P.L. is a 60-year-old woman (60 kg) recently initiated on gentamicin and clindamycin. After the first gentamicin dose of 110 mg (infused from 6:00 p.m. to 6:30 p.m.), serum gentamicin concentrations are drawn. They are 3.6 mg/L at 7:30 p.m. and 0.9 mg/L at 11:30 p.m. Which is the best assessment of this patient's gentamicin pharmacokinetic parameters?

    A. The half-life is about 2 hours.

    B. The half-life is about 3 hours.

    C. The maximum concentration (Cmax) is about 3.8 mg/L.

    D. The Vd is about 11.6 L.

3. R.O. is a 74-year-old woman initiated on gentamicin 100 mg intravenously every 24 hours for pyelonephritis. On admission, her serum creatinine (SCr) is 1.8 mg/dL. She also has congestive heart failure and is fluid overloaded because of her diminished renal function, and she is nonadherent to her angiotensin-converting enzyme inhibitor and diuretic. A few days into her hospitalization, her SCr is down to 1.1 mg/dL, and she is reinitiated on furosemide and enalapril. Which most likely happened to the gentamicin half-life in R.O. during her hospitalization?

    A. Her clearance increased, which increased her Vd and decreased her half-life.

    B. Her clearance increased, which increased her elimination rate constant and decreased her half-life.

    C. Her Vd decreased, which increased her clearance and decreased her half-life.

    D. Her Vd decreased, which increased her elimination rate constant and increased her half-life.

4. A patient receives vancomycin 1000 mg intravenously every 24 hours and has a trough concentration, drawn 30 minutes before the next dose, of 6 mg/L. Which regimen is best for this patient if the goal trough concentration is 10–15 mg/L?

    A. Maintain the dose at 1000 mg intravenously every 24 hours.

    B. Lower the dose to 500 mg, but keep the interval at every 24 hours.

    C. Keep the dose at 1000 mg, but shorten the interval to every 12 hours.

    D. Lower the dose to 500 mg, and shorten the interval to every 12 hours.

5. R.K., a 39-year-old man who is human immunodeficiency virus (HIV)-positive, receives a diagnosis of cryptococcal meningitis and begins taking amphotericin B and flucytosine. You want to keep flucytosine peak concentrations between 50 and

100 mcg/mL. Assuming a trough concentration of 25 mcg/ mL, dosing every 6 hours, and 100% bioavailability, which is the best dose to achieve a peak concentration within the desired range (flucytosine volume of distribution of 0.7 L/kg and half-life of 3 hours)?

A. 12.5 mg/kg.

B. 37.5 mg/kg.

C. 75 mg/kg.

D. 150 mg/kg.

6. L.R. is a 49-year-old patient with diabetes mellitus and renal failure. He was recently in a car accident and sustained a head trauma. He currently receives phenytoin 100 mg intravenously three times/day, and his most recent concentration was 5.6 mcg/mL. You are asked to suggest a new dose to achieve a concentration within the therapeutic range. Laboratory results include sodium 145 mEq/L, potassium 3.9 mEq/L, chloride 101 mEq/L, carbon dioxide 26 mEq/L, blood urea nitrogen (BUN) 95 mg/dL, SCr 5.4 mg/dL, glucose 230 mg/dL, and albumin (Alb) 2.8 g/dL. Which is the best recommendation?

A. Increase the dose to 200 mg intravenously three times/day.

B. Increase the dose to 200 mg intravenously two times/day.

C. Decrease the dose to 100 mg intravenously two times/day.

D. Keep the dose the same.

7. You are asked how the fluorescence polarization immunoassay (TDx) and enzyme multiplied immunoassay technique (EMIT) assays compare with each other. Which statement is most accurate?

A. Although both are immunoassays, one labels antibody, whereas the other labels antigen.

B. Although both are immunoassays, one uses antibody as a marker, whereas the other uses a radioisotope.

C. Although both are immunoassays, one uses an enzyme label, whereas the other uses a fluorescent label.

D. They are both names for the same assay technique.

8. An older adult is seen in the morning medicine clinic for a routine follow-up. Medication history includes digoxin 0.25 mg/day by mouth, furosemide 40 mg/day by mouth, and potassium chloride 10 mEq/day by mouth. All doses were last taken at 8:00 a.m. today at home. The patient has vague complaints of stomach upset, which began 2 days ago, but is otherwise in no apparent distress. A serum digoxin concentration drawn today at 10:00 a.m. is 2.5 mcg/L. Which statement best describes what should be done next?

A. Admit the patient for administration of digoxin Fab.

B. Tell the patient to skip tomorrow's dose of digoxin and begin 0.125 mg/day by mouth.

C. Administer a dose of activated charcoal.

D. Do nothing today about the digoxin.

9. A research group is analyzing the relationship between various independent patient demographics (e.g., age, height, weight, Alb, creatinine clearance [CrCl]) and phenytoin pharmacokinetics. Which is the best statistical test to use in assessing the relationship?

A. One-way analysis of variance.

B. Analysis of covariance.

C. Multiple regression.

D. Spearman rank correlation.

10. N.T. is a 24-year-old woman receiving valproic acid for tonic-clonic seizures. Her most recent trough valproic acid concentration was 22 mg/L. Her most recent Alb concentration was 4.1 g/dL. Given this Alb, which recommendation is best regarding her dose?

A. Continue with the current dose; the concentration is close enough to the therapeutic range.

B. Assess adherence and increase her dose; the concentration is below the therapeutic range.

C. Decrease her dose; the concentration is slightly above the therapeutic range.

D. Assess adherence and then check a free valproic acid concentration and adjust accordingly.

Patient Cases

1. H.R. is receiving vancomycin for a methicillin-resistant *Staphylococcus aureus* bacteremia. H.R. has chronic renal failure. A 1-g intravenous dose of vancomycin is given at noon on March 21. A concentration drawn at 2:00 p.m. on March 21 is 23.8 mcg/mL. A concentration drawn at 2:00 p.m. on March 24 is 12.1 mcg/mL. If you were to give a dose at 4:00 p.m. on March 24 and your goal trough concentration was 10–15 mg/L, which would be the best time to give the next dose?

    A. 1 day after the dose on the 24th.

    B. 3 days from the dose on the 24th.

    C. 6 days from the dose on the 24th.

    D. Insufficient information to calculate when to redose.

2. After the administration of 100 mg of a drug intravenously and 200 mg of the same drug by mouth, the areas under the curves (AUCs) are 50 and 25 mg/L/hour. Which best describes the bioavailability of this drug?

    A. 25%.

    B. 37.5%.

    C. 50%.

    D. 100%.

3. L.B. is receiving tobramycin for a resistant *Pseudomonas aeruginosa* pneumonia. L.B. has chronic renal failure. A loading dose of 160 mg is given at noon over 1 hour. A concentration is drawn at 6:00 p.m., which is 6.5 mg/L, and again at 6:00 am the next day, which is 5.4 mg/L. When L.B.'s concentration is 1 mg/L, which dose will be best to achieve a peak of 9 mg/L?

    A. 140 mg.

    B. 160 mg.

    C. 180 mg.

    D. 200 mg.

I. BASIC PHARMACOKINETIC RELATIONSHIPS

Table 12 contains definitions of terms.

A. Absorption
$$F = \frac{\text{dose}_{iv} * \text{AUC}_{ev}}{\text{dose}_{ev} * \text{AUC}_{iv}}$$

B. Distribution

Rapid intravenous (or oral) bolus:
$$Vd = \frac{F * \text{dose}}{C_0}$$

Continuous intravenous infusion at steady state:
$$Vd = \frac{R_0}{k * C_{ss}}$$

Continuous intravenous infusion before steady state: $Vd = \dfrac{R_0}{C*k}(1-e^{-kt_i})$ and $C = \dfrac{R_0}{V_d*k}(1-e^{-kt_i})$

Multiple intravenous bolus at steady state: $Vd = \dfrac{dose}{C_{ss\,max}*(1-e^{-k\tau})}$

Multiple intermittent intravenous infusion at steady state: $Vd = \dfrac{R_0}{k} * \dfrac{1-e^{-kt}}{C_{max}-(C_{min}*e^{-kt'})}$

$C_{ss\,max} = \dfrac{R_0*(1-e^{-kt'})}{V_d*k*(1-e^{-k\tau})}$ $\qquad C_{ss\,min} = C_{ss\,max} = * \; e^{-k(\tau-t')}$

C. Clearance

$Clearance = \dfrac{dose}{AUC} \qquad k = \dfrac{Cl}{V_d} \qquad k = \dfrac{(\ln C_1 - \ln C_2)}{(t_2 - t_1)} \qquad t_{1/2} = \dfrac{0.693}{k}$

Continuous intravenous infusion at steady state: $\qquad Clearance = \dfrac{R_0}{C_{ss}}$

Continuous intravenous infusion before steady state: $\qquad Clearance = \dfrac{R_0}{C} * (1 - e^{-kt_i})$

Multiple intravenous (or oral) bolus at steady state: $\qquad Clearance = \dfrac{\dfrac{F*dose}{\tau}}{C_{ss,avg}}$

$\tau = \dfrac{(\ln C_{max} - \ln C_{min})}{k} \qquad C_1 = C_0 * e^{-kt}$

II. ABSORPTION

A. First-Pass Effect
1. Blood that perfuses almost all the gastrointestinal (GI) tissues passes through the liver by means of the hepatic portal vein.
   a. Fifty percent of the rectal blood supply bypasses the liver (middle and inferior hemorrhoidal veins).
   b. Drugs absorbed in the buccal cavity bypass the liver.
2. Examples of drugs with significant first-pass effect

Amitriptyline	Labetalol	Nitroglycerin
Desipramine	Lidocaine	Pentazocine
Diltiazem	Metoprolol	Propoxyphene
Doxepin	Morphine	Propranolol
Imipramine	Nicardipine	Verapamil
Isosorbide dinitrate	Nifedipine	

B. Enterohepatic Recirculation
   1. Drugs are excreted through the bile into the duodenum, metabolized by the normal flora in the GI tract, and reabsorbed into the portal circulation.
   2. Occurs with drugs that have biliary (hepatic) elimination and good oral absorption
   3. Drug is concentrated in the gallbladder and expelled on sight, smell, or ingestion of food.

Table 1. Examples of Compounds Excreted in Bile and Subject to Enterohepatic Cycling

Compound	Entity in Bile
Chloramphenicol	Glucuronide conjugate
Digoxin	Parent
Estrogens	Parent
Imipramine	Parent and desmethyl metabolite
Indomethacin	Parent and glucuronide
Nafcillin	Parent
Rifampin	Parent
Sulindac	Glucuronides of parent and metabolites
Testosterone	Conjugates
Tiagabine	Glucuronide conjugate
Valproic acid	Glucuronide conjugates
Vitamin A	Conjugates

Patient Case

4. Which statement best describes P-glycoprotein?

   A. It is a plasma protein that binds basic drugs.

   B. It transfers drugs through the GI mucosa, increasing absorption.

   C. It diminishes the effect of cytochrome P450 3A4 (CYP3A4) in the GI mucosa.

   D. It is an efflux pump that decreases GI mucosal absorption.

C. P-Glycoprotein
   1. P-glycoprotein is an efflux pump (located in the esophagus, stomach, and small and large intestines) that pumps drugs back into the GI lumen; it is a more important factor in drug absorption drug interactions than intestinal CYP3A4.
   2. Both CYP3A4 and P-glycoprotein are located in small intestinal enterocytes and work together to decrease the absorption of xenobiotics.
   3. Most CYP3A4 substrates are also P-glycoprotein substrates.
   4. Many CYP3A4 inhibitors/inducers also inhibit/induce P-glycoprotein, leading to increases or decreases in bioavailability.
   5. Examples of P-glycoprotein absorption drug interactions
      a. Dabigatran is affected by rifampin, St. John's wort, quinidine, ketoconazole, verapamil, amiodarone, and dronedarone.
      b. Digoxin is affected by St. John's wort, quinidine, verapamil, amiodarone, and dronedarone or dabigatran.
      c. Human immunodeficiency virus protease inhibitors are affected by rifampin and St. John's wort.

III. DISTRIBUTION

A. Definition: Apparent Vd: Proportionality constant that relates the amount of drug in the body to an observed concentration of drug

B. Protein Binding

Table 2. Common Proteins Involved in Drug Protein Binding

Protein	Types of Drugs Bound	Molecular Weight	Normal Concentrations	
			g/L	mcmol
Albumin	Acidic	65,000	35–50	500–700
α-1-Acid glycoprotein	Basic	44,000	0.4–1.0	9–23
Lipoprotein	Lipophilic and basic	200,000–3,400,000	Variable	Variable

C. P-Glycoprotein
   1. Functions as an efflux pump on the luminal surface of the blood-brain barrier, limiting entry to the central nervous system
   2. It may be especially important with opioids: Induction of P-glycoprotein by chronic use of opioids may decrease the opioid effect (tolerance).
   3. P-glycoprotein is also found in tumor cells, resulting in the efflux of chemotherapeutic agents from the cell and, ultimately, multidrug resistance.

IV. CLEARANCE

Table 3. Enzymes Involved in Drug Metabolism

Oxygenases	**Hydrolytic enzymes**
CYPs	Esterases
Monoamine oxygenases	Amidases
Alcohol dehydrogenases	Epoxide hydrolases
Aldehyde dehydrogenases	Dipeptidases
Xanthine dehydrogenases	
Conjugating enzymes	
Uridine diphosphate–glucuronyl transferases	
Glutathione *S*-transferase	
Acetyltransferases	
Methyltransferases	

CYP = cytochrome P450.

Table 4. Drug Transport Proteins

Transport Protein Superfamily	Transport Protein (*Gene* [Protein])	Location and Function	Drugs Affected by Transport Protein
SLC	*SLC01A2* [OATP-A]	Hepatocyte: Bile acid uptake	Digoxin Levofloxacin Methotrexate Statins
	SLCO1B1 [OATP1B1]	Hepatocyte: Hepatic uptake of drugs	Pravastatin Rifampin Simvastatin Valsartan
	SLCO1B3 [OATP1B3]	Hepatocyte: Hepatic uptake of drugs	Digoxin Fexofenadine Rifampin Statins
	SLC22A1, SLC22A2, SLC22A6, SLC22A8 [OAT and OCT]	Hepatocyte: Hepatic uptake of drugs Renal tubule (interstitial side): Secretion of drugs	Salicylate[a] Methotrexate[a] Zidovudine[a] Tetracycline[a] Organic anions and cations[b]
	SLCO2B1 [OATP2B1]	Hepatocyte: Hepatic uptake of drugs	Fexofenadine Glyburide Statins
	SLC15A1, SLC15A2 [PEPT1, PEPT2]	Renal tubule Intestinal enterocytes	Cephalexin Captopril Enalapril Valacyclovir
	SLC47A1, SLC47A2 [MATE1, MATE2-K]	Renal tubule	Metformin
ABC	*ABCB11* [BSEP]	Hepatocyte: Bile acid excretion into bile	Pravastatin
	ABCC2, 3, 4, and *5* [MRP2, 3, 4, and 5]	Hepatocyte: Excreting water-soluble drugs and metabolites into blood Renal tubule (luminal side): Secretion of drugs	Glucuronide, sulfate, and glutathione metabolites[a] Methotrexate[a] Pravastatin[a] Rifampin[a]
	ABCB1 [MDR1] (P-glycoprotein)	Hepatocyte: See text in handout Renal tubule (luminal side): See text in handout	See text
	ABCB4 [MDR3]	Hepatocyte	Digoxin Paclitaxel Vinblastine
	ABCG2 [BCRP]	Hepatocyte: Biliary excretion	Daunorubicin Doxorubicin Imatinib Methotrexate Mitoxantrone Statins Topotecan

[a]Drugs affected by transport proteins in hepatocytes.

[b]Drug affected by transport proteins in the renal tubule.

Patient Case

5. A renal transplant patient receiving cyclosporine is given a diagnosis of community-acquired pneumonia. The patient is admitted to the hospital and initiated on ceftriaxone and a macrolide. A physician asks you to choose a macrolide that will not interact with the patient's cyclosporine. Which macrolide is the best choice to meet the physician's criteria?

    A. Erythromycin.

    B. Clarithromycin.

    C. Azithromycin.

    D. Any macrolide (all macrolides inhibit CYP3A4).

A. Cytochrome P450
   1. Introduction
      a. A group of heme-containing enzymes responsible for phase 1 metabolic reactions
      b. Characteristic absorbance of light at 450 nm (thus, CYP450)
      c. Located primarily in the membranes of the smooth endoplasmic reticulum in liver; small intestine; and brain, lung, and kidney
      d. Encoded by a supergene family and subfamily; separate genes code for different isoenzymes
      e. Drugs generally have a high affinity for one particular CYP, but most drugs also have secondary pathways.
      f. Nomenclature

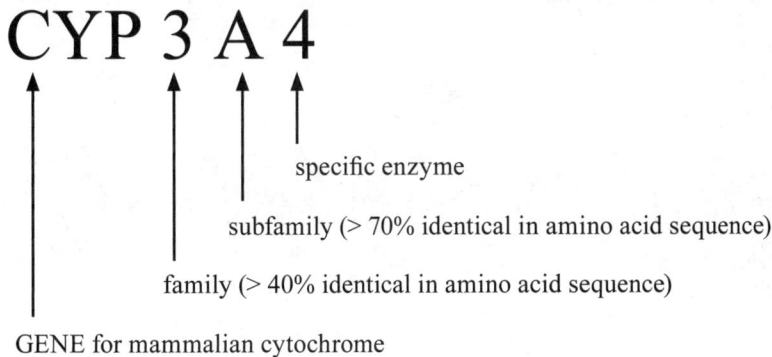

CYP 3 A 4

↑ ↑ ↑ ↑

specific enzyme

subfamily (> 70% identical in amino acid sequence)

family (> 40% identical in amino acid sequence)

GENE for mammalian cytochrome

Figure 1. Nomenclature.

2. Distribution of CYP isoenzymes in human liver

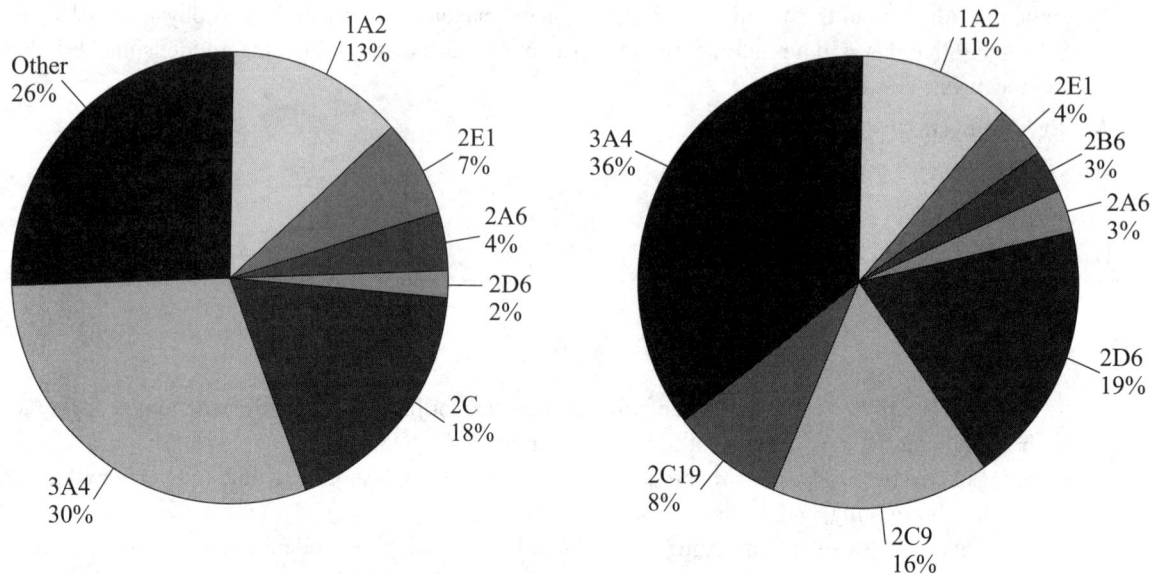

Figure 2. Distribution of CYP isoenzymes in human liver.

3. Distribution of CYP isoenzymes in human GI tract

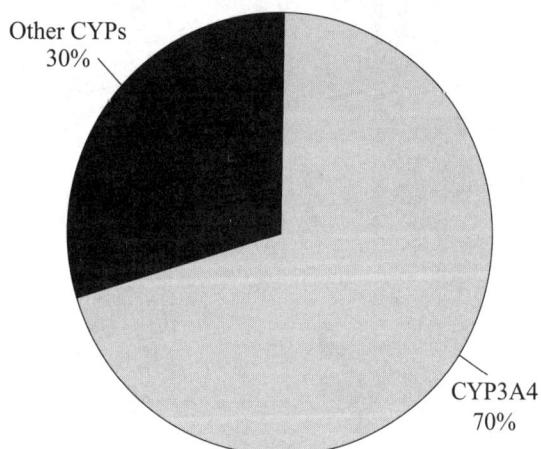

Figure 3. Distribution of CYP isoenzymes in human gastrointestinal tract.

4. Characteristics of CYP metabolism
   a. Inhibition is substrate-independent.
   b. Some substrates are metabolized by more than one CYP (e.g., tricyclic antidepressants [TCAs], selective serotonin reuptake inhibitors [SSRIs]).
   c. Enantiomers may be metabolized by a different CYP (e.g., R- vs. S-warfarin).
   d. Differences in inhibition may exist within the same class of agents (e.g., fluoroquinolones, azole antifungals, macrolides, calcium channel blockers, histamine-2 blockers).

    e.   Substrates can also be inhibitors (e.g., erythromycin, verapamil, diltiazem).

    f.   Most inducers and some inhibitors can affect more than one isozyme (e.g., cimetidine, ritonavir, fluoxetine, erythromycin).

    g.   Inhibitors may affect different isozymes at different doses (e.g., fluconazole inhibits CYP2C9 at doses of 100 mg/day or greater and inhibits CYP3A4 at doses of 400 mg/day or greater).

B. P-Glycoprotein
    1.   P-glycoprotein is an efflux pump that pumps drugs into the bile; the clinical effect of P-glycoprotein drug interactions in the bile is unknown.

    2.   P-glycoprotein pumps drugs from renal tubules into the urine; it also potentially limits the degree of reabsorption.

    3.   Examples of drug interactions: quinidine/digoxin, cyclosporine/digoxin, and propafenone/digoxin

C. Pharmacogenetics and Polymorphic Drug Metabolism and Transport
    1.   Population in general is divided into poor, intermediate, extensive, and ultrarapid metabolizers; therefore, metabolism is considered polymorphic.

    2.   Definition of polymorphism: Coexistence of more than one genetic variant (alleles), which are stable components in the population (more than 1% of population)

    3.   Clear antimode results

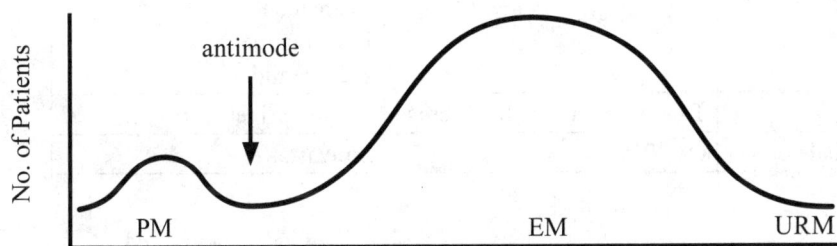

Metabolic ratio of unchanged drug to metabolite → (increasing metabolic capacity)

Figure 4. Distribution of patients in a drug that follows polymorphic metabolism.

EM = extensive metabolizer; PM = poor metabolizer; URM = ultrarapid extensive metabolizer.

    4.   Phenotype: Expression of the trait; interaction of gene with environment
        a.   Manifestation of the trait clinically
        b.   Not necessarily constant
    5.   Genotype: Genetic makeup

Table 5. Metabolic Pathways Showing Polymorphism

Pathway	Prototypical Substrate	Enzyme or Transporter	Drug Examples
Oxidation	Debrisoquine, dextromethorphan	CYP2D6	Tertiary amines Fluoxetine Flecainide Propafenone Metoprolol Propranolol Timolol Codeine Tamoxifen
Oxidation	Warfarin	CYP2C9	Amitriptyline Phenytoin Warfarin
Oxidation	Mephenytoin	CYP2C19	Clopidogrel Tertiary amines (diazepam) Phenytoin Omeprazole
Acetylation	Isoniazid, caffeine	N-acetyltransferase	Clonazepam Dapsone Hydralazine Inamrinone Procainamide Sulfonamides
Methylation	Thiopurines	Thiopurine methyltransferase	Azathioprine
Transport	Bromosulfophthalein	OATP1B1	Simvastatin

CYP = cytochrome P450.

6. Clinical Pharmacogenetics Implementation Consortium (CPIC)
   a. Designed to facilitate translation of pharmacogenetics information from research to clinical practice
   b. Developing guidelines for use of pharmacogenetic tests results in drug dosing
   c. Focused on specific drug-gene pairs (Table 6)

Table 6. CPIC Clinical Recommendations for Drug-Gene Pairs

Drug	Gene	Recommendation
Thiopurines (azathioprine, 6-mercaptopurine, thioguanine)	TMPT	Dosing recommendations for each drug based on TMPT genotype (normal/high, intermediate, and low activity)
Clopidogrel	CYP2C19	Normal dosing for ultrarapid metabolizer; alternative antiplatelet therapy in intermediate or poor metabolizers
Warfarin	VKORC1/CYP2C9	Use available table or algorithms to initiate warfarin dosing based on VKORC1 and CYP2C9 genotypes
Codeine	CYP2D6	Avoid using codeine because of potential toxicity or lack of efficacy in ultrarapid and poor metabolizers

Specific dosing recommendations for extensive and intermediate metabolizers |
| Abacavir | HLA-B | Avoid using because of increased incidence of hypersensitivity reactions in patients with the HLA-B*57:01 allele |
| Simvastatin | SLCO1B1 | Dosing recommendations based on genotype at rs4149056 in SLCO1B1, including starting at lower doses or using alternative statins |
| Allopurinol | HLA-B | Severe cutaneous adverse reactions associated with carriers of the HLA-B*58:01 allele

Avoid using allopurinol in these patients |
| Tricyclic antidepressants | CYP2D6, CYP2C19 | Dosing recommendations for depression based on metabolizer status (ultrarapid, extensive, intermediate, poor)

Limited recommendations when using for peripheral neuropathy |
| Carbamazepine | HLA-B | Avoid using because of increased incidence of severe cutaneous adverse reactions in patients with the HLA-B*15:02 allele |
| Capecitabine/5-fluorouracil/tegafur | DPYD | Increased risk of serious or fatal toxicity in patients with reduced or absent dihydropyrimidine dehydrogenase activity |
| Phenytoin | HLA-B | Reduce initial dose by 25% in CYP2C9 in intermediate metabolizers and 50% in poor metabolizers

Severe cutaneous adverse reactions associated with carriers of the HLA-B*58:01 allele

Use an alternative anticonvulsant |
Rasburicase	G6PD	Contraindicated in those with G6PD deficiency
Peginterferon	IFNL3	Patients with the favorable response IFNL3 genotype (rs12979860 CC) have increased likelihood of response to PEG-interferon-alpha-containing regimens
Ivacaftor	CFTR	Only recommended for cystic fibrosis patients who are either homozygous or heterozygous for the G551D-CFTR variant
SSRIs	CYP2D6, CYP2C19	TBA

Table 6. CPIC Clinical Recommendations for Drug-Gene Pairs *(continued)*

Drug	Gene	Recommendation
Irinotecan	*UGT1A1*	TBA
Oxycodone/tramadol	*CYP2D6*	TBA
Tacrolimus	*CYP3A5*	TBA
Aripiprazole/risperidone	*CYP2D6*	TBA
Atomoxetine	*CYP2D6*	TBA
Ondansetron	*CYP2D6*	TBA
Celecoxib	*CYP2C9*	TBA
Fluoroquinolones	*G6PD*	TBA
Dapsone	*G6PD*	TBA
Trimethoprim/ sulfamethoxazole	*G6PD*	TBA
Sulfasalazine	*G6PD*	TBA
Proton pump inhibitors	*CYP2C19*	TBA
Mirtazapine/venlafaxine	*CYP2D6*	TBA
Tamoxifen	*CYP2D6*	TBA
Voriconazole	*CYP2C19*	TBA

TBA = recommendations to be announced.

V. NONLINEAR PHARMACOKINETICS

Patient Case

6. C.M. is a 55-year-old man who is initiated on phenytoin after a craniotomy. His current steady-state phenytoin concentration is 6 mg/L at a dose of 200 mg/day by mouth. If his affinity constant (Km) is calculated to be 5 mg/L, which is most likely to occur if the dose is doubled (to 400 mg/day by mouth)?

   A. His concentration will double because phenytoin clearance is linear above the Km.

   B. His concentration will more than double because phenytoin clearance is nonlinear above the Km.

   C. His concentration will stay the same because phenytoin is an autoinducer, and clearance increases with time.

   D. His concentration will increase by only 50% because phenytoin absorption decreases significantly with doses greater than 300 mg.

A. Michaelis-Menten Pharmacokinetics

$$velocity = \frac{V_{max} * S}{K_m + S}$$

V_{max} = capacity constant (amount/time)

K_m = affinity constant (amount/volume)

S = substrate concentration (amount/volume)

B. Nonlinear Elimination

1. Saturation or partial saturation of the elimination pathway

$$\text{rate of elimination (dose)} = \frac{V_{max} * C}{K_m + C}$$

V_{max} = maximum rate of elimination (amount/time)

K_m = concentration where elimination is ½ V_{max} (affinity constant)

C = drug concentration

2. Note: Nonlinearity occurs when concentration is at or above K_m.
Example: Phenytoin

   a. V_{max} normal = 7 mg/kg/day

   b. K_m normal = 5.6 mg/L

   c. 50% variability between individuals

VI. NONCOMPARTMENTAL PHARMACOKINETICS

A. Why Noncompartmental Pharmacokinetics?
   1. Identification of the "correct" model is often impossible.
   2. A compartmental view of the body is unrealistic.
   3. Linear regression is unnecessary; it is easier to automate analysis.
   4. Requires fewer and less stringent assumptions
   5. More general methods and equations
   6. There is no need to match all data sets to the same compartmental model.

B. Definitions
   1. Zero moment concentration versus time curve
      • Area under the curve (AUC)

$$AUC = \sum \frac{(C_{n+1} + C_n)}{2} * (t_{n+1} - t_n)... + \frac{C_{last}}{k}$$

   2. First moment concentration * time versus time curve
      • Area under the first moment curve (AUMC)

$$AUMC = \sum \frac{(C_{n+1} * t_{n+1} + C_n * t_n)}{2} * (t_{n+1} - t_n)... + \frac{C_{last} * t_{last}}{k} + \frac{C_{last}}{k^2}$$

   3. Mean residence time (MRT)

$$MRT = \frac{AUMC}{AUC}$$

   4. Mean absorption time (MAT)

$$MAT = MRT_{ev} - MRT_{iv}$$

C. Pharmacokinetic Parameter Estimation
1. Clearance

$$\text{Clearance} = \frac{\text{dose}}{\text{AUC}}$$

2. Vd at steady state

$$V_{ss} = \frac{\text{dose} * \text{AUMC}}{\text{AUC}^2}$$

3. Elimination rate constant

$$k = \frac{1}{\text{MRT}}$$

4. Absorption rate constant

$$k_a = \frac{1}{\text{MAT}}$$

5. Bioavailability

$$F = \frac{D_{iv} * \text{AUC}_{ev}}{D_{ev} * \text{AUC}_{iv}}$$

VII. DATA COLLECTION AND ANALYSIS

Patient Case

7. R.K. is a 54-year-old woman with a history of diabetes mellitus and end-stage renal disease. She is receiving gentamicin for P. aeruginosa pneumonia. A gentamicin concentration is ordered after dialysis. Which is the best approach to obtaining this sample?

A. Obtain the concentration immediately after hemodialysis.

B. Wait a few hours to obtain the concentration because it will decrease significantly within the first few hours after hemodialysis.

C. Wait a few hours to obtain the concentration because it will increase significantly within the first few hours after hemodialysis.

D. Wait until the next day so that all the effects of hemodialysis will have abated.

A. Timing of Collection
1. Ensure completion of absorption and distribution phases (especially digoxin [8–12 hours] and vancomycin [30–60 minutes after 60-minute infusion]).
2. Ensure completion of redistribution after dialysis (especially aminoglycosides [3–4 hours after hemodialysis]).

B. Specimen Requirements
1. Whole blood: Use anticoagulated tube. Examples: cyclosporine, amiodarone
2. Plasma: Use anticoagulated tube and centrifuge; clotting proteins and some blood cells are maintained.
3. Serum: Use red top tube, allow to clot, and centrifuge. Examples: most analyzed drugs including aminoglycosides, vancomycin, phenytoin, and digoxin

---

Patient Case

8. A drug assay is touted as having high specificity but low sensitivity. Which statement best describes what this means?

A. The assay will not be able to distinguish the drug from like products, but it will be able to detect extremely low concentrations.

B. The assay will not be able to distinguish the drug from like products, and it will not be able to detect extremely low concentrations.

C. The assay will be able to distinguish the drug from like products and will be able to detect extremely low concentrations.

D. The assay will be able to distinguish the drug from like products but will not be able to detect extremely low concentrations.

C. Assay Terminology
1. Precision (reproducibility): Closeness of agreement among the results of repeated analyses performed on the same sample
   a. Standard deviation (SD): Average difference of the individual values from the mean
   b. Coefficient of variation (CV): SD as a percentage of the mean (relative rather than absolute variation)

$$CV = \frac{SD}{Mean}$$

2. Accuracy: Closeness with which a measurement reflects the true value of an object
   • Correlation coefficient: Strength of the relationship between two variables
3. Predictive performance (measure of accuracy): Precision: a.k.a. root mean squared error (RMSE)

$$MSE = \frac{1}{N}\sum_{i=1}^{N} pe_i^2 \qquad RMSE = \sqrt{mse}$$

Bias: a.k.a. mean prediction error (ME)

$$ME = \frac{1}{N}\sum_{i=1}^{N} pe_i$$

   • Prediction error (pe) is the prediction minus the true value.

4. Sensitivity: Ability of an assay to quantitate low drug concentrations accurately; usually the lowest concentration an assay can differentiate from zero.
5. Specificity (cross-reactivity): Ability of an assay to differentiate the drug in question from like substances

D. Assay Methodology
    1. Immunoassays
        a. Radioimmunoassay
            i.   Advantages: Extremely sensitive (picogram range)
            ii. Disadvantages: Radioimmunoassay kits have limited shelf life because of the short half-life of labels, radioactive waste, and cross-reactivity.
                - Clinical use for assaying digoxin and cyclosporine
        b. Enzyme immunoassay; e.g., enzyme multiplied immunoassay technique (EMIT)
            i.   Advantages: Simple, automated, highly sensitive, inexpensive and stable reagents, inexpensive and widely available equipment, no radiation hazards
            ii. Disadvantages: Measuring enzyme activity more complex than radioisotopes, enzyme activity may be affected by plasma constituents, less sensitive than radioimmunoassays
        c. Fluorescence immunoassay: TDx (e.g., fluorescence polarization immunoassay (FPIA)): Most common therapeutic drug monitoring assay
            i.   Advantages: Simple, automated, highly sensitive, inexpensive and stable reagents, inexpensive and widely available equipment, no radiation hazards
            ii. Disadvantages: Background interference attributable to endogenous serum fluorescence
    2. High-pressure liquid chromatography
    3. Gas chromatography–mass spectrometry and liquid chromatography–mass spectrometry
    4. Flame photometry
    5. Bioassay

E. Population Pharmacokinetics in Therapeutic Drug Monitoring
    1. Population pharmacokinetics useful when:
        a. Drug concentrations are obtained during complicated dosing regimens.
        b. Drug concentrations are obtained before steady state.
        c. Only a few drug concentrations are feasibly obtained (limited sampling strategy).
    2. Bayesian pharmacokinetics
        a. Prior population information is combined with patient-specific data to predict the most probable individual parameters.
        b. When patient-specific data are limited, there is greater influence from population parameters; when patient-specific data are extensive, there is less influence.
        c. With a small amount of individual data, Bayesian forecasting generally yields more precise results.

Patient Cases

9. K.M., an 80-year-old white woman (52 kg, 64 inches), is admitted to the hospital for pyelonephritis with sepsis. She has a history of myocardial infarction × 2, congestive heart failure, hypertension, osteoporosis, rheumatoid arthritis, and cerebrovascular accident. On admission, her BUN is 25 mg/dL, SCr is 0.92 mg/dL, and Alb is 2.9 g/dL. K.M. is initiated on the following drugs: trimethoprim/sulfamethoxazole intravenously, 240 mg of trimethoprim every 12 hours, lisinopril 10 mg/day by mouth, digoxin 0.125 mg/day by mouth, furosemide 40 mg/day by mouth, cimetidine 400 mg by mouth two times/day, acetaminophen 650 mg by mouth every 6 hours, calcium carbonate 500 mg by mouth three times/day, and carvedilol 6.25 mg by mouth two times/day. Which is the best assessment of K.M.'s renal function?

   A. Her SCr is in the normal range, and no dosage adjustments need to be madeare necessary.

   B. Because of her age, K.M. will have some degree of renal dysfunction, and doses may need to be adjusted.

   C. Because of the pyelonephritis, K.M. will have renal dysfunction, and doses may need to be adjusted.

   D. Her SCr is in the normal range but her BUN is elevated, so doses may need to be adjusted.

10. Which of K.M.'s drug combinations is most likely to alter her SCr concentrations?

   A. Lisinopril and digoxin.

   B. Trimethoprim/sulfamethoxazole and cimetidine.

   C. Furosemide and calcium carbonate.

   D. Acetaminophen and carvedilol.

VIII. PHARMACOKINETICS IN RENAL DISEASE

A. Estimation of Kidney Function Through Glomerular Filtration Rate (GFR)/Creatinine Clearance
   1. Creatinine production and elimination
      a. Creatine is produced in the liver.
      b. Creatinine is the product of creatine metabolism in skeletal muscle; formed at a constant rate for any one person
      c. Creatinine is filtered at the glomerulus, where it undergoes limited secretion.
      d. CrCl is useful in approximating GFR because:
         i. At normal concentrations of creatinine, secretion is low.
         ii. The creatinine assay picks up a noncreatinine chromogen in the blood but not in the urine.
   2. CrCl calculation to estimate GFR

      • CrCl is calculated from a 24-hour urine collection and the following equation:

$$\text{CrCl (mL/minute/1.73 m}^2) = \frac{\text{volume of urine/1440 minutes} \times \text{urine creatinine concentration}}{\text{serum creatinine concentration}}$$

      • Normal CrCl
         Healthy young men = 125 mL/minute/1.73 m^2
         Healthy young women = 115 mL/minute/1.73 m^2

      • After age 30, 1% of GFR is lost per year.

3. CrCl estimation to estimate GFR
   a. Factors affecting SCr concentrations
      i. Sex
      ii. Age
      iii. Weight/muscle mass
      iv. Renal function. Caveats: CrCl estimations worsen as renal function worsens (usually an overestimation).
   b. Jeliffe

$$CrCl \ (mL/minute/1.73 \ m^2) = \frac{98 - 0.8 \ (age - 20)}{SCr}$$

Women: Use 90% of the above equation.

   • Limitations:
      SCr concentration must be stable.
      Adults 20–80 years of age
      Controversy: Rounding up SCr in patients with low concentrations (less than 0.7–1 mg/dL)

   c. Cockcroft-Gault

$$CrCl \ (mL/min) = \frac{(140 - Age) * (weight)}{72 * Scr}$$

Women: Use 85% of the above equation.
   • For "weight": Use actual body weight (ABW) in patients with body mass index (BMI) less than 18.5 kg/m², ideal body weight (IBW) in patients with BMI 18.5–25 kg/m², and IBW plus 40% of (ABW – IBW) in patients with BMI greater than 25 kg/m².

      Ideal body weight (IBW) (men) = 50 kg + 2.3 kg for each inch over 5 feet
      IBW (women) = 45.5 kg + 2.3 kg for each inch over 5 feet
   • Limitations:
      SCr concentration must be stable. Developed for adults only
      Not corrected for creatinine standardization (results in lower estimations)
      Controversy: Rounding up SCr in patients with low concentrations (less than 0.7–1 mg/dL)

   d. Modification of Diet in Renal Disease study equation
   Full equation:

GFR (mL/minute/1.73 m²) = 161.5 * $(SCr)^{-0.999}$ * (age in years)$^{-0.176}$ * 1.180 (if patient is African American) * 0.762 (if patient is a woman) * $(BUN)^{-0.170}$ * $(Alb)^{+0.318}$

Simplified four-variable equation:

GFR (mL/minute/1.73 m²) = 175 * $(SCr)^{-1.154}$ * (age in years)$^{-0.203}$ * 1.212 (if patient is African American) * 0.742 (if patient is a woman)

      i. These equations directly estimate GFR (*not* CrCl) and were developed using standardized creatinine concentrations to stage kidney function.
      ii. These equations are recommended by the American Kidney Foundation and the European Renal Association to estimate renal function.

      iii. Not as accurate when GFR is greater than 60 mL/minute/1.73 m^2

      iv. If used for drug dosing, convert value from milliliters per minute per 1.73 m^2 to milliliters per minute.

      v. If used for drug dosing and significantly different from Cockcroft-Gault, use clinical judgment and optimize risk versus benefit.

  e. Chronic Kidney Disease Epidemiology Collaboration equation (CKD-Epi)

      i. These equations directly estimate GFR (not CrCl).

      ii. These equations are more accurate than Modification of Diet in Renal Disease at higher GFRs (i.e., greater than 60 mL/minute/1.73 m^2).

Table 7. Chronic Kidney Disease Epidemiology Collaboration Equation

Race and Sex	Serum Creatinine (mg/dL)	Equation
African American		
Female	<0.7	GFR = 166 * (SCr/0.7) – 0.329 * (0.993) Age
	>0.7	GFR = 166 * (SCr/0.7) – 1.209 * (0.993) Age
Male	<0.9	GFR = 163 * (SCr/0.9) – 0.411 * (0.993) Age
	>0.9	GFR = 163 * (SCr/0.9) – 1.209 * (0.993) Age
White or other		
Female	<0.7	GFR = 144 * (SCr/0.7) – 0.329 * (0.993) Age
	>0.7	GFR = 144 * (SCr/0.7) – 1.209 * (0.993) Age
Male	<0.9	GFR = 141 * (SCr/0.9) – 0.411 * (0.993) Age
	>0.9	GFR = 141 * (SCr/0.9) – 1.209 * (0.993) Age

GFR = glomerular filtration rate; SCr = serum creatinine.

  f. Pediatric formulas. Do not round up low SCr values in pediatric patients.

Schwartz:

$$\text{GFR (mL/minute/1.73 m}^2) = \frac{K * ht \text{ (cm)}}{SCr}$$

Table 8. Schwartz Equation Constants

Age	K
Low birth weight ≤1 year	0.33
Full term ≤1 year	0.45
1–13 years	0.55
13- to 18-year-old adolescent female	0.55
13- to 18-year-old adolescent male	0.7

Note: $K = 0.413$ for 1–13 years old and 13- to 18-year-old adolescent females when using standardized creatinine concentrations (other K values have not been updated); this is known as the bedside Chronic Kidney Disease in Children (CKiD) equation.

Counahan-Barratt:

$$\text{GFR (mL/minute/1.73 m}^2) = \frac{0.43 * ht \text{ (cm)}}{SCr}$$

4. Factors influencing CrCl estimates
    a. Patient characteristics
        i. Age (↓ production of creatinine with age)
        ii. Female sex (↓ production of creatinine)
        iii. Race (↑ production of creatinine in African Americans)
    b. Disease states and clinical conditions
        i. Spinal cord injuries (↓ muscle mass; ↓ creatinine)
        ii. Amputations (↓ muscle mass; ↓ creatinine)
        iii. Cushing syndrome (↓ muscle mass; ↓ creatinine)
        iv. Muscular dystrophy (↓ muscle mass; ↓ creatinine)
        v. Guillain-Barré syndrome (↓ muscle mass; ↓ creatinine)
        vi. Rheumatoid arthritis (↓ muscle mass; ↓ creatinine)
        vii. Liver disease (↓ creatine; ↓ creatinine)
        viii. Glomerulopathic disease (greater amount of creatinine secretion in relation to filtration)
        ix. Hydration status (dehydration vs. fluid overload)
    c. Diet
        i. High-meat protein diets (↑ creatinine ingestion)
        ii. Vegetarians (↓ creatinine ingestion)
        iii. Protein calorie malnutrition (↓ creatinine ingestion)
    d. Drugs and endogenous substances
        i. Laboratory interaction: Kinetic alkaline picrate method
            (a) Noncreatinine chromogens: In blood but not in urine
            (b) Cephalosporins (especially cefoxitin): Chromogenic, causing false elevations that are much greater in urine than in blood
            (c) Acetoacetate (elevated in fasting individuals, patients with diabetic ketoacidosis): Chromogenic, causing false elevations
        ii. Pharmacokinetic interaction: Drugs compete with creatinine for renal secretion (causing false elevations), trimethoprim, cimetidine, fibric acid derivatives (other than gemfibrozil), and dronedarone.

B. Drug Dosing in Renal Disease
    1. Loading dose
        a. In general, no alteration is necessary, but it should be given to hasten the achievement of therapeutic drug concentrations.
        b. Alterations in loading dose must occur if the Vd is altered secondary to renal dysfunction. Example: digoxin
    2. Maintenance dose: Alterations should be made in either the dose or the dosing interval.
        a. Changing the dosing interval
            i. Use when the goal is to achieve similar steady-state concentrations.
            ii. Less costly
            iii. Ideal for limited-dosage forms (i.e., oral medications)
        b. Changing the dose
            i. Use when the goal is to maintain a steady therapeutic concentration.
            ii. More costly
        c. Changing the dose and the dosing interval
            i. Often necessary for substantial dosage adjustment with limited-dosage forms
            ii. Often necessary for narrow therapeutic index drugs with target concentrations
                (a) If a drug is given more than once daily, then adjust the interval.
                (b) If a drug is given once daily or less often, then adjust the dose.

Patient Case

11. S.J. is a 55-year-old man with hepatic dysfunction and fungemia caused by Candida krusei. He has a small amount of ascites but is not encephalopathic. He is initiated on caspofungin, and the package insert states that doses should be decreased in patients with a Child-Pugh score of 7–9. If he has the following hepatic laboratory values, which best estimates his Child-Pugh score?

    Aspartate transaminase = 85 U/L, alanine transaminase = 56 U/L, alkaline phosphatase = 190 U/L, total bilirubin = 1.8 mg/dL, Alb = 2.9 g/dL, lactic dehydrogenase = 270 U/L, prothrombin time/international normalized ratio = 14.6/1.7, γ-glutamyl transferase = 60 U/L

    A. 3.

    B. 5.

    C. 8.

    D. 11.

IX. PHARMACOKINETICS IN HEPATIC DISEASE

   A. Dosage Adjustment in Hepatic Disease
      1. Clinical response is the most important factor in adjusting doses in hepatic disease.
      2. Low hepatic extraction ratio drugs
         a. Adjustment of maintenance dose is necessary only when hepatic disease alters the intrinsic clearance (Cl_{int})
         b. Alterations in protein binding alone do not require alteration of maintenance dose, even though total drug concentrations decline.
         c. Loading doses may require reduction.
      3. High hepatic extraction ratio drugs
         a. Intravenous administration
            i. Usually necessary to decrease maintenance dose rate as hepatic blood flow changes
            ii. Consider effect of hepatic disease on protein binding as it alters free concentrations.
         b. Oral administration: Similar to low hepatic extraction ratio drugs; necessary to decrease maintenance dose rate when hepatic disease alters Cl_{int}

   B. Rules for Dosing in Hepatic Disease
      1. Hepatic elimination of high extraction ratio drugs is more consistently affected by liver disease than hepatic elimination of low extraction ratio drugs.
      2. The clearance of drugs that are exclusively conjugated is not substantially altered in liver disease.

Table 9. Child-Pugh Classification for Liver Disease

	Points		
	1	**2**	**3**
Encephalopathy	0	1 or 2	3 or 4
Ascites	0	+	++
Bilirubin (mg/dL)	<1.5	1.5–2.3	>2.3
Alb (g/dL)	>3.5	2.8–3.5	<2.8
Prothrombin time (seconds over control)	0–4	4–6	>6

Pugh score: 5 = normal; 6 or 7 = mild (A); 8 or 9 = moderate (B); >9 = severe (C). Alb = albumin.

X. PHARMACODYNAMICS

Patient Case

12. Which is the most likely reason that a drug will follow clockwise hysteresis?

    A. Formation of an active metabolite.

    B. Delay in equilibrium between the blood and the site of action.

    C. Tolerance.

    D. Increased sensitivity with time.

A. Definition: Relationship Between Drug Concentrations and the Pharmacologic Response

B. Hill equation

$$E = \frac{E_{max} * C^y}{EC_{50}{}^y + C^y}$$

E = pharmacologic response

E_{max} = maximum drug effect

EC_{50} = concentration producing half of the maximum drug effect

γ = Hill coefficient that accommodates the shape of the curve

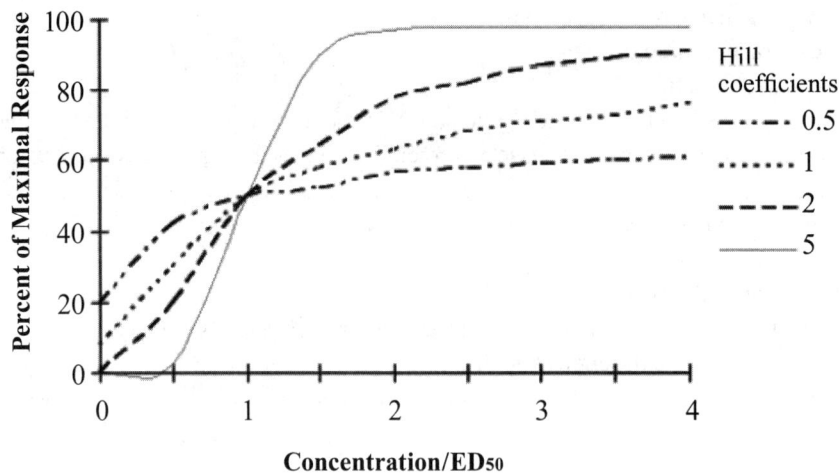

Figure 5. Concentration response plot.

C. Hysteresis Loops. Definition: Concentrations late after a dose produce an effect different from that produced by the same concentration soon after the dose.

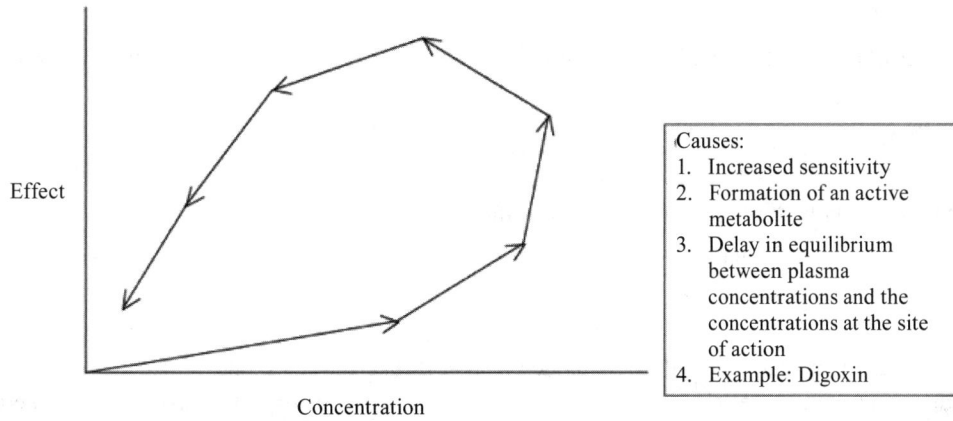

Figure 6. Counterclockwise hysteresis.

Causes:
1. Increased sensitivity
2. Formation of an active metabolite
3. Delay in equilibrium between plasma concentrations and the concentrations at the site of action
4. Example: Digoxin

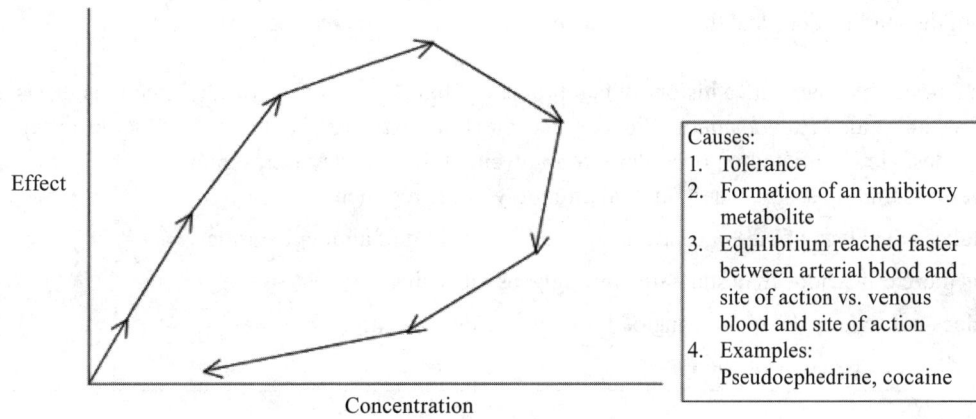

Figure 7. Clockwise hysteresis.

Causes:
1. Tolerance
2. Formation of an inhibitory metabolite
3. Equilibrium reached faster between arterial blood and site of action vs. venous blood and site of action
4. Examples: Pseudoephedrine, cocaine

Patient Cases

13. P.L., a 45-year-old man with chronic renal failure, is receiving phenytoin 400 mg/day for a history of tonic-clonic seizures. His phenytoin concentration today is 13.6 mg/L, and his Alb concentration is 4.2 g/dL. Based on his current concentrations, which change should be recommended?

    A. Make no changes to his drug regimen.

    B. Keep the total daily dose the same, but change the regimen to 200 mg two times/day.

    C. Increase the dose for better seizure control.

    D. Decrease the dose to prevent toxicity.

14. N.R. is a 63-year-old man with renal insufficiency who comes to the emergency department in atrial fibrillation with a ventricular rate of 120 beats/minute. Because of his history of ventricular dysfunction, it is decided to initiate him on digoxin for rate control. Which is the best dosing for this patient?

    A. The loading dose should remain the same, but the maintenance dose should be decreased.

    B. The loading dose should be decreased, and the maintenance dose should remain the same.

    C. Neither the loading dose nor the maintenance dose should be adjusted.

    D. Both the loading dose and the maintenance dose should be decrease

15. P.P. is a 34-year-old man with a history of cerebral palsy and chronic urinary tract infections. He is admitted to the hospital with a *Pseudomonas* urinary tract infection that is resistant to all antibiotics except for aminoglycosides. He is initiated on once-daily tobramycin at 400 mg/day intravenously. Which statement best describes this high-dose, extended-interval aminoglycoside regimen?

    A. It takes advantage of the concentration-dependent killing of aminoglycoside.

    B. It is more efficacious than standard aminoglycoside dosing.

    C. It does not require the monitoring of aminoglycoside concentrations.

    D. It will not cause nephrotoxicity.

Table 10. Specific Drugs

Drug	Therapeutic Range	Sampling Issues	Comments
Aminoglycosides	Cp = 4–10 mg/L maximum Amikacin = 20–30 mg/L Cp < 2 mg/L minimum Amikacin < 10 mg/L	Duration of infusion, timing of first sample after infusion (generally should be ½–1 hour)	Be familiar with Sawchuk-Zaske method and high-dose, extended-interval dosing
Vancomycin	Cp = 10–15 mg/L minimum (15–20 mg/L for certain infections, including pneumonia, meningitis, and osteomyelitis)	Controversial whether to obtain peaks or concentrations altogether	Be familiar with changes in trough concentration recommendations
Phenytoin	10–20 mg/L Free: 1–2 mg/L	In general, obtain trough concentrations	Percentage free increases with renal failure and hypoalbuminemia Equations to correct: Changes in albumin: $$Cp = \frac{Cp'}{(0.9 * \frac{Alb}{4.4})} + 0.1$$ Renal failure: $$Cp = \frac{Cp'}{0.5}$$ Renal failure with change in albumin: $$Cp = \frac{Cp'}{(0.48 * 0.9 * \frac{Alb}{4.4}) + 0.1}$$ Induces liver enzymes; susceptible to metabolic drug interactions
Carbamazepine	4–12 mg/L		Autoinduction; active metabolite 10,11 epoxide
Phenobarbital	15–40 mg/L		Enzyme inducer
Valproic acid	50–100 mg/L		Saturable protein binding; percentage free increases with renal failure and hypoalbuminemia
Digoxin	0.8–2.0 mcg/L	Prolonged distribution period necessitates sampling >6–12 hours after dose	Vd decreases in renal disease; susceptible to drug interactions
Cyclosporine	100–250 mcg/L	Whole blood samples	Many drug interactions
Lithium	0.3–1.3 mmol/L	Prolonged distribution necessitates sampling 12 hours after dose	
Theophylline	10–20 mg/L		Treat as continuous infusion with sustained-release dosage forms

Cp = concentration of drug in plasma.

Table 11. CYP Drug Interactions

Gene Designation	CYP1A2	CYP2C9/10	CYP2C19	CYP2D6	CYP3A4	
Substrates	Acetaminophen	Amitriptyline	Amitriptyline	(norfluoxetine)	Alfentanil	Maraviroc
	Amitriptyline	Celecoxib	Cilostazol	Amitriptyline	Alprazolam	Methadone
	Caffeine	Diclofenac	Citalopram	Aripiprazole	Amiodarone	Midazolam
	Clomipramine	Etravirine	Clomipramine	Atomoxetine	Amlodipine	Mirtazapine
	Clozapine	Fluoxetine	Clopidogrel	Carvedilol	Aprepitant	Nateglinide
	Cyclobenzaprine	Fluvastatin	Diazepam	Clomipramine	Atazanavir	Nefazodone
	Estradiol	Glimepiride	Etravirine	Clozapine Codeine	Atorvastatin	Nelfinavir
	Fluvoxamine	Glipizide	Imipramine	Debrisoquine	Boceprevir	Nevirapine
	Haloperidol	Glyburide	Lansoprazole	Desipramine	Buspirone	Nifedipine
	Imipramine	Ibuprofen	Naproxen	Dextromethorphan	Carbamazepine	Quetiapine
	Mirtazapine	Indomethacin	Nelfinavir	Donepezil	Cilostazol	Quinidine
	Olanzapine	Irbesartan	Omeprazole	Duloxetine	Citalopram	Rabeprazole
	Riluzole	Losartan	Pantoprazole	Flecainide	Clarithromycin	Repaglinide
	Ropinirole	Phenytoin	Phenobarbital	Fluoxetine	Cyclosporine	Rifabutin
	R-warfarin	Piroxicam	Phenytoin	Fluvoxamine	Dapsone	Ritonavir
	Theophylline	Rosuvastatin	Propranolol	Haloperidol	Darunavir	R-warfarin
	Zolmitriptan	S-warfarin	Rabeprazole	Hydrocodone	Delavirdine	Saquinavir
		Tamoxifen	(minor)	Imipramine	Diazepam	Sertraline
				Metoprolol	Diltiazem	Sibutramine
				Mirtazapine	Donepezil	Sildenafil
				Nebivolol	Efavirenz	Simvastatin
				Nortriptyline	Eplerenone	Sirolimus
				Oxycodone	Erlotinib	Sorafenib
				Paroxetine	Erythromycin	Sunitinib
				Propafenone	Ethinyl estradiol	Tacrolimus
				Propranolol	Etravirine	Telaprevir
				Risperidone	Felodipine	Tertiary amines
				Tamoxifen	Fentanyl	(amitriptyline,
				Thioridazine	Finasteride	clomipramine,
				Timolol	Fosamprenavir	imipramine)
				Tramadol	Gefitinib	Tiagabine
				Trazodone	Gleevec	Tipranavir
				Venlafaxine	Imatinib	Trazodone
					Indinavir	Triazolam
					Irinotecan	Vardenafil
					Itraconazole	Verapamil
					Ketoconazole	Voriconazole
					Lapatinib	Zaleplon
					Lidocaine	Ziprasidone
					Lopinavir	Zolpidem
					Lovastatin	Zonisamide
Induction	Char-grilled	Phenobarbital	Carbamazepine		Carbamazepine	Pioglitazone
	meat Cigarettes	Phenytoin	Phenobarbital		Efavirenz	Rifabutin
	Nafcillin	Rifampin	Prednisone		Etravirine	Rifampin
	Omeprazole	Rifapentine	Rifampin		Nevirapine	Rifapentine
	Rifampin				Oxcarbazepine	St. John's wort
					Phenobarbital	Tipranavir
					Phenytoin	

Table 11. CYP Drug Interactions *(continued)*

Gene Designation	CYP1A2	CYP2C9/10	CYP2C19	CYP2D6	CYP3A4	
Inhibition	Amiodarone	Amiodarone	Cimetidine	Amiodarone	Amiodarone	Indinavir
	Cimetidine	Etravirine	Etravirine	Bupropion	Aprepitant	Itraconazole
	Ciprofloxacin	Fluconazole	Felbamate	Celecoxib	Atazanavir	Ketoconazole
	Diltiazem	Fluoxetine	Fluoxetine	Chlorpheniramine	Boceprevir	Lopinavir
	Erythromycin	Fluvoxamine	Fluvoxamine	Cimetidine	Cimetidine	Nefazodone
	Fluvoxamine	Isoniazid	Ketoconazole	Cinacalcet	Clarithromycin	Nelfinavir
	Mexiletine	Leflunomide	Lansoprazole	Citalopram	Darunavir	Norfluoxetine
	Norfloxacin	Omeprazole	Modafinil	Diphenhydramine	Delavirdine	Ritonavir
	Ticlopidine	Sertraline	Omeprazole	Duloxetine	Diltiazem	Saquinavir
		Sulfamethoxazole	Oxcarbazepine	Escitalopram	Erythromycin	Synercid
		Trimethoprim	Pantoprazole	Fluoxetine	Fluconazole	Telaprevir
		Voriconazole	Rabeprazole	Haloperidol	(large doses)	Tipranavir
			Ticlopidine	Metoclopramide	Fluvoxamine	Verapamil
			Topiramate	Paroxetine	Fosamprenavir	Voriconazole
				Propafenone	Grapefruit juice	
				Quinidine	Imatinib	
				Ritonavir		
				Sertraline		
				Terbinafine		
				Thioridazine		

CYP = cytochrome P450.

Table 12. PK Term Definitions

AUC	Area under the curve
AUC_{ev}	Area under the curve after an extravascular dose
AUC_{iv}	Area under the curve after an intravenous dose
Cmax	Maximum concentration
Cmin	Minimum concentration
C_0	Concentration at time zero
C_{ss}	Concentration at stead state
$C_{ss\,avg}$	Average concentration at steady state
C_{ss} max	Maximum concentration at steady state
DoseEV	Dose given extravascularly
DoseIV	Dose given intravenously
F	Bioavailability
k	Elimination rate constant
R_0	Rate of infusion
τ	Dosing interval
t	Time of the infusion
ti	Time from initiation of the infusion
Vd	Volume of distribution

REFERENCES

1. Bauer LA. Applied Clinical Pharmacokinetics, 2nd ed. New York: McGraw-Hill Medical, 2008.

2. Bauer LA. Clinical pharmacokinetics and pharmacodynamics. In: DiPiro JT, Talbert RL, Yee GC, et al., eds. Pharmacotherapy: A Pathophysiologic Approach, 8th ed. New York: McGraw-Hill Medical, 2011:chap 8.

3. Burton ME, Shaw LM, Schentag JJ, eds. Applied Pharmacokinetics & Pharmacodynamics: Principles of Therapeutic Drug Monitoring, 4th ed. Baltimore: Lippincott Williams & Wilkins, 2006.

4. International Transporter Consortium. Membrane transporters in drug development. Nat Rev Drug Discov 2010;9:215-36.

5. Johnson JA. Pharmacogenetics in clinical practice: how far have we come and where are we going? Pharmacogenomics 2013;14:835-43.

6. Lee CK, Swinford RD, Cerda RD, et al. Evaluation of serum creatinine concentration–based glomerular filtration rate equations in pediatric patients with chronic kidney disease. Pharmacotherapy 2012;32:642-8.

7. Matheny CJ, Lamb MW, Brouwer KLR, et al. Pharmacokinetic and pharmacodynamic implications of P-glycoprotein modulation. Pharmacotherapy 2001;21:778-96.

8. Nyman HA, Dowling TC, Hudson JQ, et al. Comparative evaluation of the Cockcroft-Gault equation and the Modification of Diet in Renal Disease (MDRD) study equation for drug dosing: an opinion of the Nephrology Practice and Research Network of the American College of Clinical Pharmacy. Pharmacotherapy 2011;31:1130-44.

9. Winter ME. Basic Clinical Pharmacokinetics, 5th ed. Baltimore: Lippincott Williams & Wilkins, 2010.

ANSWERS AND EXPLANATIONS TO PATIENT CASES

1. Answer: C
In 6 days (2 half-lives), the concentration will decrease from 35.9 mg/L to about 9 mg/L; now is the time to redose. A 1-g dose given on March 24 will increase the concentration in the blood from 12.1 mg/L to 35.9 mg/L (12.1 + 23.8 mg/L). Given that the half-life is about 3 days, it will take longer than 1 day to reach a concentration of about 10 mg/L. In 3 days (1 half-life), the concentration will decrease from 35.9 mg/L to about 18 mg/L—still too early to redose CYP = cytochrome P450. Redosing can be determined because plenty of information exists about how to calculate when to redose.

2. Answer: A
F = (100 mg * 25 mg/L/hour)/(200 mg * 50 mg/L/hour) = 25%.

3. Answer: C
The elimination rate constant equals (ln 6.5 mg/L − ln 5.4 mg/L)/12 hours = 0.015/hour. The concentration at the end of the infusion equals 6.5 mg/L/e − (0.015 * 5) = 7 mg/L. The patient's Vd = dose/change in concentration or 160 mg/7 mg/L = 22.9 L. If you desire a change in concentration from 1 mg/L to 9 mg/L (or 8 mg/L), then dose = 22.9 L * 8 mg/L = 183.2 mg. Therefore, a dose of 180 mg is appropriate.

4. Answer: D
P-glycoprotein is an efflux pump that pumps drugs back into the GI lumen. P-glycoprotein is not a plasma protein, and it does not transfer drugs through the GI mucosa; rather, it pumps drugs back into the GI lumen. In addition, P-glycoprotein acts in concert with CYP3A4 to diminish oral absorption.

5. Answer: C
Azithromycin does not inhibit CYP3A4. Erythromycin and clarithromycin are potent inhibitors of CYP3A4 and would be expected to increase cyclosporine concentrations. Cytochrome P450 inhibition is not a drug class effect.

6. Answer: B
By definition, clearance becomes nonlinear once the concentration exceeds the K_m; therefore, the concentrations will more than double. Phenytoin is not a significant autoinducer. Although phenytoin absorption

decreases as the dose is increased, it is not clinically significant until a single dose exceeds 400 mg.

7. Answer: C
The correct answer, because of redistribution, is to wait a few hours to obtain the concentration because it will increase significantly within the first few hours after hemodialysis. Waiting a full 24 hours is not necessary.

8. Answer: D
The correct answer is that the assay will be able to distinguish the drug from like products but will not be able to detect extremely low concentrations. High specificity means the assay can distinguish the drug from like products, and low sensitivity means the assay cannot detect extremely low concentrations.

9. Answer: B
Although her SCr is in the normal range, her renal function is decreased because of her age. After age 30, patients lose around 1 mL/minute/year of CrCl. Therefore, her CrCl needs to be calculated to assess drug dosing. Patients with pyelonephritis do not have a decrease in their renal function. Her elevated BUN is probably a sign of prerenal azotemia caused by dehydration associated with her infection. The BUN measurement is generally not used to assess renal function for drug dosing purposes.

10. Answer: B
Both trimethoprim/sulfamethoxazole and cimetidine compete with creatinine for secretion in the kidneys, increasing SCr concentrations. Although angiotensin-converting enzyme inhibitors may transiently increase SCr concentrations, digoxin does not affect renal function. Although furosemide may secondarily affect SCr concentrations, calcium carbonate does not affect renal function. Acetaminophen and carvedilol generally will not affect SCr concentrations.

11. Answer: C
This patient has 1 point for not being encephalopathic, 2 points for mild ascites, 2 points for the bilirubin concentration, 2 points for the Alb concentration, and 1 point for the prothrombin time value, for a total of 8 points. Normal patients have a Child-Pugh score of 5, which means no hepatic dysfunction.

12. Answer: C
Tolerance leads to a decrease in effect with time; this is clockwise hysteresis. The formation of an active metabolite, a delay in equilibrium between the blood and site of action, and the increased sensitivity with time would lead to an increase in effect with time; this is counterclockwise hysteresis.

13. Answer: D
The dose should be decreased to prevent toxicity. In renal failure, acidic byproducts build up in the blood and compete with phenytoin for protein binding. Total concentrations must be corrected, and this correction leads to a doubling of the concentration. Therefore, the current concentration is too high, and the dose should be decreased. Single doses of 400 mg are fine (doses higher than 400 mg should be divided).

14. Answer: D
Both the loading dose and the maintenance dose should be decreased. In general, loading doses need not be altered in renal dysfunction because they are dependent primarily on the Vd. However, the digoxin Vd is decreased in renal dysfunction. Because digoxin is eliminated renally, the maintenance dose needs to be decreased.

15. Answer: A
Aminoglycosides show concentration-dependent killing, and a high-dose, extended-interval aminoglycoside dose takes advantage of this characteristic. However, it has not proved more efficacious than traditional dosing. Aminoglycoside concentrations still need to be monitored with high-dose, extended-interval therapy. In addition, high-dose, extended-interval aminoglycoside dosing can still cause nephrotoxicity (although the incidence is generally diminished).

ANSWERS AND EXPLANATIONS TO SELF-ASSESSMENT QUESTIONS

1. Answer: B
With two concentrations, there are enough data to calculate an elimination rate constant and, therefore, a half-life. In addition, the Vd can be calculated by back extrapolation to the Cmax and use of appropriate equations (because this was the first dose, and therefore it is known that the tobramycin concentration was 0 mg/L before the dose was given).

2. Answer: A
The half-life is about 2 hours. The Cmax is about 5 mg/L, and the Vd is about 20 L.

3. Answer: B
Her clearance increased because of the improvement in renal function, which increased her elimination rate constant and decreased her half-life. The Vd would not be altered by changes in clearance (they are independent). With the diuresis and angiotensin-converting enzyme inhibitor, her Vd probably decreased, but clearance would not be altered by changes in Vd (they are independent). In addition, if her Vd decreased, her half-life would decrease, not increase.

4. Answer: C
Because the trough is too low, the interval will have to be shortened to increase the concentration. Changes in dose will have the greatest effect on the peak concentration, and changes in interval will have the greatest effect on the trough concentration.

5. Answer: B
To achieve flucytosine peak concentrations between 50 and 100 mcg/mL (assuming a trough concentration of 25 mcg/mL, dosing every 6 hours, and 100% bioavailability; flucytosine volume of distribution of 0.7 L/kg; half-life of 3 hours), the concentration must be changed by 25–75 mcg/mL. Using the equation $\Delta Cp = dose/V$, a dose of 12.5 mg/kg would increase the concentration by only 17.8 mcg/mL. A dose of 75 mg/kg would increase the concentration by 107 mcg/mL, whereas a dose of 150 mg/ kg would increase the concentration by 214 mcg/mL. The correct dose is 37.5 mg/kg because it would increase the concentration by 53.6 mcg/mL.

6. Answer: D
Because of the patient's renal failure and low Alb, the total concentration must be corrected. The patient's corrected phenytoin concentration is 14.7 mcg/mL. Therefore, no changes should be made to the dose.

7. Answer: C
Both of these are immunoassays. A brand name for the Abbott fluorescence polarization immunoassay is TDx, which uses a fluorescent label. The term *EMIT* stands for enzyme multiplied immunoassay technique, which is an immunoassay that uses an enzyme label.

8. Answer: D
The digoxin concentration was drawn too close to the 8:00 a.m. dose. The digoxin had not yet had a chance to complete its distribution phase. Once distribution is complete (generally 6–12 hours after the dose), the concentration will be lower and probably within the therapeutic range. Therefore, there is no need for the digoxin antibody, activated charcoal, or lowering of the dose.

9. Answer: C
The correct statistical test is multiple regression. Multiple regression is used to describe the relationship between a dependent variable and two or more independent variables when both the dependent and independent variables are numeric. Analysis of variance is used to describe the relationship between a dependent variable and two or more independent variables when the dependent variable is numeric and the independent variables are nominal. Likewise, analysis of covariance is used to describe the relationship between a dependent variable and two or more independent variables when the dependent variable is numeric and the independent variables are nominal with confounding factors. Spearman rank correlation is a nonparametric test used to describe the relationship between one dependent and one independent variable when the data are ordinal or numeric and not normally distributed.

10. Answer: B

Assessing adherence and increasing her dose, because the concentration is below the therapeutic range, is the correct answer. The valproic acid therapeutic range is 50–100 mg/L, and she is well below this concentration. Although some patients are controlled at lower concentrations, this concentration is most likely too low. She definitely does not need a decrease in dose. Although total valproic acid concentrations are affected by changes in Alb, her Alb is normal, and obtaining a free concentration is unnecessary.

Biostatistics: A Refresher

Kevin M. Sowinski, Pharm.D., FCCP

Purdue University College of Pharmacy
Indiana University School of Medicine
West Lafayette and Indianapolis, Indiana

BIOSTATISTICS: A REFRESHER

KEVIN M. SOWINSKI, PHARM.D., FCCP

PURDUE UNIVERSITY COLLEGE OF PHARMACY
INDIANA UNIVERSITY SCHOOL OF MEDICINE
WEST LAFAYETTE AND INDIANAPOLIS, INDIANA

Learning Objectives

1. Describe differences between descriptive and inferential statistics.
2. Identify different types of data (nominal, ordinal, continuous [ratio and interval]) to determine an appropriate type of statistical test (parametric vs. nonparametric).
3. Describe strengths and limitations of different types of measures of central tendency (mean, median, and mode) and data spread (standard deviation, standard error of the mean, range, and interquartile range).
4. Describe the concepts of normal distribution and the associated parameters that describe the distribution.
5. State the types of decision errors that can occur when one is using statistical tests and the conditions under which they can occur.
6. Describe hypothesis testing and state the meaning of and distinguish between p-values and confidence intervals.
7. Describe areas of misuse or misrepresentation that are associated with various statistical methods.
8. Select appropriate statistical tests on the basis of the sample distribution, data type, and study design.
9. Interpret statistical significance for results from commonly used statistical tests.
10. Describe the similarities and differences between statistical tests; state how to apply them appropriately.
11. Identify the use of survival analysis and different ways to perform and report it.

Self-Assessment Questions

Answers and explanations to these questions can be found at the end of the chapter.

1. A randomized controlled trial assesses the effects of heart failure treatment on global functioning in three groups of adults after 6 months of treatment. Investigators wanted to assess global functioning with the New York Heart Association (NYHA) functional classification, an ordered scale from I to IV, and to compare the patient classification after 6 months of treatment. Which statistical test is most appropriate to assess differences in functional classification between the groups?

A. Kruskal-Wallis.
B. Wilcoxon signed rank test.
C. Analysis of variance (ANOVA).
D. Analysis of covariance (ANCOVA).

2. You are evaluating a randomized, double-blind, parallel-group controlled trial that compares four antihypertensive drugs for their effect on blood pressure. The authors conclude that hydrochlorothiazide is better than atenolol ($p<0.05$) and that enalapril is better than hydrochlorothiazide ($p<0.01$), but no difference is observed between any other drugs. The investigators used an unpaired (independent samples) t-test to test the hypothesis that each drug was equal to the other. Which statement is most appropriate?

A. Investigators used the appropriate statistical test to analyze their data.
B. Enalapril is the most effective of these drugs.
C. ANOVA would have been a more appropriate test.
D. A paired t-test is a more appropriate test.

3. In the results of a randomized, double-blind, controlled clinical trial, it is reported that the difference in hospital readmission rates between the intervention group and the control group is 6% ($p=0.01$), and it is concluded that there is a statistically significant difference between the groups. Which statement is most consistent with this finding and conclusions?

A. The chance of making a type I error is 5 in 100.
B. The trial does not have enough power.
C. There is a high likelihood of having made a type II error.
D. The chance of making an alpha error is 1 in 100.

4. You are reading a manuscript that evaluates the impact of obesity on enoxaparin pharmacokinetics. The authors used an unpaired t-test to compare the baseline values of body mass index (BMI) in normal subjects and obese subjects. You are evaluating the use of an unpaired t-test to compare the BMI between the two groups. Which choice

represents the most appropriate criteria to be met to use this parametric test?

A. The sample sizes in the normal and obese subjects should be equal to allow the use of a t-test.

B. A t-test is not appropriate because BMI data are ordinal.

C. The variance of the BMI data needs must be similar in each group.

D. The pre-study power should be at least 90%.

5. You are evaluating the results and discussion of a journal club article to present to the pharmacy residents at your institution. The randomized, prospective, controlled trial evaluated the efficacy of a new controller drug for asthma. The primary end point was the morning forced expiratory volume in 1 second (FEV_1) in two groups of subjects (men and women). The difference in FEV_1 between the two groups was 15% (95% confidence interval [CI], 10%–21%). Which statement is most appropriate, given the results?

A. Without the reporting of a p-value, it is not possible to conclude whether these results were statistically significant.

B. There is a statistically significant difference between the men and women ($p<0.05$).

C. There is a statistically significant difference between the men and women ($p<0.01$).

D. There is no statistically significant difference between the men and women.

6. An early-phase clinical trial of 40 subjects evaluated a new drug known to increase high-density lipoprotein cholesterol (HDL-C) concentrations. The objective of the trial was to compare the new drug's ability to increase HDL-C with that of lifestyle modifications (active control group). At the beginning of the study, the mean baseline HDL-C was 37 mg/dL in the active control group and 38 mg/dL in the new drug group. At the end of the 3-month trial, the mean HDL-C for the control group was 44 mg/dL and for the new drug group, 49 mg/dL. The p-value for the comparison at 3 months was 0.08. Which statement provides the best interpretation of these results?

A. An a priori α of less than 0.10 would have made the study more clinically useful.

B. The new drug and active control appear to be equally efficacious in increasing HDL-C.

C. The new drug is better than lifestyle modifications because it increases HDL-C to a greater extent.

D. This study is potentially underpowered.

7. Researchers planned a study to evaluate the percentage of subjects who achieved less than a target blood pressure (less than 140/90 mm Hg) when initiated on two different doses of amlodipine. In the study of 100 subjects, the amlodipine 5-mg group (n=50) and the amlodipine 10-mg group (n=50) were compared. The investigators used a blood pressure goal as their primary end point, defined as the percentage of subjects who successfully achieved the blood pressure goal at 3 months. Which is the most appropriate statistical test to answer such a question?

A. Independent samples t-test.

B. Chi-square or Fisher exact test.

C. Wilcoxon signed rank test.

D. One-sample t-test.

8. An investigational drug is being compared with an existing drug for the treatment of anemia in patients with chronic kidney disease. The study is designed to detect a minimum 20% difference in response rates between the groups, if one exists, with an a priori α of 0.05 or less. The investigators are unclear whether the 20% difference between response rates is too large and think a smaller difference might be more clinically meaningful. In revising their study, they decide they want to be able to detect a minimum 10% difference in response. Which change in the study parameters is most appropriate?

A. Increase the sample size.

B. Select an α of 0.001 as a cutoff for statistical significance.

C. Select an α of 0.10 as a cutoff for statistical significance.

D. Decrease the sample size.

9. You are designing a new computer alert system to investigate the impact of several factors on the risk of QTc prolongation. You want to develop a model to predict which patients are most likely to experience QTc prolongation after the administration of certain drugs or the presence of certain conditions. You plan to assess the presence or absence of several different variables. Which technique will be most useful in completing such an analysis?

    A. Correlation.

    B. Kaplan-Meier curve.

    C. Regression.

    D. Confidence intervals.

I. INTRODUCTION TO STATISTICS

A. Method for Collecting, Classifying, Summarizing, and Analyzing Data

B. Useful Tool for Quantifying Clinical and Laboratory Data in a Meaningful Way

C. Assists in Determining Whether and by How Much a Treatment or Procedure Affects a Group of Patients

D. Why Pharmacists Need to Know Statistics

E. As Statistics Pertains to Most of You:
   1. *Pharmacotherapy Specialty Examination content outline*
      - Domain 2: Retrieval, Generation, Interpretation, and Dissemination of Knowledge in Pharmacotherapy (25%)
      - Interpret biomedical literature with respect to study design and methodology, statistical analysis, and significance of reported data and conclusions.
      - Knowledge of biostatistical methods, clinical and statistical significance, research hypothesis generation, research design and methodology, and protocol and proposal development

F. Several articles have investigated the various types of statistical tests used in the biomedical literature; the data from one of these articles are illustrated below.

Table 1. Statistical Content of Original Articles in *The New England Journal of Medicine,* 2004–2005

Statistical Procedure	% of Articles Containing Methods	Statistical Procedure	% of Articles Containing Methods
No statistics or descriptive statistics	13	Adjustment and standardization	1
t-tests	26	Multiway tables	13
Contingency tables	53	Power analyses	39
Nonparametric tests	27	Cost-benefit analysis	<1
Epidemiologic statistics	35	Sensitivity analysis	6
Pearson correlation	3	Repeated-measures analysis	12
Simple linear regression	6	Missing data methods	8
Analysis of variance	16	Noninferiority trials	4
Transformation	10	Receiver operating characteristics	2
Nonparametric correlation	5	Resampling	2
Survival methods	61	Principal component and cluster analyses	2
Multiple regression	51	Other methods	4
Multiple comparisons	23		

Table 2. Statistical Content of Original Articles from Six Major Medical Journals from January to March 2005 (n=239 articles).

Statistical Test	No. (%)	Statistical Test	No. (%)
Descriptive statistics (mean, median, frequency, SD, and IQR)	219 (91.6)	Others	
Simple statistics	120 (50.2)	Intention-to-treat analysis	42 (17.6)
Chi-square analysis	70 (29.3)	Incidence or prevalence	39 (16.3)
t-test	48 (20.1)	Relative risk or risk ratio	29 (12.2)
Kaplan-Meier analysis	48 (20.1)	Sensitivity analysis	21 (8.8)
Wilcoxon rank sum test	38 (15.9)	Sensitivity or specificity	15 (6.3)
Fisher exact test	33 (13.8)		
Analysis of variance	21 (8.8)		
Correlation	16 (6.7)		
Multivariate analysis	164 (68.6)		
Cox proportional hazards	64 (26.8)		
Multiple logistic regression	54 (22.6)		
Multiple linear regression	7 (2.9)		
Other regression analysis	38 (15.9)		
None	5 (2.1)		

IQR = interquartile range; SD = standard deviation.

Articles published in American Journal of Medicine, Annals of Internal Medicine, BMJ, JAMA, Lancet, and The New England Journal of Medicine. Table modified from JAMA 2007;298:1010-22.

II. TYPES OF VARIABLES AND DATA

    A. Definition: Random variables—A variable with observed values that may be considered outcomes of an experiment and whose values cannot be anticipated with certainty before the experiment is conducted

    B. Two Types of Random Variables
        1. Discrete variables (e.g., dichotomous, categorical)
        2. Continuous variables

    C. Discrete Variables
        1. Can take only a limited number of values within a given range
        2. Nominal: Classified into groups in an unordered manner and with no indication of relative severity (e.g., male/female sex, mortality [dead or alive], disease presence [yes or no], race, marital status). These data are often expressed as a frequency or proportion.
        3. Ordinal: Ranked in a specific order but with no consistent level of magnitude of difference between ranks (e.g., New York Heart Association [NYHA] functional class describes the functional status of patients with heart failure, and subjects are classified in increasing order of symptoms: I, II, III, IV; Likert-type scales)
        4. Common error: Measure of central tendency—In most cases, means and standard deviations (SDs) should not be reported with ordinal data. What is a common incorrect use of means and SDs to show ordinal data?

D. Continuous Variables, Sometimes Called Counting Variables
   1. Continuous variables can take on any value within a given range.
   2. Interval: Data are ranked in a specific order with a consistent change in magnitude between units; the zero point is arbitrary (e.g., degrees Fahrenheit).
   3. Ratio: Like interval but with an absolute zero (e.g., degrees Kelvin, heart rate, blood pressure, time, distance)

III. TYPES OF STATISTICS

A. Descriptive Statistics: Used to summarize and describe data that are collected or generated in research studies. This is done both visually and numerically.
   1. Visual methods of describing data
      a. Frequency distribution
      b. Histogram
      c. Scatterplot
   2. Numerical methods of describing data: Measures of central tendency
      a. Arithmetic mean (i.e., average)
         i. Sum of all values divided by the total number of values
         ii. Should generally be used only for continuous and normally distributed data
         iii. Very sensitive to outliers and tend toward the tail, which has the outliers
         iv. Most commonly used and most understood measure of central tendency
         v. Geometric mean
      b. Median
         i. Midpoint of the values when placed in order from highest to lowest. Half of the observations are above and below. When there are an even number of observations, it is the mean of the two middle values.
         ii. Also called 50th percentile
         iii. Can be used for ordinal or continuous data (especially good for skewed populations)
         iv. Insensitive to outliers
      c. Mode
         i. Most common value that occurs in a distribution
         ii. Can be used for nominal, ordinal, or continuous data
         iii. Sometimes, there may be more than one mode (e.g., bimodal, trimodal).
         iv. Does not help describe meaningful distributions with a large range of values, each of which occurs infrequently
   3. Numerical methods of describing data: Measures of data spread or variability
      a. Standard deviation
         i. Measure of the variability around the mean; most common measure used to describe the spread of data
         ii. Square root of the variance (average squared difference of each observation from the mean), so the SD is reported in the original units (nonsquared).
         iii. Appropriately applied only to continuous data that are normally or near-normally distributed or that can be transformed to be normally distributed
         iv. By the empirical rule, 68% of the sample values are found within ±1 SD, 95% are found within ±2 SD, and 99% are found within ±3 SD.
         v. The coefficient of variation relates the mean and the SD (SD/mean × 100%).

b. Range
   i. Difference between the smallest and largest value in a data set; does not give a tremendous amount of information by itself
   ii. Easy to compute (simple subtraction)
   iii. Size of range is very sensitive to outliers.
   iv. Often reported as the actual values rather than the difference between the two extreme values
c. Percentiles
   i. The point (value) in a distribution in which a value is larger than some percentage of the other values in the sample; can be calculated by ranking all data in a data set
   ii. The 75th percentile lies at a point at which 75% of the other values are smaller.
   iii. Does not assume the population has a normal distribution (or any other distribution)
   iv. The interquartile range (IQR) is an example of the use of percentiles to describe the middle 50% values. The IQR encompasses the 25th–75th percentile.

4. Presenting data using only measures of central tendency can be misleading without some idea of data spread. Studies that report only medians or means without their accompanying measures of data spread should be closely scrutinized. What are the measures of spread that should be used with means and medians?

5. Example data set

Table 3. Twenty Baseline HDL-C Concentrations from an Experiment Evaluating the Impact of Green Tea on HDL-C

64	60	59	65	64	62	54
54	68	67	79	55	48	65
59	65	87	49	46	46	

HDL-C = high-density lipoprotein cholesterol.

a. Calculate the mean, median, and mode of the above data set.
b. Calculate the range, SD (will not have to do this by hand), and standard error of the mean (SEM) of the above data set (we will describe this later).
c. Evaluate the visual presentation of the data.

B. Inferential Statistics
1. Conclusions or generalizations made about a population (large group) from the study of a sample of that population
2. Choosing and evaluating statistical methods depend, in part, on the type of data used.
3. An educated statement about an unknown population is commonly referred to in statistics as an inference.
4. Statistical inference can be made by estimation or hypothesis testing.

IV. POPULATION DISTRIBUTIONS

A. Discrete Distributions
   1. Binomial distribution
   2. Poisson distribution

B. Normal (Gaussian) Distribution
   1. Most common model for population distributions
   2. Symmetric or bell-shaped frequency distribution
   3. Landmarks for continuous, normally distributed data
      a. μ: Population mean
      b. σ: Population SD
      c. x and s represent the sample mean and SD.
   4. When measuring a random variable in a large-enough sample of any population, some values will occur more often than will others.
   5. A visual check of a distribution can help determine whether it is normally distributed (whether it appears symmetric and bell shaped). Need the data to perform these checks:
      a. Frequency distribution and histograms (visually look at the data; you should do this anyway)
      b. Median and mean will be about equal for normally distributed data (most practical and easiest to use).
      c. Formal test: Kolmogorov-Smirnov test
      d. More challenging to evaluate this when we do not have access to the data (when we are reading an article), because most articles do not present all data or both the mean and median
   6. The parameters mean and SD completely define a normally distributed population.
   7. Probability: The likelihood that any one event will occur given all the possible outcomes
   8. Estimation and sampling variability
      a. One method that can be used to make an inference about a population parameter
      b. Separate samples (even of the same size) from a single population will give slightly different estimates.
      c. The distribution of means from these separate random samples approximates a normal distribution.
         i. The mean of this "distribution of means" = the unknown population mean, μ.
         ii. The SD of the means is estimated by the SEM, which conceptually represents the variability of the distribution of means.
         iii. As in any normal distribution, 95% of the sample means lie within ±2 SEM of the population mean.
      d. The distribution of means from these random samples is about normal regardless of the underlying population distribution (central limit theorem). You will get slightly different mean and SD values each time you repeat this experiment.
      e. The SEM is estimated for a single sample by dividing the SD by the square root of the sample size (n). The SEM quantifies uncertainty in the estimate of the mean, not variability in the sample. Important for hypothesis testing and 95% CI estimation
      f. Why is all of this information about the difference between the SEM and SD worth knowing?
         i. Calculation of CIs (95% CI is about mean ± 2 times the SEM)
         ii. Hypothesis testing
         iii. Deception (e.g., makes results look less "variable," especially when used in graphic format)
   9. Recall the previous example about HDL-C and green tea. From the calculated values in section III, do these data appear to be normally distributed?

V. CONFIDENCE INTERVALS

A. Commonly Reported as a Way to Estimate a Population Parameter
1. In the medical literature, 95% CIs are the most commonly reported CIs. In repeated samples, 95% of all CIs include true population value (i.e., the likelihood or confidence [or probability] that the population value is contained within the interval). In some cases, 90% or 99% CIs are reported.
2. Why are 95% CIs most often reported?
   a. Assume a baseline birth weight in a group n = 13 with a mean ± SD of 1.18 ± 0.4 kg.
   b. 95% CI is about equal to the mean ± 1.96 × SEM (or 2 × SEM). In reality, it depends on the distribution being used and is a bit more complicated.
   c. What is the 95% CI? It is (1.07–1.29), meaning there is 95% certainty that the true mean of the entire population studied is between 1.07 and 1.29 kg.
   d. What is the 90% CI? The 90% CI is calculated to be (1.09–1.27). Of note, the 95% CI will always be wider than the 90% CI for any given sample. Therefore, the wider the CI, the more likely it is to encompass the true population mean.
3. The differences between the SD, SEM, and CIs should be noted when interpreting the literature because they are often used interchangeably. Although it is common for CIs to be confused with SDs, the information each provides is quite different and must be assessed correctly.
4. Recall the previous example about HDL-C and green tea. What is the 95% CI of the data set, and what does that mean?

B. CIs can also be used for any sample estimate. Estimates derived from categorical data such as risk, risk differences, and risk ratios are often presented with the CI and will be discussed later.

C. CIs Instead of Hypothesis Testing
1. Hypothesis testing and calculation of p-values tell us (ideally) whether there is or is not a statistically significant difference between groups, but they do not tell us anything about the magnitude of the difference.
2. CIs help us determine the importance of a finding or findings, which we can apply to a situation.
3. CIs give us an idea of the magnitude of the difference between groups and the statistical significance.
4. CIs are a "range" of data, together with a point estimate of the difference.
5. Wide CIs
   a. Many results are possible, either larger or smaller than the point estimate provided by the study.
   b. All values contained in the CI are statistically plausible.
6. If the estimate is the difference between two continuous variables, a CI that includes zero (no difference between two variables) can be interpreted as not statistically significant (a p-value of 0.05 or greater). There is no need to show both the 95% CI and the p-value.
7. The interpretation of CIs for odds ratios and relative risks is somewhat different. In that case, a value of 1 indicates no difference in risk, and if the CI includes 1, there is no statistical difference. (See the discussions of case-control and cohort in other sections for how to interpret CIs for odds ratios and relative risks.)

VI. HYPOTHESIS TESTING

A. Null and Alternative Hypotheses (See Table 4 for other types of examples.)
1. Null hypothesis (H_0): Example: No difference between groups being compared (treatment A = treatment B)
2. Alternative hypothesis (Ha): Example: Opposite of null hypothesis; states that there is a difference (treatment A ≠ treatment B)
3. The structure or the manner in which the hypothesis is written dictates which statistical test is used. Two-sample t-test: H_0: mean 1 = mean 2
4. Used to assist in determining whether any observed differences between groups can be explained by chance
5. Tests for statistical significance (hypothesis testing) determine whether the data are consistent with H_0 (no difference).
6. The results of the hypothesis testing will indicate whether enough evidence exists for H_0 to be rejected.
   a. If H_0 is rejected = statistically significant difference between groups (unlikely attributable to chance)
   b. If H_0 is not rejected = no statistically significant difference between groups (any "apparent" differences may be attributable to chance). Note that we are not concluding that the treatments are equal.
7. Types of hypothesis testing. These are situations in which two groups are being compared. There are numerous other examples of situations these procedures could be applied to.

Table 4. Types of Hypothesis Testing   *Take a look at differences*

	Question	Hypothesis	Method
Non-directional			
Difference	Are the means different?	H_0: Mean$_1$ = Mean$_2$ H_A: Mean$_1$ ≠ Mean$_2$ OR H_0: Mean$_1$ − Mean$_2$ = 0 H_A: Mean$_1$ − Mean$_2$ ≠ 0	Traditional 2-sided t-test Confidence intervals
Equivalence	Are the means practically equivalent?	H_0: Mean$_1$ − Mean$_2$ ≥ Δ H_A: Mean$_1$ − Mean$_2$ < Δ	Two 1-sided t-test procedures Confidence intervals
Directional			
Superiority	Is mean 1 > mean 2? (or some other similarly worded question)	H_0: Mean$_1$ ≤ Mean$_2$ H_A: Mean$_1$ > Mean$_2$ or H_0: Mean$_1$ − Mean$_2$ ≤ 0 H_A: Mean$_1$ − Mean$_2$ > 0	Traditional 1-sided t-test Confidence intervals
Noninferiority	Is mean 1 no more than a certain amount lower than mean 2?	H_0: Mean$_1$ − Mean$_2$ ≥ Δ H_A: Mean$_1$ − Mean$_2$ < Δ	Confidence intervals

B. To Determine What Is Sufficient Evidence to Reject H_0: Set the a priori significance level (α) and generate the decision rule.
    1. Developed after the research question has been stated in hypothesis form
    2. Used to determine the level of acceptable error caused by a false positive (also known as level of significance)
        a. Convention: A priori α is usually 0.05.
        b. Critical value is calculated, capturing how extreme the sample data must be to reject H_0.

C. Perform the Experiment and Estimate the Test Statistic.
    1. A test statistic is calculated from the observed data in the study, which is compared with the critical value.
    2. Depending on this test statistic's value, H_0 is not rejected (often called fail to reject) or rejected.
    3. In general, the test statistic and critical value are not presented in the literature; instead, p-values are generally reported and compared with a priori α values to assess statistical significance. p-Value: Probability of obtaining a test statistic and critical value as extreme, or more extreme, than the one actually obtained
    4. Because computers are used in these tests, this step is often transparent; the p-value estimated in the statistical test is compared with the a priori α (usually 0.05), and the decision is made.

VII. STATISTICAL TESTS AND CHOOSING A STATISTICAL TEST

A. Which Tests Do You Need to Know?

B. Choosing the Appropriate Statistical Test Depends on
    1. Type of data (nominal, ordinal, or continuous)
    2. Distribution of data (e.g., normal)
    3. Number of groups
    4. Study design (e.g., parallel, crossover)
    5. Presence of confounding variables
    6. One-tailed versus two-tailed
    7. Parametric versus nonparametric tests
        a. Parametric tests assume:
            i.   Data being investigated have an underlying distribution that is normal or close to normal or, more correctly, randomly drawn from a parent population with a normal distribution.
            ii. Data measured are continuous data, measured on either an interval or a ratio scale.
            iii. Parametric tests assume that the data being investigated have variances that are homogeneous between the groups investigated. This is often called homoscedasticity.
        b. Nonparametric tests are used when data are not normally distributed or do not meet other criteria for parametric tests (e.g., discrete data).d

C. Parametric Tests
    1. Student t-test: Several different types
        a. One-sample test: Compares the mean of the study sample with the population mean

Group 1	Known population mean

   b. Two-sample, independent samples, or unpaired test: Compares the means of two independent samples. This is an independent samples test.

Group 1	Group 2

     i. Equal variance test
        (a) Rule for variances: If the ratio of larger variance to smaller variance is greater than 2, we generally conclude the variances are different.
        (b) Formal test for differences in variances: F test
        (c) Adjustments can be made for cases of unequal variance.
     ii. Unequal variance
   c. Paired test: Compares the mean difference of paired or matched samples. This is a related samples test.

Group 1	
Measurement 1	Measurement 2

   d. Common error: Use of multiple t-tests with more than two groups.
  2. Analysis of variance (ANOVA): A more generalized version of the t-test that can apply to more than two groups
   a. One-way ANOVA: Compares the means of three or more groups in a study. Also known as single-factor ANOVA. This is an independent samples test.

Group 1	Group 2	Group 3

   b. Two-way ANOVA: Additional factor (e.g., age) added

Young groups	Group 1	Group 2	Group 3
Old groups	Group 1	Group 2	Group 3

   c. Repeated-measures ANOVA: This is a related samples test.

	Related Measurements		
Group 1	Measurement 1	Measurement 2	Measurement 3

   d. Several more complex factorial ANOVAs can be used.
   e. Many comparison procedures are used to determine which groups actually differ from each other. Post hoc tests: Tukey HSD (honestly significant difference), Bonferroni, Scheffé, Newman-Keuls
  3. Analysis of covariance (ANCOVA): Provides a method to explain the influence of a categorical variable (independent variable) on a continuous variable (dependent variable) while statistically controlling for other variables (confounding)

D. Nonparametric Tests
  1. These tests may also be used for continuous data that do not meet the assumptions of the t-test or ANOVA.
  2. Tests for independent samples
   a. Wilcoxon rank sum, Mann-Whitney U test, or Wilcoxon-Mann-Whitney Test: Compare two independent samples (related to a t-test)

      b.   Kruskal-Wallis one-way ANOVA by ranks
         i.   Compares three or more independent groups (related to one-way ANOVA)
        ii.   Post hoc testing
   3.   Tests for related or paired samples
      a.   Sign test and Wilcoxon signed rank test: Compares two matched or paired samples (related to a paired t-test)
      b.   Friedman ANOVA by ranks: Compares three or more matched or paired groups

E.   Nominal Data
   1.   Chi-square (χ^2) test: Compares expected and observed proportions between two or more groups
      a.   Test of independence
      b.   Test of goodness of fit
   2.   Fisher exact test: Specialized version of the chi-square test for small groups (cells) containing less than five predicted observations
   3.   McNemar: Paired samples
   4.   Mantel-Haenszel: Controls for the influence of confounders

F.   Correlation and Regression (see section IX)

G.   Choosing the Most Appropriate Statistical Test: Example 1
   1.   A trial was conducted to determine whether rosuvastatin was better than simvastatin at lowering low-density lipoprotein cholesterol (LDL-C) concentrations. The trial was designed such that the subjects' baseline characteristics were as comparable as possible with each other. *The intended primary end point for this 3-month trial was the difference in LDL-C between the two drugs.* The results of the trial are reported as follows:

Table 5. Rosuvastatin and Simvastatin Effect on LDL-C

	Rosuvastatin (n=25)	Simvastatin (n=25)
Men/women	12/13	10/15
Smokers	10	13
Baseline LDL-C (mg/dL)	152 ± 5	151 ± 4
Final LDL-C (mg/dL)	138 ± 7	135 ± 5

LDL-C = low-density lipoprotein cholesterol.

   2.   Which is the appropriate statistical test to determine baseline differences in:
      a.   Sex distribution?
      b.   LDL-C?
      c.   Percentage of smokers and nonsmokers?
   3.   Which is the appropriate statistical test to determine:
      a.   The effect of rosuvastatin on LDL-C?
      b.   The primary end point?
   4.   The authors concluded that rosuvastatin is similar to simvastatin. What else would you like to know in evaluating this study?

VIII. DECISION ERRORS

Table 6. Summary of Decision Errors

Test Result	Underlying "Truth" or Reality	
	H_0 *Is True* (No difference)	H_0 *Is False* (Difference)
Accept H_0 (no difference)	No error (correct decision)	Type II error (beta error)
Reject H_0 (difference)	Type I error (alpha error)	No error (correct decision)

H_0 = null hypothesis.

A. Type I Error: The probability of making this error is defined as the significance level α.
   1. Convention is to set the α to 0.05, effectively meaning that, 1 in 20 times, a type I error will occur when the H_0 is rejected. So, 5.0% of the time, a researcher will conclude that there is a statistically significant difference when one does not actually exist.
   2. The calculated chance that a type I error has occurred is called the p-value.
   3. The p-value tells us the likelihood of obtaining a given (or a more extreme) test result if the H_0 is true. When the α level is set a priori, H_0 is rejected when p is less than α. In other words, the p-value tells us the probability of being wrong when we conclude that a true difference exists (false positive).
   4. A lower p-value does not mean the result is more important or more meaningful but only that it is statistically significant and not likely to be attributable to chance.

B. Type II Error: The probability of making this error is called β.
   1. Concluding that no difference exists when one truly does (not rejecting H_0 when it should be rejected)
   2. It has become a convention to set β to between 0.20 and 0.10.

C. Power (1 − β)
   1. The probability of making a correct decision when H_0 is false; the ability to detect differences between groups if one actually exists
   2. Dependent on the following factors:
      a. Predetermined α
      b. Sample size
      c. The size of the difference between the outcomes you want to detect, called the effect size. Often not known before the experiment is conducted, so to estimate the power of your test, you will have to specify how large a change is worth detecting.
      d. The variability of the outcomes that are being measured
      e. Items c and d are generally determined from previous data or the literature.
   3. Power is decreased by (in addition to the above criteria):
      a. Poor study design
      b. Incorrect statistical tests (use of nonparametric tests when parametric tests are appropriate)
   4. Statistical power analysis and sample size calculation
      a. Related to above discussion of power and sample size
      b. Sample size estimates should be performed in all studies a priori.
      c. Necessary components for estimating appropriate sample size
         i. Acceptable type II error rate (usually 0.10–0.20)
         ii. Observed difference in predicted study outcomes that is clinically significant

iii. The expected variability in item ii

iv. Acceptable type I error rate (usually 0.05)

v. Statistical test that will be used for primary end point

5. Statistical significance versus clinical significance

a. As stated earlier, the size of the p-value is not necessarily related to the clinical importance of the result. Smaller values mean only that chance is less likely to explain observed differences.

b. Statistically significant does not necessarily mean clinically significant.

c. Lack of statistical significance does not mean that results are not clinically important.

d. When considering nonsignificant findings, consider sample size, estimated power, difference study was powered to detect, and observed variability and observed variability.

IX. CORRELATION AND REGRESSION

A. Introduction: Correlation Versus Regression

1. Correlation examines the strength of the association between two variables. It does not necessarily assume that one variable is useful in predicting the other.

2. Regression examines the ability of one or more variables to predict another variable.

B. Pearson Correlation

1. The strength of the relationship between two variables that are normally distributed, ratio or interval scaled, and linearly related is measured with a correlation coefficient.

2. Often referred to as the degree of association between the two variables

3. Does not necessarily imply that one variable is dependent on the other (regression analysis will do that)

4. Pearson correlation (r) ranges from -1 to $+1$ and can take any value in between:

-1	0	$+1$
Perfect negative linear relationship	No linear relationship	Perfect positive linear relationship

5. Hypothesis testing is performed to determine whether the correlation coefficient is different from zero. This test is highly influenced by sample size.

C. Pearls About Correlation

1. The closer the magnitude of r to 1 (either + or $-$), the more highly correlated the two variables. The weaker the relationship between the two variables, the closer r is to 0.

2. There is no agreed-on or consistent interpretation of the value of the correlation coefficient. It is dependent on the environment of the investigation (laboratory vs. clinical experiment).

3. Pay more attention to the magnitude of the correlation than to the p-value because it is influenced by sample size.

4. Crucial to the proper use of correlation analysis is interpretation of the graphic representation of the two variables. Before using correlation analysis, it is essential to generate a scatterplot of the two variables to visually examine the relationship.

D. Spearman Rank Correlation: Nonparametric test that quantifies the strength of an association between two variables but does not assume a normal distribution of continuous data. Can be used for ordinal data or nonnormally distributed continuous data

E. Regression
1. A statistical technique related to correlation. There are many different types; for simple linear regression, one continuous outcome (dependent) variable and one continuous independent (causative) variable
2. Two main purposes of regression: (1) development of prediction model and (2) accuracy of prediction
3. Prediction model: Making predictions of the dependent variable from the independent variable; $Y = mx + b$ (dependent variable = slope × independent variable + intercept)
4. Accuracy of prediction: How well the independent variable predicts the dependent variable. Regression analysis determines the extent of variability in the dependent variable that can be explained by the independent variable.
   a. Coefficient of determination (r^2) measured describing this relationship. Values of r^2 can range from 0 to 1.
   b. An r^2 of 0.80 could be interpreted as saying that 80% of the variability in Y is explained by the variability in X.
   c. This does not provide a mechanistic understanding of the relationship between X and Y but rather a description of how clearly such a model (linear or otherwise) describes the relationship between the two variables.
   d. Like the interpretation of r, the interpretation of r^2 depends on the scientific arena (e.g., clinical research, basic research, social science research) to which it is applied.
5. For simple linear regression, two statistical tests can be used.
   a. To test the hypothesis that the y-intercept differs from zero
   b. To test the hypothesis that the slope of the line is different from zero
6. Regression is useful in constructing predictive models. The literature is full of examples of predictions. The process involves developing a formula for a regression line that best fits the observed data.
7. There are many different types of regression analysis.
   a. Multiple linear regression: One continuous independent variable and two or more continuous dependent variables
   b. Simple logistic regression: One categorical response variable and one continuous or categorical explanatory variable
   c. Multiple logistic regression: One categorical response variable and two or more continuous or categorical explanatory variables
   d. Nonlinear regression: Variables are not linearly related (or cannot be transformed into a linear relationship). This is where our pharmacokinetic equations come from.
   e. Polynomial regression: Any number of response and continuous variables with a curvilinear relationship (e.g., cubed, squared)
8. Example of regression
   a. The following data are taken from a study evaluating enoxaparin use. The authors were interested in predicting patient response (measured as antifactor Xa concentrations) from the enoxaparin dose in the 75 subjects who were studied.

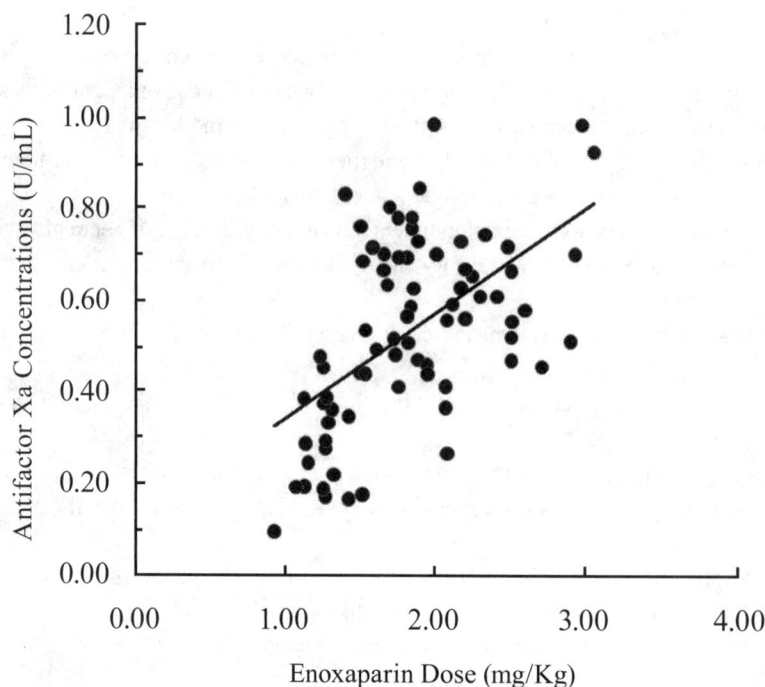

Figure 1. Relationship between antifactor Xa concentrations and enoxaparin dose.

b. The authors performed regression analysis and reported the following: slope, 0.227; y-intercept, 0.097; $p<0.05$; $r^2 = 0.31$.
c. Answer the following questions:
  i. What are the necessary assumptions to use regression analysis?
  ii. Provide an interpretation of the coefficient of determination.
  iii. Predict antifactor Xa concentrations at enoxaparin doses of 2 and 3.75 mg/kg.
  iv. What does the $p<0.05$ value indicate?

X. SURVIVAL ANALYSIS

A. Studies the Time Between Entry in a Study and Some Event (e.g., death, myocardial infarction)
  1. Censoring makes survival methods unique; considers that some subjects leave the study for reasons other than the event (e.g., lost to follow-up, end of study period).
  2. Considers that all subjects do not enter the study at the same time
  3. Standard methods of statistical analysis such as t-tests and linear or logistic regression may not be appropriately applied to survival data because of censoring.

B. Estimating the Survival Function
  1. Kaplan-Meier method
    a. Uses survival times (or censored survival times) to estimate the proportion of people who would survive a given length of time under the same circumstances
    b. Allows the production of a table ("life table") and a graph ("survival curve")
    c. We can visually evaluate the curves, but we need a test to evaluate them formally.

2. Log-rank test: Compare the survival distributions between two or more groups.
   a. This test precludes an analysis of the effects of several variables or the magnitude of difference between groups or the CI (see below for Cox proportional hazards model).
   b. H_0: No difference in survival between the two populations
   c. Log-rank test uses several assumptions:
      i. Random sampling and subjects chosen independently
      ii. Consistent criteria for entry or end point
      iii. Baseline survival rate does not change as time progresses.
      iv. Censored subjects have the same average survival time as uncensored subjects.
3. Cox proportional hazards model
   a. Most popular method to evaluate the impact of covariates; reported (graphically) like Kaplan-Meier
   b. Investigates several variables at a time
   c. Actual method of construction and calculation is complex.
   d. Compares survival in two or more groups after other variables are adjusted for
   e. Allows calculation of a hazard ratio (and CI)

XI. SELECTED REPRESENTATIVE STATISTICAL TESTS

Table 7. Representative Statistical Tests

Type of Variable	2 Samples (independent)	2 Samples (related)	>2 Samples (independent)	>2 Samples (related)
Nominal	χ^2 or Fisher exact test	McNemar test	χ^2	Cochran Q
Ordinal	Wilcoxon rank sum Mann-Whitney U test Wilcoxon-Mann-Whitney	Wilcoxon signed rank Sign test	Kruskal-Wallis (MCP)	Friedman ANOVA
Continuous No factors	Equal variance t-test Unequal variance t-test	Paired t-test	1-way ANOVA (MCP)	Repeated-measures ANOVA
1 factor	ANCOVA	2-way repeated-measures ANOVA	2-way ANOVA (MCP)	2-way repeated-measures ANOVA

ANCOVA = analysis of covariance; ANOVA = analysis of variance; MCP = multiple comparisons procedure.

REFERENCES

1. Crawford SL. Correlation and regression. Circulation 2006;114:2083-8.

2. Davis RB, Mukamal KJ. Hypothesis testing: means. Circulation 2006;114:1078-82.

3. DeYoung GR. Understanding biostatistics: an approach for the clinician. In: Zarowitz B, Shumock G, Dunsworth T, et al., eds. Pharmacotherapy Self-Assessment Program, 5th ed. Kansas City, MO: ACCP, 2005:1-20.

4. DiCenzo R, ed. Clinical Pharmacist's Guide to Biostatistics and Literature Evaluation. Lenexa, KS: ACCP, 2010.

5. Gaddis ML, Gaddis GM. Introduction to biostatistics. Part 1, basic concepts. Ann Emerg Med 1990;19:86-9.

6. Gaddis ML, Gaddis GM. Introduction to biostatistics. Part 2, descriptive statistics. Ann Emerg Med 1990;19:309-15.

7. Gaddis ML, Gaddis GM. Introduction to biostatistics. Part 3, sensitivity, specificity, predictive value, and hypothesis testing. Ann Emerg Med 1990;19:591-7.

8. Gaddis ML, Gaddis GM. Introduction to biostatistics. Part 4, statistical inference techniques in hypothesis testing. Ann Emerg Med 1990;19:820-5.

9. Gaddis ML, Gaddis GM. Introduction to biostatistics. Part 5, statistical inference techniques for hypothesis testing with nonparametric data. Ann Emerg Med 1990;19:1054-9.

10. Gaddis ML, Gaddis GM. Introduction to biostatistics. Part 6, correlation and regression. Ann Emerg Med 1990;19:1462-8.

11. Harper ML. Biostatistics for the clinician. In: Zarowitz B, Shumock G, Dunsworth T, et al., eds. Pharmacotherapy Self-Assessment Program, 4th ed. Kansas City, MO: ACCP, 2002:183-200.

12. Hayney MS, Meek PD. Essential clinical concepts of biostatistics. In: Carter BL, Lake KD, Raebel MA, et al., eds. Pharmacotherapy Self-Assessment Program, 3rd ed. Kansas City, MO: ACCP, 1999:19-46.

13. Jones SR, Carley S, Harrison M. An introduction to power and sample size estimation. Emerg Med J 2003;20:453-8.

14. Kier KL. Biostatistical methods in epidemiology. Pharmacotherapy 2011;31:9-22.

15. Kusuoka H, Hoffman JIE. Advice on statistical analysis for circulation research. Circ Res 2002;91:662-71.

16. Larson MG. Descriptive statistics and graphical displays. Circulation 2006;114:76-81.

17. Larson MG. Analysis of variance. Circulation 2008;117:115-21.

18. Overholser BR, Sowinski KM. Biostatistics primer. Part 1. Nutr Clin Pract 2007;22:629-35.

19. Overholser BR, Sowinski KM. Biostatistics primer. Part 2. Nutr Clin Pract 2008;23:76-84.

20. Rao SR, Schoenfeld DA. Survival methods. Circulation 2007;115:109-13.

21. Rector TS, Hatton RC. Statistical concepts and methods used to evaluate pharmacotherapy. In: Zarowitz B, Shumock G, Dunsworth T, et al., eds. Pharmacotherapy Self-Assessment Program, 2nd ed. Kansas City, MO: ACCP, 1997:130-61.

22. Strassels SA. Biostatistics. In: Dunsworth TS, Richardson MM, Chant C, et al., eds. Pharmacotherapy Self-Assessment Program, 6th ed. Lenexa, KS: ACCP, 2007:1-16.

23. Sullivan LM. Estimation from samples. Circulation 2006;114:445-9.

24. Tsuyuki RT, Garg S. Interpreting data in cardiovascular disease clinical trials: a biostatistical toolbox. In: Richardson MM, Chant C, Cheng JWM, et al., eds. Pharmacotherapy Self-Assessment Program, 7th ed. Lenexa, KS: ACCP, 2010:241-55.

25. Windish DM, Huot SJ, Green ML. Medicine resident's understanding of the biostatistics and results in the medical literature. JAMA 2007;298:1010-22.

26. Horton NJ, Switzer SS. Statistical methods in the journal. N Engl J Med. 2005;353:1977-79.

ANSWERS AND EXPLANATIONS TO SELF-ASSESSMENT QUESTIONS

1. Answer: A

The NYHA functional class is an ordinal scale from I (no symptoms) to IV (severe symptoms). Neither ANOVA nor ANCOVA is appropriate for ordinal or noncontinuous data (Answer C and Answer D are incorrect). The Wilcoxon signed rank test is an appropriate nonparametric test to use for paired ordinal data, such as the change in NYHA functional class over time on the same person (Answer B is incorrect). The Kruskal-Wallis test is the nonparametric analog of a one-way ANOVA and is appropriate for this analysis (Answer A is correct).

2. Answer: C

You cannot determine which finding is more important (in this case, the best drug) on the basis of the p-value (i.e., a lower p-value does not mean more important) (Answer B is incorrect). All statistically significant results are interpreted as significant without respect to the size of the p-value. This trial had four independent samples, and use of the unpaired (independent samples) t-test is not appropriate because it requires several unnecessary tests and increases the chances of making a type I error (Answer A is incorrect). In this setting, ANOVA is the correct test (Answer C is correct), followed by a multiple comparisons procedure to determine where the actual differences between groups lie. A paired t-test is inappropriate because this is a parallel-group trial (Answer D is incorrect). The use of ANOVA in this case assumes a normal distribution and equal variance in each of the four groups.

3. Answer: D

The typical a priori alpha error (type I rate) rate is 5% (i.e., when the study was designed, the error rate was designed to be 5% or less) (Answer D is correct). The actual type I error rate is reported in the question as 0.01 (1%) (Answer A is incorrect). Answer B and Answer C are related; the study did have enough power because a statistically significant difference was observed. Similarly, a type II error was not made because this error has to do with not finding a difference when one truly exists. In this question, the type I error rate is 1%, the value of the p-value.

4. Answer: C

Sample sizes need not be equal for a t-test to be appropriate (Answer A is incorrect). Body mass index data are not ordinal but rather continuous; thus, a t-test is appropriate (Answer B is incorrect). The assumption of equal variances is necessary to use any parametric test (Answer C is correct). A specific value for power is not necessary to use a test (Answer D is incorrect).

5. Answer: B

Many think reporting the mean difference and CI is a superior means of presenting the results from a clinical trial because it describes both precision and statistical significance versus a p-value, which distills everything into one value, making Answer A incorrect. The presentation of the data in this manner clearly shows all the necessary information for making the appropriate conclusion. To assess statistical significance by use of CIs, the 95% CI (corresponding to the 5% type I error rate used in most studies) may not contain zero (signifying no difference between men and women) for the mean difference, making Answer D incorrect. Answer B is correct because the p-value of less than 0.05 corresponds to the 95% CI in that item. To evaluate Answer C, we would need to know the 99% CI.

6. Answer: D

Answer A is incorrect because it uses unconventional approaches to determine statistical significance. Although this can be done, it is unlikely to be accepted by other readers and investigators. This study observed a nonsignificant increase in HDL-C between the two groups. With a small sample size, such as the one used in this study, there is always concern about adequate power to observe a difference between the two treatments. A difference may exist between these two drugs, but the number of subjects studied may be too small to detect it statistically. Answer D is correct because, given the lack of information provided in this narrative, it is not possible to estimate power; thus, more information is needed. Answer B may be correct, but without first addressing the question of adequate power, it would be an inappropriate conclusion to draw. Answer C is incorrect because even though the new drug increased HDL-C more than the other treatment, it is inappropriate to conclude that it is better because, statistically, it is not.

7. Answer: B

The primary end point in this study, the percentage of subjects at or below the target blood pressure, is nominal data. Subjects at target blood pressure (less than 140/90 mm Hg) are defined as having reached the target. This type of data requires either a chi-square test or a Fisher exact test (depending on the sample size or, more accurately, the number of counts in the individual contingency table cells) (Answer B is correct). An independent samples t-test is not appropriate because actual blood pressure values are not being compared (at least not in this question or this end point) (Answer A is incorrect). If we were comparing the actual blood pressure between the two groups, the test might be appropriate, if parametric assumptions were met. The Wilcoxon signed rank test is the appropriate nonparametric test when paired samples are compared (usually in a crossover trial) (Answer C is incorrect). Finally, a one-sample t-test is used to compare the mean of a single group with the mean of a reference group. This is also incorrect in this situation because two groups are being compared (Answer D is incorrect).

8. Answer: A

Detecting the smaller difference between the treatments requires more power. Power can be increased in several different ways. Answer A is correct because the most common approach is to increase the sample size, which is expensive for the researchers. Answer D is incorrect because smaller sample sizes decrease a study's ability to detect differences between groups. Power can also be increased by increasing α, but doing so increases the chances of a type I error. Answer B decreases α, thus making it more difficult to detect differences between groups. Answer C certainly makes it easier to detect a difference between the two groups; however, it uses an unconventional α value and is thus not the most appropriate technique.

9. Answer: C

Regression analysis is the most effective way to develop models to predict outcomes or variables (Answer C is correct). There are many different types of regression, but all share the ability to evaluate the impact of multiple variables simultaneously on an outcome variable. Correlation analysis is used to assess the association between two (or more) variables, not to make predictions (Answer A is incorrect). Kaplan-Meier curves are used to graphically depict survival curves or time to an event (Answer B is incorrect). Confidence intervals are not used to make predictions (Answer D is incorrect).

Study Designs:
Fundamentals of Interpretation

Kevin M. Sowinski, Pharm.D., FCCP

Purdue University College of Pharmacy
Indiana University School of Medicine
West Lafayette and Indianapolis, Indiana

STUDY DESIGNS: FUNDAMENTALS OF INTERPRETATION

KEVIN M. SOWINSKI, PHARM.D., FCCP

PURDUE UNIVERSITY COLLEGE OF PHARMACY
INDIANA UNIVERSITY SCHOOL OF MEDICINE
WEST LAFAYETTE AND INDIANAPOLIS, INDIANA

Learning Objectives

1. Define and compare the concepts of internal and external validity, bias, and confounding in clinical study design.
2. Identify potential sources of bias in clinical trials; select strategies to eliminate or control for bias.
3. Outline the hierarchy of evidence generated by various study designs.
4. Compare the advantages and disadvantages of various study designs (e.g., prospective, retrospective, case-control, cohort, cross-sectional, randomized controlled clinical trials, systematic review, meta-analysis). Delineate the difference between parallel and crossover study designs.
5. Select from various biostatistical measures to appropriately compare groups or their assessments from various study designs and use their findings/output to interpret results.
6. Define and evaluate odds, odds ratios, risk and incidence rates, risk ratios and relative risks (RRs), and other risk estimates. Compute and evaluate number needed to treat and number needed to harm. Define and calculate terms such as point and period prevalence, incidence rate, prevalence rate, absolute risk difference, and RR difference.
7. Define and calculate terms such as true positive, false positive, true negative, false negative, sensitivity, specificity, positive predictive value, negative predictive value, positive likelihood ratio, and negative likelihood ratio.

Self-Assessment Questions

Answers and explanations to these questions can be found at the end of the chapter.

Questions 1 and 2 pertain to the following case:
A recently released statin is associated with less myopathy than other currently available statins. After 2 years of use, a retrospective case-control study was undertaken by the manufacturer after 20 different reports of severe myopathy were sent to the U.S. Food and Drug Administration (FDA) MedWatch program. Risk factors for statin-induced myopathy were not assessed; however, both the cases and the controls of this study had identical diagnostic evaluations and were stratified according to the duration of statin use before the onset of myopathy.

1. Which type of bias is this study design most susceptible to?
   A. Confounding by indication.
   B. Recall bias.
   C. Diagnostic bias.
   D. Misclassification.

2. Which factor will be most affected by the type of bias likely to occur in this study?
   A. External validity.
   B. Internal validity.
   C. Assessment of exposure.
   D. Number of patients needed for the study.

3. When describing the results of a randomized controlled clinical trial, the investigators report using an intention-to-treat analysis to analyze their data. The results of their investigation comparing two diuretics for heart failure show no difference in the number of hospitalizations for decompensated heart failure between the treatment groups. Given their method of data analysis, which statement is most appropriate?
   A. May be susceptible to issues of a lack of power.
   B. Provides a good measure of effectiveness under typical clinical conditions.
   C. Cannot provide an estimate of the method's effectiveness.
   D. May overestimate the actual treatment effect.

4. A prospective randomized study compared once-daily enoxaparin with twice-daily enoxaparin for treating patients with venous thromboembolism (VTE). One of the study end points was the recurrence of VTE. The following table summarizes recurrence rates in all patients.

	Once Daily	**Twice Daily**
All patients, *n* (%)	13/298 (4.4)	9/312 (2.9)

The 95% confidence interval (CI) for the difference in recurrence rates between the two groups was –1.5% to 4.5%. Which conclusion is most appropriate?

A. The difference in recurrence rates between the two treatments is statistically significant.

B. The difference in recurrence rates between the two treatments is not statistically significant.

C. Because twice-daily therapy causes fewer recurrences, clinicians should feel comfortable using that dosing scheme for their patients with VTE.

D. No conclusion can be drawn because p-values are unavailable.

5. According to the data in the previous question and the result obtained, which best represents the number of patients who would need to be treated with twice-daily enoxaparin to prevent the recurrence of one VTE?

   A. 7.

   B. 23.

   C. 67.

   D. Number needed to treat (NNT) should not be calculated because the result was nonsignificant.

Questions 6 and 7 pertain to the following case:
A multicenter, double-blind, placebo-controlled trial randomly assigned 4837 patients to treatment with margarine supplemented with the omega-3 fatty acid ALA (margarine with ALA) or a placebo margarine. The primary combined end point was the rate of cardiovascular events, defined as fatal and nonfatal cardiovascular events and percutaneous coronary interventions. Data were analyzed according to intention-to-treat analysis with the use of a Cox proportional hazards model. The 95% hazard ratio (HR) and 95% CI for the margarine with ALA group were 0.91 and 0.78–1.05, respectively. In the prespecified subgroup of women, margarine with ALA was associated with an HR of 0.73 (95% CI, 0.51–1.03).

6. Which statement is most appropriate?

   A. Margarine with ALA statistically significantly reduced the risk of cardiovascular events ($p < 0.05$).

   B. Margarine with ALA statistically significantly reduced the risk of cardiovascular events ($p < 0.01$).

   C. Margarine with ALA did not significantly reduce the risk of cardiovascular events ($p > 0.05$).

   D. Without a p-value, it is not possible to determine whether margarine with ALA affected cardiovascular events.

7. When the study was being designed, which choice describes the outcome for which the study was most likely to have been powered?

   A. Differences in the rate of the composite outcome, cardiovascular events.

   B. Differences in the rate of percutaneous coronary interventions.

   C. Differences in the rate of the composite outcome in women.

   D. Differences in the rate of the composite outcome in men.

8. In a meta-analysis of randomized controlled trials examining the effects of several antihypertensive drugs, the odds ratio (OR) for treatment with low-dose diuretics compared with calcium channel blockers for cardiovascular disease events was 0.84 (95% CI, 0.75–0.95). Which statement is the most appropriate interpretation of these findings?

   A. Treatment of hypertension with low-dose diuretics was more effective in preventing cardiovascular disease events than treatment with calcium channel blockers.

   B. Treatment of hypertension with calcium channel blockers was more effective in preventing cardiovascular disease events than treatment with low doses of diuretics.

   C. The difference observed between treatment with calcium channel blockers and low doses of diuretics is not statistically significant.

   D. The odds of developing cardiovascular events when treating hypertension with low doses of diuretics are lower than when using calcium channel blockers.

I. INTRODUCTION

A. Why Do Pharmacists Need to Know About Study Design and Interpretation?

B. Online Statistical and Study Design Tools (www.graphpad.com/quickcalcs/)

C. As It Pertains to Most of You:
   Pharmacotherapy Specialty Examination Content Outline
   - Domain 2: Retrieval, Generation, Interpretation, and Dissemination of Knowledge in Pharmacotherapy (25%)
   - Interpret biomedical literature with respect to study design and methodology, statistical analysis, and significance of reported data and conclusions.
   - Knowledge of biostatistical methods, clinical and statistical significance, research hypothesis generation, research design and methodology, and protocol and proposal development.

II. VARIOUS ISSUES IN STUDY DESIGN

A. Research Design Classification
   1. Study purpose: Descriptive versus analytical
   2. Time orientation: Prospective versus retrospective design
      a. Prospective: Begin in the present and progress forward, collecting data from subjects whose outcome lies in the future.
      b. Retrospective: Begin and end in the present; however, this design involves a major backward look to collect information about events that occurred in the past.
   3. Investigator orientation: Interventional versus quasiexperimental
   4. Experimental setting
      a. Randomized controlled trials
      b. Observational trials

B. Relative Strength of Evidence: Hierarchy of Study Designs

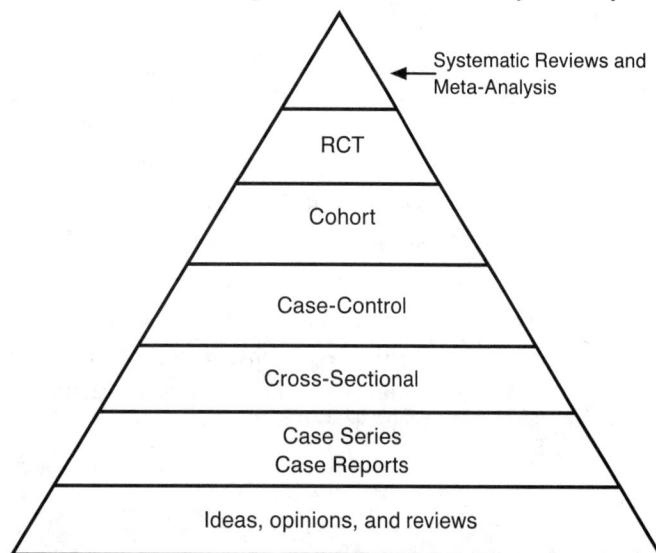

Figure 1. Hierarchy of Clinical Study Design.
RCT = randomized controlled clinical trial.

C. Validity in Study Design
   1. Internal validity
      a. Validity within the confines of the study methods
      b. Does the study design adequately and appropriately test or measure what it purports?
      c. Does the study adequately and appropriately address bias, confounding, and measurement of end points?
   2. External validity
      a. Validity related to generalizing the study results outside the study setting
      b. Can the results be applied to other groups, patients, or systems?
      c. Addresses issues of generalizability and representativeness.

D. Bias in Study Design
   1. Definition: Systematic, nonrandom variation in study methods and conductance, ultimately introducing error in outcome interpretation. Bias can occur in all aspects of the study design.
   2. Examples of bias
      a. Selection bias: An error in the selection or sampling of individuals for a clinical study. A classic example would be the situation in which the subjects chosen for the case and control groups differ in one or more characteristics that alter the outcome of a study.
      b. Observational or information bias: An error in the recording of individual factors of a study, such as inaccurate recording of a patient's risk factor, inaccurate recording of the timing of a blood sample
      c. Recall bias: Classic example: Studies of birth defects secondary to medications
      d. Interviewer bias: Classic example: Interviews are not conducted in a uniform manner (or by the same person) for all study participants.
      e. Misclassification bias
         i. Differential
         ii. Nondifferential
   3. Controlling for bias
      a. Design: For example, selection of study population
      b. Means of collecting data
      c. Sources of information (about disease and exposure)
      d. Analysis: May be difficult to interpret

E. Confounding in Study Design
   1. A variable that affects the independent or dependent variable, altering the ability to determine the true effect on the measured outcome. These factors may hide or exaggerate a true association.
   2. To minimize the potential for missing a confounding variable, all relevant information should be collected and evaluated.
   3. Controlling for confounding
      a. During the design of a study
         i. Randomization
         ii. Restriction
         iii. Matching
      b. Analysis
         i. Stratification
         ii. Multivariate analysis

F. Causality
  1. Temporality: Cause before effect
  2. Strength: Plausibility increases with strength of relationship
  3. Biological gradient: Dose-response?
  4. Consistency: Observations over numerous settings
  5. Specificity: Single cause for effect
  6. Plausibility: Biologically plausible
  7. Coherence: Consistency with existing knowledge
  8. Analogy: Preclinical expectation applied to clinical testing
  9. Experiment: Randomized controlled trials

III. CASE REPORTS AND CASE SERIES

A. Document and Describe Experiences, Novel Treatments, and Unusual Events. Allows hypothesis generation that can be tested with other study designs. Note that the title does not state "study."
  1. Possible adverse drug reactions in one or more patients: QT interval prolongation associated with fluoroquinolone antibiotics
  2. Case report: One patient
  3. Case series: More than one patient with a similar experience or many case reports combined into a descriptive review
  4. Reports should provide sufficient detail to allow readers to recognize same or similar cases at their center or practice.

B. Advantages and Disadvantages
  1. Advantages: Hypotheses are formed, which may be the first step in describing an important clinical problem. Easy to perform and inexpensive
  2. Disadvantages: Does not provide explanation other than conjecture and does not establish causality or association

IV. OBSERVATIONAL STUDY DESIGNS

A. Design Does Not Involve Investigator Intervention, Only Observation. It is essential to remember that observational study designs investigate associations, not, in most cases, causes.

B. Case-Control Study: Study Exposure in Those With and Without the Outcome of Interest

Classify and Compare ◄——— Begin

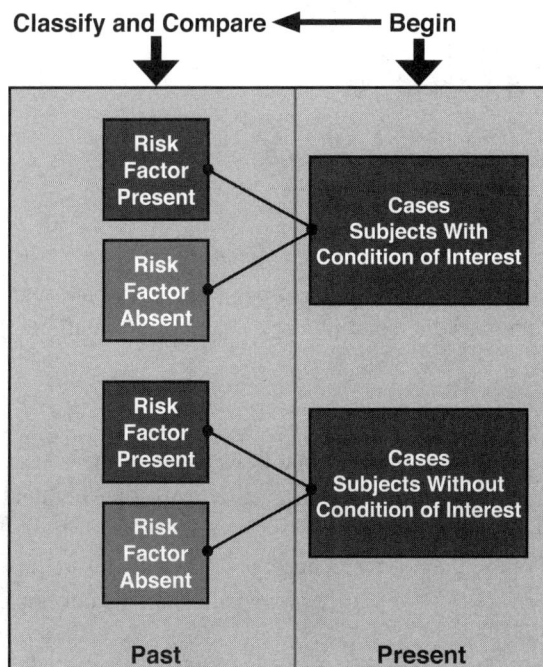

Figure 2. Case-control study design.

1. Determine the association between exposures or risk factors and disease or condition. Classic example: Aspirin use and Reye syndrome
2. Also called retrospective studies
3. Useful method (and perhaps the only practical way) to study exposures in rare diseases or diseases that take long periods to develop
4. Critical assumptions to minimize bias
   a. Cases are selected to be representative of those who have the disease.
   b. Controls are representative of the general population that does not have the disease and are as identical as possible to the cases, minus the presence of the disease.
   c. Information is collected from cases and controls in the same way.
5. Examples
   a. Psaty BM, Heckbert SR, Koepsell TD, et al. The risk of myocardial infarction associated with antihypertensive drug therapies. JAMA 1995;274:620-5.
   b. Kernan WN, Viscoli CM, Brass LM, et al. Phenylpropanolamine (PPA) and the risk of hemorrhagic stroke. N Engl J Med 2000;343:1826-32. Purpose of study:
      i. To estimate in women the association between hemorrhagic stroke and the use of appetite suppressants containing phenylpropanolamine (PPA)
      ii. To estimate the association between any use of PPA (in appetite suppressant or cough or cold remedy) and hemorrhagic stroke
      iii. To estimate in men and women the association between hemorrhagic stroke and the type of exposure to PPA
      iv. Disease: Hemorrhagic stroke (several types). Exposure: PPA
      v. Cases: Symptomatic subarachnoid or intracerebral hemorrhage (n=702). Controls: Matched by sex, race, and age (n=1376)
      vi. Exposure assessed by structured questionnaire, product photographs, and ingredient confirmation

6. Advantages
   a. Inexpensive and can be conducted quickly
   b. Allows investigation of several possible exposures or associations
7. Disadvantages
   a. Confounding must be controlled for.
   b. Observational and recall bias: Looking back to recall exposures and their possible levels
   c. Selection bias: Case selection and control matching are difficult.
8. Measure of association: The odds ratio (OR): In some cases, this can be an estimate of the relative risk or risk ratio (RR). The OR is interpreted as the odds (and its ratio) of exposure to a factor in those with a condition or disease compared with those who do not have the condition or disease. Interpretation of these concepts will be presented later in the chapter.

C. Cohort Study
   1. Determines the association between exposures or factors and disease or condition development. Allows an estimation of the risk of outcome (and the RR between the exposure groups). Study outcome of interest in those with and without the exposure of interest. Classic examples:
      a. Framingham Study. A cohort of subjects from Framingham, Massachusetts, were (and are) studied over time to evaluate the relationship between a variety of conditions (exposures) on the development of cardiovascular disease.
      b. Nurses' Health Study: Investigated the potential long-term consequences of the use of oral contraceptives
   2. Describes the incidence or natural history of a disease or condition and measures it in time sequence
   3. Retrospective: Begins and ends in the present but involves a major backward look to collect information about events that occurred in the past

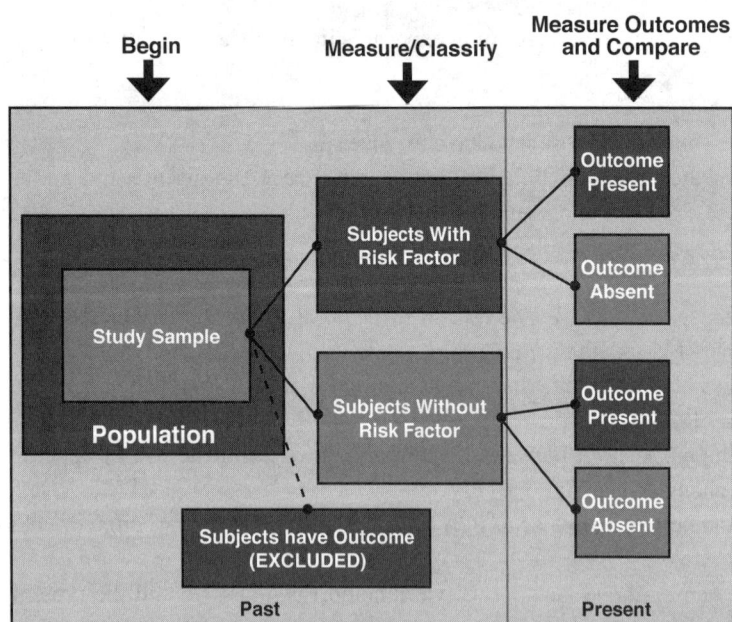

Figure 3. Retrospective cohort study design.

   a. Advantages: Less expensive and time-consuming; no loss to follow-up, ability to investigate issues not amenable to a clinical trial or ethical or safety issues
   b. Disadvantages: Only as good as the data available, little control of confounding variables through nonstatistical approaches, recall bias

4. Prospective or longitudinal: Begin in the present and progress forward, collecting data from subjects whose outcome lies in the future.

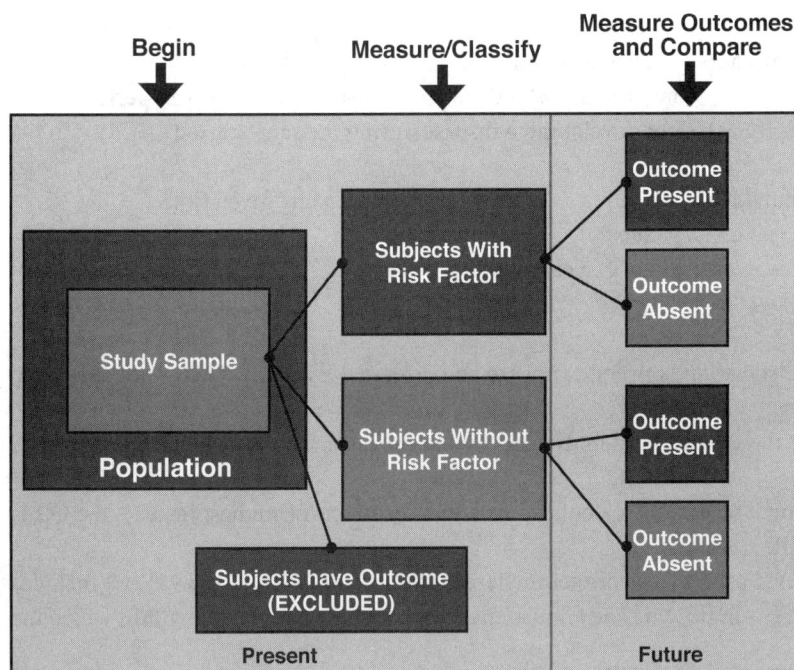

Figure 4. Prospective cohort study design.

       a. Example: Grodstein F, Manson JE, Stampfer MJ. Postmenopausal hormone use and secondary prevention of coronary events in the Nurses' Health Study. A prospective, observational study. Ann Intern Med 2001;135:1-8.

       b. Advantages: Able to control for confounding factors to a greater extent, easier to plan for data collection

       c. Disadvantages: More expensive and time-intensive, loss of subject follow-up, difficult to study rare diseases or conditions at a reasonable cost

5. Measure of association: RR: The risk of an event or development of a condition relative to exposure; the risk of someone developing a condition when exposed compared with someone who has not been exposed

D. Cross-sectional (a.k.a. prevalence study)
   1. Identify the prevalence or characteristics of a condition in a group of individuals.
   2. Examples:
       a. Reidy A, et al. Prevalence of serious eye disease and visual impairment in a north London population: population based, cross sectional study. BMJ 1998;316:1643-7.
       b. Nezvalova K, et al. Maternal characteristics and migraine pharmacotherapy during pregnancy: cross sectional analysis of data from a large cohort study. Cephalgia 2009;29:1267-76.
   3. Advantages: Easy design, snapshot in time, all data collected at one time, studies are accomplished by questionnaire, interview, or other available biomedical information (e.g., laboratory values)
   4. Disadvantages: Does not allow the study of a factor (or factors) in individual subjects over time, just at the time of assessment; difficult to study rare conditions

V. INCIDENCE, PREVALENCE, RELATIVE RISK OR RISK RATIOS, AND ODDS RATIOS

A. Incidence
   1. Measure of the probability of developing a disease
   2. Incidence rate: Number of new cases of disease per population in a specified time
   3. Calculated by dividing the number of individuals who develop a disease during a given period by the number of individuals who were at risk of developing a disease during the same period

B. Prevalence
   1. Measure of the number of individuals who have a condition or disease at any given time
   2. Point prevalence: Prevalence on a given date
   3. Period prevalence: Prevalence in a period (e.g., year, month)

C. Interpreting RRs and ORs
   1. Estimate the magnitude of association between exposure and disease. Key point: This is not cause and effect; it is an association.
   2. The incidence of disease in the exposed group divided by the incidence of disease in the unexposed group
   3. The RR (a.k.a. risk ratio) cannot be directly calculated for most case-control studies; instead, the OR is usually an estimate of the RR.
   4. The RR and OR are interpreted on the basis of their difference from unity (1.0). If the 95% CI includes unity, no statistical difference is indicated. The CI also gives us an idea of the spread within which the true effect lies.
   5. Interpretation of the index of risk
      a. Direction of risk

Table 1. Direction of Risk Associated With OR and RR

RR	OR	Interpretation
<1	<1	Negative association RR: Risk of disease is lower in the exposed group OR: Odds of exposure is lower in the diseased group
1	1	No association RR: Risk of disease in the 2 groups is the same OR: Odds of exposure in the 2 groups is the same
>1	>1	Positive association RR: Risk of disease is greater in the exposed group OR: Odds of exposure is greater in the diseased group

OR = odds ratio; RR = relative risk or risk ratio.

      b. Magnitude of risk

Table 2. Magnitude of Risk Associated With OR and RR

RR	OR	Interpretation
0.75	0.75	25% reduction in the risk or odds
1.0	1.0	No difference in risk or odds
1.5	1.5	50% increase in the risk or odds
3.0	3.0	3-fold (or 200%) increase in the risk or odds

OR = odds ratio; RR = relative risk or risk ratio.

6. Calculating RR, OR, and contingency tables

Table 3. Contingency Table for Estimating RR and OR

		Disease?	
		Yes	No
Exposure?	Yes	*A*	*B*
	No	*C*	*D*

a. $RR = \dfrac{A/(A+B)}{C/(C+D)}$

b. $OR = \dfrac{\dfrac{A}{C}}{\dfrac{B}{D}}$ or $= (A \times D)/(B \times C)$

7. Example: From Kernan WN, et al. N Engl J Med 2000;343:1826-32: PPA study

Table 4. Contingency Table From "Phenylpropanolamine (PPA) and the Risk of Hemorrhagic Stroke"

		Disease? Hemorrhagic stroke in women	
		Yes	No
Exposure? Appetite suppression use	Yes	6	377
	No	1	749

a. OR = (6/1)/(377/749) = 12.
b. Data from the PPA study above related to appetite suppressant and development of hemorrhagic stroke

Table 5. Use of PPA and Appetite Suppressants and the Risk of Developing Hemorrhagic Stroke

	Cases (with hemorrhagic stroke) n=383	**Controls** (without hemorrhagic stroke) n=750	**Adjusted OR** (95% CI)
Appetite suppressant: Women	6	1	16.6 (1.51–182)
Appetite suppressant: Men	0	0	—
Appetite suppressant: Either	6	1	15.9 (1.38–184)
PPA: Women	21	20	1.98 (1.00–3.90)
PPA: Men	6	13	0.62 (0.20–1.92)
PPA: Either	27	33	1.49 (0.84–2.64)

CI = confidence interval; OR = odds ratio; PPA = phenylpropanolamine.

      c. What do these numbers mean?

      d. Can you interpret the point estimate and 95% CI in all cases?

         i. What does the point estimate mean?

         ii. What does the CI mean?

         iii. Which ones are statistically significant?

8. Presenting or evaluating data related to interpreting magnitude of risk

      a. Example: Four new drugs have been compared with placebo to determine their ability to prevent a first myocardial infarction (MI) in men with high low-density lipoprotein cholesterol (LDL-C).

      b. After a median follow-up of 5 years, the following was observed:

         i. Drug A reduced the rate of first MI by 30%.

         ii. Drug B resulted in an absolute reduction in deaths of 2.4%.

         iii. Drug C showed that 42 men are needed to undergo treatment to prevent a single first MI.

         iv. Drug D reduced first MI from 7.9% of patients (placebo group) to 5.5% of patients (drug D group) at 5 years.

      c. Which one of the above provides the most appropriate description of the effect?

D. Causation

    1. Remember: In general, we do not prove or show causality with observational studies, but there is some general guidance to consider when evaluating them. It is important to recognize that, in many situations, the conduct of studies to establish causality is not possible, practical, or ethical.

    2. Types of causality

      a. Sufficient cause

      b. Necessary cause

      c. Risk factor

    3. Questions used to evaluate causality

      a. Was statistical significance observed?

      b. What was the strength of the association, as measured by the OR or the RR?

      c. Were dose-response relationships evaluated?

      d. Was there a temporal relationship between exposure and disease or outcome?

      e. Have the results been consistently shown?

      f. Is there biologic plausibility to the association?

      g. Is there any experimental (e.g., animal, in vitro) evidence?

VI. RANDOMIZED CONTROLLED TRIAL DESIGN

A. Characteristics

    1. Type of study can be experimental or interventional. The investigator makes intervention and evaluates cause and effect. Can examine etiology, cause, efficacy, and so forth, using comparative groups.

    2. Some previous background information or studies should exist to suggest that the intervention will probably be beneficial.

    3. Design allows assessment of causality.

      a. Sufficient cause

      b. Necessary cause

      c. Risk factor

    4. Minimizes bias through randomization or stratification

      a. Randomization

      b. Block randomization

     c. Stratification

     d. Cluster randomization

5. Treatment controls

     a. Placebo control

     b. Active control

     c. Historical control

6. Blinding methods

     a. Single-blind: Either subjects or investigators are unaware of subject assignment to active or control.

     b. Double-blind: Both subjects and investigators are unaware of subject assignment to active or control.

     c. Triple-blind: Both subjects and investigators are unaware of subject assignment to active or control; in addition, an analysis group is also unaware.

     d. Double-dummy: Two placebos necessary to match active and control therapies

     e. Open label

7. May use parallel or crossover design (see additional information below)

     a. Crossover provides practical and statistical efficiency.

     b. Crossover is not appropriate for certain types of treatment questions. Effect of treatment on a disease that worsens quickly over time or worsens during the study period

8. Factorial design: Designed to answer two separate research questions in a single group of subjects

9. Examples:

     a. Clinical trial: Comparison of two drugs, comparison of two behavioral modifications

     b. Educational intervention: Online course versus lecture class format

     c. Health care intervention: Pharmacist-based health care team versus non–pharmacist-based health care team

B. Randomized Controlled Trial: Parallel Design

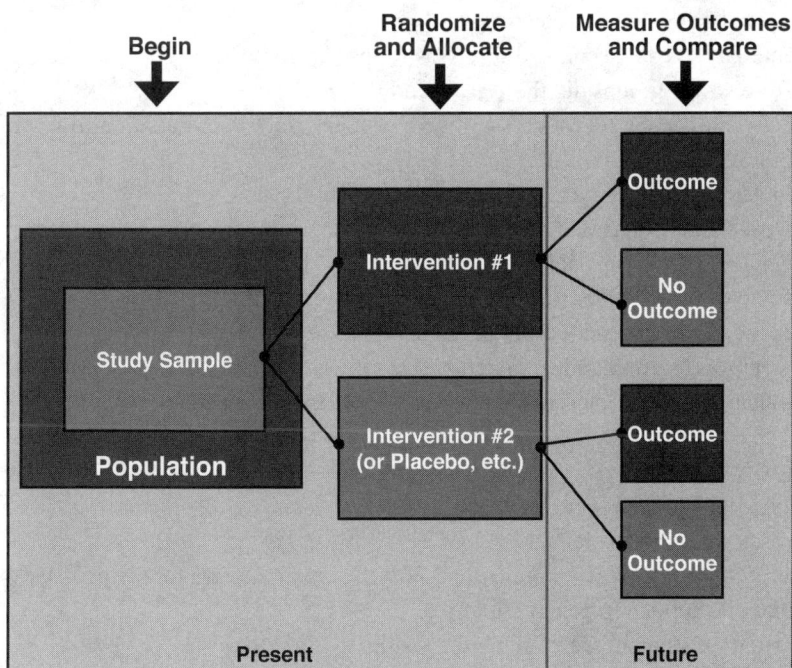

Figure 5. Randomized controlled trial: Parallel design.

C. Randomized Controlled Trial: Crossover Design

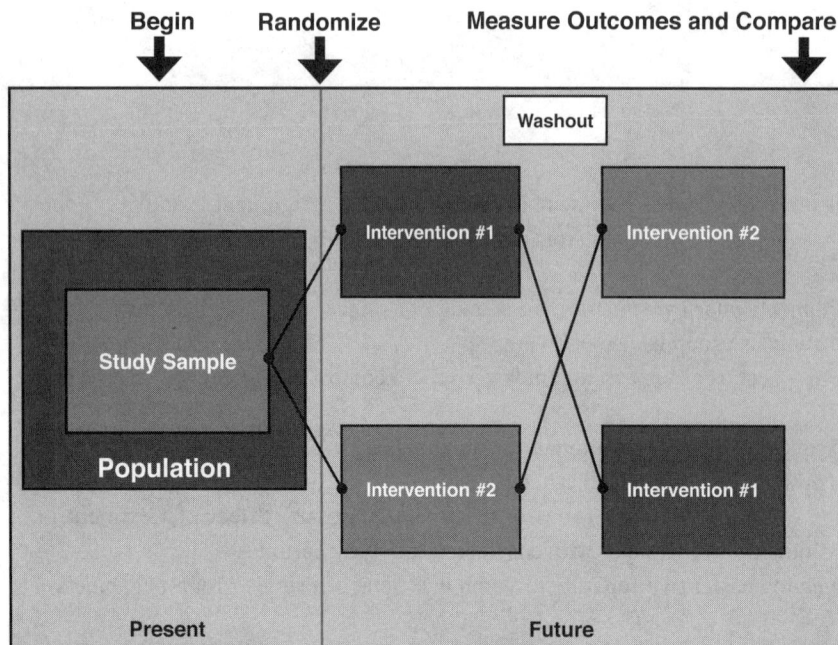

Figure 6. Randomized controlled trial: Crossover design.

D. Examples of Considerations for Controlled Trials
   1. Are the results of the study valid?
      a. Were the subjects randomly assigned, and what was the randomization technique? Did the randomization process result in equal baseline characteristics?
      b. Were all subjects who entered the trial accounted for? Was follow-up complete? If not, how many were lost to follow-up, from which groups did they leave, and why?
      c. Were subjects analyzed in the groups to which they were randomized? Was intention-to-treat, per-protocol, or actual treatment analysis used?
      d. How was blinding conducted (e.g., subject, investigator), if applicable?
      e. Were the inclusion and exclusion criteria appropriate, or were they too restrictive or inclusive? Were the groups similar at the start of the trial?
      f. Was the sample size sufficient, and was a power calculation included?
      g. Were the groups handled the same way, aside from the interventions?
      h. Were the statistical tests appropriate and understandable?
      i. What was assessed: Surrogate markers or true outcomes? Were a priori subgroup analyses performed?
   2. What were the results?
      a. How large was the treatment effect?
      b. How precise was the effect (how precise were the CIs)?
      c. Did the authors properly interpret the results?
   3. Can I apply the results of this study to my patient population? Will they help me care for my patients?
      a. Can the results of this study be applied to general practice?
      b. Was a representative population studied? Can I apply the results to my setting?
      c. Do the patients I care for fill the enrollment criteria for this study?
      d. Do the patients I care for fill the subgroup criteria evaluated?
      e. Do the expected benefits outweigh the expected or unanticipated risks?

VII. OTHER ISSUES TO CONSIDER IN CONTROLLED TRIALS

A. Subgroup Analysis
   1. Important part of controlled clinical trials (if set a priori)
   2. Many times, they are overused and overinterpreted, leading to unnecessary research, misinterpretation of results, or suboptimal patient care.
   3. Many potential pitfalls in identifying and interpreting
      a. Failure to consider several comparisons or to adjust p-values
      b. Problems with sample size (power), classification, and lack of assessment of interaction

B. Composite End Points
   1. The primary end point is one of the most important decisions to make in the design of a clinical study.
   2. A composite end point combines several end points.
      a. For example, cardiovascular death, nonfatal MI, and cardiac arrest with resuscitation
      b. Usually combines measures of morbidity and mortality
      c. What does the following statement mean? Our findings show that ramipril reduces the rates of death, MI, stroke, revascularization, cardiac arrest, heart failure, complications related to diabetes, and new cases of diabetes in a broad spectrum of high-risk patients. Treating 1000 patients with ramipril for 4 years prevents about 150 events in about 70 patients.
         i. Was there a reduction in all the end points or just in some?
         ii. Are all the outcomes just as likely to occur?
         iii. Why would the investigators of this trial have been interested in all these outcomes?
   3. What are the positives for using composite end points?
      a. No single primary outcome
      b. Alleviates problems of multiple testing
      c. Increases number of events, which decreases sample size and cost
   4. What are the problems?
      a. Difficulties in interpreting composite end points; consider our earlier example
      b. Misattribution of statistically beneficial effects of composite measure to each of its component end points
      c. Dilution of effects: Negative results for common component of composite end point hide real differences in other end points. Undue influence exerted on composite end point by "softer" component end points
      d. Averaging of overall effect, problems when component end points move in opposite directions
      e. Should all end points be weighed the same, or should death weigh more?
   5. The results for each end point should be reported together with the results for the composite.

C. Surrogate End Points
   1. Parameters thought to be associated with clinical outcomes
      a. Blood pressure and stroke prevention
      b. LDL-C reduction and cardiovascular death reduction
         i. Statins: Yes
         ii. Hormone replacement therapy: No
      c. Premature ventricular contraction suppression and reduced mortality
   2. Surrogate outcomes do not always predict clinical outcomes.
   3. Short-duration studies that evaluate surrogate end points may not be large enough to detect uncommon adverse events.

D. Superiority Versus Equivalence Versus Noninferiority
1. A superiority trial is designed to detect a difference between experimental treatments. This is the typical design in a clinical trial.
2. An equivalence trial is designed to confirm the absence of meaningful differences between treatments. The key is the definition of the specified margin. What difference is important? One example is a bioequivalence trial.
3. A noninferiority trial is designed to investigate whether a treatment is not clinically worse (no less effective, or inferior) than an existing treatment. The noninferiority difference or point drives the design of the study and must be evaluated for appropriateness.
    a. It may be the most effective, or it may have a similar effect.
    b. Useful when placebo administration is not possible for ethical reasons
    c. ONTARGET (The Ongoing Telmisartan Alone and in Combination With Ramipril Global Endpoint Trial)
        i. Designed to evaluate telmisartan, ramipril, or the combination of them in patients with a high risk of vascular disease
        ii. Objective was to determine whether telmisartan was noninferior to ramipril in the incidence of cardiovascular deaths.
        iii. Noninferior difference was defined as 13% or less.
    d. Essentials of noninferiority design
        i. Control group must be effective.
        ii. Current study similar to previous study with control and with equal doses, clinical conditions, and design used.
        iii. Adequate power is essential, and usually larger sample sizes are necessary.

VIII. CONTROLLED CLINICAL TRIALS: ANALYSIS

A. Controlled Clinical Trial: Application (Hulley S, et al. JAMA 1998;280:605-13)
1. Randomized trial of estrogen plus progestin for secondary prevention of coronary heart disease (CHD) in postmenopausal women
2. Objective: To determine whether estrogen plus progestin therapy alters the risk of CHD in postmenopausal women with established CHD
3. Randomized blinded placebo controlled
    a. Two treatment arms: ERT-P (conjugated equine estrogen 0.625 mg/day plus medroxyprogesterone acetate 2.5 mg/day) and placebo; n=2763 with coronary artery disease younger than 80 years; mean age = 66.7 years.
    b. Follow-up averaged 4.1 years; 82% of hormone replacement therapy patients still taking at the end of 1 year; 75% at the end of 3 years
4. End points
    a. Primary: Nonfatal MI, CHD death
    b. Secondary: Many, including all-cause mortality. Are these composite outcomes appropriate?
5. Statistical analysis
    a. Baseline characteristics: t-test and chi-square: Is comparing baseline characteristics necessary in this type of trial?
    b. Power analysis and sample size calculation
    c. Kaplan-Meier with Cox proportional hazards model, intention to treat
6. Surrogate end point: LDL-C lowered
7. Results (Table 6)

Table 6. Death and Secondary End Points by Treatment Group

	ERT-P	Placebo	HR (95% CI)
Primary CHD events	12.4	12.7	0.99 (0.80–1.22)
CHD death	5.1	4.2	1.24 (0.81–1.75)
Any thromboembolic event	2.5	0.9	2.89 (1.50–5.58)
Gallbladder disease	6.1	4.5	1.38 (1.00–1.92)

CHD = coronary heart disease; CI = confidence interval; ERT-P = conjugated equine estrogen 0.625 mg/day plus medroxyprogesterone acetate 2.5 mg/day; HR = hazard ratio.

8. Significant time trend: More CHD events in the treatment group than in placebo in year 1 and fewer in years 4 and 5

9. Conclusions

B. Questions to Consider in Evaluating and Interpreting a Clinical Trial
1. Study design
   a. Was the studied sample representative of the population or the individual to whom the results were being applied?
   b. Were the inclusion and exclusion criteria appropriate, or were they overly restrictive or inclusive?
   c. Sufficient sample size, power, and so forth? Was a power analysis included?
   d. Was a study objective or hypothesis provided?
   e. Was the study blinded and to whom? (Subject, investigator, study personnel, or all?)
   f. Was a run-in phase included? If so, why? Did it affect the interpretation of the trial?
   g. What type of randomization method was performed? Did the randomization process produce equal baseline characteristics between all groups?
2. Outcomes/assessments
   a. Were the primary and/or secondary outcomes identified, were they reasonable, and did they apply to clinical practice?
   b. Was a composite outcome employed, and were all the individual components identified and clearly stated in the methods and results?
   c. Were surrogate markers employed instead of (or in addition to) clinically relevant outcomes?
3. Analysis
   a. What analysis technique was used: Intention-to-treat, actual treatment, or per-protocol?
   b. Were the statistical tests appropriate?
4. Interpretation: Was the author's interpretation appropriate and within the confines of the study design?
5. Extrapolation
   a. Are you applying the results to similar patients in a similar setting?
   b. Are there possible additional adverse effects that were not measured in this study?

IX. COMMON APPROACHES TO ANALYZING CLINICAL TRIALS

A. Intention-to-Treat Analysis
   1. Compares outcomes on the basis of initial group assignment or as randomized. The allocation to groups was how they were intended to be treated, even though they may not have taken the medication for the duration of the study, they dropped out, and so forth.
   2. Determines effect of treatment under usual conditions of use. Analogous to routine clinical practice in which a patient receives a prescription but may not adhere to the drug

3. Gives a conservative estimate of differences in treatments; may underestimate treatment benefits
4. Most common approach to assessing clinical trial results

B. Per-Protocol Analysis
   1. Subjects who do not adhere to allocated treatment are not included in the final analysis; only those who completed the trial and adhered to the protocol (based on some predetermined definition [e.g., 80% adherence])
   2. Provides additional information about treatment effectiveness and provides more generous estimates of differences between treatments
   3. Subject to several problems because of factors such as lower sample size and definitions of adherence. Results are more difficult to interpret.

C. As-Treated Analysis
   1. Subjects are analyzed by the actual intervention received. If subjects were in the active treatment group but did not take active treatment, the data would be analyzed as if they were in the placebo group.
   2. This analysis essentially ignores the randomization process for those who did not adhere to the study design.

X. SYSTEMATIC REVIEW AND META-ANALYSIS

A. Introduction
   1. Dramatic increase in the number of these types of papers
   2. First meta-analysis probably published in 1904: Assessment of typhoid vaccine effectiveness

B. Systematic Review
   1. Summary that uses explicit methods to perform a comprehensive literature search, critically appraise it, and synthesize the world literature on a specific topic. Instead of the subjects being human subjects, the individual studies are the "study subjects" (i.e., the subjects are studies).
   2. Differs from a standard literature review: The study results are more comprehensively synthesized and reviewed.
   3. As with a controlled clinical trial (or other studies), the key is a well-documented and well-described systematic review.
   4. Some systematic reviews will attempt to statistically combine results from many studies.
   5. Differs from other reviews, which combine evaluation with opinions

C. Meta-analysis
   1. Systematic review that uses mathematical and statistical techniques to summarize the results of the evaluated studies
   2. These techniques may improve on:
      a. Calculation of effect size
      b. Increase in statistical power
      c. Interpretation of disparate results
      d. Reduction in bias
      e. Answers to questions that may not be addressable with individual studies
   3. Issues related to meta-analysis
   4. Reliant on criteria for inclusion of previous studies and statistical methods to ensure validity. Details of included studies are essential.

5. Elements of trial methods
    a. Research question
    b. Identification of available studies
    c. Criteria for trial inclusion and exclusion
    d. Data collection and presentation of findings
    e. Calculation of summary estimate: Ideally with Forest plot (Figure 7)
    f. Assessment of heterogeneity
        i. Statistical heterogeneity
        ii. Chi-square and Cochran Q are common tests for heterogeneity.
    g. Assessment of publication bias: funnel plot
    h. Sensitivity analysis

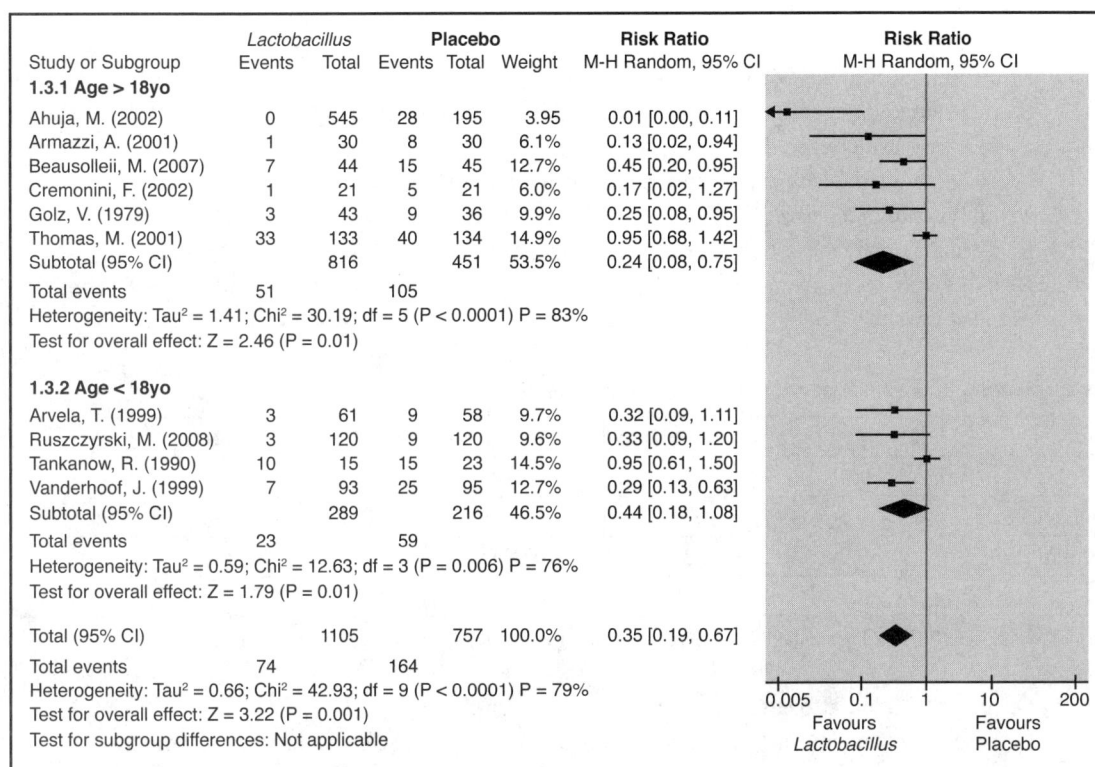

Figure 7. Forest plots (Pharmacotherapy 2010;30:119-26).

D. Meta-analysis: Application (Koshman SL, et al. Pharmacist care of patients with heart failure. A systematic review of randomized trials. *Arch Intern Med* 2008;168;687-94)

XI. SUMMARY MEASURES OF EFFECT

A. Absolute and Relative Differences
    1. Absolute differences or absolute changes
    2. Relative differences or relative changes
    3. Absolute differences are more important than relative differences, although the authors of many clinical studies highlight the differences observed in their trials with relative differences because they are larger. Why? Larger numbers are more convincing to practitioners and patients. Most drug advertisements (both directly to patients and to health care professionals) quote relative differences.

B. Number Needed to Treat
1. Characteristics
a. Another means to characterize changes or differences in absolute risk
b. Definition: The reciprocal of the absolute risk reduction (ARR)
i. NNT = 1/(ARR).
ii. Rounded to the next highest whole number is the most conservative approach.
c. Applied to clinical outcomes with dichotomous data (e.g., yes/no, alive/dead, MI/no MI)
d. Cautions: Assumes the baseline risk is the same for all patients (or that it is unrelated to RR)
e. Extrapolation beyond studied time points
f. NNTs should be provided only for significant effects because it is difficult to interpret the CIs for nonsignificant results.
g. Number needed to harm
2. NNT application
a. HOPE study (N Engl J Med 2000;342:145-53)
b. Study evaluated the effect of ramipril on cardiovascular events in high-risk patients.
c. Prospective randomized double-blind study
i. 9297 high-risk patients received ramipril or matching placebo once daily for an average follow-up of 5 years.
ii. Primary outcome: Composite of MI, stroke, or death from cardiovascular causes
d. Results (data taken from above-referenced paper). NNTs = 1/(0.178 − 0.140) = 1/0.038 = 26.3, rounded up to 27.

Table 7. Risk of Primary and Secondary End Points by Treatment Group

Outcome	Ramipril (%)	Placebo (%)	Relative Risk	RRR	ARR	NNT
Combined	14.0	17.8	0.79	0.21	0.038	27
Death from CV causes	6.1	8.1	0.74	0.25	0.02	50
Myocardial infarction	9.9	12.3	0.80	0.20	0.024	42
Stroke	3.4	4.9	0.68	0.31	0.015	67

ARR = absolute risk reduction; CV = cardiovascular; NNT = number needed to treat; RRR = relative risk reduction.

e. Online calculator: http://araw.mede.uic.edu/cgi-bin/nntcalc.pl
f. OR to NNT calculator: http://ktclearinghouse.ca/cebm/practise/ca/calculators/ortonnt

XII. REPORTING GUIDELINES FOR CLINICAL STUDIES

A. The Consolidated Standards of Reporting Trials (CONSORT)
1. Initially published in 1996 and updated several times since, most recently in 2010
2. Created in an effort to improve, standardize, and increase the transparency of the reporting of clinical trials and to facilitate the improvement of literature evaluation
3. Available at www.consort-statement.org/
4. The CONSORT statement has been endorsed by numerous publications and published in these journals.
5. The CONSORT statement
a. The checklist: 25-item checklist pertaining to the content of the following
i. Title
ii. Abstract
iii. Introduction
iv. Methods

    v. Results

    vi. Discussion

    vii. Other information

   b. The flow diagram: Intended to depict the passage of study participants through the randomized controlled trial

  6. Extensions of the CONSORT statement

   a. Design extensions

    i. Cluster trials

    ii. Noninferiority and equivalence trials

    iii. Pragmatic trials

   b. Intervention extension

    i. Herbal medicinal interventions

    ii. Nonpharmacologic interventions

    iii. Acupuncture interventions

   c. Data extensions

    i. Patient-reported outcomes

    ii. Harms

    iii. Abstracts

B. Strengthening the Reporting of Observational Studies in Epidemiology (STROBE) Statement

 1. Initially published in 2007

 2. "An international, collaborative initiative of epidemiologists, methodologists, statisticians, researchers and journal editors involved in the conduct and dissemination of observational studies"

 3. Available at www.strobe-statement.org

 4. Endorsed by numerous publications and published in these journals

 5. The STROBE checklist: 22-item checklist, same basic concepts as the CONSORT checklist, with alterations germane to observational trials

C. Preferred Reporting Items for Systematic Reviews and Meta-Analyses (PRISMA)

 1. Established in 1996 (as QUOROM), renamed in 2009

 2. Evidence-based minimum set of items for reporting systematic reviews and meta-analyses

 3. Available at www.prisma-statement.org/

  a. The PRISMA checklist: 27-item checklist with alterations germane to systematic reviews and meta-analyses

  b. The PRISMA flow diagram: Four-stage diagram, depicting the flow of information through the systematic review

  c. The PRISMA explanation and elaboration document: Intended to enhance the use and understanding of the PRISMA statement

D. Enhancing the Quality and Transparency of Health Research (EQUATOR) Network

 1. International initiative to improve the reliability and value of medical research literature by promoting transparent and accurate reporting of research studies

 2. Does not have its own statements but promotes the use of key reporting guidelines

 3. Many other statements about study types not addressed in the discussion related to CONSORT, STROBE, and PRISMA are listed on the EQUATOR network Web site (www.equator-network.org).

XIII. PHARMACOECONOMIC STUDIES

A. Cost Minimization Analysis
   1. Outcome: Equal, only cost is addressed
   2. Determines the lest expensive alternative

B. Cost-benefit Analysis
   1. Outcome: Monetary; is a treatment worth the cost?
   2. Determines the greatest net benefit alternative

C. Cost-effectiveness Analysis
   1. Clinical units
   2. Determines the most cost-effective alternative

D. Cost-utility Analysis
   1. Utility
   2. Determines the greatest benefit alternative

XIV. SENSITIVITY, SPECIFICITY, AND PREDICTIVE VALUES

A. Sensitivity: Proportion of True Positives That Are Correctly Identified by a Test

B. Specificity: Proportion of True Negatives That Are Correctly Identified by a Test

C. Positive Predictive Value: Proportion of Patients With a Positive Test Who Are Given a Correct Diagnosis

D. Negative Predictive Value: Proportion of Patients With a Negative Test Who Are Given a Correct Diagnosis

E. Example: Relationship Between Test and Correct Diagnosis Identified by Disease (data from J Nucl Med 1972;13:908-15)

Table 8. Relationship Between Test and Correct Diagnosis Identified by Disease

Test	Disease		
	Positive Disease	Negative Disease	Total
Positive	231 (true positive)	32 (false positive)	263
Negative	27 (false negative)	54 (true negative)	81
Total	258	86	344

REFERENCES

1. Altman DG, Bland JM. Diagnostic tests 1: sensitivity and specificity. BMJ 1994;308:1552.

2. Altman DG, Bland JM. Diagnostic tests 2: predictive values. BMJ 1994;309:102.

3. Clancy MJ. Overview of research designs. Emerg Med J 2002;19:546-9.

4. Dasgupta A, Lawson KA, Wilson JP. Evaluating equivalence and noninferiority trials. Am J Health Syst Pharm 2010;67:1337-43.

5. DiCenzo R, ed. Clinical Pharmacist's Guide to Biostatistics and Literature Evaluation. Lenexa, KS: ACCP, 2010.

6. DiPietro NA. Methods in epidemiology: observational study designs. Pharmacotherapy 2010;30:973-84.

7. Koretz RL. Methods of meta-analysis: an analysis. Curr Opin Clin Nutr Metab Care 2002;5:467-74.

8. Lagakos SW. The challenge of subgroup analyses: reporting without distorting. N Engl J Med 2006;354:1667-9.

9. Lesaffre E. Superiority, equivalence and noninferiority trials. Bull Hosp Jt Dis 2008;66:150-4.

10. Mann CJ. Observational research methods. Research design II: cohort, cross sectional and case-control studies. Emerg Med J 2003;20:54-60.

11. Moher D, Liberati A, Tetzlaff J, et al.; The PRISMA Group. Preferred reporting items for systematic reviews and meta-analyses: the PRISMA statement. Ann Intern Med 2009;151:264-9.

12. Neely JG, Magit AE, Rich JT, et al. A practical guide to understanding systematic reviews and meta-analysis. Otolaryngol Head Neck Surg 2010;142:6-14.

13. Quilliam BJ, Barbour MM. Evaluating drug-induced cardiovascular disease: a pharmacoepidemiologic perspective. In: Richardson MM, Chant C, Cheng JWM, et al., eds. Pharmacotherapy Self-Assessment Program, 7th ed. Lenexa, KS: ACCP, 2010:225-39.

14. Reporting of noninferiority and equivalence randomized trials, an extension of the CONSORT statement. JAMA 2006;295:1152-60.

15. Schulz KF, Altman DG, Moher D; CONSORT Group. CONSORT 2010 statement: updated guidelines for reporting parallel group randomized trials. Ann Intern Med 2010;152:726-32.

16. Shermock KM. Secondary data analysis/observational research. In: Dunsworth TS, Richardson MM, Chant C, et al., eds. Pharmacotherapy Self-Assessment Program, 5th ed. Kansas City, MO: ACCP, 2005:43-63.

17. Shields KM, DiPietro NA, Kier KL. Principles of drug literature evaluation for observational study designs. Pharmacotherapy 2011;31:115-27.

18. Smith GH, Mays DA. Clinical study design and literature evaluation. In: Zarowitz B, Shumock G, Dunsworth T, et al., eds. Pharmacotherapy Self-Assessment Program, 4th ed. Kansas City, MO: ACCP, 2002:203-31.

19. Strassels SA, Wilson JP. Pharmacoepidemiology. In: Dunsworth TS, Richardson MM, Chant C, et al., eds. Pharmacotherapy Self-Assessment Program, 6th ed. Lenexa, KS: ACCP, 2007:17-31.

20. Tomlinson G, Detsky AS. Composite endpoints in randomized trials: there is no free lunch. JAMA 2010;303:267-8.

21. Tsuyuki RT, Garg S. Interpreting data in cardiovascular disease clinical trials: a biostatistical toolbox. In: Richardson MM, Chant C, Cheng JWM, et al., eds. Pharmacotherapy Self-Assessment Program, 7th ed. Lenexa, KS: ACCP, 2010:241-55.

22. von Elm E, Altman DG, Egger M, et al. The Strengthening the Reporting of Observational Studies in Epidemiology (STROBE) statement: guidelines for reporting observational studies. Ann Intern Med 2007;147:573-7.

23. Windish DM, Huot SJ, Green ML. Medicine resident's understanding of the biostatistics and results in the medical literature. JAMA 2007;298:1010-22.

ANSWERS AND EXPLANATIONS TO SELF-ASSESSMENT QUESTIONS

1. Answer: B

Recall bias is always a potential concern for case-control studies because of the amount of time that passes between the study and the treatment. Because risk factors were not included in the study design, this is of concern (Answer B is correct). Although a study may be susceptible to many types of bias, the other choices would not pose as much risk (if any) compared with recall bias.

2. Answer: B

Internal validity is greatly jeopardized because the study is not designed to protect against this possible bias. In a sense, this design flaw jeopardizes external validity (how well does a study apply to other patients with this condition or disease?), but a lack of internal validity is most affected (Answer B is correct). The other answers can be adequately controlled for in the design and conduct of the study.

3. Answer: B

Intention-to-treat analysis generally considers the approach, which gives the best estimate of use effectiveness (use under typical clinical trial conditions), whereas per-protocol analysis gives a better estimate of method effectiveness (use under ideal conditions) (Answer B is correct and Answer C is incorrect). Intention-to-treat analysis is the most common approach to data analysis for randomized controlled trials and may underestimate the treatment effect (Answer D is incorrect). A per-protocol analysis discards data from patients who do not adhere to the treatment to which they were initially randomized; therefore, it is susceptible to a loss of power to detect differences between groups (Answer A is incorrect). This loss of power occurs as patients are removed from the analysis completely because of non-adherence, which decreases the sample size of the study and thus the power to detect differences.

4. Answer: B

The CI of the difference in recurrence rate between the two groups includes zero; thus, there is no statistically significant difference between the two groups (Answer B is correct). Answer A is incorrect because the 95% CI contains zero and therefore is not statistically significant. Answer C is incorrect because twice-daily

therapy did not have fewer recurrences. Because of the lack of statistical significance, it is unreasonable to conclude that twice-daily therapy would be more appropriate in this or any other patient population. Answer D is incorrect because all the above information can be determined without the benefit of reported p-values.

5. Answer: D

Answer A and Answer B are incorrect calculations. Calculating the NNT to prevent one recurrence using twice-daily therapy is as follows: $0.044 - 0.029 = 0.015$, and $1/0.015 = 66.7$, rounded to 67; however, the NNT should not be calculated when the end point of interest is nonsignificant (Answer C is incorrect; Answer D is correct).

6. Answer: C

Answer A and Answer B are incorrect because the margarine with ALA did not significantly reduce the risk of cardiovascular events (the 95% CI includes 1 [no difference in risk]). Answer D is incorrect because the p-value is not necessary for interpreting statistical significance when the 95% CI is provided. Answer C is correct because the p-value corresponds to the 95% CI.

7. Answer: A

Clinical trials are usually adequately powered to compare primary end points (Answer A is correct). Because Answer B is part of the composite outcomes, the study was probably not powered to detect this outcome independently. Similarly, even though the subgroup analysis was determined a priori, the study is not typically designed to have sufficient power to make this comparison (Answer C and Answer D are incorrect).

8. Answer: D

Answer A and Answer B are incorrect because each implies that one drug is more effective than the other. In this type of study design, neither drug is more or less effective. Answer C is incorrect because the CI of the OR does not include 1; thus, the finding is statistically significant at the 5% level, making Answer D correct.

Neurology

Melody Ryan, Pharm.D., MPH, BCPS

University of Kentucky
Lexington, Kentucky

NEUROLOGY

MELODY RYAN, PHARM.D., MPH, BCPS

UNIVERSITY OF KENTUCKY
LEXINGTON, KENTUCKY

Learning Objectives

1. Differentiate between various seizure medications on the basis of use and adverse effects.
2. Develop a treatment strategy for status epilepticus.
3. Identify appropriate treatment strategies for primary and secondary stroke prevention.
4. Determine the appropriateness of treatment with tissue plasminogen activator for acute stroke.
5. Examine common adverse effects associated with the treatment of Parkinson disease.
6. Differentiate between regimens for acute and prophylactic treatment of migraine, tension, and cluster headaches.
7. Identify common adverse effects of disease-modifying therapies for multiple sclerosis.

Self-Assessment Questions

Answers and explanations to these questions can be found at the end of this chapter.

1. T.L. is a 35-year-old man with complex partial seizures. He is otherwise healthy. He was placed on phenytoin after a seizure about 2 months ago. He currently takes phenytoin 100 mg 3 capsules orally every night. During his clinic visit, he tells you he has had no seizures, and he has no signs of toxicity. He is allergic to sulfa drugs. His phenytoin serum concentration is 17.7 mcg/mL. Which is the best interpretation of this concentration?

    A. It is too low.

    B. It is too high.

    C. It is just right.

    D. A serum albumin concentration is necessary to interpret this concentration.

2. B.V. is a 28-year-old woman brought to your emergency department for treatment of status epilepticus. She receives lorazepam 4 mg intravenously with subsequent seizure cessation. Which medication is the best next treatment step for B.V.?

    A. Topiramate.

    B. Phenytoin.

    C. Zonisamide.

    D. Diazepam.

3. J.H. is a 42-year-old man with complex partial seizures for which he was prescribed topiramate. He has been increasing the topiramate dose every other day according to instructions from his primary care provider. He comes to the pharmacy where you work but seems a little confused and has difficulty finding the words to have a conversation with you. Which is the best assessment of J.H.'s condition?

    A. Discontinue topiramate; he is having an allergic reaction.

    B. Increase the topiramate dose; he is having partial seizures.

    C. Slow the rate of topiramate titration; he is having psychomotor slowing.

    D. Get a topiramate serum concentration; he is probably supratherapeutic.

Questions 4 and 5 pertain to the following case:
R.H. is a 59-year-old man who presents to the emergency department for new-onset left-sided weakness that began 6 hours ago. He has a history of hypertension and coronary artery disease. His medication list includes atenolol 50 mg/day orally, hydrochlorothiazide 25 mg/day orally, and aspirin 325 mg/day orally. His vital signs include blood pressure (BP) 160/92 mm Hg, heart rate 92 beats/minute, respiratory rate 14 breaths/minute, and temperature 38°C. The treatment team assesses this patient for treatment with tissue plasminogen activator and asks for your opinion.

4. Which reply is best, given this information?

    A. R.H. should be treated with tissue plasminogen activator.

    B. R.H. should not be treated with tissue plasminogen activator because the onset of his stroke symptoms was 6 hours ago.

    C. R.H. should not be treated with tissue plasminogen activator because he has hypertension.

    D. R.H. should not be treated with tissue plasminogen activator because he takes aspirin.

5. R.H. survives his stroke. As part of his discharge treatment plan, you evaluate his risk factors for a second stroke. His aspirin therapy is discontinued. Which medication for secondary stroke prevention is best to initiate at this time?

   A. Dipyridamole.

   B. Enoxaparin.

   C. Heparin.

   D. Clopidogrel.

Questions 6 and 7 pertain to the following case:
C.P. is a 69-year-old man given a diagnosis of Parkinson disease 7 years ago. He states that he is most bothered by his bradykinesia symptoms. On examination, he also has a pronounced tremor, postural instability, and masked facial expression. He currently takes carbidopa/levodopa/entacapone 25 mg/100 mg/200 mg orally four times daily, ropinirole 1 mg orally three times daily, and selegiline 5 mg orally twice daily. He has no drug allergies. He also describes a worsening of his Parkinson disease symptoms, which fluctuate randomly during the day. He has developed a charting system for his symptoms during the day, and no relationship seems to exist with the time he is scheduled to take his carbidopa/levodopa/entacapone doses.

6. Which condition best describes C.P.'s fluctuating Parkinson disease symptoms?

   A. Wearing off.

   B. On-off.

   C. Dyskinesia.

   D. Dystonia.

7. For his symptoms, C.P. is given a prescription for apomorphine. Which statement about this drug is most accurate?

   A. He must be trained on self-injection techniques with saline, but he can administer his first dose of apomorphine at home when he needs it.

   B. He should not take apomorphine if he is allergic to penicillin.

   C. If he does not take a dose for more than 1 week, he should begin with a loading dose with his next injection.

   D. It may cause severe nausea and vomiting.

8. W.S. is a 57-year-old man initiated on rasagiline for treatment of his newly diagnosed Parkinson disease. He develops a cough, body aches, and nasal congestion. Which medication is best to treat W.S.'s symptoms?

   A. Guaifenesin.

   B. Dextromethorphan.

   C. Tramadol.

   D. Pseudoephedrine.

Questions 9 and 10 pertain to the following case:
R.M. is a 47-year-old woman with long-standing migraine headaches. Her headache pain is easily relieved with sumatriptan 100 mg orally as the occasion requires. However, with her last dose she experienced substernal chest pain radiating to her left arm. She reported to her local emergency department, where she had a complete workup. Her final diagnoses were coronary artery disease and hypertension. For these conditions, she was placed on hydrochlorothiazide 25 mg orally every morning.

9. Which drug is best for R.M. to use for her migraine headaches?

   A. Frovatriptan.

   B. Zolmitriptan.

   C. Dihydroergotamine.

   D. Naproxen.

10. If R.M. requires a drug for migraine prophylaxis, which agent is best to recommend?

    A. Propranolol.

    B. Valproic acid.

    C. Amitriptyline.

    D. Gabapentin.

Questions 11–13 pertain to the following case:
L.M. is a 43-year-old man who received a diagnosis of progressive-relapsing multiple sclerosis 2 years ago. He has been taking glatiramer acetate since then. However, no discernible difference exists in the number of exacerbations he has experienced. He has spasticity in his legs, which has caused several falls during the past month, and he experiences fatigue that worsens as the day progresses.

11. Which drug therapy is best for L.M.'s multiple sclerosis?

    A. Cyclophosphamide.

    B. Methylprednisolone.

    C. Azathioprine.

    D. Fingolimod.

12. Which drug is best to treat L.M.'s spasticity?

    A. Diazepam.

    B. Baclofen.

    C. Carisoprodol.

    D. Metaxalone.

13. Which drug is best to treat L.M.'s fatigue?

    A. Propranolol.

    B. Lamotrigine.

    C. Amantadine.

    D. Ropinirole.

I. EPILEPSY

A. Epidemiology
   1. Ten percent of the population will have a seizure.
   2. About 50 million people worldwide have epilepsy.
   3. About 50% of patients with a new diagnosis become seizure free on their first treatment, with up to 70% becoming seizure free after treatment adjustment.

B. Classification of Seizures: Seizures are generally classified according to the International League Against Epilepsy (ILAE) scheme, adopted in 1981, with modifications in 2001 and 2010 (Berg AT, Berkovic SF, Brodie MJ, et al. Revised terminology and concepts for organization of seizures and epilepsies: report of the ILAE Commission on Classification and Terminology, 2005-2009. Epilepsia 2010;51:676-85).
   1. Focal seizures are conceptualized as originating at some point within networks limited to one hemisphere.
      a. No specific classification within focal seizures is recommended.
      b. The terms *simple partial seizure, complex partial seizure,* and *secondarily generalized seizure* have been eliminated from classification; however, they are still used to describe seizures.
   2. Generalized seizures are conceptualized as originating at some point within and rapidly engaging bilaterally distributed neural networks.
      a. Absence: Typical absence seizures are brief and abrupt, last 10–30 seconds, and occur in clusters. Absence seizures usually result in a short loss of consciousness, or the patient may stare, be motionless, or have a distant expression on his or her face. Electroencephalograms (EEGs) performed during seizure activity usually show three Hz spike-and-wave complexes. Absence seizures can be further classified as typical, atypical, myoclonic absence, and eyelid myoclonia.
      b. Myoclonic: Consist of brief, lightning-like jerking movements of the entire body or the upper and occasionally lower extremities. Myoclonic seizures can be further classified as myoclonic, myoclonic atonic, or myoclonic tonic.
      c. Tonic-clonic: Typically, there are five phases of a primary tonic-clonic seizure: flexion, extension, tremor, clonic, and postictal. During the flexion phase, the patient's mouth may be held partly open, and the patient may experience upward eye movement, involvement of the extremities, and loss of consciousness. In the extension phase, the patient may be noted to extend his or her back and neck; experience contraction of thoracic and abdominal muscles; be apneic; and have flexion, extension, and adduction of the extremities. The patient may cry out as air is forced from the lungs in this phase. The tremor phase occurs as the patient goes from tonic rigidity to tremors and then to a clonic state. During the clonic phase, the patient will experience rhythmic jerks. The length of the entire seizure is usually 1–3 minutes. After the seizure, the patient may be postictal. During this time, the patient can be difficult to arouse or very somnolent. Before the seizure, a patient may experience a prodrome but not an aura.
      d. Clonic: Only the clonic phase of a tonic-clonic seizure; rhythmic, repetitive, jerking muscle movements
      e. Tonic: Only the flexion or extension phases of a tonic-clonic seizure
      f. Atonic: Characterized by a loss of muscle tone. Atonic seizures are often described as drop attacks, in which a patient loses tone and falls to the ground.
   3. Status epilepticus is any seizure that lasts more than 20 minutes or recurrent seizures of sufficient frequency that the patient does not regain consciousness between episodes. Mortality is up to 20% for status epilepticus.
   4. Nonepileptic seizures are paroxysmal nonepileptic episodes resembling epileptic seizures that can be organic or psychogenic.

5. Other associated symptoms
   a. Prodrome: Awareness of an impending seizure before it occurs. The prodrome may consist of headache, insomnia, irritability, or feeling of impending doom.
   b. Aura: A focal seizure, without loss of consciousness, consisting of sensory or autonomic symptoms that may precede evolution to a bilateral, convulsive seizure. Patients may experience feelings of fear, embarrassment, or déjà vu. Automatic behavior (automatism) and psychic symptoms may occur. Automatisms may include lip smacking, chewing, swallowing, abnormal tongue movements, scratching, thrashing of the arms or legs, fumbling with clothing, and snapping the fingers. Psychic symptoms include illusions, hallucinations, emotional changes, dysphasia, and cognitive problems.

C. Diagnosis
   1. Physical examination should be performed with special attention to neurologic findings. The neurologic examination may include examination of the head, vision, cranial nerves, motor function, cerebellar function, and sensory function.
   2. Laboratory tests are based on the history and physical examination results; a full diagnostic onslaught is unnecessary in many patients. Because metabolic causes of seizures are common, serum glucose, electrolytes, calcium, complete blood cell counts, and renal function tests may be necessary. A toxicology screen may also be prudent.
   3. EEGs are used to help confirm the diagnosis, classify seizures, locate the site of the seizures, and select the best seizure medication. The best time to perform an EEG is while the patient is having seizures. If it is not possible to perform the EEG during seizures, it should be performed as soon after the seizure as possible. Depending on the clinical situation, an EEG may be obtained under normal conditions, when the patient is sleep deprived, or when the patient is asleep. Patients whose seizures are difficult to diagnose or control may require prolonged closed-circuit video-EEG monitoring. Keep in mind that an interictal (when the patient is not having clinical seizures) EEG may be normal but that this does not preclude the diagnosis of epilepsy.
   4. Magnetic resonance imaging is the neuroimaging technique of choice for epilepsy. Computed tomography (CT) scanning can be useful in finding brain lesions when magnetic resonance imaging cannot be performed in a timely fashion.

D. Treatment
   1. Medications (see Tables 1–4)
      a. Benzodiazepines
         i. Mechanism of action: Augment γ-aminobutyric acid–mediated chloride influx
         ii. Tolerance may develop: Usually used as adjunctive, short-term therapy
         iii. Most commonly used drugs: Chlorazepate (Tranxene), clobazam (Onfi), clonazepam (Klonopin), diazepam (Valium), and lorazepam (Ativan)
         iv. All benzodiazepines are controlled substances, scheduled as C-IV.
         v. Nonepileptic indications: Chlorazepate (anxiety disorders, anxiety), clonazepam (panic disorder with or without agoraphobia), lorazepam (anxiety disorders, anxiety)
      b. Carbamazepine (Carbatrol, Epitol, Equetro, Tegretol, Teril)
         i. Mechanism of action: Fast sodium channel blocker
         ii. Pharmacokinetics: Enzyme inducer, autoinduction
         iii. Adverse effects: Rash (occurs after a delay of 2–8 weeks), syndrome of inappropriate antidiuretic hormone release, aplastic anemia, thrombocytopenia, anemia, leukopenia

    iv. Extended-release tablets (Tegretol XR) 100, 200, and 400 mg; extended-release capsules (Carbatrol) 100, 200, and 300 mg available. Dosing is still twice daily. Do not crush or chew. Extended-release capsules (Carbatrol) can be opened and sprinkled on food. Ghost tablets can be seen in the stool with the extended-release tablets (Tegretol XR).

    v. Patients with the *HLA-B*1502* allele are at a 10-fold elevated risk of Stevens-Johnson syndrome.

        (a) Testing is recommended for Asians (including Indians).

        (b) More than 15% of populations in Hong Kong, Malaysia, the Philippines, and Thailand have this allele.

    vi. Patients with the *HLA-A*3101* allele are also at a 12-fold elevated risk of hypersensitivity syndrome and a 3-fold elevated risk of maculopapular exanthema.

        (a) The prevalence of this allele is 2%–5% in northern European populations and 9.1% of Japanese populations.

        (b) No recommendations for testing for this allele have been issued.

    vii. Nonepileptic indication: Trigeminal neuralgia

c. Eslicarbazepine acetate (Aptiom)

    i. Mechanism of action: Fast sodium channel blocker

    ii. Prodrug for S(+)-licarbazepine, an active metabolite of oxcarbazepine

    iii. Adjust dose if creatinine clearance (CrCl) is less than 50 mL/minute.

d. Ethosuximide (Zarontin)

    i. Mechanism of action: T-type calcium current blocker

    ii. Useful only for absence seizures

e. Ezogabine (Potiga)

    i. Mechanism of action: Potassium channel opener

    ii. Adverse effects: Urinary retention, hallucinations, QT prolongation, pigment changes in retina, or blue discoloration of the lips, nail beds, face, legs, sclera, and conjunctiva

    iii. Monitoring recommendations: Baseline and periodic eye examinations (every 6 months) with visual acuity testing and dilated fundus photography

    iv. Ezogabine is a schedule V controlled substance

f. Felbamate (Felbatol)

    i. Mechanism of action: Blocks glycine site on *N*-methyl-D-aspartate receptor

    ii. Serious adverse effects: Hepatotoxicity, aplastic anemia. Patient or guardian must sign consent form. Used only when seizures are severe and refractory to other medications and when the benefit clearly outweighs the potential adverse effects

g. Fosphenytoin (Cerebyx)

    i. Mechanism of action: Prodrug for phenytoin; fast sodium channel blocker

    ii. Uses: Parenteral formulation for loading or maintenance dosing in place of phenytoin; status epilepticus

    iii. Pharmacokinetics: Enzyme inducer, nonlinear kinetics

    iv. Dosing: Phenytoin equivalents are used; 1 mg of phenytoin = 1.5 mg of fosphenytoin = 1 mg of phenytoin equivalent. Intramuscular or intravenous dosing is appropriate.

    v. Adverse effects: Hypotension, perianal itching, other adverse effects of phenytoin

    vi. Advantages over phenytoin

        (a) Intramuscular or intravenous dosing

        (b) Phlebitis is minimized.

        (c) Infusion can be up to 150 mg of phenytoin equivalents per minute.

        (d) Can deliver in normal saline solution or D_5W (5% dextrose [in water] injection)

h. Gabapentin (Neurontin)

    i. Mechanism of action: Inhibition of $\alpha2\delta$ subunit of voltage-dependent calcium channels

    ii. Pharmacokinetics: Not metabolized, eliminated renally; adjustments may be necessary for renal dysfunction and hemodialysis

    iii. Nonepileptic indication: Postherpetic neuralgia pain

    iv. Doses often exceed product information maximum of 3600 mg/day.

    v. Extended-release tablets (Gralise) 300 and 600 mg are available. Their indication is for postherpetic neuralgia, not epilepsy.

    vi. Gabapentin enacarbil (Horizant) extended-release tablets 300 and 600 mg are available. This agent is a prodrug for gabapentin and is indicated for postherpetic neuralgia and restless legs syndrome, not epilepsy.

i. Lacosamide (Vimpat)

    i. Mechanism of action: Slow sodium channel blocker

    ii. Maximal dose of 300 mg/day with a CrCl of 30 mL/minute or less or with mild to moderate hepatic impairment

    iii. Adverse effects: PR interval prolongation or first-degree atrioventricular block; baseline and steady-state electrocardiogram recommended in patients with known cardiac conduction problems, taking medications known to induce PR interval prolongation, or with severe cardiac disease

    iv. Controlled substance schedule V because of euphoric effects

    v. Parenteral formulation: Has a U.S. Food and Drug Administration (FDA) indication only for replacement of oral formulation

j. Lamotrigine (Lamictal)

    i. Mechanism of action: Decreases glutamate and aspartate release, delays repetitive firing of neurons, blocks fast sodium channels

    ii. Rash is a primary concern; lamotrigine must be titrated slowly to avoid a rash.

    iii. Valproic acid decreases lamotrigine metabolism; this interaction requires even slower titration and lower final doses.

    iv. Estrogen-containing oral contraceptives increase lamotrigine clearance, so twice the amount of lamotrigine may be necessary.

    v. Extended-release tablets (Lamictal XR) are available (25 mg, 50 mg, 100 mg, 200 mg, 250 mg, 300 mg).

    vi. Nonepileptic indications: Maintenance treatment of bipolar I mood disorder

k. Levetiracetam (Keppra)

    i. Mechanism of action: May prevent hypersynchronization of epileptiform burst firing and propagation of seizure activity

    ii. Pharmacokinetics: Not metabolized largely, adjust dose in renal dysfunction, no drug interactions with other seizure medications

    iii. Parenteral use: Currently indicated by the FDA only for replacement of oral dosing; however, sometimes used for status epilepticus

    iv. Extended-release tablets (500 mg, 750 mg) are available for once-daily dosing.

l. Oxcarbazepine (Trileptal)

    i. Mechanism of action: Fast sodium channel blocker

    ii. Pharmacokinetics: Active metabolite 10-monohydroxy oxcarbazepine; enzyme inducer, no autoinduction

    iii. Adverse effects: Hyponatremia more common than with carbamazepine (increased dose and increased age increase risk of hyponatremia); blood dyscrasias less common than with carbamazepine; 25%–30% of patients with hypersensitivity to carbamazepine will have hypersensitivity to oxcarbazepine; rash

    iv. Extended-release tablets (Oxtellar XR) are available (150 mg, 300 mg, 600 mg).

m. Perampanel (Fycompa)

    i. Mechanism of action: Noncompetitive antagonist of the inotropic α-amino-3-hydroxy-5-methyl-4-isoxazole propionic acid (AMPA) glutamate receptor

    ii. Pharmacokinetics: 95%–96% protein bound to albumin and α_1-acid glycoprotein; metabolized by cytochrome P450 (CYP) 3A4 and 3A5; 105-hour half-life

    iii. Adverse effects: Neuropsychiatric effects (irritability, aggression, anger, anxiety), dizziness, gait disturbance, weight gain

    iv. Perampanel is a Schedule III controlled substance

n. Phenobarbital (Luminal)

    i. Mechanism of action: Increases γ-aminobutyric acid–mediated chloride influx

    ii. Pharmacokinetics: Enzyme inducer

    iii. Adverse effects: Hyperactivity, cognitive impairment

    iv. Phenobarbital is a schedule IV controlled substance

    v. Nonepileptic use: Anxiety

o. Phenytoin (Dilantin, Phenytek)

    i. Mechanism of action: Fast sodium channel blocker

    ii. Pharmacokinetics: Enzyme inducer, nonlinear kinetics

    iii. Administration considerations

        (a) Intravenous formulation: Very basic product. Phlebitis and extravasation are concerns; hypotension; maximal infusion rate of 50 mg/minute. Can prepare only in normal saline solution

        (b) Oral suspension: Must be shaken well; adheres to feeding tubes and is bound by enteral nutrition products

    iv. Dose-related adverse effects: Nystagmus, ataxia, drowsiness, cognitive impairment

    v. Non–dose-related adverse effects: Gingival hyperplasia, hirsutism, acne, rash, hepatotoxicity, coarsening of facial features

p. Pregabalin (Lyrica)

    i. Mechanism of action: Inhibition of α2δ subunit of voltage-dependent calcium channels

    ii. Pharmacokinetics: Not metabolized, renally excreted, reduce dose in renal dysfunction

    iii. Adverse effects: Drowsiness, blurred vision, weight gain, edema, angioedema, creatine kinase elevations (three reports of rhabdomyolysis), rash

    iv. Schedule V controlled substance: Insomnia, nausea, headache, diarrhea reported after abrupt discontinuation

    v. Nonepileptic indications: Neuropathic pain associated with diabetic neuropathy, postherpetic neuralgia, and fibromyalgia

Table 1. Medication Selection for Various Seizure Types[a]

Drug	Focal	Generalized Tonic-Clonic	Absence	Atypical Absence	Atonic	Myoclonic	Infantile Spasms	Status Epilepticus	Lennox-Gastaut Syndrome
Acetazolamide	4	4	3	3	—	—	—	—	—
Carbamazepine	1	1	—	—	4	4	—	—	—
Clobazam	4	4	3	—	—	3	—	—	1
Clonazepam	3	3	2	2	1	2	2	—	1
Corticotropin	—	—	—	—	—	—	1	—	—
Diazepam	—	—	—	4	—	4	4	1	2
Eslicarbazepine	4	—	—	—	—	—	—	—	—
Ethosuximide	—	—	1	1	—	4	—	—	—
Ezogabine	4	—	—	—	—	—	—	—	—
Felbamate	5	5	5	—	—	5	—	—	5
Gabapentin	1	2	—	—	—	—	—	—	—
Lacosamide	1	—	—	—	—	—	—	3	—
Lamotrigine	1	1	2	4	3	3	—	—	1
Levetiracetam	1	1	4	—	—	3	—	3	—
Lorazepam	3	3	3	3	—	3	—	1	—
Oxcarbazepine	1	1	—	—	3	3	—	—	—
Perampanel	4	—	—	—	—	—	—	—	—
Phenobarbital	2	2	2	—	—	3	—	2	—
Phenytoin	2	2	—	—	—	3	—	1	—
Pregabalin	4	—	—	—	—	—	—	—	—
Primidone	2	2	2	—	—	—	—	—	—
Rufinamide	4	3	3	—	3	—	—	—	1
Tiagabine	4	—	—	—	4	4	—	—	—
Topiramate	1	1	3	—	3	1	—	—	—
Valproic acid	2	1	1	1	1	1	1	2	—
Vigabatrin	5	5	—	—	—	—	5	—	—
Zonisamide	1	3	3	—	—	4	—	—	—

[a]Not all uses are U.S. Food and Drug Administration (FDA)-approved indications. 1 = first-line drug; 2 = second-line drug; 3 = some therapeutic effect; 4 = adjunctive therapy; 5 = used only when benefits outweigh risks.

Table 2. Selected Interactions Between Seizure Medications

Antiepileptic Drug	Added Seizure Medication	Change in Serum Concentration of the Initial Seizure Medication	Mechanism
Carbamazepine	Ethosuximide	Decreased	Increased metabolism
	Felbamate	Decreased, increased epoxide (active component of carbamazepine)	Inhibits epoxide degradation
	Phenytoin	Decreased	Increased metabolism
	Phenobarbital	Decreased	Increased metabolism
	Primidone	Decreased	Increased metabolism
	Rufinamide	Decreased	Increased metabolism
Clobazam	Eslicarbazepine	Increased	Decreased metabolism
Eslicarbazepine	Carbamazepine	Decreased	Increased metabolism
	Phenobarbital	Decreased	Increased metabolism
	Phenytoin	Decreased	Increased metabolism
Ezogabine	Carbamazepine	Decreased	Probable increased metabolism
	Phenytoin	Decreased	Probable increased metabolism
Felbamate	Carbamazepine	Decreased	Increased metabolism
	Phenytoin	Decreased	Increased metabolism
Lamotrigine	Carbamazepine	Decreased	Increased metabolism
	Phenobarbital	Decreased	Increased metabolism
	Phenytoin	Decreased	Increased metabolism
	Primidone	Decreased	Increased metabolism
	Rufinamide	Decreased	Increased metabolism
	Valproic acid	Increased	Decreased metabolism
Oxcarbazepine	Carbamazepine	Decreased	Increased metabolism
	Phenobarbital	Decreased	Increased metabolism
	Phenytoin	Decreased	Increased metabolism
	Valproic acid	Decreased	Unknown
Perampanel	Carbamazepine	Decreased	Increased metabolism
	Oxcarbazepine	Decreased	Increased metabolism
	Phenytoin	Decreased	Increased metabolism
Phenobarbital	Oxcarbazepine	Increased	Decreased metabolism
	Phenytoin	Increased	Unknown
	Rufinamide	Increased	Decreased metabolism
	Valproic acid	Increased	Inhibition of metabolism
Phenytoin	Carbamazepine	Decreased	Increased metabolism
	Eslicarbazepine	Increased	Decreased metabolism
	Oxcarbazepine	Increased or no change	Unknown
	Phenobarbital	Increased or decreased	Decreased or increased metabolism
	Rufinamide	Increased	Unknown
	Topiramate	Increased	Decreased metabolism
	Valproic acid	Decreased total; increased free	Displacement from binding sites
	Vigabatrin	Decreased	Increased metabolism

Table 2. Selected Interactions Between Seizure Medications (*continued*)

Antiepileptic Drug	Added Seizure Medication	Change in Serum Concentration of the Initial Seizure Medication	Mechanism
Primidone	Carbamazepine	Increased phenobarbital concentration	Unknown
	Phenytoin	Increased phenobarbital concentration	Unknown
Rufinamide	Carbamazepine	Decreased	Increased metabolism
	Phenobarbital	Decreased	Increased metabolism
	Phenytoin	Decreased	Increased metabolism
	Primidone	Decreased	Increased metabolism
	Valproic acid	Increased	Decreased clearance
Topiramate	Carbamazepine	Decreased	Increased metabolism
	Lamotrigine	Decreased	Unknown
	Phenytoin	Decreased	Increased metabolism
	Valproic acid	Decreased	Increased metabolism
Valproic acid	Carbamazepine	Decreased	Increased metabolism
	Felbamate	Increased	Unknown
	Oxcarbazepine	Decreased	Unknown
	Phenobarbital	Decreased	Increased metabolism
	Phenytoin	Decreased	Increased metabolism
	Primidone	Decreased	Increased metabolism
	Topiramate	Decreased	Increased metabolism
Zonisamide	Carbamazepine	Decreased	Increased metabolism
	Phenobarbital	Decreased	Increased metabolism
	Phenytoin	Decreased	Increased metabolism

Table 3. Selected Interactions of Non-AEDs on Seizure Medications

Seizure Medication	Other Drug	Effect on the Seizure Medication	Mechanism
Carbamazepine	Cimetidine	Increased serum concentration	Inhibition of carbamazepine metabolism
	Diltiazem	Increased serum concentration	Inhibition of carbamazepine metabolism
	Erythromycin	Increased serum concentration	Inhibition of carbamazepine metabolism
	Isoniazid	Increased serum concentration	Inhibition of carbamazepine metabolism
	Nefazodone	Increased serum concentration	Inhibition of carbamazepine metabolism
	Theophylline	Decreased serum concentration	Increased carbamazepine metabolism
	Troleandomycin	Increased serum concentration	Inhibition of carbamazepine metabolism
	Verapamil	Increased serum concentration	Inhibition of carbamazepine metabolism
Clobazam	Fluconazole	Increased serum concentration	Inhibitor of CYP2C19
	Fluvoxamine	Increased serum concentration	Inhibitor of CYP2C19
	Omeprazole	Increased serum concentration	Inhibitor of CYP2C19
	Ticlopidine	Increased serum concentration	Inhibitor of CYP2C19
Gabapentin	Antacids	Decreased serum concentration	Decreased bioavailability

Table 3. Selected Interactions of Non-AEDs on Seizure Medications *(continued)*

Seizure Medication	Other Drug	Effect on the Seizure Medication	Mechanism
Lamotrigine	Estrogen-containing contraceptives	Decreased serum concentration	Possibly induction of glucuronidation of lamotrigine
	Rifampin	Decreased serum concentration	Possibly induction of glucuronidation of lamotrigine
Perampanel	Ethanol and other CNS depressants	CNS additive or supra-additive effects	Additive CNS depression
	Rifampin	Decreased serum concentration	Increased metabolism
	St. John's wort	Decreased serum concentration	Increased metabolism
Phenobarbital; primidone	Ethanol	Acute ethanol ingestion may cause CNS additive effects and respiratory depression; chronic ethanol ingestion may result in variable effects	Additive CNS depression and decreased barbiturate metabolism with acute ethanol ingestion
Phenytoin	Anticoagulants, oral	May increase phenytoin serum concentration; decreased or increased anticoagulant effects	Complex mechanism
	Antineoplastics (bleomycin, cisplatin, vinblastine, methotrexate, carmustine)	Decreased pharmacologic effect	Unknown, possible decreased absorption caused by antineoplastic mucosal damage
	Chloramphenicol	Increased phenytoin serum concentration; decreased or increased chloramphenicol serum concentration	Inhibition of phenytoin metabolism; effect on chloramphenicol unknown
	Cimetidine	Increased serum concentration	Inhibition of phenytoin metabolism
	Diazoxide	Decreased pharmacologic effect; decreased serum concentration	Increased phenytoin metabolism
	Diltiazem	Increased serum concentration	Inhibition of phenytoin metabolism
	Disulfiram	Increased serum concentration	Inhibition of phenytoin metabolism
	Folic acid	Decreased serum concentration	Complex mechanism
	Isoniazid	Increased serum concentration	Inhibition of phenytoin metabolism
	Phenylbutazone	Increased serum concentration	Inhibition of phenytoin metabolism; plasma protein displacement
	Rifampin	Decreased serum concentration	Increased phenytoin metabolism
	Sulfonamides	Increased serum concentration	Inhibition of phenytoin metabolism
	Trimethoprim	Increased serum concentration	Inhibition of phenytoin metabolism
Topiramate	Hydrochlorothiazide	Increased serum concentration	Unknown
Valproic acid	Estrogen-containing oral contraceptives	Decreased serum concentration	Possibly induction of glucuronidation of lamotrigine
	Meropenem	Decreased serum concentration	Increased valproic acid metabolism
	Rifampin	Decreased serum concentration	Increased valproic acid metabolism
	Salicylates	Increased pharmacologic effect	Plasma protein displacement; increased free valproic concentration

AED = antiepileptic drug; CNS = central nervous system; CYP = cytochrome P450.

Table 4. Pharmacokinetic Parameters of Seizure Medications When Used as Monotherapy

Drug	Therapeutic Serum Concentration (mcg/mL)	Bioavail-ability (%)	Plasma Protein Binding (%)	Vd (L/kg)	Eliminated Unchanged (%)	Clinically Active Metabolites	Half-life (hours)
Acetazolamide	10–14	100	>90	0.23	100	None	48–96 10–15 (children)
Carbamazepine	4–12	>70	40–90	0.8–1.9 1.5 (neonates) 1.9 (children)	Little, if any	10,11-epoxide	12–17 8–14 (children)
Clobazam	Not established	100	80–90	100	3	N-desmethylclobazam	36–2 71–82 (N-desmethylclobazam)
Clonazepam	20–80 ng/mL	100	47–80	3.2	Low percentage	7-amino, low activity	19–50 22–33 (children)
Eslicarbazepine	Not established	90	<40	0.87	90	R-licarbazepine, oxcarbazepine	13–20
Ethosuximide	40–100	100	0	0.6–0.7	10–20	None	52–60 24–36 (children)
Ezogabine	Not established	60	80	2–3	36	NAMR	7–11
Felbamate	30–60[a]	>90	22–36	0.74–0.85	40–50	None	11–20 13–23 (children)
Gabapentin	2–20[a]	Dose-dependent	<3	0.65–1.04	75–80	None	5–7
Lacosamide	Not established	100	<15	0.6	40	None	13
Lamotrigine	1–13	98	55	0.9–1.2	10	None	12–55 24–30 (children)
Levetiracetam	12–46[a]	100	<10	0.5–0.7	66	None	7 5 (children)
Oxcarbazepine	3–35[a]	100[f]	67	0.7	<1	10-monohydroxy	9[f]
Perampanel	Not established	100	95–96	—	20–36	None	105
Phenobarbital	15–40	80–100	40–60	0.7–1	25	None	80–100 45–173 (neonates) 37–73 (children)
Phenytoin	10–20	85–95	>90	0.6–0.8	<5	None	~20b 10–140 (neonates)b 5–18 (children)b
Pregabalin	Not established	≥90	0	0.5	90	None	6
Primidone	4–12 (20)[c]	90–100	80	0.6	20–40	Phenobarbital PEMA	10–15; 17 (PEMA) 4.5–18 (children) 10–36 (PEMA; children)
Rufinamide	Not established	85	34	50d	2	None	6–10
Tiagabine	0.02–0.2[a]	90–95	96	1.2	—	None	3.2–5.7
Topiramate	5–20[a]	80	13–17	0.6–0.8	70	None	12–21
Valproic acid	40–100 (150)[c]	100	>90[e]	0.2	<5	Unknown	8–17 4–14 (children)
Vigabatrin	Not established	100	0	1.1	80	None	7.5 5.7 (infants)
Zonisamide	10–40	50	40	1.45	35	None	63

[a]Therapeutic serum concentrations not well established.

[b]Michaelis-Menten pharmacokinetics; half-life varies with serum concentration; therefore, it might be better to express phenytoin elimination in the length of time it takes to clear 50% of the drug from the body, for example.

[c]Upper end of the serum concentration range is not definitely established.

[d]Depends on dose.

[e]May vary with serum concentration.

[f]Bioavailability decreased in children younger than 8 years and in older adults; clearance is 80% higher in children 2–4 years and 40% higher in children 4–12 years compared with adults.

NAMR = N-acetyl metabolite of ezogabine; PEMA = phenylethylmalonamide; Vd = volume of (drug) distribution.

q. Primidone (Mysoline)

    i. Mechanism of action: Increases γ-aminobutyric–mediated chloride influx

    ii. Metabolized to phenobarbital and phenylethylmalonamide

    iii. Primidone, phenobarbital, and phenylethylmalonamide all have antiepileptic action.

    iv. Pharmacokinetics: Enzyme inducer

    v. Also used for essential tremor

r. Rufinamide (Banzel)

    i. Mechanism of action: Fast sodium channel blocker

    ii. Pharmacokinetics: Absorption increased by food (should be administered with food); metabolized by hydrolysis rather than through CYP enzymes

    iii. Decreases concentrations of ethinyl estradiol and norethindrone

    iv. Has an FDA indication only for Lennox-Gastaut syndrome

    v. Slightly shortens the QT interval and therefore should not be used in patients with familial short QT syndrome

    vi. Available as an oral solution

s. Tiagabine (Gabitril)

    i. Mechanism of action: Blocks γ-aminobutyric reuptake in the presynaptic neuron

    ii. Associated with new-onset seizures and status epilepticus in patients without epilepsy

t. Topiramate (Topamax)

    i. Mechanism of action: Fast sodium channel blocker, enhances γ-aminobutyric activity, and antagonizes AMPA/kainate activity, weak carbonic anhydrase inhibitor

    ii. Pharmacokinetics: Not extensively metabolized, eliminated in urine

    iii. Adverse effects: Drowsiness, paresthesias, psychomotor slowing (titrate slowly), weight loss, renal stones, acute angle closure glaucoma, metabolic acidosis, and hyperthermia (associated with decreased perspiration, or oligohidrosis)

    iv. Extended-release formulation (Trokendi XR)

    v. Nonepileptic indication: Prophylaxis of migraine headaches

u. Valproic acid (Depacon, Depakene, Depakote, Stavzor)

    i. Mechanism of action: Blocks T-type calcium currents, blocks sodium channels, increases γ-aminobutyric production

    ii. Pharmacokinetics: Enzyme inhibitor

    iii. Parenteral use: Has FDA indication only for replacement of oral dosing; however, sometimes used for status epilepticus, especially if absence status epilepticus

    iv. Adverse effects: Hepatotoxicity, nausea and vomiting, weight gain, interference with platelet aggregation, pancreatitis, alopecia, tremor

    v. Available in immediate-release (valproic acid [Depakene]) capsules for three- or four-times-daily dosing; delayed-release (enteric coated) (divalproex sodium [Depakote], valproic acid [Stavzor]) capsules and tablets for twice-daily dosing (if patient on enzyme inducer, drug is dosed more frequently); and extended-release (divalproex sodium [Depakote ER]) tablets for once-daily dosing

    vi. Nonepileptic indications: Manic episodes associated with bipolar disorder, prophylaxis of migraine headaches

v. Vigabatrin (Sabril)

    i. Mechanism of action: Irreversible inhibition of γ-aminobutyric acid transaminase

    ii. Pharmacokinetics: Induces CYP2C9; renal elimination

    iii. Adverse effects: Fatigue, somnolence, nystagmus, tremor, blurred vision, vision impairment, weight gain, arthralgia, abnormal coordination, and confusional state

    iv. Serious adverse effect: Vision loss; increased risk with higher total dose and duration; periodic vision testing necessary; restricted distribution program

    v. Available as oral powder for solution

w. Zonisamide (Zonegran)

    i. Mechanism of action: Fast sodium channel blocker, blocks T-type calcium currents, weak carbonic anhydrase inhibitor

    ii. Nonacrylamine sulfonamide: Avoid in sulfa-sensitive patients; it is sometimes used in patients with nonserious sulfa allergies, particularly when nonacrylamides (i.e., sulfonylureas) have been used successfully.

    iii. Pharmacokinetics: Long half-life

    iv. Adverse effects: Depression, rash, psychomotor slowing, paresthesias, kidney stones, blood dyscrasias, hyperthermia (associated with decreased perspiration, or oligohidrosis)

Table 5. Starting and Maximal Adult Seizure Medicine Doses

Drug	Starting Dose	Usual Maximal Dose
Carbamazepine	200 mg twice daily	1600 mg/day
Clobazam	10 mg/day	40 mg/day
Clonazepam	0.5 mg three times/day	20 mg/day
Eslicarbazepine	400 mg/day	1200 mg/day
Ethosuximide	250 mg twice daily	1.5 g/day
Ezogabine	100 mg three times/day	1200 mg/day
Felbamate	400 mg three times/day	3600 mg/day
Gabapentin	300 mg three times/day	3600 mg/day
Lacosamide	50 mg twice daily	400 mg/day
Lamotrigine	With valproic acid: 25 mg every other day Without carbamazepine, phenytoin, phenobarbital, primidone, or valproic acid: 25 mg/day With carbamazepine, phenytoin, phenobarbital, primidone, and not with valproic acid: 50 mg/day	With valproic acid: 200 mg/day Without carbamazepine, phenytoin, phenobarbital, primidone, or valproic acid: 375 mg/day With carbamazepine, phenytoin, phenobarbital, primidone, and not with valproic acid: 500 mg/day
Levetiracetam	500 mg twice daily	3000 mg/day
Oxcarbazepine	300 mg twice daily	2400 mg/day
Perampanel	With enzyme-inducing seizure medications: 4 mg/day Without enzyme-inducing seizure medications: 2 mg/day	With enzyme-inducing seizure medications: 12 mg/day Without enzyme-inducing seizure medications: 8 mg/day
Phenobarbital	1–3 mg/kg/day	300 mg/day
Phenytoin	100 mg three times/day	600 mg/day
Pregabalin	75 mg twice daily	600 mg/day
Primidone	100 mg at bedtime	2000 mg/day
Rufinamide	200–400 mg twice daily	3200 mg/day

Table 5. Starting and Maximal Adult Seizure Medicine Doses *(continued)*

Drug	Starting Dose	Usual Maximal Dose
Tiagabine	With carbamazepine, phenytoin, primidone, phenobarbital: 4 mg/day Without carbamazepine, phenytoin, primidone, phenobarbital: 2 mg/day	With carbamazepine, phenytoin, primidone, phenobarbital: 56 mg/day
Topiramate	25–50 mg/day	1000 mg/day
Valproic acid	10–15 mg/kg/day	60 mg/kg/day
Vigabatrin	500 mg twice daily	3000 mg/day
Zonisamide	100 mg/day	600 mg/day

2. Surgery: Surgery can sometimes drastically reduce the number of seizures; possible surgical procedures include removal of the seizure focus, corpus callosotomy, or vagus nerve stimulators.
3. Status epilepticus
   a. Treatment principles
      i. Ascertain ABCs (airway, breathing, and circulation).
      ii. Laboratory values (fingerstick blood glucose, complete blood cell count, basic metabolic panel, calcium, magnesium, and seizure medicine serum concentrations, if applicable) are sent to determine any reversible causes of status epilepticus.
      iii. Give an emergent medication to stop the seizure immediately.
      iv. Follow with an urgent medication to prevent the recurrence of seizures.
      v. In general, all drugs for status epilepticus should be given parenterally.
      vi. Neuromuscular-blocking drugs do not stop seizures; they stop only the muscular response to the brain's electrical activity.
   b. Emergency medications
      i. Lorazepam: Drug of choice
         (a) Rapid onset (2–3 minutes)
         (b) Dosage 0.1 mg/kg (up to 4 mg/dose) at rate of up to 2 mg/minute; may repeat every 5–10 minutes
      ii. Diazepam
         (a) Rapid onset, short duration
         (b) Dosage 0.15 mg/kg (up to 10 mg/dose) at rate of up to 5 mg/minute. May repeat every 5 minutes
         (c) Rectal gel formulation can be given in absence of intravenous access.
      iii. Midazolam: Preferred for intramuscular administration
         (a) Rapid onset, short duration
         (b) Dosage 0.2 mg/kg (up to 10 mg/dose). Can be given intramuscularly, intranasally, or buccally
   c. Urgent medications
      i. Phenytoin: Dosage 20 mg/kg; administration rate less than 50 mg/minute
      ii. Fosphenytoin: Administration rate less than 150 mg of phenytoin equivalent per minute
      iii. Phenobarbital: Dosage 20 mg/kg at 50–100 mg/minute
      iv. Valproic acid: Dosage 20–40 mg/kg at up to 6 mg/kg/minute; does not have FDA-labeled approval for status epilepticus
      v. Levetiracetam: 20-30 mg/kg over 15 minutes; does not have FDA-labeled approval for status epilepticus

      vi. Lacosamide: 200- to 400-mg bolus over 15 minutes; does not have FDA-labeled approval for status epilepticus

   d. Refractory status epilepticus medications

      i. Pentobarbital: Load 5–15 mg/kg up to 50 mg/minute; follow with a 0.5- to 5-mg/kg/hour infusion

         (a) May have severe hypotension, requiring treatment with vasopressors; should have continuous blood pressure (BP) measurement

         (b) Must be on ventilator

      ii. Thiopental: Load 2–7 mg/kg up to 50 mg/minute; follow with 0.5- to 5-mg/kg/hour infusion.

         (a) May have severe hypotension, respiratory depression, cardiac depression

         (b) Must be on ventilator

      iii. Midazolam: Load 0.2-mg/kg infused up to 2 mg/minute; follow with a 0.05- to 2-mg/kg/hour infusion.

         (a) May have hypotension, respiratory depression

         (b) May experience tachyphylaxis

      iv. Propofol: Load a 1- to 2-mg/kg intravenous bolus for 30–60 seconds; follow with a 20- to 200-mcg/kg/minute infusion.

         (a) Significant source of lipids

         (b) Some reports of seizure exacerbation with propofol

         (c) Must be on ventilator

4. Special populations

   a. Older adults: Pharmacokinetic changes in older adults that may affect seizure medications include the following:

      i. Carbamazepine: Decreased clearance

      ii. Phenytoin: Decreased protein binding if hypoalbuminemic or in renal failure

      iii. Valproic acid: Decreased protein binding

      iv. Diazepam: Increased half-life

      v. Phenylethylmalonamide (active metabolite of primidone): Decreased clearance if CrCl is decreased

      vi. Lamotrigine: Decreased clearance

      vii. Seizure medications with renal elimination must be adjusted according to the CrCl value.

   b. Women's health

      i. During their reproductive years, women with epilepsy should:

         (a) Take the best drug for their seizure type.

         (b) Be treated with monotherapy, if possible.

         (c) Discuss the possible decrease in hormonal contraceptive effectiveness if taking enzyme-inducing medications (Table 6).

         (d) Use folic acid supplementation with no less than 0.4 mg/day.

      ii. Three practice guidelines exist regarding epilepsy during pregnancy (relevant material excerpted below).

         (a) Avoiding valproic acid monotherapy or polytherapy during the first trimester of pregnancy should be considered to decrease the risk of major congenital malformations, particularly neural tube defects, facial clefts, hypospadias, and poor cognitive outcomes. Valproic acid use has now been associated with lower IQ scores at ages 3 and 4½ (Meador KJ et al. Effects of fetal antiepileptic drug exposure: outcomes at age 4.5 years. Neurology 2012;78:1207-14).

(b) To reduce the risk of major congenital malformations and poor cognitive outcomes, avoiding the use of seizure medication polytherapy during pregnancy, if possible, should be considered.

(c) Limiting the dose of valproic acid or lamotrigine during the first trimester, if possible, should be considered to lessen the risk of major congenital malformations.

(d) Avoiding the use of phenytoin, carbamazepine, and phenobarbital, if possible; may be considered to reduce the risk of cleft palate (phenytoin), posterior cleft palate (carbamazepine), cardiac malformations (phenobarbital), and poor cognitive outcomes (phenytoin, phenobarbital).

(e) Women with epilepsy taking seizure medications during pregnancy probably have an elevated risk of small-for-gestational-age babies and 1-minute Apgar scores less than 7.

(f) Monitoring of lamotrigine, carbamazepine, and phenytoin serum concentrations during pregnancy should be considered.

(g) Having levetiracetam and oxcarbazepine (as the monohydroxylated derivative [MHD]) serum concentrations monitored during pregnancy may be considered.

Table 6. Effect of Seizure Medications on Hormonal Contraceptives

Seizure Medication	Oral Contraceptives, Contraceptive Patch, Contraceptive Vaginal Ring, Progestogen Implant	Medroxyprogesterone Acetate Depot Injection, Levonorgestrel-Releasing Intrauterine System
Carbamazepine Clobazam Eslicarbazepine Felbamate Lamotrigine Oxcarbazepine Perampanel Phenobarbital Phenytoin Primidone Rufinamide Topiramate[a]	Decrease effectiveness	No effect
Benzodiazepines Ethosuximide Gabapentin Lacosamide Levetiracetam Pregabalin Tiagabine Valproic acid Vigabatrin Zonisamide	No effect	No effect

[a]Above doses of 200 mg/day.

E. Other Issues
   1. Driving: All states place driving restrictions on people with epilepsy; some require mandatory physician reporting to the state department of transportation.
   2. Medication discontinuation
       a. The American Academy of Neurology (AAN) has a practice guideline (Practice parameter: a guideline for discontinuing antiepileptic drugs in seizure-free patients—a summary statement. Neurology 1996;47:600-2. Available at http://aan.com/professionals/practice/pdfs/gl0007.pdf) with the following criteria for withdrawal:
           i.   Patient should be seizure free for 2–5 years on seizure medication.
           ii. Patient should have a single type of partial or primary generalized tonic-clonic seizures.
           iii. Patient should have a normal neurologic examination and normal IQ.
           iv. Patient's EEG should have become normalized with seizure medication treatment.
       b. If a drug is discontinued, it is usually tapered for several months; a typical regimen would reduce the dose by one-third for 1 month, reduce it by another one-third for 1 month, and then discontinue it.
   3. Monitoring
       a. Number of seizures: The goal number of seizures is always zero.
       b. Signs of toxicity
       c. Laboratory values: Specific for each drug
       d. Blood concentrations: Available for many of the medications, commonly used for carbamazepine, phenobarbital, phenytoin, and valproic acid. The International League Against Epilepsy has a position paper on therapeutic drug monitoring, giving situations in which serum concentrations are most likely to be of benefit:
           i.   When a person has attained the desired clinical outcome, to establish an individual therapeutic concentration that can be used subsequently to assess potential causes for a change in drug response
           ii. As an aid in the diagnosis of clinical toxicity
           iii. To assess adherence, particularly in patients with uncontrolled seizure or breakthrough seizures
           iv. To guide dosage adjustment in situations associated with increased pharmacokinetic variability (e.g., children, older adults, patients with associated diseases, drug formulation changes)
           v.   When a potentially important pharmacokinetic change in anticipated (e.g., in pregnancy, or when an interacting drug is added or removed)
           vi. To guide dose adjustments for seizure medications with dose-dependent pharmacokinetics, particularly phenytoin
   4. Sexual dysfunction
       a. Described in 30%–60% of men and women with epilepsy
       b. Includes hyposexuality, orgasmic dysfunction, and erectile dysfunction
       c. Mechanism may be induction of CYP isoenzymes to increase testosterone metabolism, increased hepatic synthesis of sex hormone binding globulin, or induction of aromatase, which converts free testosterone to estradiol.
       d. Sexual dysfunction has been reported with carbamazepine, phenobarbital, phenytoin, pregabalin, topiramate, and zonisamide.
       e. Improved sexual functioning has been reported with lamotrigine and oxcarbazepine.
   5. Bone health
       a. Osteopenia or osteoporosis is found in 38%–60% of patients in tertiary epilepsy clinics.
       b. Increased fractures in patients with epilepsy and with seizure medication use

    c.   Risk is increased with increased treatment duration; there is a dose-response relationship; the medications most often associated with poor bone health are carbamazepine, clonazepam, phenobarbital, and valproic acid. However, there is now evidence that all seizure medications may contribute to osteopenia or osteoporosis.

    d.   Proposed mechanisms: Hepatic induction of CYP isoenzymes leads to increased vitamin D catabolism, impaired calcium absorption, calcitonin deficiency, vitamin K interference, and direct detrimental effect on bone cells.

    e.   Proposed treatments: High-dose vitamin D (4000 international units/day for adults and 2000 international units/day for children) improves bone mineral density compared with low doses; estrogen may be helpful for women but may also trigger seizures in some women.

6. Suicidality

    a.   Meta-analysis of 199 placebo-controlled clinical trials of 11 drugs (n=43,892 patients older than 5 years) showed patients who received seizure medications had about twice the risk of suicidal behavior or ideation (0.43%) compared with patients receiving placebo (0.22%), and there were four completed suicides in the treatment group versus zero in the placebo group.

       i.   Risk increased at 1 week and continued through week 24.

      ii.   Patients with epilepsy (RR = 3.6), psychiatric disorders (RR = 1.6), or other conditions (RR = 2.3) were all at elevated risk of suicidality; no differences between drugs; no differences between age groups

    b.   An FDA alert was issued on January 31, 2008. Beginning December 16, 2008, the FDA required a warning and a medication guide for all seizure medications.

    c.   A more recent cohort study was performed that showed no increased risk of suicide or suicide attempts with the use of seizure medications in patients with epilepsy compared with patients with epilepsy who were not taking seizure medications.

    d.   An expert consensus statement was released in 2013 making the following points:

       i.   Although some (but not all) antiepileptic drugs can be associated with treatment-emergent psychiatric problems that may lead to suicidal ideation and behavior, the actual suicidal risk is yet to be established; however, it seems to be very low. The risk of discontinuing antiepileptic drugs or refusing to initiate them is significantly worse and can actually result in serious harm, including death to the patient.

      ii.   Suicidality in epilepsy is multifactorial. Primary operant variables include postictal suicidal ideation; a history of psychiatric disorders, particularly mood and anxiety disorders (and above all, when associated with prior suicidal attempts); and a family history of mood disorder complicated by suicide attempts.

     iii.   When starting or switching antiepileptic drugs, patients should be advised to report any changes in mood and suicidal ideation.

Patient Cases

Questions 1–3 pertain to the following case:

T.M. is an 18-year-old new patient in the pharmacy where you work. He presents a prescription for carbamazepine 100 mg 1 orally twice daily with instructions to increase to 200 mg 1 orally three times daily. Currently, he does not take any medications and does not have any drug allergies. During your counseling session, T.M. tells you he must have blood drawn for a test in 3 weeks.

1. Which common potential adverse effect of carbamazepine is best assessed through a blood draw?
    A. Leukopenia.
    B. Renal failure.
    C. Congestive heart failure.
    D. Hypercalcemia.

2. One month later, T.M. returns to your pharmacy with a new prescription for lamotrigine 25 mg with instructions to take 1 tablet daily for 2 weeks, followed by 1 tablet twice daily for 2 weeks, followed by 2 tablets twice daily for 2 weeks, and then 3 tablets twice daily thereafter. He tells you that he is discontinuing carbamazepine because he developed a rash a few days ago. Which response is best?
    A. The rash is probably caused by carbamazepine because carbamazepine rash often has delayed development.
    B. The rash is unlikely to be caused by carbamazepine because carbamazepine rash usually presents after the first dose.
    C. The rash is probably not caused by carbamazepine; it is probably attributable to carbamazepine-induced liver failure.
    D   The rash is probably not caused by carbamazepine; it is probably attributable to carbamazepine-induced renal failure.

3. T.M. wants to know why it is necessary to increase the dose of lamotrigine so slowly. Which reply is best?
    A. It causes dose-related psychomotor slowing.
    B. It causes dose-related renal stones.
    C. It causes dose-related paresthesias.
    D. It causes dose-related rash.

4. J.G. is a 34-year-old patient who has been maintained on carbamazepine extended release 400 mg orally twice daily for the past 2 years. She has had no seizures for the past 4 years. She presents to the emergency department in status epilepticus. Which drug is best to use first?
    A. Diazepam.
    B. Lorazepam.
    C. Phenytoin.
    D. Phenobarbital.

Patient Cases *(continued)*

5. S.R. is a 37-year-old patient who began taking phenytoin 100 mg 3 capsules orally at bedtime 6 months ago. He has experienced several seizures since then, the most recent of which occurred 7 days ago. At that time, his phenytoin serum concentration was 8 mcg/mL. The treating physician increased his dose to phenytoin 100 mg 3 capsules orally twice daily. Today, which best represents his expected serum concentration?

    A. 10 mcg/mL.

    B. 14 mcg/mL.

    C. 16 mcg/mL.

    D. 20 mcg/mL.

6. S.S. is a 22-year-old woman who has always had episodes of "zoning out." Recently, one of these episodes occurred after an examination while she was driving home. She had a noninjury accident, but it prompted a visit to a neurologist. She is given a diagnosis of absence seizures. Which drug is best to treat this type of epilepsy?

    A. Phenytoin.

    B. Tiagabine.

    C. Carbamazepine.

    D. Ethosuximide.

7. J.B. is a 25-year-old man with a history of seizure disorder. He has been treated with phenytoin 200 mg orally twice daily for 6 months, and his current phenytoin concentration is 6.3 mcg/mL. His neurologist decides to increase his phenytoin dose to 300 mg twice daily. Which adverse effect is J.B. most likely to experience related to the dose increase?

    A. Drowsiness.

    B. Acne.

    C. Gingival hyperplasia.

    D. Rash.

8. M.G., a 15-year-old boy with a diagnosis of juvenile myoclonic epilepsy, has been prescribed sodium divalproate. On which adverse effect is it best to counsel M.G.?

    A. Oligohidrosis.

    B. Renal stones.

    C. Alopecia.

    D. Word-finding difficulties.

Patient Cases *(continued)*

Questions 9 and 10 pertain to the following case:

G.Z., a 26-year-old woman, presents with a 6-month history of "spells." The spells are all the same, and all start with a feeling in the abdomen that is difficult for her to describe. This feeling rises toward the head. The patient believes that she will then lose awareness. After a neurologic workup, she is given a diagnosis of focal seizures evolving to a bilateral, convulsive seizure. The neurologist is considering initiating either carbamazepine or oxcarbazepine.

9. Which is the most accurate comparison of carbamazepine and oxcarbazepine?

    A. Oxcarbazepine causes more liver enzyme induction than carbamazepine.

    B. Oxcarbazepine does not cause rash.

    C. Oxcarbazepine does not cause hyponatremia.

    D. Oxcarbazepine does not form an epoxide intermediate in its metabolism.

10. When you see G.Z. 6 months later for a follow-up, she tells you she is about 6 weeks pregnant. She has had no seizures since beginning drug therapy. Which strategy is best for G.Z.?

    A. Discontinue her seizure medication immediately.

    B. Discontinue her seizure medication immediately and give folic acid.

    C. Continue her seizure medication.

    D. Change her seizure medication to phenobarbital.

II. ISCHEMIC STROKE

  A. Epidemiology
    1. Updated definitions
      a. Central nervous system (CNS) infarction: Brain, spinal cord, or retinal cell death attributable to ischemia, based on pathologic evidence, imaging, or other objective evidence of cerebral, spinal cord, or retinal focal ischemic injury in a defined vascular distribution, *or* clinical evidence of cerebral, spinal cord, or retinal focal ischemic injury, based on symptoms persisting for 24 hours or more or until death, and other etiologies excluded
      b. Ischemic stroke: An episode of neurologic dysfunction caused by focal cerebral, spinal, or retinal infarction
    2. Third or fourth most common cause of death in all developed countries
    3. More than 795,000 cases per year in the United States (128,842 deaths)
    4. Most common cause of adult disability
    5. Risk factors
      a. Nonmodifiable
        i. Age: Stroke risk doubles each decade after 55 years.
        ii. Race: Risk for Native Americans is greater than for African Americans, whose risk is greater than for whites.
        iii. Sex: Risks are greater for men than for women; however, about half of strokes occur in women.
        iv. Low birth weight: Odds of stroke for those with birth weights less than 2500 g are twice has high as the odds for those weighing more than 4000 g.
        v. Family history: Parental history increases risk; some coagulopathies (e.g., protein C and S deficiencies, factor V Leiden mutations) are inherited.

   b.   Somewhat modifiable: Diabetes mellitus increases risk 1.8–6 times; risk reduction has not been shown for glycemic control.
   c.   Modifiable
      i.   Hypertension increases risk 1.4–8 times; 32% risk reduction with control
      ii.   Smoking increases risk 1.9 times; 50% risk reduction in 1 year, baseline risk at 5 years with smoking cessation; exposure to environmental cigarette smoke also increases risk.
      iii.   Oral contraceptives with less than 50 mcg of estrogen double risk of stroke; those with more than 50 mcg of estrogen increase risk 4.5 times; risk increases with age; adding smoking to oral contraceptive use increases risk of stroke 7.2 times; obesity and hypertension also increase the risk with oral contraceptives.
      iv.   Postmenopausal hormone therapy increases risk 1.4 times.
      v.   Atrial fibrillation increases risk 2.6–4.5 times; 68% risk reduction with warfarin
      vi.   Coronary heart disease increases risk 1.55 times (women) to 1.73 times (men).
      vii.   Asymptomatic carotid stenosis increases risk 2 times; about a 50% risk reduction with endarterectomy
      viii.   Dyslipidemia: High total cholesterol increases risk 1.5 times; low high-density lipoprotein cholesterol (less than 35 mg/dL) increases risk 2 times; 27%–32% risk reduction with statins in patients with coronary heart disease, hypertension, or diabetes. Twenty-five percent risk reduction with high-dose statins compared with low-dose statins
      ix.   Obesity (especially abdominal body fat) increases risk 1.75–2.37 times; risk reduction with weight loss is unknown.
      x.   Physical inactivity increases risk 2.7 times; risk reduction with increased activity is unknown.
      xi.   Sickle cell disease increases risk 200–400 times; 91% risk reduction with transfusion therapy
      xii.   Peripheral artery disease increases risk 3 times; impact of risk reduction strategies is unknown.
      xiii.   Pregnancy increases risk 2.4 times over nonpregnant women; the risk remains elevated for the first 6 weeks postpartum.
      xiv.   Patent foramen ovale increases the risk of stroke in young patients (younger than 55 years).
      xv.   Depression increases the risk of stroke 1.35 times compared with nondepressed people.
   d.   Less well documented: Alcohol abuse (5 or more drinks a day), hyperhomocystinemia, drug abuse (cocaine, amphetamines, and heroin), hypercoagulability, periodontal disease, inflammation and infection, sleep-disordered breathing (sleep apnea and snoring), metabolic syndrome, and migraine with aura

B.   Primary Prevention
   1.   Reduction in risk factors (e.g., control of hypertension, smoking cessation, control of diabetes, cholesterol reduction)
   2.   Patient education: Patients should be educated about stroke warning signs and instructed to seek emergency care if they experience any of them. Warning signs: Sudden numbness or weakness of the face, arm, or leg, especially on one side of the body; sudden confusion; trouble speaking or understanding; sudden trouble seeing in one or both eyes; sudden trouble walking; dizziness, loss of balance or coordination; sudden, severe headache with no known cause
   3.   Treatment of atrial fibrillation: Up to 70% of cases are inappropriately treated.
      a.   Recommendations based on Lansberg MG, O'Donnell MJ, Khatri P, et al. Antithrombotic and thrombolytic therapy for ischemic stroke: Antithrombotic Therapy and Prevention of Thrombosis, 9th ed. American College of Chest Physicians Evidence-Based Clinical Practice Guidelines. Chest 2012;141:e601S-36S. Available at http://journal.publications.chestnet.org/pdfaccess.ashx?Resource ID=6568275&PDFSource=13. Accessed September 17, 2014; You JJ, Singer DE, Howard PA, et al. Antithrombotic and thrombolytic therapy for atrial fibrillation: Antithrombotic Therapy and Prevention of Thrombosis, 9th ed. American College of Chest Physicians Evidence-Based

Clinical Practice Guidelines. Chest 2012;141:e531S-75S. Available at http://journal.publications. chestnet.org/pdfaccess.ashx?ResourceID=6568280&PDFSource=13. Accessed September 17, 2014; Culebras A, Messe SR, Caturvedi S, et al. Summary of evidence-based guideline update: prevention of stroke in nonvalvular atrial fibrillation. Neurology 2014;82:716-24. Available at www.neurology. org/content/82/8/716.full. Accessed September 17, 2014; and Meschia JF, Bushnell C, Boden-Albala B., et al. Guidelines for primary prevention of stroke. A statement for healthcare professionals from the American Heart Association/American Stroke Association. Stroke 2014;45:3754-3832. Available at http://stroke.ahajournals.org/content/45/12/3754. Accessed February 17, 2015.

b. CHA_2DS_2-VASc is used for risk stratification.
   i. Assign 1 point each for congestive heart failure, hypertension, age 65-74 years, diabetes, vascular disease, or female sex.
   ii. Assign 2 points for previous stroke or TIA or age 75 years or older.
   iii. Total for the CHA_2DS_2-VASc score
       (a) If 0, give no therapy.
       (b) If 1, give no therapy, aspirin, or oral anticoagulant.
       (c) If 2 or more, give oral anticoagulant.

c. Dabigatran (Pradaxa)
   i. When oral anticoagulation is recommended, current guidelines suggest dabigatran 150 mg twice daily over warfarin (target international normalized ratio [INR] of 2.5). Dabigatran had similar rates of hemorrhage, but intracranial hemorrhage was less likely with dabigatran and gastrointestinal hemorrhage was more likely.
   ii. Mechanism of action: Direct thrombin inhibitor
   iii. Dose: 150 mg twice daily; dose reduction needed in severe renal dysfunction
   iv. Dose reduction to 75 mg twice daily is recommended when administered with dronedarone or systemic ketoconazole in patients with a CrCl of 30–50 mL/minute.
   v. Avoid the use of dabigatran and P-glycoprotein (P-gp) inhibitors in patients with a CrCl of 15–30 mL/minute.
   vi. Avoid use in patients with a CrCl less than 15 mL/minute or advanced liver disease.
   vii. Avoid use in patients with mechanical heart valves.
   viii. The capsule should not be opened because it increases bioavailability by 75%.

d. Rivaroxaban (Xarelto) is probably as effective as warfarin with similar risk of major bleeding. Higher risk of gastrointestinal bleeding and lower risk of intracranial hemorrhage and fatal bleeding.
   i. Mechanism of action: Direct factor Xa inhibitor
   ii. Dose: 20 mg/day with evening meal; dose reduction needed in renal dysfunction
   iii. Metabolized by CYP3A4/5, CYP2J2, P-gp, and *ABCG2;* avoid concomitant use with strong inhibitors or inducers.

e. Apixaban (Eliquis) is probably more effective than warfarin, with similar risk of stroke and less risk of bleeding and mortality.
   i. Mechanism of action: Direct, competitive factor Xa inhibitor
   ii. Dose: 5 mg twice daily; dose reduction needed in renal dysfunction
   iii. Metabolized by CYP3A4 and P-gp; reduce dose if given with inhibitors (e.g., ketoconazole, itraconazole, ritonavir, clarithromycin); avoid with strong inducers (e.g., rifampin, carbamazepine, phenytoin, St. John's wort)

f. Warfarin (Coumadin) is probably more effective than clopidogrel plus aspirin, but intracranial bleeding is more common.
   i. INR range 2–3
   ii. Give warfarin if patient has atrial fibrillation and mitral stenosis or prosthetic heart valve.

C. Treatment of Acute Event
  1. Heparin
     a. Good data on outcomes unavailable; generally not recommended for stroke treatment at therapeutic doses; increases risk of hemorrhagic transformation; heparin is often used for deep venous thrombosis prevention at a dose of 10,000–15,000 units/day.
     b. Avoid in hemorrhagic stroke.
  2. Streptokinase: Should be avoided because of excess mortality
  3. Tissue plasminogen activator (Activase)
     a. Within 4½ hours of symptom onset
     b. Three-month outcome significantly improved (decreased disability)
     c. Intracerebral hemorrhage increased but no increase in mortality
     d. Dose 0.9 mg/kg intravenously (maximum is 90 mg), with 10% as a bolus and the remainder over 1 hour.
     e. Exclusion criteria
        i. Minor or rapidly improving stroke signs or symptoms
        ii. Intracranial or subarachnoid bleeding (or history)
        iii. Other active internal bleeding
        iv. Intracranial surgery, head trauma, stroke within 3 months
        v. Major surgery or serious trauma within 2 weeks
        vi. Gastrointestinal (GI) or urinary tract hemorrhage within 3 weeks
        vii. Blood pressure greater than 185/110 mm Hg or aggressive treatment required to lower blood pressure
        viii. Glucose less than 50 mg/dL or greater than 400 mg/dL
        ix. Arterial puncture at a noncompressible site or lumbar puncture within 1 week
        x. Seizure at stroke onset
        xi. Intracranial neoplasm, arteriovenous malformation, aneurysm
        xii. Active treatment with warfarin (INR greater than 1.7), heparin (elevated activated partial thromboplastin time), or platelet count less than 100,000 cells/mm^3
        xiii. Postmyocardial infarction pericarditis
        xiv. Pregnancy
        xv. Additional criteria for the 3- to 4½-hour period
           (a) Taking any oral anticoagulant
           (b) Baseline National Institutes of Health Stroke Scale score greater than 25
           (c) Previous stroke combined with diabetes
           (d) Age older than 80
  4. Initiate aspirin (160- to 325-mg initial dose with 50- to 100-mg maintenance dose) within 48 hours of stroke onset in patients not eligible for tissue plasminogen activator.

D. Secondary Prevention
  1. Reduction in all modifiable risk factors (specific changes below based on Kernan WN, Ovbiagele B, Black HR, et al. Guidelines for the prevention of stroke in patients with stroke and transient ischemic attack: a guideline for healthcare professionals from the American Heart Association/American Stroke Association. Stroke 2014;45:2160-236. Available at http://stroke.ahajournals.org/content/45/7/2160.full.pdf+html?sid=0efbdc13-bba8-4e90-b197-d58dd042f816. Accessed September 17, 2014.)
     a. Hypertension: Goal <140/<90 mm Hg. With lacunar stroke, may target <130 mm Hg systolic
     b. Hyperlipidemia: High-intensity statin therapy should be initiated or continued as first-line therapy in women and men less than 75 years of age who have had stroke or TIA.

2. Carotid endarterectomy if 70%–99% stenosis. For 50%–69% stenosis, carotid endarterectomy recommendation depends on age, sex, and comorbidities; use aspirin 50–100 mg/day and statin therapy before and after the procedure.

3. Carotid angioplasty and stenting may be an alternative to carotid endarterectomy in some patients, particularly younger patients.

4. Antiplatelet therapy: Each agent has shown efficacy in reducing secondary stroke risk. Guidelines differ slightly on their recommendations. The American Stroke Association suggests that aspirin, aspirin/extended-release dipyridamole, and clopidogrel are all options after a first stroke or TIA, and the combination of aspirin and clopidogrel might be considered for initiation within 24 hours of a minor ischemic stroke or TIA or in the setting of intercranial atherosclerotic disease and continued for 90 days; however, long-term treatment increases risk of hemorrhage. The American Association of Chest Physicians recommends clopidogrel or aspirin/dipyridamole over aspirin or cilostazol.

    a. Aspirin
        i. Dose: Between 75 and 100 mg/day
        ii. If the patient has an additional stroke while taking aspirin, there is no evidence that increasing the aspirin dose will provide additional benefit.

    b. Aspirin/dipyridamole (Aggrenox)
        i. Capsule contains dipyridamole extended-release pellets (200 mg) and aspirin tablet (25 mg).
        ii. Dose: 1 capsule orally twice daily
        iii. Most common adverse effects: Headache, nausea, and dyspepsia; can increase liver enzymes

    c. Clopidogrel (Plavix)
        i. Inhibits adenosine diphosphate–induced platelet aggregation
        ii. Dose: 75 mg/day orally
        iii. Very low incidence of neutropenia (0.04% severe)
        iv. Rarely, thrombotic thrombocytopenic purpura has been reported.
        v. Partly metabolized by CYP2C19; there may be interactions with inhibitors of CYP2C19, notably proton pump inhibitors, or with genetic polymorphisms of this enzyme. The FDA has issued an alert on this topic (www.fda.gov/Drugs/DrugSafety/PostmarketDrugSafety InformationforPatientsandProviders/DrugSafetyInformationforHeathcareProfessionals/ ucm190787.htm).

    d. Cilostazol (Pletal)
        i. Inhibits cyclic adenosine monophosphate phosphodiesterase type 3–inducted platelet aggregation
        ii. Dose: 100 mg orally twice daily on an empty stomach
        iii. Metabolized extensively by CYP3A4 and CYP2C19
        iv. Adverse effects: Headache, palpitation, diarrhea, and dizziness; rarely, thrombocytopenia or agranulocytosis. Contraindicated in patients with congestive heart failure
        v. Monitoring: Complete blood cell count with differential every 2 weeks for 3 months, periodically thereafter. Thus, used infrequently

5. Anticoagulation: Warfarin (Athrombin-K, Coumadin, Jantoven, Panwarfin)
    a. Prevention of second ischemic event, if patient has atrial fibrillation, rheumatic mitral valve disease, mechanical prosthetic heart valves, bioprosthetic heart valves, or left ventricular mural thrombus formation
    b. Target INR of 2.5 (3.0 for mechanical prosthetic heart valves)

Patient Cases

Questions 11–13 pertain to the following case:

L.R. is a 78-year-old man who presents to the emergency department for symptoms of right-sided paralysis. He states that these symptoms began about 5 hours ago and have not improved since then. He also has hypertension, benign prostatic hypertrophy, diabetes mellitus, erectile dysfunction, and osteoarthritis.

11. Which is the most accurate list of L.R.'s risk factors for stroke?

    A. Erectile dysfunction, age, osteoarthritis.

    B. Sex, diabetes mellitus, osteoarthritis.

    C. Benign prostatic hypertrophy, diabetes mellitus, age, sex.

    D. Age, diabetes mellitus, sex, hypertension.

12. Is L.R. a candidate for tissue plasminogen activator for treatment of stroke?

    A. Yes.

    B. No, he is too old.

    C. No, his stroke symptoms began too long ago.

    D. No, his diabetes mellitus is a contraindication for tissue plasminogen activator.

13. L.R. was previously taking no drugs at home. Which choice is the best secondary stroke prevention therapy for this patient?

    A. Sildenafil.

    B. Celecoxib.

    C. Aspirin.

    D. Warfarin.

14. You are the pharmacist at a community pharmacy and receive a call from M.W., a 60-year-old man recently given a diagnosis of atrial fibrillation. He is concerned about his risk of having a stroke because his friend, who also has atrial fibrillation, asked him which dose of warfarin he is taking. M.W. called you because he is not taking warfarin and wants to know whether he should. He has no other medical conditions and takes atenolol 50 mg/day orally for ventricular rate control. After encouraging M.W. to discuss this with his physician, what should you tell him?

    A. You need warfarin treatment to prevent a stroke.

    B. You do not need warfarin, but you should take aspirin and clopidogrel.

    C. You do not need drug therapy at this time.

    D. Because you have atrial fibrillation, nothing can reduce your risk of stroke.

15. L.S. is a 72-year-old woman with a medical history of hypertension, type 2 diabetes mellitus, renal failure, and atrial fibrillation. She presents to the anticoagulation clinic for her initial visit. Which best reflects her target INR?

    A. 1.5.

    B. 2.0.

    C. 2.5.

    D. 3.0.

III. PARKINSON DISEASE

A. Epidemiology
   1. Prevalence is 160 in 100,000.
   2. Onset usually between 40 and 70 years of age, with peak onset in sixth decade
   3. Slightly more common in men
   4. Observed in all countries, ethnic groups, and socioeconomic classes

B. Signs/Symptoms
   1. Cardinal signs
      a. Akinesia/hypokinesia
      b. Rigidity
      c. Tremor
      d. Posture/gait abnormalities
   2. Secondary signs
      a. Cognitive dysfunction
      b. Autonomic dysfunction
      c. Speech disturbances
      d. Micrographia
      e. Masked facies

C. Treatment
   1. General treatment principles
      a. No treatment has been unequivocally shown to prevent progression of Parkinson disease; therefore, treatment is based on symptoms.
      b. In patients who require the initiation of dopaminergic treatment, either levodopa or a dopamine agonist may be used. The choice depends on the relative impact of improving motor disability (better with levodopa) compared with the lessening of motor complications (better with dopamine agonists) for each individual patient.
      c. Treatment may be initiated with rasagiline as well, but the effects are not robust.
      d. Treatment with several different classes of medications simultaneously is common.
   2. Medications
      a. Monoamine oxidase type B (MAO-B) inhibitors
         i. Selegiline (Eldepryl, Zelapar)
            (a) Loses selectivity for MAO-B at doses greater than 10 mg/day
            (b) Contraindicated with meperidine because of serotonin syndrome risk.
            (c) Dose: 5 mg orally twice daily (tablets; usually morning and noon); 1.25–2.5 mg/day (orally disintegrating tablets)
            (d) Adverse effects: Nausea, hallucinations, orthostatic hypotension, insomnia (metabolized to amphetamine)
            (e) Dosage forms: Tablets, orally dissolving tablets, and patches. The patches are FDA indicated for depression; they should not usually be used to treat Parkinson disease.
         ii. Rasagiline (Azilect)
            (a) Selectivity for MAO-B has not been definitively established.
               (1) Contraindicated with meperidine because of serotonin syndrome risk.
               (2) Do not administer with tramadol, methadone, dextromethorphan, sympathomimetics, fluoxetine, or fluvoxamine because of serotonin syndrome risk.
               (3) Ciprofloxacin can double the concentration of rasagiline (through CYP1A2 inhibition).
            (b) Dose: 0.5–1 mg/day orally

b. Levodopa
   i. Improvement in disability and possibly mortality
   ii. Greatest effect on bradykinesia and rigidity; less effect on tremor and postural instability
c. Carbidopa
   i. Combined in fixed ratios with levodopa
   ii. Prevents some of the peripheral conversion of levodopa to dopamine by inhibiting peripheral dopamine decarboxylase; therefore, levodopa is available to cross the blood-brain barrier
   iii. 75 mg/day is usually required to inhibit peripheral decarboxylase activity.
d. Carbidopa/levodopa (Carbilev, Parcopa, Sinemet)
   i. Pharmacokinetic considerations
      (a) High-protein diets decrease absorption.
      (b) Immediate-release half-life 60–90 minutes
      (c) Orally disintegrating tablet available; not absorbed sublingually
      (d) Slow-release considerations: Fewer daily doses; less plasma fluctuations; delay to effect; cannot crush; can divide. No measurable effect on "freezing"
   ii. Acute adverse effects: Nausea/vomiting, orthostatic hypotension, cardiac arrhythmias, confusion, agitation, hallucinations
   iii. Long-term adverse effects: Wearing-off and on-off phenomena, involuntary movements (dyskinesias)
      (a) Wearing-off phenomenon is the return of Parkinson disease symptoms before the next dose. Treatment of wearing-off includes adding a dopamine agonist, adding a MAO-B inhibitor, adding a catechol-O-methyl transferase inhibitor or increasing the frequency/dose of levodopa.
      (b) On-off phenomenon is a profound, unpredictable return of Parkinson disease symptoms without respect to the dosing interval. Treatment of on-off includes adding entacapone, rasagiline, pramipexole, ropinirole, apomorphine, and selegiline or redistributing dietary protein.
      (c) Dyskinesias are drug-induced involuntary movements including chorea and dystonia. Treatment of dyskinesias includes decreasing the levodopa dose or adding amantadine as an antidyskinetic drug.
   iv. Therapy initiation
      (a) Standard formulation: 25 mg/100 mg 1 tablet orally three times daily; also available as orally disintegrating tablet
      (b) Controlled-release formulation: 1 tablet orally two or three times daily
      (c) Titration always necessary
      (d) A combination of formulations may be required (e.g., ½ tablet of Sinemet 25 mg/100 mg on awakening and 1 tablet of Sinemet CR 25/100 three times daily).
e. Direct dopamine agonists
   i. Drugs: Apomorphine (Apokyn), bromocriptine (Parlodel), pramipexole (Mirapex), ropinirole (Requip), rotigotine (Neupro)
   ii. Bromocriptine is an ergot-derived product: Very rarely, adverse effects such as retroperitoneal, pleuropulmonary, or cardiac fibrosis have been attributed to it; regular monitoring of the electrocardiogram is recommended.
   iii. Rotigotine is a transdermal system. With the initial formulation, problems occurred with crystallization of the medication. The product was withdrawn from the market and has since been reformulated.
   iv. Dosing: Always titrate to final dose.

Table 7. Usual Dosage Range for Dopamine Agonists

Agent	Usual Dosage Range (mg/day)
Bromocriptine	5–40
Pramipexole	1.5–4.5
Ropinirole	0.75–24
Rotigotine	6–8

    v. Adverse effects: Nausea, vomiting, postural hypotension, hallucinations, hypersexuality, compulsive behaviors, falling asleep during activities of daily living

    vi. Pramipexole and ropinirole also have FDA indications for restless legs syndrome.

    vii. Ropinirole and pramipexole are available as extended-release formulations.

    viii. Apomorphine: Short-acting dopamine receptor agonist

       (a) Indication: Acute, intermittent treatment of "off" episodes associated with advanced Parkinson disease

       (b) Contraindications: Its use with 5-hydroxytryptamine-3 antagonists (ondansetron, granisetron, dolasetron, palonosetron, and alosetron) causes profound hypotension; sulfite sensitivity/allergy

       (c) Pharmacokinetics: When given orally, poorly bioavailable and extensive first-pass metabolism; used as subcutaneous injection in a pen self-injector

       (d) Adverse effects

          (1) Severe nausea and vomiting

            (A) Treat with trimethobenzamide 300 mg three times daily for 3 days before initiating treatment and for at least 6 weeks during treatment.

            (B) About 50% of patients can discontinue trimethobenzamide after 2 months.

            (C) Thirty-one percent nausea and 11% vomiting WITH trimethobenzamide

          (2) Hypotension

          (3) Hallucinations

          (4) Injection site reactions

          (5) Dyskinesias

       (e) Dosing

          (1) Must be titrated in a setting where BP can be monitored

          (2) In the "off" state, the patient should be given a 0.2-mL (2 mg) test dose.

          (3) Supine and standing BP taken before dose; 20, 40, and 60 minutes after dose

          (4) If tolerated, begin with a 0.2-mL dose as needed; increase by 0.1 mL if necessary.

          (5) Doses greater than 0.6 mL, more than five times daily, or greater than 20 mg/day have limited experience.

          (6) If first dose is ineffective, do not re-dose.

          (7) If patients do not dose for more than 1 week, reinitiate at a 0.2-mL dose.

  f. Anticholinergics

    i. Drugs: Trihexyphenidyl (Artane), benztropine (Cogentin)

    ii. Most useful for tremor

    iii. Initial dosing

       (a) Trihexyphenidyl 0.5 mg 1 tablet orally twice daily

       (b) Benztropine 0.5 mg 1 tablet orally twice daily

    iv. Adverse effects: Dry mouth, urinary retention, dry eyes, constipation, confusion

g. Amantadine (Symmetrel)
   i. Has symptomatic benefits and may reduce dyskinesias caused by levodopa or dopamine agonists
   ii. Dosing: 100 mg 1 tablet orally two or three times daily; caution in renal dysfunction
   iii. Adverse effects: Dizziness, insomnia, anxiety, livedo reticularis, nausea, nightmares
h. Catechol-O-methyl transferase inhibitors
   i. Prevent breakdown of dopamine, more levodopa available to cross blood-brain barrier
   ii. Tolcapone (Tasmar): Severely restricted because of hepatotoxicity; must sign consent form
   iii. Entacapone (Comtan)
      (a) Increased area under the curve, increased half-life; no change in Cmax or Tmax of levodopa
      (b) Dosing: 1 tablet with each carbidopa/levodopa dose; maximum of eight times daily; one dosage form (Stalevo) includes carbidopa, levodopa, and entacapone 200 mg
      (c) Must use with carbidopa/levodopa
      (d) Adverse effects: Dyskinesias, nausea, diarrhea (may be delayed for up to 2 weeks after initiation or dose increase), urine discoloration (orange), hallucinations/vivid dreams

3. Surgery: Several types of surgery are performed for Parkinson disease.
   a. Thalamotomy: Ablation of portions of the thalamus to control tremor
   b. Pallidotomy: Ablation of structures in the globus pallidus for the treatment of Parkinson disease
   c. Fetal transplants: Transplantation of dopaminergic tissue into the striatum; considered experimental
   d. Trophic factors: Glial-derived nerve growth factor and neurturin have been delivered directly to the striatum or substantia nigra; considered experimental
   e. Deep brain stimulation
      i. Most frequently performed surgery for Parkinson disease
      ii. Thought to work by stimulating areas of the basal ganglia to reversibly block the neuronal activity in the area
      iii. Patient selection focuses on patients with
         (a) Motor fluctuations and/or dyskinesias that are not adequately controlled with optimized medical therapy
         (b) Medication-refractory tremor
         (c) Intolerance of medical therapy
         (d) Some centers will not perform the surgery in patients older than 70 years.
      iv. Two areas are targeted.
         (a) Globus pallidum
            (1) Reduces off-time
            (2) Reduces dyskinesias
            (3) Thought to have fewer cognitive adverse effects than subthalamic nucleus stimulation
         (b) Subthalamic nucleus
            (1) Reduces off-time
            (2) Reduces dyskinesias
            (3) Thought to be more effective than globus pallidum stimulation

4. Special situations
   a. Hallucinations/psychosis may be caused by either Parkinson disease or treatment.
      i. Discontinue/reduce Parkinson disease medications as tolerated.
      ii. If an antipsychotic is required, use quetiapine or clozapine as the first choice.
      iii. Avoid typical antipsychotics, risperidone, and olanzapine because they may worsen Parkinson symptoms.

b. Cognitive disorders
   i. Discontinue/reduce Parkinson disease medications as tolerated.
   ii. Rivastigmine has an FDA indication for treatment; other cholinesterase inhibitors may have efficacy.
c. Sleep disorders, depression, agitation, anxiety, constipation, orthostatic hypotension, seborrhea, and blepharitis can be seen in Parkinson disease; treat as usual.

Patient Cases

Questions 16 and 17 pertain to the following case:

L.S. is taking carbidopa/levodopa 25 mg/100 mg orally four times daily and trihexyphenidyl 2 mg orally three times daily for Parkinson disease. L.S.'s wife reports that he is often confused and experiences constipation; he has trouble talking because of his dry mouth.

16. Which change is best to resolve these symptoms?
    A. Increase carbidopa/levodopa.
    B. Increase trihexyphenidyl.
    C. Decrease carbidopa/levodopa.
    D. Decrease trihexyphenidyl.

17. Six months later, L.S. returns to the clinic concerned that his carbidopa/levodopa dose is wearing off before his next dose is due. Which recommendation is best?
    A. Increase the carbidopa/levodopa dose.
    B. Decrease the carbidopa/levodopa dose.
    C. Increase the dosing interval.
    D. Decrease the dosing interval.

18. P.J. is a 57-year-old man with an 8-year history of Parkinson disease. His current drugs include carbidopa/levodopa 50 mg/200 mg orally four times daily, entacapone 200 mg orally four times daily, and amantadine 100 mg three times daily. He presents to the clinic with a reddish blue discoloration on his lower arms and legs. Which, if any, of his drugs is the most likely cause of this condition?
    A. Carbidopa/levodopa.
    B. Entacapone.
    C. Amantadine.
    D. None; probably represents venous stasis.

19. L.L. is a 47-year-old man with Parkinson disease. He takes carbidopa/levodopa 50 mg/200 mg orally four times daily. He recently noticed an involuntary twitching movement of his left foot. Which is the best therapy for L.L.'s dyskinesia?
    A. Add ropinirole.
    B. Add selegiline.
    C. Increase the carbidopa/levodopa dose.
    D. Decrease the carbidopa/levodopa dose.

Patient Cases *(continued)*

20. C.A., a 57-year-old white man who just retired from the New York City Fire Department, has been experiencing tremors in his right hand that have become progressively worse for the past 6 months. He has difficulty walking. He also has backaches and no longer plays golf. In addition, he is losing his sense of taste. He is given a diagnosis of Parkinson disease. Which is the best treatment for this man?

   A. Trihexyphenidyl.

   B. Entacapone.

   C. Apomorphine.

   D. Ropinirole.

IV. HEADACHE

A. Definitions
   1. Classic migraine: At least two attacks with at least three of the following: One or more fully reversible aura symptoms, at least one aura symptom for more than 4 minutes, or two or more symptoms occurring in succession; no single aura symptom lasts more than 60 minutes; headache follows aura within 60 minutes.
   2. Migraine without aura: At least five attacks of headache lasting 4–72 hours with at least two of the following: Unilateral location, pulsating quality, intensity moderate or severe, aggravation by walking stairs or similar routine physical activity. During headache, at least one of the following: Nausea or vomiting, photophobia, phonophobia
   3. Tension: At least 10 previous headaches, each lasting from 30 minutes to 7 days, with at least two of the following: Pressing or tightening (nonpulsating) quality, intensity mild to moderate, bilateral location, no aggravation with physical activity
   4. Cluster: Several episodes, short-lived but severe, of unilateral, orbital, supraorbital, or temporal pain. At least one of the following must occur: Conjunctival injection, lacrimation, nasal congestion, rhinorrhea, facial sweating, miosis, ptosis, or eyelid edema.
   5. Analgesic rebound headache: If patients use analgesics often (usually defined as more than three times weekly), they may develop analgesic rebound headache. Patients with this condition usually present with a chronic daily headache, for which they take simple or narcotic analgesics. Treatment consists of the withdrawal of all analgesics (but not prophylactic medications).

B. Epidemiology
   1. Migraine: 15%–17% of women, 5% of men
   2. Tension: 88% of women, 69% of men
   3. Cluster: 0.01%–1.5% of population; ratio of men to women is 6:1.

C. Treatment
   1. Migraine
      a. Prophylaxis should be considered if any of the following criteria are met: Migraines are recurrent and interfere with daily routine, migraines are frequent, patient experiences inefficacy or inability to use acute therapy, patient prefers prophylaxis as therapy, cost of acute medications is problematic, adverse effects with acute therapies occur, or migraine presentation is uncommon.
         i. General principles
            (a) Use lowest effective dose.
            (b) Give adequate trial (2–3 months).

(c) If patient has a coexisting condition, consider prophylaxis choice (e.g., β-blockers are contraindicated in patients with asthma but beneficial in hypertension).

ii. Medications with established efficacy

(a) Frovatriptan (for menstrually associated migraine, short-term prophylaxis only)

(b) Metoprolol

(c) Petasites (butterbur extract)

(d) Propranolol

(e) Timolol

(f) Topiramate

(g) Valproic acid

iii. Medications with probable efficacy

(a) Amitriptyline

(b) Atenolol

(c) Fenoprofen

(d) Histamine, subcutaneous

(e) Ibuprofen

(f) Ketoprofen

(g) Magnesium

(h) MIG-99 (feverfew extract)

(i) Nadolol

(j) Naproxen/naproxen sodium

(k) Naratriptan (for menstrually associated migraine, short-term prophylaxis only)

(l) Riboflavin

(m) Venlafaxine

(n) Zolmitriptan (for menstrually associated migraine, short-term prophylaxis only)

iv. Medications with possible efficacy

(a) Candesartan

(b) Carbamazepine

(c) Clonidine

(d) Coenzyme Q10

(e) Cyproheptadine

(f) Estrogen

(g) Flurbiprofen

(h) Guanfacine

(i) Lisinopril

(j) Mefenamic acid

(k) Nebivolol

(l) Pindolol

v. Medications with conflicting or inadequate evidence of efficacy: Acetazolamide, aspirin, bisoprolol, fluoxetine, fluvoxamine, gabapentin, hyperbaric oxygen, indomethacin, nicardipine, nifedipine, nimodipine, omega-3, protriptyline, verapamil

vi. Medications that are possibly ineffective, probably ineffective, or ineffective: Acebutolol, botulinum toxin, clomipramine, clonazepam, lamotrigine, montelukast, nabumetone, oxcarbazepine, telmisartan

b. Acute treatment

i. Triptans (see Table 8)

(a) Sumatriptan and zolmitriptan have nonoral administration routes (subcutaneous [sumatriptan] and intranasal [sumatriptan and zolmitriptan]) that should be considered for patients with nausea or vomiting.

(b) Orally disintegrating tablets are available for zolmitriptan and rizatriptan if patients do not have access to water; however, they do not work faster than oral tablets and are not absorbed sublingually.

(c) All are contraindicated in patients with or at risk of coronary artery disease, stroke, uncontrolled hypertension, peripheral vascular disease, ischemic bowel disease, and pregnancy; they should not be used in patients with hemiplegic or basilar migraines.

(d) Drug interactions: Contraindicated within 2 weeks of MAO inhibitors; do not use within 24 hours of ergotamines; caution with other serotonin-active medications. Propranolol increases serum concentrations of rizatriptan; thus, a 5-mg dose should be used with propranolol, and the dose should not exceed 15 mg/day.

  ii. Ergots

(a) Dihydroergotamine has nonoral administration routes (subcutaneous, intravenous, and intranasal) that should be considered for patients with nausea or vomiting.

(b) All are contraindicated in patients with, or at risk of, coronary artery disease, stroke, uncontrolled hypertension, peripheral vascular disease, ischemic bowel disease, and pregnancy; they should not be used in patients with hemiplegic or basilar migraines.

  iii. Nonsteroidal anti-inflammatory drugs: Usually effective for only mild to moderate headache pain

  iv. Opioids: Butorphanol has a nonoral administration route (intranasal) that should be considered for patients with nausea or vomiting.

  v. Isometheptene combination products: Conflicting evidence about efficacy

  vi. Antiemetics: Prochlorperazine, metoclopramide, and chlorpromazine are most commonly used; there is some suggestion that they have independent antimigraine action; all are available in nonoral routes.

  vii. Status migrainosus: Attack of migraine, with headache phase lasting more than 72 hours despite treatment. Headache-free intervals of less than 4 hours (sleep not included) may occur.

(a) Corticosteroids: Either intravenous or oral dosing

(b) Dihydroergotamine: Intravenous dosing

(c) Sodium valproate: Intravenous loading

2. Tension
  a. Prophylaxis
    i. Tricyclic antidepressants
    ii. Botulinum toxin
  b. Acute treatment
    i. Acetaminophen
    ii. Nonsteroidal anti-inflammatory drugs

3. Cluster
  a. Prophylaxis
    i. Verapamil
    ii. Melatonin
    iii. Suboccipital injection of betamethasone
    iv. Lithium: May be efficacious at serum concentrations as low as 0.3 mmol/L
  b. Treatment
    i. Triptans: Subcutaneous and intranasal sumatriptan and intranasal zolmitriptan are effective. Oral formulations usually do not act quickly enough, but oral zolmitriptan showed efficacy in one trial.
    ii. Oxygen: 100% oxygen at 6–12 L/minute relieves pain in 50%–85% of patients.
    iii. Intranasal lidocaine: 20–60 mg as a nasal drop or spray (must be compounded)
    iv. Octreotide and 10% cocaine have been used with some effect.

Table 8. Selected Agents for Migraine Headache

	Dosage Forms	Tmax	Half-life (hours)	Dose	Maximal Dose/ 24 Hours (mg)
Triptans					
Almotriptan (Axert)	Tablets 6.25 mg, 12.5 mg	1–3 hours	2–4	1 tablet, may repeat in 2 hours	25
Eletriptan (Relpax)	Tablets 20 mg, 40 mg	1 hour	4–5	1 tablet, may repeat in 2 hours	80
Frovatriptan (Frova)	Tablets 2.5 mg	2–4 hours	26	1 tablet, may repeat in 2 hours	7.5
Naratriptan (Amerge)	Tablets 1 mg, 2.5 mg	2–3 hours	6	1 tablet, may repeat in 4 hours	5
Rizatriptan (Maxalt)	Tablets 5 mg, 10 mg	1–1.5 hours	1.8	1 tablet, may repeat in 2 hours	30
	Orally disintegrating tablets 5 mg, 10 mg	1.6–2.5 hours	1.8	1 tablet, may repeat in 2 hours	30
Sumatriptan (Imitrex)	SC injection 4 mg, 6 mg	12 minutes	1.9	1 injection, may repeat in 1 hour	12
	Intranasal 5 mg, 20 mg	30 minutes	2	1 spray in one nostril, repeat in 2 hours	40
	Tablets 25 mg, 50 mg, 100 mg	2 hours	2.5	1 tablet, may repeat in 2 hours	200
Zolmitriptan (Zomig)	Tablets 2.5 mg, 5 mg	1.5 hours	3.75	1 tablet, may repeat in 2 hours	10
	Orally disintegrating tablets 2.5 mg, 5 mg	3 hours	3.75	1 tablet, may repeat in 2 hours	10
	Intranasal 2.5 mg, 5 mg	3 hours	3	1 spray in one nostril, may repeat in 2 hours	10
Triptan/nonsteroidal anti-inflammatory combination					
Sumatriptan/naproxen sodium (Treximet)	Tablets 85 mg/500 mg	1 hour/ 5 hours	2/19	1 tablet, may repeat in 2 hours	170/1000
Ergots					
Ergotamine tartrate (Ergomar)	Sublingual tablets 2 mg	Unknown	2	1 tablet under tongue, may repeat in 1 hour	6
Dihydroergotamine (DHE 45; Migranal)	Intranasal 4-mg ampules	0.9 hour	10	1 spray (0.5 mg) in each nostril, repeat in 15 minutes	3
	IV/IM/SC 1 mg/mL 1-mL vials	SC 15–45 minutes	9	1 mL IV/IM/SC, may repeat in 1 hour	2 mg IV; 3 mg IM/SC

IM = intramuscular; IV = intravenous(ly); SC = subcutaneous.

Patient Cases

21. M.R., a 34-year-old woman, has throbbing right-sided headaches. She experiences nausea, phonophobia, and sonophobia with these headaches but no aura. She usually has headaches twice a month. She is hypertensive and morbidly obese. She takes an ethinyl estradiol/progestin combination oral contraceptive daily and hydrochlorothiazide 25 mg/day orally. She has a diagnosis of migraine headaches. Which medication is best for prophylaxis of her headaches?

    A. Propranolol.

    B. Valproic acid.

    C. Amitriptyline.

    D. Lithium.

22. S.R. is a 54-year-old female homemaker with squeezing, bandlike headaches that occur three or four times weekly. She rates the pain of these headaches as 7/10 and finds acetaminophen, aspirin, ibuprofen, naproxen, ketoprofen, and piroxicam only partly effective. She wants to take a prophylactic drug to prevent these tension headaches. Which drug is best for prophylaxis of her headaches?

    A. Propranolol.

    B. Valproic acid.

    C. Amitriptyline.

    D. Lithium.

23. D.S. is a 49-year-old male computer programmer who describes lancinating right-eye pain and tearing several times a day for 2–3 days in a row. He will have no episodes for 2–3 weeks but then will have recurrent episodes. In the office, he receives oxygen by nasal cannula during an episode, and his pain is relieved. He has a diagnosis of cluster headaches. Which drug is best for prophylaxis of his headaches?

    A. Propranolol.

    B. Valproic acid.

    C. Amitriptyline.

    D. Lithium.

24. M.K. is a 44-year-old woman with right-sided headaches of moderate intensity that are accompanied by severe nausea and vomiting. Which triptan is best to treat M.K.'s migraine headaches?

    A. Almotriptan.

    B. Naratriptan.

    C. Rizatriptan.

    D. Sumatriptan.

Patient Cases *(continued)*

25. One of the neurologists you work with read a meta-analysis of migraine treatments (Oldman AD, Smith LA, McQuay HJ, et al. Pharmacological treatment for acute migraine: quantitative systematic review. Pain 2002;91:247-57). He is most interested in the outcome of sustained relief at 24 hours, but he is confused by the number-needed-to-treat (NNT) analyses. He shows you the following table:

Drug	NNT
Ergotamine + caffeine	6.6
Eletriptan 80 mg	2.8
Rizatriptan 10 mg	5.6
Sumatriptan 50 mg	6.0

NNT = number needed to treat.

Which statement provides the best interpretation of these data?

A. Eletriptan 80 mg is the most effective agent.

B. Ergotamine plus caffeine is the most effective agent.

C. Eletriptan has the most adverse effects.

D. Ergotamine plus caffeine has the most adverse effects.

V. MULTIPLE SCLEROSIS

A. Definitions
1. Autoimmune disorder with areas of CNS demyelination and axonal transaction
2. Clinical course
   a. Clinically isolated syndrome; first clinical presentation for which the criteria of dissemination in time has not been met to diagnose multiple sclerosis (MS)
   b. Classified as relapsing or progressive disease; subclassified according to disease activity and progression
      – Relapsing-remitting: 85% of patients at diagnosis, develops into progressive disease in 50% of patients within 10 years

B. Epidemiology
1. Diagnosis usually between 20 and 50 years of age
2. Twice as many women as men develop multiple sclerosis.
3. Whites and people of northern European heritage are more likely to develop MS.
4. Risk factors: Family history of MS, autoimmune disease, or migraine; personal history of autoimmune diseases or migraine; cigarette smoke exposure (women only)

C. Treatment
1. Acute relapses are treated with corticosteroids.
   a. Intravenous methylprednisolone: The usual dose is 1 g/day as one dose or divided doses for 3–5 days.
   b. Oral prednisone: The usual dose is 1250 mg/day given every other day for five doses.
   c. Intravenous adrenocorticotropic hormone
   d. Neurologic recovery is the same with or without an oral prednisone taper.

2. Disease-modifying therapies (Table 9)
   a. Beta interferons (Avonex, Betaseron, Extavia, Plegridy, Rebif)
      i. Mechanism of action: Suppress T-cell activity, downregulate antigen presentation by major histocompatibility complex class II molecules, decrease adhesion molecules and matrix metalloproteinase 9, increase anti-inflammatory cytokines, and decrease inflammatory cytokines
      ii. Adding polyethylene glycol to interferon beta-1a decreases frequency of injections
      iii. Injection site reactions: More common in subcutaneously administered products. It may help to bring a drug to room temperature before injection, ice the injection site, and rotate injection sites.
      iv. Flulike symptoms: Usually dissipate in 2–3 months. It may help to inject the dose in the evening. Begin at the 0.25- to 0.5-mg dose and slowly increase, and use ibuprofen or acetaminophen.
      v. Neutralizing antibodies: Develop in some patients 6–18 months after treatment begins; frequency and administration route affect neutralizing antibody development; relapse rates are higher in patients with persistently high antibody titers; antibodies may disappear even during continued treatment; show cross-reactivity with other beta interferons
   b. Dimethyl fumarate (Tecfidera)
      i. Mechanism of action: Antioxidant and cytoprotective; inhibits proinflammatory cytokines, increases anti-inflammatory cytokines
      ii. Adverse effects
         (a) Skin flushing: Occurs in up to 38% of patients, usually within 30–45 minutes of dosing; involves the face, chest, and neck; dissipates after 15–30 minutes; peaks within first month of therapy and decreases thereafter; aspirin may block flushing, taking with food helps prevent
         (b) GI events: Occur in up to 41% of patients; peak within first month of therapy and decrease thereafter
         (c) Lymphocytes decrease by 30% in the first year of therapy and then stabilize.
   c. Glatiramer acetate (Copaxone)
      i. Mechanism of action: Decreases type 1 helper T cells; increases type 2 helper T cells; increases production of nerve growth factors
      ii. Injection site reactions: Icing the site before and after injection may help.
      iii. Systemic reactions: May involve flushing, chest tightness, palpitations, anxiety, and shortness of breath; this is noncardiac; recurrence is infrequent.
   d. Fingolimod (Gilenya)
      i. Mechanism of action: Binds to the S1P receptor 1 expressed on T cells, prevents activation of T cells
      ii. Contraindicated in patients with myocardial infarctions, unstable angina, stroke, TIAs, or decompensated heart failure necessitating hospitalization or class III/IV heart failure, history of Mobitz type II second- or third-degree atrioventricular block or sick sinus syndrome unless patient has a pacemaker, baseline QTc interval greater than or equal to 500 milliseconds, or treatment with class Ia or class III antiarrhythmic drugs
      iii. Patients must be monitored for bradycardia for 6 hours after the first dose; if therapy is discontinued for more than 2 weeks, patients must be remonitored.
      iv. Adverse effects
         (a) Bradycardia: Electrocardiogram is recommended within 6 months for patients using antiarrhythmics (including β-blockers and calcium channel blockers), those with cardiac risk factors, and those with slow or irregular heartbeat. Heart rate returns to baseline within 1 month of continued dosing.
         (b) Atrioventricular conduction delays: First- and second-degree block

(c) Decrease in lymphocytes: A recent complete blood cell count should be available before therapy starts. Infections may be more common. Discontinue therapy for serious infections; test patients without varicella zoster vaccine or infection history for varicella zoster virus antibodies, and immunize antibody-negative patients (wait 1 month to begin fingolimod).

(d) Macular edema: Ophthalmologic evaluation at baseline and 3–4 months after fingolimod initiation; a history of uveitis or diabetes mellitus increases risk.

(e) Respiratory effects: Decreases in forced expiratory volume over 1 second and diffusion lung capacity for carbon monoxide can be seen.

(f) Elevation of liver enzymes

(g) Hypertension: Monitor during treatment.

(h) Extended effects of drug for up to 2 months after discontinuation necessitate extended monitoring for many adverse effects.

   v. Drug interactions

(a) Ketoconazole: Increased fingolimod

(b) Vaccines: Less effective during and 2 months after fingolimod treatment; avoid live, attenuated vaccines.

   vi. Avoid pregnancy during treatment and for 2 months after treatment.

e. Mitoxantrone (Novantrone)

   i. Mechanism of action: Decreases monocytes and macrophages, inhibits T and B cells

   ii. Indicated for secondary progressive, progressive-relapsing, and worsening-relapsing-remitting multiple sclerosis

   iii. Because of the potential for toxicity, mitoxantrone is reserved for patients with rapidly advancing disease whose other therapies have failed.

   iv. Patients taking mitoxantrone should not receive live virus vaccines; other vaccines should be held for 4–6 weeks after dose.

   v. Cardiotoxicity: Echocardiograms or multiple-gated acquisition scans must be performed at baseline and before each infusion. Systolic dysfunction occurs in about 12% of patients; congestive heart failure occurs in about 0.4%. Cardiotoxicity is not dose-, sex-, or age-related. Cyclooxygenase 2 inhibitors should be avoided.

   vi. Therapy-related acute leukemia occurs in about 0.8% of patients.

   vii. Other laboratory tests (complete blood cell count, bilirubin, aspartate aminotransferase (AST), alanine aminotransferase (ALT), alkaline phosphatase, and pregnancy test) must be performed before each infusion.

   viii. Avoid pregnancy during treatment.

f. Natalizumab (Tysabri)

   i. Mechanism of action: Block T-cell entry into the CNS

   ii. Indicated for relapsing forms of multiple sclerosis but distributed through restricted distribution program because of progressive multifocal leukoencephalopathy risk (0.24%)

   iii. Adverse effects

(a) Hypersensitivity reactions: Itching, dizziness, fever, rash, hypotension, dyspnea, chest pain, anaphylaxis, usually within 2 hours of administration

(b) Progressive multifocal leukoencephalopathy: Rapidly progressive viral CNS infection; usually results in death or permanent disability. Patient selection guidelines are for patients with relapsing-remitting disease whose other treatment (efficacy or intolerability) has failed or who have an aggressive initial course; it should not be used in combination with other disease-modifying therapies. On January 20, 2012, an FDA-issued drug safety communication associated positive tests for John Cunningham virus (JCV) antibodies as a risk factor for progressive multifocal leukoencephalopathy. Thus, patients with all three of the following risk factors—presence of anti-JCV antibodies, longer duration of natalizumab treatment (especially beyond 2 years), and previous treatment with an immunosuppressant medication (mitoxantrone, azathioprine, methotrexate, cyclophosphamide, mycophenolate mofetil)—are at 1.1% chance of developing progressive multifocal leukoencephalopathy.

    (c) Antibodies to natalizumab, associated with increased relapses and hypersensitivity reactions, develop in 9%–12% of patients.

g. Teriflunomide (Aubagio)

    i. Mechanism of action: Prevents activation of lymphocytes

    ii. Indicated for relapsing forms of multiple sclerosis

    iii. Pharmacokinetics: Long half-life (8–19 days); takes about 3 months to reach steady-state concentrations; takes an average of 8 months to eliminate drug (serum concentrations less than 0.02 mcg/mL) and may take up to 2 years

    iv. Adverse effects

        (a) Hepatotoxicity may occur; teriflunomide should not be used in patients with preexisting liver disease or with ALT more than 2 times the upper limit of normal

        (b) GI effects: Diarrhea, nausea

        (c) Dermatologic effects: Alopecia, rash

        (d) Infection: Neutropenia and lymphopenia may occur; tuberculosis (TB) infections reported (negative TB skin test required at baseline); live virus vaccinations should not be administered.

        (e) Teratogenic: Pregnancy category X (based on animal studies); negative pregnancy test at baseline; adequate contraception should be ensured; if pregnancy desired for men or women, teriflunomide should be discontinued, accelerated elimination procedures should be undertaken, and two serum concentrations less than 0.02 mcg/mL taken 14 days apart should be confirmed.

    v. Accelerated elimination procedures

        (a) Cholestyramine 8 g every 8 hours for 11 days (if not tolerated, may use 4 g)

        (b) Activated charcoal powder 50 g every 12 hours for 11 days

3. Symptomatic therapies

a. Patients may experience fatigue, spasticity, urinary incontinence, pain, depression, cognitive impairment, fecal incontinence, constipation, pseudobulbar affect, and sexual dysfunction; treatment should be with standard therapies for these symptoms.

b. Fatigue: Treatment may be nonpharmacologic (rest, assistive devices, cooling strategies, exercise, stress management) or pharmacologic (amantadine, methylphenidate).

c. Spasticity: Therapies must be centrally acting.

    i. First line: Baclofen, tizanidine

    ii. Second line: Dantrolene, diazepam

    iii. Third line: Intrathecal baclofen

    iv. Focal spasticity: Botulinum toxin

d. Walking impairment: Dalfampridine (Ampyra)

    i. Indicated to improve walking in patients with multiple sclerosis by improving walking speed

    ii. Potassium channel blocker, prolongs action potentials in demyelinated neurons

    iii. Dose: 10 mg orally twice daily; extended-release tablets

    iv. Contraindicated in patients with a history of seizures or moderate or severe renal impairment

    v. Adverse effects: Seizures, urinary tract infections, insomnia

e. Pseudobulbar affect: Dextromethorphan/quinidine
   i. Affects 10% of patients
   ii. Episodes of inappropriate laughing or crying
   iii. Dextromethorphan prevents excitatory neurotransmitter release.
   iv. Low-dose quinidine blocks first-pass metabolism of dextromethorphan, thus increasing dextromethorphan serum concentrations.

Table 9. Comparison of Disease-Modifying Therapies

Drug (Brand)	Dose	Route	Frequency	Adverse Effects
Dimethyl fumarate (Tecfidera)	120 mg twice daily x 7 days; then 240 mg twice daily	PO	Twice daily	Skin flushing 38% GI events 41%
Fingolimod (Gilenya)	0.5 mg	PO	Daily	Increased AST/ALT 14% Infections 13% Diarrhea 12% Hypertension 6% Bradycardia 4% Blurred vision 4% Lymphopenia 4% Leukopenia 3%
Glatiramer acetate (Copaxone)	20 mg 40 mg	SC SC	Daily Three times/week	Injection site reaction 90% Systemic reaction 15%
Interferon beta-1a (Avonex)	30 mcg	IM	Weekly	Flulike symptoms 61% Anemia 8%
Interferon beta-1a (Rebif)	22 or 44 mcg	SC	Three times/week	Flulike symptoms 28% Injection site reactions 66% Leukopenia 22% Increased AST/ALT 17%–27%
Interferon beta-1b (Betaseron)	0.25 mg	SC	Every other day	Flulike symptoms 60%–76% Injection site reactions 50%–85% Asthenia 49% Menstrual disorder 17% Leukopenia 10%–16% Increased AST/ALT 4%–19%
Mitoxantrone (Novantrone)	12 mg/m^2 Up to 140 mg/m^2 (lifetime dose)	IV	Every 3 months	Nausea 76% Alopecia 61% Menstrual disorders 61% Urinary tract infection 32% Amenorrhea 25% Leukopenia 19% γ-Glutamyl transpeptidase increase of 15%

Table 9. Comparison of Disease-Modifying Therapies *(continued)*

Drug (Brand)	Dose	Route	Frequency	Adverse Effects
Natalizumab (Tysabri)	300 mg	IV	Every 4 weeks	Headache 38% Fatigue 27% Arthralgia 19% Urinary tract infection 20% Hypersensitivity reaction <1%
Pegylated interferon beta-1a (Plegridy)	125 mcg	SC	Every 2 weeks	Injection site reactions 62% Flulike symptoms 47% Headache 44% Myalgia 19%
Teriflunomide (Aubagio)	7 mg or 14 mg	PO	Daily	Diarrhea 15%–18% Nausea 9%–14% Alopecia 10%–13% Neutropenia 10%–15% Lymphopenia 7%–10% Elevated ALT 3%–5% Hypertension 4% Peripheral neuropathy 1%–2%

GI, gastrointestinal; IM = intramuscular; IV = intravenous; PO = by mouth; SC = subcutaneous.

Patient Cases

Questions 26–28 pertain to the following case:

S.F. is a 33-year-old African American woman of Cuban descent living in the Miami area. This morning, her right leg became progressively weaker over about 3 hours. She was previously healthy except for a broken radius when she was 13 years old and a case of optic neuritis when she was 25 years old.

26. Which method is best for treating S.F.'s exacerbation?

    A. Interferon beta-1a.

    B. Glatiramer acetate.

    C. Mitoxantrone.

    D. Methylprednisolone.

27. Which therapy is best for S.F. to prevent further exacerbations?

    A. Interferon beta-1a.

    B. Interferon beta-1b.

    C. Glatiramer acetate.

    D. Any of the above.

Patient Cases *(continued)*

28. S.F. elects to start interferon beta-1b and wants to know whether she can prevent or minimize some of the adverse effects. Which advice is best?

    A. Always give the injection at the same time of day.

    B. Lie down for 2 hours after the injection.

    C. Rotate injection sites.

    D. Use a heating pad on the injection sites.

29. B.B. is a 33-year-old woman with a recent diagnosis of multiple sclerosis. Her neurologist wants you to discuss with her potential medications to prevent exacerbations. During the discussion, you find that she and her husband are planning to have a baby in the next few years and that she is terrified of needles. Which choice is best for B.B.?

    A. Glatiramer acetate.

    B. Mitoxantrone.

    C. Teriflunomide.

    D. Dimethyl fumarate.

REFERENCES

Epilepsy

1. Brophy GM, Bell R, Claassen J, et al. Guidelines for the evaluation and management of status epilepticus. Neurocrit Care 2012;17:3-23. A review of emergency management of status epilepticus, including expert consensus opinion.

2. Glauser T, Ben-Manachem E, Bourgeois B, et al. Updated ILAE evidence review of antiepileptic drug therapy efficacy and effectiveness as initial monotherapy of epileptic seizures and syndromes. Epilepsia 2013;54:551-63. Available at www.ilae.org/Visitors/Documents/Guidelines-epilepsia-12074-2013.pdf. Accessed September 18, 2014. Reviews levels of evidence for all antiepileptic drugs for monotherapy of partial seizures in adults, children, and older adults, generalized seizures in adults and children.

3. Harden CL, Hopp J, Ting TY, et al. Practice parameter update: management issues for women with epilepsy. Focus on pregnancy (an evidence-based review): obstetrical complications and change in seizure frequency. Neurology 2009;73:126-32. Available at www.neurology.org/content/73/2/126.full.html. Accessed September 18, 2014. Provides conclusions about the influence of seizure medications on the risk of cesarean delivery, late pregnancy bleeding, premature contractions, and premature labor and delivery.

4. Harden CL, Meador KJ, Pennell PB, et al. Practice parameter update: management issues for women with epilepsy. Focus on pregnancy (an evidence-based review): teratogenesis and perinatal outcomes. Neurology 2009;73:133-41. Available at www.neurology.org/content/73/2/133.full.html. Accessed September 18, 2014. Provides conclusions about the effect of seizure medications on the risk of major congenital malformations, poor cognitive outcomes, and other adverse effects.

5. Harden CL, Pennell PB, Koppel BS, et al. Practice parameter update: management issues for women with epilepsy. Focus on pregnancy (an evidence-based review): vitamin K, folic acid, blood levels, and breastfeeding. Neurology 2009;73:142-9. Available at www.neurology.org/content/73/2/142.full.html. Accessed September 18, 2014. Provides conclusions about the use of preconception folic acid, the ability of seizure medications to cross the placenta, and the penetration of seizure medications into breast milk. Provides recommendations about the monitoring of seizure medication serum concentrations during pregnancy.

6. Mula M, Kanner AM, Schmitz B, et al. Antiepileptic drugs and suicidality: an expert consensus statement from the Task Force on Therapeutic Strategies of the ILAE Commission on Neuropsychobiology. Epilepsia 2013;54:199-203. Expert opinion paper reviewing available data on the risk of suicide and suicidal behavior while taking antiepileptics for epilepsy.

7. National Institute for Health and Clinical Excellence. The Epilepsies: The Diagnosis and Management of the Epilepsies in Adults and Children in Primary and Secondary Care. NICE Clinical Guideline 137. Issued January 2012. Available at www.nice.org.uk/guidance/CG137. Accessed September 18, 2014. Extensive review of diagnosis and treatment of seizures, including medical management.

8. Perucca E, Tomson T. The pharmacological treatment of epilepsy in adults. Lancet Neurol 2011;10:446-56. A solid review of current treatment issues and practices, including when treatment should be initiated, drugs of choice for initial treatment, management of drug-refractory patients, and discontinuation of seizure medications in seizure-free patients.

Stroke

1. Culebras A, Messe SR, Caturvedi S, et al. Summary of evidence-based guideline update: prevention of stroke in nonvalvular atrial fibrillation. Neurology 2014;82:716-24. Available at www.neurology.org/content/82/8/716.full. Accessed September 17, 2014. Detailed discussion of stroke prevention in patients with atrial fibrillation.

2. Goldstein LB, Bushnell CD, Adams RJ, et al. Guidelines for the primary prevention of stroke: a guideline for healthcare professionals from the American Heart Association/American Stroke Association. Stroke 2011;42:517-84. This is an

extremely detailed discussion of the risk factors for stroke and their influence on primary stroke occurrence.

3. Lansberg MG, O'Donnell MJ, Khatri P, et al. Antithrombotic and thrombolytic therapy for ischemic stroke: Antithrombotic Therapy and Prevention of Thrombosis, 9th ed. American College of Chest Physicians Evidence-Based Clinical Practice Guidelines. Chest 2012;141:e601S-36S. Comprehensive review of evidence for secondary stroke prevention.

4. You JJ, Singer DE, Howard PA, et al. Antithrombotic and thrombolytic therapy for atrial fibrillation: Antithrombotic Therapy and Prevention of Thrombosis, 9th ed. American College of Chest Physicians Evidence-Based Clinical Practice Guidelines. Chest 2012;141:e531S-75S. Gold standard for anticoagulation recommendations in atrial fibrillation.

Parkinson Disease

1. Horstink M, Tolosa E, Bonuccelli U, et al. Review of the therapeutic management of Parkinson's disease. Report of a joint task force of the European Federation of Neurological Societies and the Movement Disorder Society—European Section. Part I. Early (uncomplicated) Parkinson's disease. Eur J Neurol 2006;13:1170-85. Guidelines for treatment of the patient who has recently received a diagnosis of Parkinson disease.

2. Horstink M, Tolosa E, Bonuccelli U, et al. Review of the therapeutic management of Parkinson's disease. Report of a joint task force of the European Federation of Neurological Societies and the Movement Disorder Society—European Section. Part II. Late (complicated) Parkinson's disease. Eur J Neurol 2006;13:1186-202. Similar to the above reference but with an emphasis on the patient with long-standing Parkinson disease. A short review of surgical treatments is also included.

3. Miyasaki JM, Shannon K, Voon V, et al. Practice parameter: evaluation and treatment of depression, psychosis, and dementia in Parkinson disease (an evidence-based review). Report of the Quality Standards Subcommittee of the American Academy of Neurology. Neurology 2006;66:996-1002. Available at www.neurology.org/cgi/reprint/66/7/983.pdf. Accessed October 15, 2013. Reviews available evidence on depression, psychosis, and dementia. Provides more in-depth reading and summarizes most clinical trials on the subject.

4. Olanow CW, Stern MB, Sethi K. The scientific and clinical basis for the treatment of Parkinson disease (2009). Neurology 2009;72(suppl 4):S1-136. An extensive treatise on pathophysiology and treatment of Parkinson disease.

5. Pahwa R, Factor SA, Lyons KE, et al. Practice parameter: treatment of Parkinson disease with motor fluctuations and dyskinesia (an evidence-based review). Report of the Quality Standards Subcommittee of the American Academy of Neurology. Neurology 2006;66:983-95. Available at www.neurology.org/cgi/reprint/66/7/983. Accessed October 15, 2013. Reviews available evidence on motor adverse effects and their treatment. Good for more in-depth reading.

6. Zesiewicz TA, Sullivan KL, Amulf I, et al. Practice parameter: treatment of nonmotor symptoms of Parkinson disease. Report of the Quality Standards Subcommittee of the American Academy of Neurology. Neurology 2010;74:924-31. Provides detailed reading on treating symptoms other than the cardinal signs of Parkinson disease.

Headaches

1. Francis GJ, Becker WJ, Pringsheim TM. Acute and preventative pharmacologic treatment of cluster headache. Neurology 2010;75:463-73. Systematic review and meta-analysis of treatment trials for cluster headache. Endorsed by the AAN.

2. Holland S, Silberstein SD, Freitag F, et al. Evidence-based guideline update: NSAIDs and other complementary treatments for episodic migraine prevention in adults: report of the Quality Standards Subcommittee of the American Academy of Neurology and the American Headache Society. Neurology 2012;78:1346-53. Available at www.neurology.org/content/78/17/1346.full.pdf. Accessed October 15, 2013. Discussion of use of nonsteroidal anti-inflammatory drugs and complementary and alternative medicines for migraine prevention.

3. Silberstein SD, Holland S, Freitag F, et al. Evidence-based guideline update: pharmacologic treatment for episodic migraine prevention in adults: report of the Quality Standards Subcommittee of the American Academy of Neurology and the American Headache Society. Neurology 2012;78:1337-45. Available at www.neurology.org/content/78/17/1337.full. Accessed October 15, 2013. Discussion of prophylactic medications for migraine prevention, excluding nonsteroidal anti-inflammatory drugs, complimentary therapies, and botulinum toxin.

Multiple Sclerosis

1. Bendtzen K. Critical review: assessment of interferon-β immunogenicity in multiple sclerosis. J Interferon Cytokine Res 2010;30:759-66. Discussion of the known aspects of interferon-neutralizing antibodies.

2. Goodin DS, Cohen BA, O'Connor P, et al. Assessment: the use of natalizumab (Tysabri) for the treatment of multiple sclerosis (an evidence-based review). Neurology 2008;71:766-73. Available at www.neurology.org/content/71/10/766.full.pdf. Accessed October 15, 2013. A supplement to the primary guideline and a discussion of progressive multifocal leukoencephalopathy related to natalizumab administration.

3. Goodin DS, Frohman EM, Garmany GP, et al. Disease-modifying therapies in multiple sclerosis: subcommittee of the American Academy of Neurology and the MS Council for Clinical Practice Guidelines. Neurology 2002;58:169-78. Current guideline, reaffirmed July 19, 2008.

4. Marriott JJ, Miyasaki JM, Gronseth G, et al. Evidence report: the efficacy and safety of mitoxantrone (Novantrone) in the treatment of multiple sclerosis. Report of the Therapeutics and Technology Assessment Subcommittee of the American Academy of Neurology. Neurology 2010;74:1463-70. Available at www.neurology.org/cgi/reprint/74/18/1463. Accessed October 15, 2013. Review of evidence associating mitoxantrone with cardiac dysfunction and therapy-related acute leukemia.

ANSWERS AND EXPLANATIONS TO PATIENT CASES

1. Answer: A

Leukopenia is a common adverse effect of carbamazepine. Up to 10% of patients experience a transient decrease in their white blood cell count; however, the potential for serious hematologic abnormalities, including agranulocytosis and aplastic anemia, exists. Complete blood cell counts are recommended before initiation and periodically during therapy.

2. Answer: A

In general, dermatologic reactions to anticonvulsants occur after a delay of 2–8 weeks rather than immediately after medication initiation.

3. Answer: D

The rash that occurs with lamotrigine is often related to the speed of titration. Valproic acid inhibits the metabolism of lamotrigine; therefore, when these drugs are used together, the lamotrigine titration must be slowed even further. Psychomotor slowing, renal stones, and paresthesias are associated with topiramate and zonisamide.

4. Answer: B

Lorazepam is the drug of choice for status epilepticus. It is less lipophilic than diazepam; therefore, it does not redistribute from the CNS as quickly. After the seizures are stopped with lorazepam, a long-acting drug (phenytoin, fosphenytoin, or phenobarbital) should be administered to prevent further seizures.

5. Answer: D

Phenytoin shows nonlinear pharmacokinetics. A small increase in dose may result in a large increase in serum concentration. Therefore, without performing any calculations, we can surmise that an increase from 300 mg/day to 600 mg/day would more than double the serum concentration.

6. Answer: D

Ethosuximide is useful for absence seizures. The other listed medications are not used for absence seizures.

7. Answer: A

Drowsiness is a dose-related adverse effect of phenytoin. Acne, gingival hyperplasia, and rash can also be adverse effects, but they are not dose related.

8. Answer: C

Valproic acid and its derivatives are associated with alopecia. The hair will grow back if the drug is discontinued and sometimes even if the drug is continued. There are reports of the regrown hair being curly when patients previously had straight hair.

9. Answer: D

Carbamazepine forms an active epoxide intermediate (carbamazepine-10,11-epoxide), whereas oxcarbazepine does not. Carbamazepine induces more liver enzymes than oxcarbazepine. However, hyponatremia is more closely associated with oxcarbazepine than carbamazepine. Both drugs can cause allergic rashes.

10. Answer: C

Alterations to seizure treatment regimens can be made when patients present to the health system before pregnancy. In this case, a different drug may be chosen, or medications may be eliminated if the patient is taking more than one seizure medication. In addition, efforts should be made to maintain the patient on the lowest possible doses that control seizures. However, when the patient presents to the health system already pregnant, the current medications are usually continued to avoid the risk of an increase in seizures during a medication change. Again, the lowest possible doses that control seizures should be used.

11. Answer: D

Nonmodifiable risk factors for stroke include age, race, and male sex. Somewhat modifiable risk factors include hypercholesterolemia and diabetes mellitus. Modifiable stroke risk factors include hypertension, smoking, and atrial fibrillation. Less well-documented risk factors include obesity, physical inactivity, alcohol abuse, hyperhomocystinemia, hypercoagulability, hormone replacement therapy, and oral contraceptives. Modification of risk factors, if possible, may translate into reduced stroke risk, which should be a focus of all stroke prevention plans.

12. Answer: C

Contraindications to administering tissue plasminogen activator for stroke include intracranial or subarachnoid bleeding (or history), other active internal bleeding, recent intercranial surgery, head trauma, BP greater than 185/110 mm Hg, seizure at stroke onset, intracranial neoplasm, atrioventricular malformation, aneurysm, active treatment with warfarin or heparin, and platelet count less than 100,000. There is no upper limit on age. Until recently, there was a strict 3-hour limit for treating strokes. A recent study suggests this limit can be increased safely to administer tissue plasminogen activator 4½ hours after symptom onset with additional criteria.

13. Answer: C

All patients experiencing a stroke should be placed on a drug to prevent future events. Appropriate choices include aspirin, ticlopidine, cilostazol, clopidogrel, dipyridamole/aspirin, and warfarin. However, because of the risk of neutropenia, ticlopidine is usually not used first-line. If the patient has atrial fibrillation, he or she should be treated with warfarin, dabigatran, or rivaroxaban. If the patient does not have atrial fibrillation, warfarin offers no benefit but has considerable risk compared with aspirin. Otherwise, any of these drugs are reasonable choices.

14. Answer: C

No therapy is an appropriate choice for this patient (CHA_2DS_2-VASc score of 0) because he is younger than 65 years and has no other risk factors such as hypertension or a prosthetic valve.

15. Answer: C

The target INR for a patient younger than 75 years with hypertension and diabetes mellitus is 2.5.

16. Answer: D

Anticholinergic drugs (benztropine and trihexyphenidyl) commonly cause adverse effects such as confusion, dry mouth, urinary retention, and constipation in older patients. Decreasing or eliminating these drugs may resolve the difficulties.

17. Answer: D

Wearing-off phenomenon is the return of Parkinson disease symptoms before the next dose. This problem can be resolved by giving doses more often, administering the controlled-release formulation of carbidopa/levodopa, or adding a catechol-O-methyl transferase inhibitor. The terms *increase the dosing interval* and *decrease the dosing interval* are often misinterpreted. To increase the dosing interval means to give the doses farther apart.

18. Answer: C

Amantadine can cause livedo reticularis, a condition in which the dilation of capillary blood vessels and the stagnation of blood within these vessels cause a mottled, reddish blue discoloration of the skin. This usually occurs on the trunk and extremities; it is more pronounced in cold weather. Although simple venous stasis could occur, livedo reticularis is more likely in this patient.

19. Answer: D

Treatment of dyskinesias includes decreasing the levodopa dose, removing selegiline or dopamine agonists from the drug regimen, or adding amantadine.

20. Answer: D

Ropinirole, a direct dopamine agonist, is a good choice for initial treatment in a patient with Parkinson disease. Trihexyphenidyl would control his tremor but would not improve his difficulty walking, which probably represents bradykinesia. Entacapone is a catechol-O-methyltransferase inhibitor; it should be used only in conjunction with carbidopa/levodopa. Apomorphine is for severe on-off symptoms.

21. Answer: A

A β-blocker is a good choice for a patient with the coexisting condition of hypertension. Valproic acid and amitriptyline could both increase weight gain in a morbidly obese patient. Lithium is used for prophylaxis of cluster headaches.

22. Answer: C

Amitriptyline is as effective as prophylaxis for tension headaches. β-Blockers and valproic acid are usually used for migraine headache prophylaxis, and lithium is used for prophylaxis of cluster headaches.

23. Answer: D

Lithium is a prophylactic agent for cluster headaches. β-Blockers and valproic acid are usually used for migraine headache prophylaxis. Amitriptyline is useful for migraine and tension headaches.

24. Answer: D

Sumatriptan is available as an injectable and as a nasal spray and would be more appropriate to use in a patient with severe nausea and vomiting. Zolmitriptan is available as a nasal spray. The other triptans are available only in oral preparations.

25. Answer: A

The NNT is a concept used to express the number of patients it would be necessary to treat to have one patient experience benefit (or to experience adverse effects, if looking at harm). It is calculated as NNT = 1/[(% improved on active therapy) − (% improved on placebo)]. The NNT is calculated for each treatment and is therefore treatment-specific. Low NNTs indicate high treatment efficacy. If an NNT of 1 were calculated, it would mean that every patient on active therapy improved and that no patient on placebo improved.

26. Answer: D

Methylprednisolone is the only option used for treating acute exacerbations. Other options are high-dose oral prednisone or adrenocorticotropic hormone. Interferon beta-1a, glatiramer acetate, and mitoxantrone are all used as disease-modifying therapies.

27. Answer: D

The beta interferons and glatiramer acetate are appropriate initial choices for disease-modifying therapy. Mitoxantrone and natalizumab would not be used as a first-line therapy because of their potential toxicities.

28. Answer: C

Rotating the injection sites for the self-injections is a good strategy for preventing injection site reactions. Other strategies that might help prevent these reactions are icing the injection site before injection and bringing the drug to room temperature. The injections should be administered at about the same time of day, but this is not a strategy for preventing adverse effects.

29. Answer: D

Patients unable to give self-injection because of their fear of needles should not be given glatiramer acetate, which is a subcutaneous injection. Mitoxantrone has significant toxicities, and it is infrequently used to treat multiple sclerosis. In addition, this drug is pregnancy category X. Teriflunomide may take up to 2 years for elimination or rapid elimination protocols before pregnancy; thus, it would not be a good choice in this patient. Dimethyl fumarate has no data in human pregnancy right now and is pregnancy category C. However, this patient should carefully plan her conception and can discontinue the medication before pregnancy. Of the available choices, dimethyl fumarate is the best answer.

ANSWERS AND EXPLANATIONS TO SELF-ASSESSMENT QUESTIONS

1. Answer: C

The therapeutic range for phenytoin is 10–20 mcg/mL. Although a serum concentration should never be interpreted without clinical information, this patient is having no seizures, nor is he experiencing toxicity. Because he is otherwise healthy, does not have known kidney dysfunction, and is not elderly, there is no need for an albumin concentration.

2. Answer: B

In general, medications to treat status epilepticus should be in parenteral formulation to facilitate rapid administration. Once the seizures of status epilepticus have been stopped, a second, long-acting drug should be initiated to prevent seizure recurrence. Medications typically used for this purpose include phenytoin, fosphenytoin, phenobarbital, and (sometimes) valproic acid. Another benzodiazepine need not be administered because this patient's seizure activity has ceased.

3. Answer: C

Psychomotor slowing is a very troublesome adverse effect for many patients initiated on topiramate. It usually manifests as difficulty concentrating, difficulty thinking, word-finding difficulties, and a feeling of slowness of movement. The usual dosage titration for topiramate calls for increasing the dose every week. This patient has been increasing the topiramate dose every other day. Because psychomotor slowing is related to the speed of titration, this makes slowing the titration rate the most probable answer. Partial seizures could present as confusion; however, they are unlikely to be a continuous condition.

4. Answer: B

Patients who can be treated within 3 hours of stroke symptom onset should be considered for tissue plasminogen activator. A recent study showed good outcomes without excess mortality in patients treated within 4½ hours of stroke onset; however, more exclusion criteria must be applied. Uncontrolled hypertension (greater than 185/100 mm Hg) is a contraindication to tissue plasminogen activator treatment. Active use of heparin (with an elevated partial thromboplastin time) or warfarin (with an elevated INR) is a contraindication, but use of aspirin is not. This patient's onset of stroke symptoms began 6 hours ago, so he is not eligible for tissue plasminogen activator treatment.

5. Answer: D

All stroke survivors require secondary stroke prevention drugs. If a patient claims to be adherent to aspirin when his first stroke occurred, a different drug is usually considered. Clopidogrel or dipyridamole/aspirin would be an acceptable choice. Heparin and enoxaparin are not suitable for long-term home use in secondary stroke prevention.

6. Answer: B

Wearing-off is the return of symptoms before the next dose. It has a definite pattern, whereas on-off is unpredictable. Dyskinesias and dystonias are long-term adverse effects of carbidopa/levodopa.

7. Answer: D

The first dose of apomorphine must be given in a clinic setting. The patient should not take apomorphine if he is allergic to metabisulfite. The dose should be retitrated if he has not taken apomorphine for 1 week. Apomorphine causes severe nausea and vomiting.

8. Answer: A

Because of the MAO inhibition induced by rasagiline, patients should not take meperidine, propoxyphene, tramadol, methadone, dextromethorphan, sympathomimetics, fluoxetine, or fluvoxamine. Guaifenesin can be safely taken in this situation.

9. Answer: D

The choice of drug for acute treatment of a patient with migraines and cardiac disease presents a difficulty. All triptans and ergotamines are contraindicated in this situation. A nonsteroidal anti-inflammatory drug is a possible choice.

10. Answer: A

When possible, a drug for migraine prophylaxis should be selected to confer additional benefit to a patient for a concomitant disease state. In the patient with coronary artery disease and hypertension, propranolol would be an excellent choice for migraine prevention.

11. Answer: D

Fingolimod is the only one of the given choices with an FDA indication for the treatment of multiple sclerosis. In addition, it has the best clinical trial evidence of efficacy. Methylprednisolone is used for treating acute multiple sclerosis exacerbations. Cyclophosphamide and azathioprine have been studied in progressive forms of multiple sclerosis, but their data are not as robust as are those for fingolimod.

12. Answer: B

Treatment of spasticity in multiple sclerosis requires the use of a centrally acting agent. Of the choices given, only diazepam and baclofen are centrally acting. Because of the significant fatigue and drowsiness occurring with diazepam, baclofen is usually a first-line therapy. Another acceptable choice would be tizanidine.

13. Answer: C

Agents used to treat multiple sclerosis–related fatigue include amantadine and methylphenidate. The other choices are not used in multiple sclerosis.

General Psychiatry

Jacintha Cauffield, Pharm.D., BCPS

Palm Beach Atlantic University
Lloyd L. Gregory School of Pharmacy
West Palm Beach, Florida

GENERAL PSYCHIATRY

JACINTHA CAUFFIELD, PHARM.D., BCPS

PALM BEACH ATLANTIC UNIVERSITY
LLOYD L. GREGORY SCHOOL OF PHARMACY
WEST PALM BEACH, FLORIDA

Learning Objectives

1. Describe pharmacotherapeutic options for managing major depression, bipolar disorder, schizophrenia, anxiety disorders, insomnia, and substance abuse.
2. Describe the drugs used to treat these disorders with respect to unique pharmacologic properties, therapeutic uses, adverse effects, and cognitive and behavioral effects.
3. Formulate a pharmacotherapeutic treatment plan when presented with a patient having major depression, bipolar disorder, schizophrenia, anxiety disorder, insomnia, or substance abuse.

Self-Assessment Questions

Answers and explanations to these questions can be found at the end of this chapter.

1. A.B. is a 25-year-old woman who presents to your practice with a depressed mood that has worsened over the past few weeks. She struggles to get out of bed in the morning. When she is not sleeping she is eating. She has gained 10 lb in the past month. She is worried about her job and does not feel like she is "pulling her weight," even though she recently received a glowing evaluation. She has passive thoughts of harming herself but no definite plan. Her past medical history includes anxiety, gastroesophageal reflux disease, and hypothyroidism. She currently takes levothyroxine 100 mcg daily, lansoprazole 30 mg every morning, and alprazolam 0.5 mg three times daily for anxiety. Which medication would best treat her symptoms?

   A. Desipramine.
   B. Fluoxetine.
   C. Mirtazapine.
   D. Paroxetine.

2. K.M. is a 56-year-old woman with recurrent major depression, diabetes type 2 with newly diagnosed neuropathy, obesity, and coronary artery disease. She is currently taking citalopram 40 mg daily, carvedilol 25 mg twice daily, lisinopril 40 mg daily, and metformin 1000 mg twice daily. She is tearful during her appointment and continues to have symptoms of depression despite initial improvement on citalopram. She wants to switch antidepressants. Which would be most beneficial?

   A. Bupropion.
   B. Duloxetine.
   C. Nortriptyline.
   D. Sertraline.

3. L.J. is a 45-year-old man who presents agitated and sweating. His right eyelid started twitching about 1 hour ago, and he cannot get it to stop. He developed cold symptoms 2 days ago and began taking dextromethorphan and pseudoephedrine. His past medical history includes depression, hypertension, and hyperlipidemia. He takes paroxetine 40 mg at bedtime, diltiazem XR 240 mg daily, and rosuvastatin 10 mg daily. Which combination of medications is contributing to his current symptoms?

   A. Cetirizine and paroxetine.
   B. Dextromethorphan and pseudoephedrine.
   C. Diltiazem and pseudoephedrine.
   D. Paroxetine and dextromethorphan.

4. H.G. is a 31-year-old man with a 5-year history of bipolar disorder type I, for which he takes lithium 300 mg twice daily. His serum concentration, taken yesterday before his morning dose of lithium, is 1.0 mEq/L. He has been without manic symptoms for the past few years. He was admitted for a suicide gesture using acetaminophen. Over the past few weeks, he has lost interest in his job and is isolating himself from other people. Which medication would best help his acute symptoms?

   A. Aripiprazole.
   B. Lamotrigine.
   C. Quetiapine.
   D. Venlafaxine.

5. H.K. is a 28-year-old woman with a history of bipolar type I. She takes lithium 450 mg twice daily. Her last serum concentration (3 months ago) was 0.7 mEq/L. She presents today for an annual examination. Her laboratory test results include sodium 138 mEq/L, potassium 4.7 mEq/L, serum creatinine concentration 0.9 mg/dL, glucose 124 mg/dL, and thyroid-stimulating hormone 24 U/mL. She is 61 inches tall, and she weighs 165 lb, 15 of which

she has gained in the past 2 months. Additional medications include olanzapine 10 mg at bedtime, Yasmin daily, and a multivitamin. Which of the following accounts for these findings?

A. Hypothyroidism.

B. Lithium concentration.

C. Olanzapine.

D. Yasmin.

6. I.T. is a 43-year-old woman with rapid-cycling bipolar disorder, hypertension, obesity, and asthma. She recently switched from lithium to divalproex sodium 500 mg daily. She additionally takes lamotrigine 150 mg twice daily, aripiprazole 30 mg daily, ramipril 10 mg daily, albuterol HFA 2 puffs every 6 hours, and Advair 250/50 twice daily, She started a prednisone taper 3 days ago for an asthma exacerbation. Today she presents with abdominal pain with rebound tenderness, nausea, and vomiting. Laboratory test results include sodium 141 mEq/L, potassium 3.3 mEq/L, chloride 95 mEq/L, carbon dioxide 26 mmol/L, serum creatinine concentration 1.0 mg/dL, glucose 72 mg/dL, cholesterol 165 mg/dL, triglycerides 188 mg/dL, aspartate aminotransferase (AST) 27 IU/L, alanine aminotransferase (ALT) 21 IU/L, amylase 456 U/L, and lipase 387 U/L. Which medication is responsible for the current clinical picture?

A. Aripiprazole.

B. Divalproex sodium.

C. Lamotrigine.

D. Prednisone.

7. N.B. is a 36-year-old man with 16-year history of schizophrenia. He was recently switched to aripiprazole from haloperidol because of gynecomastia and impotence. Today he is pacing your office. He seems anxious and agitated. He has not been sleeping well and feels uncomfortable in his skin. Which medication would help relieve his symptoms?

A. Benztropine.

B. Dantrolene.

C. Lorazepam.

D. Propranolol.

8. T.Y. is a 64-year-old woman with a 25-year history of schizophrenia. Over the past year she has developed involuntary chewing motions and abnormal blinking. It has begun interfering with her ability to eat. She is currently taking haloperidol 2.5 mg twice daily. Her symptoms improved when her haloperidol dose was decreased from 5 mg twice daily but have not resolved. She wants to switch antipsychotics. Which would offer the most relief from her symptoms?

A. Chlorpromazine.

B. Clozapine.

C. Quetiapine.

D. Risperidone.

9. U.M. is a 38-year-old woman with a 4-year history of schizophrenia. Within the past year she has been diagnosed with diabetes type 2 and dyslipidemia. Her body mass index is 32 kg/m². Her father died of a myocardial infarction (MI) at age 42. She has been treated with risperidone but has developed galactorrhea. Concomitant medications include atorvastatin, metformin, and liraglutide. Which antipsychotic would be the best choice?

A. Olanzapine.

B. Paliperidone.

C. Quetiapine.

D. Ziprasidone.

10. N.Y. is a 20-year-old woman who presents to the emergency department after experiencing trembling, sweating, chest pain, and shortness of breath accompanied by intense fear. An MI has been ruled out. Which medication regimen would effectively treat her acute symptoms?

A. Alprazolam.

B. Buspirone.

C. Hydroxyzine.

D. Paroxetine.

11. T.R. is a 55-year-old woman with generalized anxiety disorder. Concomitant medical conditions include history of breast cancer, dyslipidemia, osteoarthritis, menopausal symptoms, and osteopenia. She takes tamoxifen, simvastatin, ibuprofen, lorazepam, and alendronate. Her physician would

like her to have better control of her anxiety symptoms. He would also like to taper her off lorazepam. Which agent would be the best choice?

A. Bupropion.

B. Fluoxetine.

C. Pregabalin.

D. Venlafaxine.

12. O.P. is a 74-year-old woman who has difficulty getting to sleep. Once she falls asleep she rests comfortably throughout the night. She struggles with keeping a bedtime. This problem has been ongoing for the past few months. She has no contributing factors. Concomitant medical conditions include hypertension, arthritis, and mild cognitive impairment. She has tried diphenhydramine. She states it helped for only a few nights and "it made me loopy." She would like a medication with the least risk of hangover effect. Which medication is best?

A. Eszopiclone.

B. Ramelteon.

C. Suvorexant.

D. Zolpidem.

13. M.K. is a 23-year-old man with a history of heroin addiction. He has been successfully maintained on methadone 40 mg daily for 1 year. He would like an option that does not require him to go to a daily opioid treatment program to get his methadone dose. He is not taking other medication, nor does he abuse other substances. Which treatment regimen is appropriate?

A. Initiate supervised buprenorphine/naloxone.

B. Switch to buprenorphine x 2 days, then buprenorphine/naloxone.

C. Switch to naltrexone.

D. Taper to methadone 30 mg, then switch to buprenorphine.

14. C.H. is a 55-year-old man with a 30-year history of alcohol dependence. He drinks 1 pint of vodka daily. He has tried numerous times to quit without success. He has recently reconciled with his estranged son and wants to be sober so that he can be more present in his son's life. His liver function test results include AST 143 IU/L, ALT 74 IU/L,

albumin 4.0 g/dL, alkaline phosphatase 75 IU/L, total bilirubin 0.3 mg/dL, prothrombin time 0.9 seconds, platelet count 370 x 10^3 cells/mm³, and creatinine clearance 40 mL/min. After detoxification, which maintenance treatment is appropriate?

A. Acamprosate 666 mg three times daily.

B. Chlordiazepoxide 25 mg four times daily.

C. Disulfiram 500 mg daily.

D. Naltrexone 50 mg daily.

15. J.Z. is a 44-year-old man who is getting ready to be discharged from the hospital after an MI. He has a 25-pack-year history of smoking cigarettes and smokes 1-1/2 packs per day. He has tried twice unsuccessfully to quit. His additional past medical history includes recurrent depression. He tried quitting cold turkey the first time about 5 years ago. He resumed smoking 6 months later when he lost his job. He tried again approximately 6 months ago using nicotine gum. He used the 2-mg strength. To save money, he chewed 7 pieces daily. Which regimen would be best?

A. Bupropion.

B. Nicotine 4 mg gum.

C. Nicotine patch 21 mg/day.

D. Varenicline.

Patient Cases

Questions 1–4 pertain to the following case:

A.Z. is a 45-year-old woman with sleep apnea, hypertension, type 2 diabetes mellitus, and chronic pain. She is being seen in the clinic today for an assessment of her depressive symptoms and medication evaluation. She endorses sad mood, poor appetite (lost 15 lb), poor concentration, and feelings of hopelessness and worthlessness for the past 3 weeks. She has also stopped going to her book club because she is not motivated to get out of the house, and she has frequent nocturnal awakening. She denies suicidal or homicidal ideation. She denies any use of alcohol, tobacco, or illicit drugs. She is currently taking hydrochlorothiazide, metformin, hydrocodone/acetaminophen, and aspirin. You decide that A.Z. should receive an antidepressant in the selective serotonin reuptake inhibitor (SSRI) class to treat her depressive symptoms.

1. Which SSRI would be most likely to interact with her current medications?

    A. Citalopram.

    B. Fluvoxamine.

    C. Paroxetine.

    D. Sertraline.

2. Which antidepressant would be most appropriate for A.Z.'s depressive symptoms?

    A. Bupropion.

    B. Fluoxetine.

    C. Mirtazapine.

    D. Venlafaxine.

3. It has been 4 weeks since A.Z.'s initial visit with you, and she has been treated with citalopram 20 mg/day in the morning. She still presents with sad mood, but her insomnia, concentration, and appetite have improved. She still has feelings of hopelessness and worthlessness, lack of motivation, and anhedonia. At this point, which is the best recommendation to optimize her therapy?

    A. Continue at current dose of 20 mg/day.

    B. Increase the current dose to 40 mg/day.

    C. Add bupropion 150 mg twice daily.

    D. Switch to a different SSRI.

4. Six months later, A.Z. reports that although her depression symptoms have resolved, she has "trouble" during intercourse, which is quite disturbing to her. You determine that she has anorgasmia caused by citalopram treatment. Which is the most appropriate recommendation at this time?

    A. Discontinue citalopram.

    B. Add bupropion to treat anorgasmia.

    C. Switch to a different SSRI.

    D. Switch to mirtazapine.

I. DEPRESSION

A. Identification of Depressive Disorders. This overview is based on the *Diagnostic and Statistical Manual for Mental Disorders* (*DSM-5*); please consult the *DSM-5* for complete diagnostic criteria.
   1. Major depressive disorder (MDD), otherwise called unipolar disorder. It is diagnosed when a patient exhibits at least 5 of the following symptoms nearly every day for at least 2 weeks:
      a. The patient must have a depressed mood or anhedonia (loss of interest in pleasurable activities).
      b. Additional symptoms include sleep disturbances, changes in weight or appetite, decreased energy, feelings of guilt or worthlessness, psychomotor retardation or agitation, decreased concentration, and suicidal ideation.
      c. The symptoms must interfere with the patient's everyday ability to function.
   2. Persistent depressive disorder (dysthymia): Chronic depressed mood occurring more days than not for at least 2 years but does not meet the criteria for MDD

B. Assessment of Patients With MDD
   1. Psychiatric history: A thorough history of symptoms is compared with the diagnostic criteria, and the diagnosis is made from the collected data.
   2. Clinician rating scales: These are psychometric instruments used to identify depression and assess its severity. Common examples are the Hamilton Rating Scale for Depression (HAM-D) and the Quick Inventory of Depressive Symptoms Clinician Rated. A response is usually defined as at least a 50% reduction in the HAM-D score. "Remission" is a return to a normal state or a HAM-D of 7 or less. Scores from these scales are not required for the diagnosis, but the HAM-D is a standard instrument used to show efficacy in clinical trials for U.S. Food and Drug Administration (FDA) approval. The Clinical Global Impression scale is a clinician-rated scale that evaluates the severity and improvement of patients overall. The Montgomery-Åsberg Depression Rating Scale is another instrument that evaluates symptoms of depression. The Patient Health Questionnaire–9 is based on the *DSM-5* diagnostic criteria for major depression. It is easily administered and assessed and is thus frequently used in the primary care setting.
   3. Patient rating scales: These are patient-completed rating instruments. Answers to the questions are used to identify and assess the level of depression. The Beck Depression Inventory and the Quick Inventory of Depressive Symptoms Self-Rated are examples.
   4. Physical examination and laboratory tests: These are necessary to rule out physical causes (e.g., thyroid disorders, vitamin deficiencies) that may mimic symptoms of depression.
   5. Biologic testing: Depression is commonly associated with abnormalities in the dexamethasone suppression test and tests of the thyroid axis. However, these tests are not routinely used in clinical practice.
   6. Medications and substances (e.g., interferons, benzodiazepines, barbiturates, alcohol, central nervous system depressants, lipid-soluble β-blockers, withdrawal from stimulants, cocaine, amphetamines) can have depression as an adverse effect. Pharmacists should perform a medication and substance use review to identify possible causes.

C. Therapeutic Options
   1. Psychotherapy and exercise: Examples include interpersonal psychotherapy and cognitive-behavioral therapy (CBT). With psychotherapy, it takes longer to observe effectiveness, but when combined with pharmacotherapy, it is effective. It may have broader and longer-lasting effects. Psychotherapy is recommended as monotherapy as initial treatment in patients with mild to moderate MDD (CBT and interpersonal therapy have the best evidence).
   2. Pharmacotherapy: Medication therapy may lead to a more rapid response than psychotherapy, but when it is discontinued, there is a risk of relapse and adverse effects.

3. Electroconvulsive therapy (ECT): Option for refractory depression, depression in pregnancy, psychotic depression, and other conditions for which medications may not be optimal or effective. The usual cycle is two or three treatments per week. Temporary memory loss is common, and medications that affect seizure threshold must be withdrawn before treatment. Electroconvulsive therapy has also been recently suggested as initial treatment if symptoms are severe or life threatening (American Psychiatric Association [APA] 2010 guidelines).

D. Pharmacotherapeutic Options: Considerations and Keys to Use
   1. Selection: All antidepressants are considered to be equally efficacious. First-line medications include selective serotonin reuptake inhibitors (SSRIs), serotonin norepinephrine reuptake inhibitors (SNRIs), bupropion, and mirtazapine. Consider possible drug-drug and drug-disease interactions, concurrent illnesses, prior responses, family members' prior responses, patient preference, and cost.
   2. Onset: In general, it takes 4–6 weeks to see the full effect of antidepressants, given the correct drug, dose, and adherence, but it may take as long as 8 weeks to see a response. Remission may take up to 12 weeks. Some symptoms (e.g., sleep disturbances) may show improvement in 1–2 weeks.
   3. Adequate trial: An adequate trial includes the correct drug for the patient and a therapeutic dose for an appropriate duration. A therapeutic trial ranges from 4 to 8 weeks (2010 APA practice guideline).
   4. Response and remission: A response is usually defined as a 50% reduction in symptoms. Remission is a return to normal mood (e.g., HAM-D of 7 or less). Optimizing the dose or duration is important for achieving remission.
   5. Efficacy of antidepressants according to rigorous clinical trials is about 60%–70%, regardless of drug. Effectiveness, which is more reflective of clinical practice, is lower, about 50%–60%. The remission rate with one antidepressant is about 30%, seen in the recent Sequenced Treatment Alternatives to Relieve Depression (STAR*D trial), when the first drug is initiated.
   6. Drug interactions (Table 1): Many antidepressants inhibit cytochrome P450 (CYP) enzymes.

Table 1. Antidepressants and the CYP System

CYP Enzyme	Inhibition Potential
1A2	Fluvoxamine: high Fluoxetine: moderate
2C	Fluoxetine, fluvoxamine, sertraline: low
2D6	Fluoxetine, paroxetine: very high Duloxetine: moderate Bupropion, citalopram, escitalopram, sertraline: very low
3A4	Nefazodone: very high Fluvoxamine: moderate Fluoxetine: low Sertraline: very low
Minimal CYP inhibition	Venlafaxine, desvenlafaxine, mirtazapine, levomilnacipran

CYP = cytochrome P450.

E. Tricyclic Antidepressants
   1. Tricyclic antidepressants (TCAs) were the first antidepressants available. They are seldom used for depression, but they have several off-label uses such as treatment for pain syndromes, migraine prophylaxis, and anxiety disorders. They are effective, but adverse effects have limited their use. Now that newer agents with more tolerable adverse effect profiles are available, these agents are used less often.

2. They block the reuptake of serotonin and norepinephrine (NE). The tertiary amines are more potent for NE uptake and are metabolized to active secondary amines.
3. In addition to serotonin and NE reuptake, TCAs have α-adrenergic blockade, antihistaminic effects, and anticholinergic effects, leading to orthostasis, sedation, and anticholinergic symptoms, respectively. They also have cardiotoxic effects (Table 2).
4. TCAs can be fatal in overdose. They cause seizures and torsades de pointes. An actively suicidal patient should not receive a TCA.

Table 2. Adverse Effect Profile of the Commonly Used Tricyclic Antidepressants

Drug	Anticholinergic	Sedation	Orthostatic Hypotension	Cardiotoxicity
Tertiary amines				
Amitriptyline	High	High	Moderate	High
Imipramine	Moderate	Moderate	High	High
Secondary amines				
Desipramine	Low	Low	Moderate	Moderate
Nortriptyline	Moderate	Moderate	Low	Moderate

5. These drugs must be used cautiously in patients with cardiac disease or seizure disorders. Patients at risk of orthostatic hypotension are at elevated risk of falls if they take these agents, and appropriate caution should be taken.
6. One advantage of TCAs is that therapeutic serum concentrations can be measured. Therapeutic levels can be used to confirm adherence or toxicity. In clinical practice, this is an infrequent practice.
7. A withdrawal syndrome occurs if these drugs are discontinued too quickly. Symptoms reflect the reversal of anticholinergic effects and include lacrimation, nausea, and diarrhea, with insomnia, restlessness, and possible balance problems. Gradual dose reductions help reduce these symptoms.

F. Monoamine Oxidase Inhibitors
1. Monoamine oxidase inhibitors (MAOIs) block the enzyme responsible for the breakdown of certain neurotransmitters, such as NE. There are two forms of this enzyme (MAO-A and MAO-B), and drugs can block one or both of them. They are effective antidepressants and may be especially useful for atypical depression (hypersomnia, hyperphagia, and mood reactivity).
2. Nonselective drugs (phenelzine and tranylcypromine) are available in the United States.
3. Patients taking MAOIs must be educated and monitored to avoid foods high in tyramine (e.g., aged cheese, preserved meats) because of the potential for precipitating a hypertensive crisis. A dietary consultation can be helpful in this respect.
4. Drug interactions with MAOIs are considerable and include over-the-counter decongestants, antidepressants, stimulants, antihypertensives, and others. When switching a patient from another antidepressant to an MAOI, it is prudent to wait 2 weeks after the antidepressant is discontinued before initiating the MAOI (except for fluoxetine, in which case the waiting period should be 5–6 weeks). When a patient is changed from an MAOI to another antidepressant, a 2-week washout period is usually adequate.
5. Selegiline (MAO-B inhibitor) is available in a patch formulation called Emsam for the treatment of depression. It is available in doses of 6 mg/24 hours, 9 mg/24 hours, and 12 mg/24 hours. Once the dose reaches 9 mg/24 hours, an MAOI diet is required. How this drug compares with other antidepressants remains unknown.

G. Selective Serotonin Reuptake Inhibitors (SSRIs)

1. SSRIs selectively inhibit the reuptake of serotonin into the presynaptic neuron. There has been speculation that they also desensitize the presynaptic serotonin autoreceptor involved in the negative feedback loop that normally inhibits serotonin release. Whichever is true, the result is increased serotonin concentrations in the synapse. The FDA has approved six SSRIs for the treatment of depression: fluoxetine, sertraline, paroxetine, fluvoxamine, citalopram, and escitalopram. Fluvoxamine is indicated only for obsessive-compulsive disorder (OCD) but is an effective antidepressant.

Table 3. Characteristics of SSRIs

Characteristic	Fluoxetine	Sertraline	Paroxetine	Fluvoxamine[a]	Citalopram	Escitalopram
Half-life	1–4 days	26 hours	21 hours	15 hours	32 hours	27–32 hours
Active metabolite	Yes[b]	No	No	No	No	No
Usual dose (mg/day)	20–60	50–200	10–60	50–300	20–40	10–20
Maximal daily dose (mg)	80	200	50 (depression) 60 (anxiety)	300	40	20

[a]Indicated only for obsessive-compulsive disorder; seldom used for depression.
[b]Norfluoxetine.
SSRI = selective serotonin reuptake inhibitor.

2. The efficacy of SSRIs is equal for treatment of depression. There are slight differences in adverse effect profiles, and patients may tolerate one better than another. The STAR*D trial showed that patients who do not respond to one SSRI may respond to another.

3. Blockade of serotonin reuptake leads to an increase in serotonin overall and may influence all subtypes of serotonin receptors. Some of these (serotonin-2A, serotonin-2C, serotonin-3, and serotonin-4) may be responsible for some of the unwanted adverse effects (e.g., insomnia, restlessness, gastrointestinal [GI] complaints). Activation, agitation, anxiety, or panic may be seen in some patients, especially during the early phase of therapy. The most common adverse effects associated with this class of agents include GI complaints, insomnia, restlessness, headache, and sexual dysfunction. In general, the most activating SSRIs are fluoxetine, sertraline, and vilazodone, whereas paroxetine and fluvoxamine are the most sedating. Vortioxetine, citalopram, and escitalopram do not have appreciable sedating or activating effects. Sexual dysfunction is more common than reported in the prescribing information. Some interventions to consider for SSRI-induced sexual dysfunction include using the wait-and-see method, adding bupropion for the treatment of sexual dysfunction, lowering the dose of the SSRI, or adding an agent such as sildenafil or cyproheptadine. Of course, changing to a drug less likely to cause this problem is also reasonable.

4. Because these drugs have such potent serotonergic activity, combinations with other drugs affecting serotonin can lead to serotonin syndrome. Examples include MAOIs, dextromethorphan, meperidine, sympathomimetics, triptans, lithium, TCAs, and SNRIs. Serotonin syndrome includes symptoms from three clusters: neuromuscular hyperactivity (e.g. myoclonus, rigidity, tremors, incoordination), altered mental status (agitation, confusion, hypomania), and autonomic instability (hyperthermia, diaphoresis). It can be subtle in onset or be confused with neuroleptic malignant syndrome. Treatment includes discontinuing the offending agent, providing supportive measures such as cooling blankets and respiratory assistance, and providing clonazepam for myoclonus, anticonvulsants for seizures, and nifedipine for hypertension.

5. SSRIs have been associated with extrapyramidal symptoms (EPS), including akathisia, dystonia, and bradykinesia, but these are not common. This appears to result from an effect of serotonin on dopaminergic neurotransmission in the basal ganglia.

6. A withdrawal syndrome has been observed, especially for the drugs with shorter half-lives, so a gradual dose reduction (e.g., over 2–4 weeks) may be indicated. Symptoms include flulike symptoms, such as nausea and chills, and neurologic symptoms, such as paresthesias, insomnia, anxiety, and "electric shock"-type sensations. If the problem is severe or persists, the drug can be reinitiated and the dose gradually reduced again. It is most common with paroxetine, less so with sertraline, and even less likely with fluoxetine.

7. In 2001, the FDA ordered changes to citalopram package labeling limiting the daily dose to a maximum of 40 mg because of an elevated risk of QTc prolongation at daily doses greater than 40 mg. Patients who have risk factors for QTc prolongation (congenital long QTc syndrome, bradycardia, hypokalemia, hypomagnesemia, recent acute myocardial infarction, and uncompensated heart failure) or have concomitant medications that may increase QTc interval should not be treated with citalopram. Doses of citalopram should be lowered to 40 mg/day in patients who are receiving higher dosages unless the benefits significantly outweigh the risks. The maximal recommended dose of citalopram is 20 mg/day for patients with hepatic impairment, patients who are older than 60 years, patients who are CYP2C19 poor metabolizers, or patients who are taking concomitant cimetidine or another CYP2C19 inhibitor.

8. These drugs are not as lethal in cases of overdose as are TCAs. All SSRIs are available in generic form except for vilazodone and vortioxetine. The low cost and better tolerability of SSRIs warrant them as first-line treatment of MDD in most patients.

9. Extended dosing formulations: Fluoxetine 90 mg can be taken once weekly. It is taken only during continuation therapy rather than as initial treatment. Paroxetine controlled release may have lower rates of nausea in the first week of treatment; efficacy is comparable, and both formulations are administered once daily. The weekly and controlled release (CR) products are available generic but are higher in cost.

10. Escitalopram is the S-isomer of citalopram. It is the active component of the racemic mixture. At a 10-mg dose, it is as effective as citalopram 20 mg (or 40 mg as described in prescribing information), but at this dose, there are fewer adverse effects. At higher doses, this advantage is not as pronounced.

11. SSRIs appear to increase the risk of bleeding. Several mechanisms have been proposed, including the inhibition of serotonin activation of platelets. Case-control and cohort studies also suggest an elevated incidence of both vertebral and nonvertebral bone fractures.

H. Serotonin Norepinephrine Reuptake Inhibitors (SNRIs)
   1. Venlafaxine, desvenlafaxine, duloxetine, and levomilnacipran block the reuptake of NE and serotonin. Unlike TCAs, they have negligible effects at other receptors that cause anticholinergic or antihistaminic adverse effects, with the possible exception of duloxetine, which appears to have a slightly higher incidence of anticholinergic symptoms. Venlafaxine has a dose-related effect on NE compared with desvenlafaxine and duloxetine. At doses less than 150 mg/day, venlafaxine has primarily a serotonin effect.
   2. Levomilnacipran is a newly approved SNRI. It is the enantiomer of milnacipran, the latter of which is approved for the treatment of fibromyalgia but not depression. Levomilnacipran is not approved for the treatment of fibromyalgia. The dose must be adjusted in renal insufficiency, and its use is not recommended in end-stage renal disease. Levomilnacipran can cause hyponatremia and increase bleeding risk. The capsule should not be crushed or opened. It is metabolized through CYP3A4 (major pathway) and through CYP2C19 and CYP2D6, among others (minor pathways). Monitor signs and symptoms of potential toxicities if CYP3A4 inhibitors are used concomitantly. Both blood pressure elevations and orthostatic hypotension can occur. It is a more potent inhibitor of NE than venlafaxine or duloxetine (NE slightly preferred to serotonin).

3. Whether the dual action of venlafaxine makes it more effective than SSRIs is an area of continued research. There appear to be patients (e.g., treatment nonresponders) who benefit either from agents that affect NE and serotonin or from combinations of drugs with that effect.

4. The adverse effect profile of venlafaxine is similar to that of the SSRIs, with GI complaints being common. Of note, venlafaxine can cause increases in blood pressure, which are usually mild and not clinically significant unless the patient already has hypertension that is not well controlled. This is a dose-related phenomenon, as described earlier. All the SNRIs may produce serotonin syndrome. In overdose situations, both duloxetine and venlafaxine have been associated with higher rates of death compared with SSRIs. The risk of suicide completion with SNRIs is still lower than with TCAs.

5. Duloxetine has also been approved for the treatment of diabetic peripheral neuropathy, fibromyalgia, and chronic musculoskeletal pain caused by chronic lower back pain or osteoarthritis pain. Be careful when using this drug with CYP2D6 inhibitors. Monitor blood pressure, because increases have been observed. This drug can cause liver toxicity and should not be used in patients with hepatic insufficiency, end-stage renal disease requiring dialysis, or severe renal impairment.

6. Abrupt discontinuation of venlafaxine can lead to a withdrawal syndrome similar to that with the SSRIs.

7. Desvenlafaxine (Pristiq) is an active metabolite of venlafaxine. Whether it has any advantage over the parent compound is controversial.

8. Both desvenlafaxine and levomilnacipran doses must be adjusted downward with decreased renal function.

I. Mixed Serotonergic Medications

1. Vilazodone (Viibryd) is an SSRI with partial agonist at the serotonin-1A receptor. The clinical significance of this effect is unknown. It has a half-life of 25 hours but does not have active metabolites. Both the usual and maximum doses are 40 mg daily.

2. Vortioxetine inhibits serotonin reuptake, but its pharmacologic profile differs from that of other SSRIs. It has additional agonist activity at the serotonin-1A receptor, partial agonist activity at the serotonin-1B receptor, and antagonistic activity at the serotonin-3, serotonin-1D, and serotonin-7 receptors. The clinical significance of vortioxetine's effect on the serotonin receptors is currently unknown, but it also appears to improve measures of cognitive function that appear independent of its antidepressant effects. Vortioxetine has a half-life of 66 hours and no active metabolites. The starting and usual dose is 10 mg daily, with a maximum daily dose of 20 mg. It is metabolized by CYP2D6, and the maximal dose for poor metabolizers or patients taking a strong CYP2D6 inhibitor is 10 mg daily.

3. Trazodone is a serotonin reuptake inhibitor that also blocks serotonin-2A receptors. It does not cause anticholinergic or cardiotoxic effects, as the TCAs do, but it still causes orthostatic hypotension and sedation. Because of its sedative properties, trazodone is often used for insomnia but at lower doses than those used to treat depression. It is important to be aware of the potential for priapism, even though it is rare (0.1% or less).

4. Nefazodone is a relative of trazodone with some pharmacologic differences. It, too, is a serotonin-2A antagonist, but it also blocks the reuptake of serotonin and NE. Some have referred to this class as serotonin antagonist reuptake inhibitors (serotonin-2A antagonist/reuptake inhibitors). Unlike trazodone, it causes minimal effects on sexual function and is less likely to cause orthostatic hypotension. Some data suggest that the serotonin-2A–blocking activity makes this drug more effective for anxiety associated with depression. The short half-life makes it necessary to administer doses twice daily. The most common adverse effects of this drug include sedation, GI complaints, dry mouth, constipation, confusion, and light-headedness. Because it is a potent inhibitor of CYP3A4, caution is necessary when it is used concomitantly with drugs metabolized by this system. Because of the potential for liver toxicity and the black box warning, nefazodone is now considered a second- or third-line agent. Liver function tests must be monitored if nefazodone is used. The branded product has been withdrawn from the market. Generics remain available.

5. Mirtazapine is an antagonist of presynaptic α_2-autoreceptors and heteroreceptors, which results in an increase in NE and serotonin in the synapse. In addition, the drug blocks serotonin-2A (resulting in no sexual dysfunction, no anxiety, and sedation), serotonin-3 (no nausea and no GI disturbances), and serotonin-2C (weight gain) receptors. Although the drug is better tolerated than the TCAs, it still has a pronounced sedative effect, together with increased appetite, weight gain, constipation, and asthenia. Abnormal liver function tests may occur, and there appears to be a very small risk of neutropenia or agranulocytosis. Lower doses may be sedating, whereas higher doses may cause insomnia.

J. Bupropion
   1. This drug is primarily an inhibitor of dopamine and NE reuptake (at high doses), with minimal effects on serotonin. Its exact mechanism of action remains to be defined. The parent drug blocks dopamine reuptake, whereas the metabolite blocks NE reuptake.
   2. The most important adverse effect is increased risk of seizures. This risk can be minimized by the following:
      a. Avoid use in susceptible patients (e.g., history of seizure disorder, eating disorders).
      b. Do not give more than 150 mg/dose or 450 mg/day (immediate release), 400 mg/day (sustained release), or 450 mg/day (extended release).
      c. Avoid dosage titration any more frequently than every 4 days for sustained or extended release and every 3 days for immediate release.
      d. The sustained- and extended-release products may also cause fewer adverse effects; they have largely replaced the immediate-release tablets.
   3. The most common adverse effects include insomnia, anxiety, irritability, headache, and decreased appetite. The drug can also increase energy and cause psychosis. As noted previously, the drug may actually improve sexual function; thus, it may be useful in patients not tolerating other agents for this reason. Bupropion has also been used for attention-deficit/hyperactivity disorder and may help with concentration.

K. Antidepressants and Suicidality: Antidepressants have been associated with an increased risk of suicidal thinking and behaviors, particularly in children, adolescents, and young adults (up to 24 years of age), which has resulted in a black box warning for all antidepressants, both older and newer agents. It is important to monitor patients, especially children and adolescents, for treatment failure or worsening symptoms of depression when these drugs are initiated or the dose is increased. Other signs to watch for include suicidal ideation, agitation and anxiety (activation syndrome), and other symptoms that are unlike the presenting symptoms of depression in the patient. A medication guide must be distributed before antidepressants are dispensed.

L. Initiating, Adjusting, and Monitoring Therapy
   1. There are three phases of therapy:
      a. Short term (acute): The goal of this phase is remission, which may take 12 weeks. Remission is defined as at least 3 weeks with no symptoms of depressed mood and anhedonia and no more than 3 remaining symptoms of depression.
      b. Continuation: The goal of this phase is to keep the symptoms in remission by using full-dose therapy. This phase usually continues for 4–9 additional months to keep the patient in remission.
      c. Maintenance: Long-term therapy at full doses may be required in patients at high risk of relapse, which would include prior episodes of depression or a strong family history of relapse. The duration of this phase is determined on an individual basis.
   2. An adequate trial of any agent includes full therapeutic doses for at least 6 weeks, up to 12 weeks. If there is no response at this point, the drug can be considered a failure.

3. When one drug has failed, another agent from another class is often tried. However, some patients who do not respond to one SSRI may respond to another, and this is a reasonable option. Treatment resistance can usually be considered when two or more agents from different classes have been tried. At this point, ECT, augmentation therapy, or combination therapy can be considered, if they have not been used already.

4. Patients should be monitored for response through interviews or by repeating rating scales. In addition, patients (and their support systems, if available) should receive education about therapy and be closely monitored for adverse effects. Although most of the adverse effects are not life threatening, they do have an important effect on adherence.

5. The FDA has required that package labels for antidepressants include a statement to monitor patients for emerging suicidal thoughts and behaviors and continuing depressed mood, especially when antidepressants are initiated.

M. Antidepressant Combination Therapy

1. Drugs with different pharmacologic actions are available, and as more is learned about depression, it may be advantageous to treat different systems selectively. It is now possible to affect serotonin, NE, and dopamine differentially. Researchers are actively looking at specific symptoms of depression to determine whether certain presentations respond better to an agent that affects certain neurotransmitter systems. At this point, data are insufficient to guide treatment, but it can be expected that combinations will be used, especially for treatment-resistant depression.

2. The use of combinations with lower doses of each may lead to fewer adverse effects.

3. Using a second antidepressant may offset an adverse effect of another (e.g., using trazodone to treat SSRI-induced insomnia).

4. Adding bupropion to existing SSRI therapy is a strategy for patients who do not fully respond to the SSRI alone.

N. Augmentation Therapy

1. Patients not responding adequately have been successfully treated when nonantidepressant drugs are added to augment existing antidepressant therapy. Data indicate that many patients will respond when these agents are used.

2. Augmentation regimens include the following:

   a. Lithium: Adding lithium appears to help in treatment-resistant depression. The dosing is controversial, ranging from full doses to concentrations used for bipolar disorder to small doses.

   b. Thyroid: Adding thyroid is also effective for treatment-resistant depression. The effect is not dependent on thyroid dysfunction. T_3 appears more effective than T_4. The usual dose is 25 mcg/day.

   c. Buspirone has also been used as an augmenting agent.

   d. Second-generation antipsychotics (SGAs or atypical antipsychotics) are also being used as adjuncts to antidepressant therapy. Almost all of them have been used, but only aripiprazole and Seroquel XR have received FDA approval for this indication. Olanzapine in combination with fluoxetine is also approved for treatment-resistant depression.

O. Treatment Algorithms

1. Several algorithms for treatment exist, including the APA practice guideline on treating patients with MDD (available at www.psychiatryonline.com/pracGuide/pracGuideTopic_7.aspx. Accessed October 11, 2014).

2. The STAR*D study is a large trial sponsored by the National Institute of Mental Health, designed to evaluate the effectiveness of a sequenced approach to therapy. A series of papers were published in 2006 in the *American Journal of Psychiatry* and *The New England Journal of Medicine* describing some of the results. Highlights include the following:
   a. All patients were initially treated with citalopram monotherapy, and only about 30% achieved remission.
   b. Patients who did not achieve remission were then allowed to select a "switch" strategy or "augmentation" strategy (level 2). Options included bupropion, sertraline, venlafaxine, or cognitive therapy. There were no significant differences between strategies, but slightly higher remission rates occurred with augmentation. Bupropion and buspirone augmentation worked similarly, and the former agent was better tolerated.
   c. Patients not responding to level 2 were then allowed to change to mirtazapine or nortriptyline or to have augmentation with lithium or thyroid. Again, there were not many differences. Thyroid augmentation worked as well as lithium.
   d. Remission rates decreased at each level of treatment. Although data from this trial will continue to be analyzed, the results suggest that less than one-third of patients achieve remission with initial SSRI monotherapy, and switching or augmentation strategies are viable options, with no marked increase in efficacy with either strategy. Switching antidepressants may be a good option for patients who do not respond to or do not tolerate a drug, and augmentation may be good for partial responders. However, continued monitoring of these observations is necessary to confirm these results.
   e. For a good review of the STAR*D findings, see Rush A et al. Am J Psychiatry 2006;163:1905-17.

Patient Cases

Questions 5–7 pertain to the following case:

J.L. is a 26-year-old man with a history of type I bipolar disorder who presents to the inpatient unit with delusions that the Federal Bureau of Investigation is tracking his movements and that his thoughts are being recorded in a secret government database. He believes he has special powers to hide by making himself invisible. He is hyperverbal and has not slept in the past 48 hours. He is placed on a 72-hour hold for control of his manic symptoms. He has a history of nonadherence to medications and is currently not taking any medications. J.L.'s last hospitalization was 2 months ago, when he had significant depressive symptoms and suicidal ideation. He has three or four hospitalizations per year, and his history of medication trials includes carbamazepine, olanzapine, and lamotrigine (may be helpful but uncertain because of nonadherence). He has also received a diagnosis of hepatitis C.

5. Which statement is most applicable for selecting J.L.'s mood stabilizer at this time?
   A. Carbamazepine should be tried again because it is effective for preventing rehospitalization.
   B. Divalproex should be tried because it is good for maintenance treatment.
   C. Lithium should be tried because it can effectively treat the manic phase and prevent future episodes.
   D. Lamotrigine should be tried again because it is effective for bipolar maintenance.

6. Which adverse effects would be of most concern and would require immediate evaluation if J.L. were prescribed lithium?
   A. Hyperthyroidism.
   B. Coarse tremor.
   C. Severe acne.
   D. Weight gain.

Patient Cases *(continued)*

7. It is 3 months later, and J.L. has been stable on lithium 900 mg/day. During a clinic visit, you find that J.L. is confused and slurring his words. His other medications include lisinopril, ibuprofen, atorvastatin, and zolpidem. Which is best to recommend immediately?

    A. Discontinue lisinopril because it interacts with lithium.

    B. Discontinue zolpidem because it may increase confusion.

    C. Obtain a lithium level because J.L. may have supratherapeutic levels.

    D. Discontinue ibuprofen because it interacts with lithium.

II. BIPOLAR DISORDER

A. Overview of Bipolar Disorder
   1. The *DSM-5* defines bipolar disorder by the experience of a manic or hypomanic episode. Mania can be thought of as the affective opposite of depression. Consult the *DSM-5* for a complete description of the diagnostic criteria. A manic episode is characterized by at least 1 week of an abnormal and persistently elevated mood accompanied by an increased amount of activity. Other symptoms include inflated self-esteem, irritability, decreased need for sleep, pressured speech, flight of ideas, poor attention, increased hyperactivity or agitation, and involvement in high-risk, pleasurable activities without respect to the consequences. A hypomanic episode is a milder form mania. It must exist for 4 days or longer. Unlike mania, it is not severe enough to warrant hospitalization, does not impair social or occupational functioning, and is not associated with psychosis.
   2. The *DSM-5* includes two types of bipolar disorder:
      a. Bipolar I (BP I): Chronic disorder marked by one or more manic or mixed episodes and major depressive episodes
      b. Bipolar II (BP II): Chronic disorder marked by one or more major depressive episodes, accompanied by at least one hypomanic episode
      c. Cyclothymic disorder: Several periods of hypomania and mild depression, none of which meet the criteria for mania or major depressive episode
      d. Rapid cycling: At least 4 episodes of mania or depression in 1 year
   3. Bipolar disorder, particularly type II bipolar disorder, is often misdiagnosed as major depression. The diagnosis is important because the two conditions are treated differently.

B. Lithium for Bipolar Disorders
   1. The exact mechanism of action for lithium is unknown, but it appears to be neuroprotective.
   2. Lithium continues to be the gold standard for treating bipolar disorder type I. It is effective for the manic and depressive components. Although it is not a particularly good antidepressant as monotherapy in unipolar depression, it is effective in patients with bipolar disorder.
   3. Antimanic effects can occur in 1–2 weeks. Most clinicians use antipsychotics or benzodiazepines as adjunctive therapy during this period to cover the agitation and other symptoms. Antidepressant effects may take 6–8 weeks.
   4. Pharmacokinetics: Its half-life is 20–24 hours. It is excreted 95% unchanged by glomerular filtration, and anything that alters glomerular filtration rate affects its clearance. Pharmacokinetic methods are available for early prediction of doses, but waiting 5–6 days for steady state seems to work just as well.
   5. Initial dosing is in the range of 600–900 mg/day in divided doses and then titrated according to response and tolerability. Maintenance doses are based on serum concentrations, symptom relief, and the occurrence of adverse effects.

6. A pre-lithium workup includes a complete blood cell count, electrolytes, renal function, thyroid function tests, urinalysis, electrocardiogram (ECG), and pregnancy test for women of childbearing age.

7. Monitoring: Serum concentrations must be monitored. The half-life is about 1 day, so steady state occurs in about 5 days. Even if it is not steady state, it may be prudent to obtain a serum concentration 3 days after dosage changes. Most clinicians will aim for concentrations of 0.8–1.2 mEq/L in acute mania and 0.6–1.0 mEq/L during maintenance. Concentration-response data are based on 12-hour post-dose concentrations, so order levels in the morning 12 hours after the last evening dose. Perform renal function tests, thyroid function tests, and a urinalysis every 6–12 months.

8. Adverse effects are common with lithium and are most common during therapy initiation or after dose changes. Some points to consider are listed in Table 4.

9. Symptoms of lithium toxicity include lethargy, coarse tremor, confusion, seizures, and coma and may even result in death. Patients who present to urgent care on lithium therapy should always be monitored for lithium toxicity before any medication adjustments are made. Lithium level and sodium/renal function should be drawn so that lithium levels can be accurately estimated.

Table 4. Adverse Effects Associated With Lithium

Problem	Potential Interventions
Rash or ↑ psoriasis	Discontinue the drug temporarily or permanently
Tremor	Reduce dose (Cp); add β-blocker
CNS toxicity (e.g., agitation, confusion)	Reduce dose (Cp)
Gastrointestinal (nausea, vomiting, diarrhea)	Reduce dose; try extended-release product
Hypothyroidism	Discontinue Li or give levothyroxine
Polydipsia or polyuria	Reduce dose, manage intake, and try amiloride or HCTZ, but know that HCTZ will ↑ Li Cp; single bedtime dosing helps
Interstitial fibrosis, glomerulosclerosis	Controversial! Keep dose at lowest effective concentration
Teratogenicity	Avoid during first trimester, if possible

CNS = central nervous system; Cp = plasma concentration; HCTZ = hydrochlorothiazide; Li = lithium.

10. Situations to consider during lithium therapy are listed in Table 5.

Table 5. Situations to Consider During Lithium Therapy

Situation	Factors	Results
Drug interactions	Diuretics	
	Thiazides	↑ Li Cp; avoid use to reduce toxicity
	Furosemide	Little effect
	Amiloride	Little effect
	NSAIDs	↑ Li Cp; avoid use to reduce toxicity
	Theophylline	↓ Li Cp
	ACEIs	↑ Li Cp; avoid use to reduce toxicity
	Neuromuscular blockers	Li prolongs action
	Neuroleptics	Li may potentiate EPS
	Carbamazepine	↑ CNS toxicity
Thyroid	Li ↓ synthesis and release of thyroid hormone	Hypothyroidism
Pregnancy	↑ GFR	↓ Li Cp
Aging	↓ GFR	↓ Li requirements
	↑ Sensitivity to ADRs	Li toxicity
↓ Renal function	↓ GFR, ↑ creatinine and BUN	↑ Li Cp
Dehydration, salt restriction, and extrarenal salt loss	↑ Sodium reabsorption	↑ Li Cp

ACEI = angiotensin-converting enzyme inhibitor; ADRs = adverse drug reactions; BUN = blood urea nitrogen; CNS = central nervous system; Cp = concentration of drug plasma; EPS = extrapyramidal symptoms; GFR = glomerular filtration rate; Li = lithium; NSAIDs = nonsteroidal anti-inflammatory drugs.

C. Anticonvulsants for Bipolar Disorder: These are also considered mood-stabilizing drugs that reduce manic and depressive episodes. Refer to the Neurology chapter for additional drug-specific details.
   1. Divalproex: It is as effective as lithium in acute and prophylactic management. It appears to be good for rapid cyclers but may not be as effective during depressive episodes. It is also beneficial for patients with dysphoric mania, mixed episodes, or a history of substance abuse. Target serum concentrations range from 50 to 125 mcg/mL. The serum concentration can be checked 3–5 days after initiation or after a change of dose. Hypoalbuminemia increases the risk of increased free concentrations. Nonresponse to treatment is common if the dose is too low; however, the free fraction increases as the serum concentration is increased (above 100–125 mcg/mL). Dose-related adverse effects that occur at serum concentrations greater than 80 mcg/mL include neurotoxicity, sedation, hair loss, and thrombocytopenia. Life-threatening pancreatitis can occur but rarely (less than 5%). It can recur with reinitiation of valproate. The extended-release product has lower bioavailability than the enteric-coated preparation. The dose should be increased by 8%–20% when converting to the extended-release product.
   2. Carbamazepine: This drug also appears effective for acute mania and maintenance therapy, particularly in patients with an history of head injury. Equetro is approved by the FDA for acute manic and mixed episodes. Although the same serum concentration range as for seizures (4–12 mcg/mL) should be used, keep in mind that clinicians may push it higher on the basis of tolerability and effect. Carbamazepine can also be added to lithium for patients who have not responded to monotherapy.

3. Lamotrigine: This drug has been approved for maintenance therapy. It appears particularly effective against the depressed phase of bipolar disorder. It is less effective than other mood stabilizers in the manic phase.

   a. A Stevens-Johnson type rash occurs in about 0.3% of adults and 1% of children. Lamotrigine must be discontinued if a rash occurs and should never be rechallenged. Risk increases with rapid dose titrations, high doses, young age, and concurrent use of valproic acid. The rash most commonly occurs within the first 2–8 weeks of therapy.

   b. The dose titration must be halved if lamotrigine is given with valproate and doubled if given with carbamazepine because of increased lamotrigine metabolism. The titration period is lengthy, so the onset of therapeutic effect can be delayed. For this reason, lamotrigine is not helpful in the acute setting.

   c. Lamotrigine has been associated with aseptic meningitis in adult and pediatric patients. Patients who experience headache, fever, chills, nausea, vomiting, stiff neck, rash, abnormal sensitivity to light, drowsiness, or confusion while taking lamotrigine should contact their health care professional right away. In 15 of 40 identified cases of aseptic meningitis, symptoms returned when patients were rechallenged with lamotrigine. Symptoms have occurred 1–42 days after the drug is started, and many of the patients required hospitalization.

4. Topiramate is also being used for bipolar disorder, but comparative data with other anticonvulsants are unavailable. It should be used with caution, however, because it has been linked with depression. Other anticonvulsants, including levetiracetam and oxcarbazepine, are being used for bipolar disorder, but data about efficacy are scarce. Data for gabapentin suggest it is ineffective.

D. Antipsychotics for Bipolar Disorder: Antipsychotics, particularly atypicals or second generation, have mood stabilizing properties. They can be used alone or with anticonvulsant mood stabilizers to treat bipolar symptoms. Metabolic adverse effects associated with antipsychotic use should be considered when medications are administered long term (see Schizophrenia section).

1. Acute treatment: Antipsychotics treat acute symptoms of mania, including psychosis, aggression, or irritation. They are often combined with a traditional mood stabilizer for severe symptoms. All atypical antipsychotics have received FDA approval for use in acute mania or mixed episodes except for clozapine and iloperidone. For acute mania, the Canadian Network for Mood and Anxiety Treatments/ International Society for Bipolar Disorders (CANMAT/ISBD) guidelines include olanzapine, risperidone, quetiapine, aripiprazole, ziprasidone, asenapine, and paliperidone extended release among first-line agents.

2. Bipolar depression: Both quetiapine and lurasidone are approved for treatment of bipolar depression. Data for aripiprazole suggest it is suboptimal for the treatment of bipolar depression.

3. Maintenance treatment: Risperdal Consta and Abilify Maintena have been approved for use in bipolar maintenance as monotherapy. The CANMAT/ISBD guidelines additionally recommend olanzapine and quetiapine.

E. Benzodiazepines for Bipolar Disorder: These agents are acutely helpful for agitation but are not as helpful for the core symptoms, nor do they prevent relapses. They are particularly useful for insomnia, hyperactivity, and agitation. Lorazepam or diazepam is often used in the acute setting, but long-term therapy is not recommended.

F. Antidepressants for Bipolar Disorder:
   1. Use of these agents in bipolar disorder is controversial. There is a potential for switching to the manic phase, particularly in patients with type I bipolar disorder. The risk appears greater with TCAs and SNRIs than with SSRIs or bupropion. Because individual patients with bipolar disorder might benefit from antidepressants, the ISBD stopped short of recommending against any use of antidepressants. Antidepressants should not be used as monotherapy, and their use should be minimized in general. Antidepressants should not be used in bipolar depression if symptoms of mania are also present. The Systematic Treatment Enhanced Program for Bipolar Disorder trials found no statistically significant increased episodes of depression in patients taking mood stabilizers who discontinued their antidepressants. Patients with bipolar disorder taking mood stabilizers who received either paroxetine or bupropion were no more likely to achieve remission or have a durable recovery than those receiving placebo. They were also no more likely to experience a switch to a manic phase (Sachs GS, et al. N Engl J Med 2007;356:1711-22).
   2. Fluoxetine in combination with olanzapine is approved to treat depression associated with bipolar disorder type I.

G. Bipolar type II: The depressive phase tends to be more debilitating. Patients are usually functional during hypomanic episodes. Quetiapine is the agent of choice for depression. Lamotrigine is a reasonable alternative. Other mood stabilizers can be used but may not be as efficacious as for type I. Antidepressants are used more frequently but should never be used alone.

Patient Cases

Questions 8–11 pertain to the following case:

L.M. is a 25-year-old man recently given a diagnosis of schizophrenia, paranoid type. He often hears voices telling him that he is "stupid and worthless" and that he should "just jump off his apartment building." His parents became very concerned about his isolative behavior and brought him to the hospital. He was given haloperidol in the psychiatry unit and now presents with neck stiffness and feelings of extreme restlessness. Until now, he has not taken medications because he felt that he could control his symptoms on his own with vitamins and Red Bull drinks.

8. Which is the most appropriate treatment of L.M.'s symptoms at this time?
   A. Benztropine.
   B. Haloperidol.
   C. Olanzapine.
   D. Quetiapine.

9. You and the psychiatric team decide to recommend risperidone for L.M. Which is the most likely reason for this selection?
   A. Risperidone has less risk of causing EPS than haloperidol.
   B. Risperidone is available in a long-acting injection to increase adherence.
   C. Risperidone is effective for decreasing L.M.'s negative symptoms.
   D. Risperidone can be dosed once daily after titration to target dose.

Patient Cases (*continued*)

10. Which is the best example of an adverse effect of risperidone that would be of concern in L.M.?

    A. Sedation.

    B. Anticholinergic effects.

    C. EPS.

    D. Corrected QT (QTc) prolongation.

11. One year later, L.M. is no longer responding to risperidone, and you decide to switch him to another medication. L.M. is interested only in oral medications. Given his history, which agent is most appropriate at this time?

    A. Clozapine.

    B. Fluphenazine.

    C. Olanzapine.

    D. Quetiapine.

III. SCHIZOPHRENIA

   A. Characteristics
   1. Schizophrenia is a thought disorder characterized by a mix of symptoms. Five symptoms are involved in the diagnosis, and at least 2 of them must be present for at least 1 month. At least one of the three must be hallucinations, delusions, or disorganized speech. Patients may also have disorganized or catatonic behavior or negative symptoms.
   2. Several symptom domains have been developed for schizophrenia. Usually, symptoms are divided into two categories: positive and negative. However, other domains have also been suggested. The most common scheme is shown in Table 6.

Table 6. Categories of Schizophrenia-Associated Symptoms

Positive (presence of something that should not be there)	Negative (absence of something that should be present)	Cognitive
Traditional and Atypical Antipsychotics Effective	Atypical Antipsychotics May or May Not Be More Effective	No Current Medications Effectively Treat This
Hallucinations[a,b]	Blunted or flat affect[a,b]	Poor executive function
Delusions[a,b]	Social withdrawal (passive-apathetic)[a,b]	Impaired attention
Paranoia or suspiciousness[a,b]	Lack of personal hygiene[a]	Impaired working memory (does not learn from mistakes)
Conceptual disorganization[a,b,c]	Prolonged time to respond[a,b]	
Hostility[b]	Poor rapport[b]	
Grandiosity[b]	Poor abstract thinking[b]	
Excitement[b]	Poverty of speech (lack of spontaneity and flow of conversation)[b]	

Table 6. Categories of Schizophrenia-Associated Symptoms *(continued)*

Positive (presence of something that should not be there)	Negative (absence of something that should be present)	Cognitive
Loose associations	Emotional withdrawal[b]	
Thought broadcasting	Alogia (inability to carry on logical conversation)	
Thought insertion	Ambivalence (simultaneous, contradictory thinking); prevents decision-making	
	Autism (internally directed)	
	Amotivation (avolition)	
	Anhedonia	

[a]These symptoms can be used as a brief clinical assessment for antipsychotic response; they are known as the 4-Item Positive Symptoms Rating Scale (PSRS) and the Brief Negative Symptom Assessment (BNSA).

[b]These symptoms are used to score the positive and negative portions of the Positive and Negative Symptom Scale (PANSS).

[c]Conceptual disorganization, according to the Brief Psychiatric Rating Scale, is the "degree to which speech is confused, disconnected, vague or disorganized." This includes tangential thinking, circumstantiality, sudden topic shifts, incoherence, derailment, blocking, neologisms, clanging, word salad, and other speech disorders.

3. Terms associated with schizophrenia
   a. Delusions: These are erroneous beliefs involving misinterpretations of reality that are resistant to evidence refuting them. A fixed delusion will not change, no matter how much evidence is offered to the contrary.
   b. Hallucinations: These perceptual abnormalities can involve any sensory system. With schizophrenia, auditory hallucinations are most common. These can be persecutory (e.g., someone is going to get me), paranoid (e.g., someone is watching), or command (e.g., someone told me to do it).
   c. Thought disorder: This is manifested in several ways. "Loose associations" refers to the person going from one topic to another as though the topics were connected. "Tangential" speech refers to answers to questions that are only slightly related or totally unrelated to the question. "Word salad" refers to speech that is almost incomprehensible and is very much like receptive aphasia.

B. Course of Illness
   1. Onset is usually between adolescence and early adulthood. It occurs earlier in men (i.e., early 20s) than in women (i.e., late 20s to early 30s). The incidence is about equal between sexes.
   2. Most patients fluctuate between acute episodes and remission. Periods between episodes may include some residual symptoms.
   3. There are four phases of schizophrenia: prodromal, acute, stabilization, and stable.
      a. Prodromal phase: This phase is characterized by the gradual development of symptoms that may go unnoticed until a major symptom occurs. It may include isolation, deterioration of hygiene, loss of interest in work or school, and dysphoria.
      b. Acute phase: This is the full-blown episode of psychotic behavior. Patients may be unable to care for themselves during this phase.
      c. Stabilization phase: The acute symptoms begin to decrease, and this phase may last for several months.
      d. Stable phase: During this phase, symptoms have markedly declined and may not be present. Nonpsychotic symptoms such as anxiety and depression may be present.
   4. Complete remissions without symptoms are uncommon.

C. Causes
   1. The causes of schizophrenia are unknown. It appears to involve neurophysiological and psychological abnormalities.
   2. The primary neurotransmitters believed to be involved in the etiology are dopamine and serotonin. The exact relationship between these neurotransmitters remains unknown. It does appear that in some areas of the brain, dopamine overactivity results in some symptoms, whereas in others, underactivity may occur. Positron emission tomographic scanning shows areas of hypermetabolism and hypometabolism.
   3. Many potential risk factors for schizophrenia have been identified, including having a family history of schizophrenia, having a poor birth history, experiencing intrauterine trauma, living in an urban area, having stress, and being born during the winter.

D. Rating Scales
   1. The Brief Psychiatric Rating Scale (BPRS) is a general psychiatric rating scale that has been used to measure outcomes in clinical trials, including those involving schizophrenia.
   2. The Positive and Negative Symptom Scale (PANSS) is a 30-item, 7-point scale that was partly adapted from the BPRS. It is widely used to evaluate antipsychotic therapy in clinical trials but not in daily clinical practice. It requires a 45-minute interview with the patient. The interviewer must be specially trained to administer it.
   3. The Positive Symptoms Rating Scale (PSRS) and the Brief Negative Symptom Assessment (BNSA) are two different but complementary scales. Each consists of four items. Each of the items on the PSRS is scored from 1 (not present) to 7 (extremely severe). Each of the items on the BNSA is scored from 1 (normal) to 6 (severe). These scales were used in the Texas Algorithm Project, a large-scale clinical trial that assessed the value of algorithm-driven medication practices in the mentally ill. The PSRS and BNSA allow rapid clinical assessment.

E. First-Generation Antipsychotics (FGAs; also called typical or conventional antipsychotics) for Schizophrenia (Table 7)
   1. This class of agents includes all the older antipsychotic agents. Chlorpromazine was the first agent used clinically.
   2. These agents can be categorized according to chemical class or potency.

Table 7. Antipsychotic Agents for the Treatment of Schizophrenia by Chemical Class

Class	Agent	Degree of EPS[a]
First-generation phenothiazines (typical or conventional)	Fluphenazine	+3
	Trifluoperazine	+3
	Perphenazine	+2/+3
	Mesoridazine	+1
	Thioridazine	+1
	Chlorpromazine	+2
Butyrophenone	Haloperidol	+3
Others	Thiothixene	+3
	Loxapine	+2/+3

Table 7. Antipsychotic Agents for the Treatment of Schizophrenia by Chemical Class *(continued)*

Class	Agent	Degree of EPS[a]
Second-generation antipsychotics (atypical)	Clozapine	0
	Risperidone	+1
	Olanzapine	0/+1
	Quetiapine	0/+1
	Ziprasidone	0/+1
	Aripiprazole	0/+1
	Paliperidone	+1
	Iloperidone	0/+1
	Asenapine	0/+1
	Lurasidone	0/+1

[a]0 = none; +1 = low; +2 = moderate; +3 = high.
EPS = extrapyramidal symptoms.

3. These drugs can also be categorized by potency as antagonists at dopamine D_2 receptors. They also possess anticholinergic, antihistaminic, and α-adrenergic blocking properties and tend to be worse with low-potency agents. The high-potency agents at dopamine D_2 have less potency at the other receptors; thus, the adverse effect profiles also differ by potency (Table 8).

Table 8. Select FGAs for the Treatment of Schizophrenia by Potency

Agent	Dose Equivalent (mg)	Potency[a]	Anticholinergic[b]	Sedation[b]	↓ BP[b]	EPS
Chlorpromazine	100	Low	4	5	5	Low
Thioridazine	100	Low	5	4	5	Low
Perphenazine	10	Int.	2	2	2	Int.
Loxapine	10–15	Int.	3	3	2	Int.
Fluphenazine	2	High	2	2	2	High
Thiothixene	3–5	High	2	2	2	High
Haloperidol	2–3	High	1	2	1	High

[a]Potency = D_2 receptor affinity
[b]Scale 1–5 = low to high.
BP = blood pressure; EPS = extrapyramidal symptoms; FGA = first-generation antipsychotic; Int. = intermediate.

4. Sedation: The degree of sedation depends on the drug. If sedation occurs, it is usually worse initially and is then tolerated better with time. It tends to be dose-related.
5. Anticholinergic effects: Dry mouth, constipation, blurred vision, and urinary hesitancy can occur. Patients for whom these effects may be a problem should probably receive a high-potency agent.
6. Antiadrenergic effects: The α-adrenergic blocking effect is seen as orthostatic hypotension. Patients who are predisposed to such effects (e.g., older adults, dehydrated patients) should probably receive a high-potency agent.
7. Extrapyramidal symptoms
   a. Parkinsonism: This is manifested by symptoms such as bradykinesia, rigidity, tremor, or akinesia. It is usually responsive to anticholinergic agents such as diphenhydramine, trihexyphenidyl, and benztropine.

b. Dystonia: Examples include torticollis, laryngospasm, and oculogyric crisis. This is also treated with anticholinergics.

c. Akathisia: This is a somatic restlessness and inability to stay still or calm. Reducing the antipsychotic dose and switching to an agent with a lower incidence of akathisia are the best options but not always feasible. It responds poorly to anticholinergics. Lipophilic (fat soluble) β-blockers such as propranolol and nadolol are effective and are the agents of choice.

d. Tardive dyskinesia: Characterized by abnormal involuntary movements that occur with long-term antipsychotic therapy. It usually involves the orofacial muscles and is often insidious. If caught early, it can be reversible. With continued drug exposure, particularly at high doses, it is often irreversible. Risks are probably related to total cumulative dose. Symptoms may decrease with lowering the dose of antipsychotic or switching to an agent that is associated with less tardive dyskinesia. This dose reduction must be weighed against worsening of schizophrenic symptoms. The risk is higher with FGAs than SGAs, as well as older age. Clozapine has not been associated with tardive dyskinesia, and changing to this drug is preferred in patients with moderate to severe symptoms. The other atypical antipsychotics also appear to have a low potential to cause tardive dyskinesia. Anticholinergic agents should not be given to treat tardive dyskinesia and may actually worsen the symptoms.

8. Neuroleptic malignant syndrome: This is another serious complication. It occurs with all agents but appears more common with high-potency drugs. It is manifested by agitation, confusion, changing levels of consciousness, fever, tachycardia, labile blood pressure, and sweating. Its mortality rate is high, and it should be taken seriously. Discontinue the offending agent and give supportive therapy, including fluids and cooling. Bromocriptine and dantrolene have been used with varying success.

9. Endocrine effects: Galactorrhea and menstrual changes can occur because of hyperprolactinemia caused by antipsychotics. Prolactin secretion is blocked by dopamine. Dopamine blockers can increase prolactin concentrations (hyperprolactinemia).

10. Weight gain: This occurs in up to 40% of patients, with low-potency agents having higher risk. Important interventions include keeping the dose as low as possible and implementing dietary management. Weight gain may occur because of actions at histamine or serotonin receptors.

11. Sexual dysfunction: Erectile problems occur in 23%–54% of men. Loss of libido and anorgasmia may occur in men and women.

12. Venous thromboembolism (VTE): A published nested case-control study of older adults from the United Kingdom showed that FGAs and SGAs were associated with greater risk of deep VTE or pulmonary embolism than matched controls (Parker C et al. BMJ 2010;341:c4245). Patients from primary care with schizophrenia, bipolar disorder, or dementia who had been prescribed antipsychotics in the past 24 months had a 32% elevated risk of VTE (odds ratio = 1.32 [95% confidence interval, 1.23–1.42]) and a 56% elevated risk if the treatment had been in the past 3 months. Second-generation antipsychotics had a higher risk of VTE than did first-generation drugs (73% vs. 28%, respectively). The study was limited by possible confounders such as smoking status and body mass index, although these factors were deemed not to have considerably altered the results.

13. Miscellaneous: Low-potency agents such as thioridazine and chlorpromazine can cause pigmentary deposits on the retina and corneal opacity. Many of the typical agents can cause serious changes on the ECG (e.g., prolongation of the QTc interval). These changes can lead to arrhythmias and death.

14. Therapy initiation: In the past, acute episodes were treated very aggressively with high doses, and the process was called neuroleptization. Because neuroleptization can lead to adverse effects and is probably no more effective than starting with full therapeutic doses, it is no longer advocated. Dosing during the stabilization phase may be less aggressive, but a very low dose increases the risk of relapse.

15. Administration route: Oral therapy is most common; however, parenteral drugs can be used acutely if the patient does not adhere to therapy or is agitated and will not take oral medications. Haloperidol can be given intramuscularly. Intravenous haloperidol has been linked to toxicity including torsades de pointes and should not be given. Depot forms of haloperidol and fluphenazine are available, providing sustained concentrations for about 1 month for haloperidol and 2–3 weeks for fluphenazine. These are indicated only for chronic therapy in patients who have trouble adhering to oral therapy. Fluphenazine decanoate requires "bridging" with oral therapy when treatment is begun.

16. Therapy duration: Continuation of therapy during the stable phase is of concern because of the risk of adverse effects (e.g., the tardive dyskinesia associated with the older agents). This is of less concern with the newer drugs. Relapse rates are more than 50% during the first year or so after discontinuing these agents for both first-episode patients and patients who relapse; thus, maintaining the antipsychotic at the minimal effective dose continuously may be the best approach for most patients. Some first-episode patients may be tried off drugs after being symptom free for 2 years. Those with a history of episodes should probably be symptom free for 5 years before discontinuation is considered. Long-term therapy should include monitoring for metabolic complications such as diabetes, weight gain, and lipid abnormalities.

F. Second-Generation Antipsychotics for Schizophrenia
   1. SGAs (or atypical antipsychotics) were developed to reduce EPS adverse effects and tardive dyskinesia and to improve efficacy. The characteristics that define "atypicality" are not all agreed on, but in general, they all share at least three characteristics: The risk of EPS is lower than with typical antipsychotics at usual clinical doses, the risk of tardive dyskinesia is reduced, and the ability to block serotonin-2 receptors is present. This third property may improve activity for the negative symptoms of schizophrenia and reduce the risk of EPS. Many clinicians see atypical drugs as first-line agents, despite the higher acquisition costs of the brand name agents. Atypical agents (particularly clozapine and olanzapine) have been associated with new-onset diabetes mellitus and metabolic syndrome. All patients prescribed atypical antipsychotics should be monitored for weight, blood pressure, fasting glucose, lipids, and waist circumference at baseline and periodically thereafter.
   2. Clozapine (Clozaril): Clozapine is a less potent dopamine blocker than typical antipsychotics and is a serotonin-2 antagonist. Some of its action may be attributable to D_1 antagonism. It is as effective as typical agents, is not associated with EPS or tardive dyskinesia, and may lead to an improvement in negative symptoms more effectively than typical drugs. It is also effective for many patients who have not responded to typical agents. It appears to affect brain regions selectively, particularly those that control the cognitive and affective states altered in people with schizophrenia (i.e., the mesolimbic A10 tract, but not the A9 tract, which modulates movement). Adverse effects have limited the use of this agent.
      a. Agranulocytosis: This is manifested as a reduction in white blood cell count, and it increases the risk of serious or fatal infections. It is contraindicated if the white blood cell count is less than 3500 cells/mm^3 (Table 9). The incidence is about 1%–2% and is highest during the first 4–6 months of therapy. Because of this risk, patients must have a weekly complete blood cell count for 6 months and then every 2 weeks after that while taking the drug. The frequency can be decreased to monthly after 1 year if the white blood cell count is greater than 3500 cells/mm^3 and the absolute neutrophil count is greater than 2000 cells/mm^3. If the white blood cell count is significantly decreased during therapy (less than 3000 cells/mm^3), the drug should be discontinued. Patients must be enrolled in a Clozaril registry program (Clozaril National Registry, Teva Clozapine National Registry), which monitors the reporting of absolute neutrophil and white blood cell counts.

Table 9. Hematologic Monitoring for Clozapine

Situation	Hematologic Values for Monitoring	Frequency of WBC and ANC Monitoring
Initiation of therapy	WBC ≥3500 cells/mm³ ANC ≥2000 cells/mm³ Note: Do not initiate in patients with (1) history of myeloproliferative disorder or (2) clozapine-induced agranulocytosis or granulocytopenia	Weekly for 6 months
6–12 months of therapy	All results for WBC ≥3500 cells/mm³ and ANC ≥2000 cells/mm³	Every 2 weeks for 6 months
12 months of therapy	All results for every WBC ≥3500 cells/mm³ and ANC ≥2000 cells/mm³	Every 4 weeks ad infinitum
Immature forms present	N/A	Repeat WBC and ANC
Therapy discontinuation	N/A	Weekly for at least 4 weeks from day of discontinuation or until WBC ≥ 3500 cells/mm³ and ANC > 2000 cells/mm³
Substantial drop in WBC or ANC	Single drop or cumulative drop within 3 weeks of WBC ≥3000 cells/mm³ or ANC ≥1500 cells/mm³	1. Repeat WBC and ANC 2. If repeat values are 3000 cells/mm³ ≤ WBC ≥ 3500 cells/mm³ and ANC < 2000 cells/mm³, then monitor twice weekly
Mild leukopenia, mild granulocytopenia	3500 cells/mm³ > WBC ≥ 3000 cells/mm³ or 2000 cells/mm³ > ANC ≥ 1500 cells/mm³	Twice weekly until WBC > 3500 cells/mm³ and ANC > 2000 cells/mm³, then return to previous monitoring frequency
Moderate leukopenia, moderate granulocytopenia	3000 cells/mm³ > WBC ≥ 2000 cells/mm³ or 1500 cells/mm³ > ANC ≥ 1000 cells/mm³	1. Interrupt therapy 2. Daily until WBC > 3000 cells/mm³ and ANC > 1500 cells/mm³ 3. Twice weekly until WBC > 3500 cells/mm³ and ANC > 2000 cells/mm³ 4. May rechallenge when WBC > 3500 cells/mm³ and ANC > 2000 cells/mm³ 5. If rechallenged, monitor weekly for 1 year before returning to the usual monitoring schedule of every 2 weeks for 6 months and then every 4 weeks ad infinitum
Severe leukopenia, severe granulocytopenia	WBC <2000 cells/mm³ or ANC <1000 cells/mm³	1. Discontinue treatment and do not rechallenge patient 2. Monitor until normal and for at least 4 weeks from day of discontinuation as follows: • Daily until WBC > 3000 cells/mm³ and ANC > 1500 cells/mm³ • Twice weekly until WBC > 3500 cells/mm³ and ANC > 2000 cells/mm³ • Weekly after WBC > 3500 cells/mm³

Table 9. Hematologic Monitoring for Clozapine *(continued)*

Situation	Hematologic Values for Monitoring	Frequency of WBC and ANC Monitoring
Agranulocytosis	ANC ≤500 cells/mm³	1. Discontinue treatment and do not rechallenge patient 2. Monitor until normal and for at least 4 weeks from day of discontinuation as follows: • Daily until WBC > 3000 cells/mm³ and ANC > 1500 cells/mm³ • Twice weekly until WBC > 3500 cells/mm³ and ANC > 2000 cells/mm³ • Weekly after WBC > 3500 cells/mm³

ANC = absolute neutrophil count; WBC = white blood cell count.

    b.   Common adverse effects: These include weight gain, sedation, hypersalivation, rapid heart rate, orthostatic hypotension, and fever. Note that the presence of fever should alert the clinician to the possibility of infection and agranulocytosis. There are also black box warnings for seizures (more frequent at higher doses) and myocarditis, orthostatic hypotension, and respiratory arrest. If the drug is discontinued for 48 hours or more, retitration is required to avoid orthostatic hypotension.

3.   Aripiprazole (Abilify): This drug's pharmacology differs from that of other atypical agents. It is a dopamine D_2/serotonin-1 partial agonist and a serotonin-2 antagonist, sometimes called a dopamine-serotonin–stabilizing agent. It has a low risk of most forms of EPS, including tardive dyskinesia. It is associated with a high incidence of akathisia.

4.   Asenapine (Saphris) is available in a sublingual formulation. It appears to have a lower risk of metabolic effects and EPS; however, it has been associated with a high risk of orthostasis and sedation. There has also been a warning about the risk of hypersensitivity reactions with asenapine.

5.   Iloperidone (Fanapt) appears to have a lower risk of metabolic effects. It also has a higher risk of orthostasis but a lower risk of EPS, anticholinergic symptoms, and sedation. Short- and long-term studies have also shown an association with QTc prolongation similar to that of haloperidol and ziprasidone.

6.   Lurasidone (Latuda) has a low risk of metabolic and cardiac effects together with a low EPS risk. It has potent antagonistic activity at serotonin-7 and a high affinity to serotonin-1A receptors, which is theorized to have beneficial cognitive and anxiolytic effects. The maximal daily dose has recently been increased to 160 mg/day, and it should be taken with food. The recommended starting dose for moderate and severe renal impairment and when used with a moderate CYP3A4 inhibitor (e.g., diltiazem) is 20 mg, and the maximal dose is 80 mg. The recommended starting dose for moderate and severe hepatic impairment is 20 mg, and the maximal dose is 80 mg in moderate hepatic impairment and 40 mg in severe hepatic impairment.

7.   Olanzapine (Zyprexa): This drug is structurally similar to clozapine and has a similar pharmacology. Unlike clozapine, however, it has not been associated with agranulocytosis. Olanzapine may affect only the A10 tract of the mesolimbic system. In one study, negative symptoms responded better than with haloperidol. Along with clozapine, olanzapine carries the highest risk for diabetes. For this reason, the PORT guidelines do not consider it a first-line treatment.

8.   Paliperidone (Invega) is an active metabolite of risperidone (see below). Paliperidone palmitate is also available as a monthly depot injection.

9.   Quetiapine (Seroquel): offers a low incidence of EPS. Quetiapine is also the preferred antipsychotic if psychosis occurs in a patient with Parkinson disease.

10. Risperidone (Risperdal): This drug is a potent dopamine D_2 antagonist and a serotonin-2 antagonist. It has limited anticholinergic activity. At doses of up to 6 mg/day, the incidence of EPS has been no higher than with placebo in clinical studies. However, EPS is a dose-related phenomenon that may occur in patients taking the drug even at usual doses. Patients often tolerate risperidone better than haloperidol. It probably has no advantage in patients requiring high doses of antipsychotics. Adverse effects include sedation, orthostatic hypotension, weight gain, sexual dysfunction, and hyperprolactinemia. A long-acting intramuscular formulation (risperidone [Risperdal Consta]) is available that is better tolerated than the other intramuscular depot forms of antipsychotics. It is administered every 2 weeks and requires a 3-week bridge therapy with oral risperidone. It is generally used only after the patient is known to tolerate oral therapy. Like with long-acting risperidone, tolerability with oral therapy should be established before starting it.

11. Ziprasidone (Geodon): Use caution if combining it with other drugs (e.g., TCAs or antiarrhythmics) that can also increase the QTc interval. It is also available in a parenteral formulation for acute agitation. The drug must be taken with food to increase absorption. Electrocardiographic changes occur with antipsychotics. QTc prolongation can predispose the patient to ventricular arrhythmias including torsades de pointes syndrome. The risk appears highest with thioridazine, clozapine, ziprasidone, and iloperidone, although the other agents may do this to a lesser extent. Patients must be assessed for predisposing factors such as preexisting ECG abnormalities, electrolyte disturbances, and concurrent therapy with other drugs that prolong the QTc interval.

Table 10 summarizes the adverse effects associated with SGAs.

Table 10. Adverse Effects of SGAs

Drug (generic/ brand)	Metabolic Syndrome			Cardiac (clinically significant)	Sedation	Misc. Clinically Significant Side Effects
	Weight gain	DM	Dyslipidemia			
Fast Facts		Cases: 60% occur w/i 1st 6mos.		OH: tolerance builds over 2-3 mos.	Tolerance usually develops	Hyperprolactinemia: no tolerance develops
Aripiprazole (Abilify)	Little to none	No	Little to none	None	Low	Decreases prolactin levels; akathisia
Asenapine (Saphris)	Little to None	Little to None	Little to none	Possible QTc prolongation, OH	Low	Dose-dependent EPS (akathisia)
Clozapine (Clozaril)	Highest	Yes	High	OH, prolonged QTc tachycardia	High (antichol)	Seizures (dose-dependent), sialorrhea, neutropenia/ agranulocytosis
Iloperidone (Fanapt)	Moderate	Low	Low	QTc prolongation, OH	Low	QTc prolongation comparable with ziprasidone
Lurasidone (Latuda)	Low	Low	Low to none	None	Moderate	Dose-dependent EPS (akathisia, pseudo-parkinsonism)
Olanzapine (Zyprexa)	Highest	Yes	High	None	High (antichol)	

Table 10. Adverse Effects of SGAs *(continued)*

Drug (generic/ brand)	Metabolic Syndrome			Cardiac (clinically significant)	Sedation	Misc. Clinically Significant Side Effects
	Weight gain	DM	Dyslipidemia			
Paliperidone (Invega)	Low	Low	None	Possible QTc prolongation	Low	Hyperprolactine mia; daily doses >9 mg can cause EPS
Quetiapine (Seroquel)	Moderate	Moderate	Moderate	OH	High (antichol)	Agent of choice in patients with Parkinson's disease
Risperidone (Risperdal)	Moderate	Moderate	Less	OH	Low	Hyperprolactinemia; daily doses > 6 mg/ day can cause EPS
Ziprasidone (Geodon)	Little	No	Less	Prolonged QTc	Low	QTc prolongation~ 15.9 msec;* QTc >500 msec (increased risk for torsade des pointes) rare; no increase in rate of sudden cardiac death over other agents

* Compared with thioridazine (30 msec), a FGA which is not used often due to its potential to cause torsade des pointes.

Key: EPS= extrapyramidal symptoms. OH=orthostatic hypotension

G. Adjunctive Medications
1. Lithium: This agent may augment antipsychotic action.
2. Anticonvulsants (carbamazepine and valproic acid): These agents may augment antipsychotics, but their role in therapy remains undetermined. They may be useful in patients with agitated or violent behavior.
3. Benzodiazepines: These may be useful during the acute phase for agitation or anxiety, but they are less effective for treatment of psychotic symptoms. These drugs must also be used with caution in patients with schizophrenia because this population is at high risk of substance abuse.

H. Comparisons of FGAs and SGAs
1. Almost all treatment guidelines now suggest that SGAs are the preferred first-line agents to typical drugs because most clinicians believe they are better tolerated and pose less risk. However, studies have questioned this conclusion. In these trials, the older agents appeared to do as well in efficacy and tolerability; however, they were not conclusive. Some issues with the study design limit the findings. Some clinicians may wish to use typical agents. There is certainly pressure from a cost standpoint. The results of a study named the Cost Utility of the Latest Antipsychotic Drugs in Schizophrenia Study were published in the October 2006 issue of *Archives of General Psychiatry* (Jones PB, et al. Arch Gen Psychiatry 2006;63:1079-87). The findings of this study suggest that the differences in the effect of FGAs and SGAs are not as much as had been thought.
2. The Clinical Antipsychotic Trials of Intervention Effectiveness study (CATIE, sponsored by NIMH) compared several SGAs with the older agent perphenazine. Here are some of the findings:
    a. Discontinuation
        i. High in all groups: 74% of all patients discontinued before 18 months

      ii. Olanzapine = 64%

      iii. Perphenazine = 75%

      iv. Quetiapine = 82%

      v. Risperidone = 74%

      vi. Ziprasidone = 79%

  b. Time to discontinuation

      i. All causes: Longest for olanzapine (significantly longer than for quetiapine and risperidone, not the others)

      ii. Lack of efficacy: Longest for olanzapine (significantly longer than perphenazine, quetiapine, and risperidone, but not ziprasidone)

  c. Duration of successful treatment: Longest for olanzapine (significantly longer than for quetiapine, risperidone, and perphenazine, as well as for risperidone compared with quetiapine)

  d. Efficacy: Positive and Negative Syndrome Scale (PANSS) scores

      i. Scores improved in all groups as time progressed.

      ii. Initially, more improvement with olanzapine, but improvement diminished with time

  e. Adverse drug reactions

      i. Olanzapine: More often associated with weight gain and metabolic adverse effects

      ii. Perphenazine: More often associated with EPS

3. Two meta-analyses of comparison trials were conducted. The first analysis of FGAs and SGAs suggested that clozapine, risperidone, and olanzapine were more effective than the FGAs evaluated. Other SGAs were not superior to FGAs. Further research is needed to resolve this issue (Leucht S, et al. Lancet 2009;373:31-41). In the second meta-analysis, SGAs were compared for the change in total PANSS score (Leucht S, et al. Am J Psychiatry 2009;166:152-63). Olanzapine was significantly more efficacious than aripiprazole (p=0.002), quetiapine (p<0.001), risperidone (p=0.006), and ziprasidone (p<0.001). Most of the efficacy differences were caused by improvement in positive, not negative, symptoms.

Patient Cases

Questions 12–15 pertain to the following case:

C.P. is a recent Iraq war veteran who has been treated successfully with paroxetine for his major depression for the past 3 weeks. He presents to the clinic experiencing nightmares, "feeling on edge all the time," and having flashbacks of his time in the war. He is evaluated and given a diagnosis of posttraumatic stress disorder (PTSD). He has no history of substance dependence and has no significant medical history.

12. Which recommendation is most appropriate at this time?
    A. Continue paroxetine because it treats both PTSD and major depression.
    B. Discontinue paroxetine and initiate sertraline, which treats both PTSD and major depression.
    C. Continue paroxetine and add lorazepam for the anxiety symptoms.
    D. Discontinue paroxetine and initiate buspirone for the anxiety symptoms.

13. C.P. has been adherent to the medication you recommended earlier, but he still feels very irritable and has been aggressive at times at work toward others. Which adjunctive medication is most appropriate in this patient?
    A. Buspirone.
    B. Clonazepam.
    C. Divalproex.
    D. Lithium.

Patient Cases (*continued*)

14. After 8 months of treatment, C.P. is not responding to the medication you recommended. Having heard a lot about buspirone, he wonders whether this medication might be helpful for his conditions. Which is the most accurate statement for this patient?
    A. Buspirone may be helpful for the nightmares.
    B. Buspirone may work as quickly as 3 days.
    C. Buspirone is convenient because of its once-daily dosing.
    D. Buspirone does not have much dependence potential.

15. C.P. returns to the clinic and states that his depressive and anxiety symptoms are much improved. However, he is concerned that his girlfriend, who has OCD, is not doing well on her treatment with lorazepam. If you were also treating the girlfriend, which is the most appropriate medication you would initiate?
    A. Clomipramine.
    B. Amitriptyline.
    C. Imipramine.
    D. Nortriptyline.

IV. ANXIETY DISORDERS

A. Overview of Anxiety Disorders
   1. Generalized anxiety disorder (GAD) is characterized by 6 months or more of excessive worry or anxiety, generally with an unidentified cause.
   2. Panic disorder is characterized by discrete periods of sudden, intense fear or terror and feelings of impending doom. Usually, the precipitating cause is unknown, but the patient can become conditioned to believe it is attributable to some environmental cause.
   3. Agoraphobia: Intense fear in 2 or more settings (mostly in the open or in public). These settings include: using public transportation, being in open spaces, being in enclosed spaces, standing in line or being in a crowd, and being outside the home alone.
   4. OCD is characterized by obsessive or intrusive thoughts that cannot be controlled and that are repetitive. Compulsions are ritualistic behaviors (e.g., washing the hands, combing the hair, cleaning the house).
   5. PTSD follows a traumatic event. It is characterized by increased arousal and avoidance of stimuli that approximate the original traumatic event.
   6. Social anxiety disorder is characterized by marked and persistent fear and anxiety in social or performance situations that are recognized as excessive or unreasonable. These situations are either avoided or endured with intense anxiety.
   7. Specific phobias are characterized by intense fear or anxiety induced by a specific object.

B. Pharmacotherapeutic Options for Anxiety Disorders
   1. Benzodiazepines: These drugs have anxiolytic properties, and some have preventive efficacy for panic attacks. Depending on the choice of agent, the onset can be very rapid, as outlined below. The high-potency, short half-life agents are the most rapidly acting. They are effective for treating the acute somatic and autonomic symptoms of anxiety, but do not adequately address the underlying cognitive and psychologically pathology.

a. Pharmacologically, they share, to various degrees, five properties: (1) anxiolytic, (2) hypnotic, (3) muscle relaxation, (4) anticonvulsant, and (5) amnesic actions. Tolerance of the anxiolytic action is uncommon. Benzodiazepines are differentiated by their half-life (plus or minus active metabolites) and potency. If they are thought of as short half-life/high-potency versus long half-life/lower-potency drugs, the following distinctions can be made:

   i. Short half-life/high potency: These are usually more rapid-acting agents that provide quicker control of the symptoms. However, tolerance of the hypnotic effect develops rapidly, withdrawal problems are common, and interdose breakthrough symptoms can occur. These are often used for acute management and later replaced with longer half-life agents.

   ii. Long half-life/low potency: These drugs produce longer-lasting effects throughout the day, and although withdrawal symptoms may be less pronounced, they do occur. Interdose breakthrough symptoms are less likely; however, more "hangover" symptoms occur in the morning. These agents can accumulate in elderly patients.

   iii. Table 11 compares the half-lives and potencies of the five main/most commonly prescribed benzodiazepines.

Table 11. Half-lives and Potency of the Most Commonly Prescribed Benzodiazepines

Agent	Half-life (hours)	Dose (mg)
Alprazolam (Xanax)	6–12	0.5
Chlordiazepoxide (Librium)	5–30 (act. met.)	25
Clonazepam	20–50	0.5
Diazepam (Valium)	20–100 (act. met.)	10
Lorazepam (Ativan)	10–18	1

act. met. = active metabolite.

b. The primary issues associated with benzodiazepines are tolerance and dependence. Tolerance of the hypnotic actions occurs within days. Dependence occurs within weeks to months of continued use. Abrupt cessation can lead to withdrawal problems. For this reason, it is generally recommended that treatment periods be restricted to 3–4 months, or about the time of an adequate trial on an antidepressant. After this time, the patient is tapered off the drug to avoid withdrawal and supplementation with other agents. Benzodiazepine tapers can take months to more than 1 year to complete. In practice, many of these patients go on to use these drugs for long periods. Often, these patients are not in remission, despite treatment with maintenance medications. In patients with a history of substance abuse or risk factors for substance abuse, the situation is different. In these patients, try to avoid the use of benzodiazepines because patients may begin to show an abusive pattern of use.

2. Antidepressants: SSRIs are also effective for several anxiety disorders. They are the agents of choice for long term treatment of anxiety disorders. Venlafaxine has been approved for the treatment of generalized anxiety and social anxiety disorders. Duloxetine is also approved for GAD. Some initial symptoms may be improved within days, but the full benefit of treatment may take weeks, as for depression treatment. Tricyclic antidepressants have preventive efficacy for panic disorder and anxiolytic activity. **Important note:** About 25% of these patients experience a hyper-stimulatory response to antidepressants, which can be confused with a worsening of the anxiety symptoms. This response is more common when therapy is first begun. Using low doses at first can help. Antidepressants can also be helpful for anxiety that accompanies depression.

3. Buspirone: This drug has anxiolytic properties, but clinicians' opinions are divided on its real value in treating GAD. It has little efficacy for other anxiety disorders. The main drawback to buspirone is its long onset of action (weeks). In the meantime, the anxiety must be covered with another agent. Some clinicians will use short-term benzodiazepines as a bridge until buspirone takes effect.

4. Miscellaneous agents
   a. β-Blockers are sometimes used to block the peripheral symptoms of panic disorder or performance anxiety.
   b. MAOIs can be effective for the treatment of panic disorder when the patient also has atypical depression. However, these drugs are seldom used because of the potential for serious adverse effects.
   c. Antihistamines with sedating properties (e.g., hydroxyzine) can help reduce physical symptoms of anxiety
   d. Barbiturates are seldom used. They are often less effective and can be lethal if taken in overdose.
   e. Antipsychotics are not considered first-line agents for the treatment of anxiety disorders. Selected SGAs can be useful as add-on therapy for OCD, GAD, and PTSD.

5. CBT should be an integral part of any therapeutic plan for treating anxiety disorders.

C. Recommended Therapy for Specific Anxiety Disorders
   1. Generalized anxiety disorder
      a. Antidepressants: These are considered first-line agents. These include the SSRIs (escitalopram, paroxetine, and sertraline), the SNRIs (duloxetine and venlafaxine), and imipramine
      b. Benzodiazepines: This class of drugs is rapidly effective; if possible, try to discontinue in 3–4 months, or once the patient has remittance of symptoms. Long-term therapy is common but not recommended. Benzodiazepines can be taken in combination with either antidepressants or buspirone as a bridge until these drugs start to take effect. They are more effective against somatic symptoms than against the underlying psychic pathology.
      c. Buspirone: Good when benzodiazepines should be avoided (e.g., in patients with a history of substance abuse); takes 2–4 weeks to be effective
      d. Pregabalin: Considered a second-line agent behind antidepressants. Limited data suggest comparable efficacy with venlafaxine and benzodiazepines.
      e. CBT or another type of psychotherapy should generally be included with pharmacotherapy.
      f. In treatment-refractory patients, augmentation with quetiapine, olanzapine, or risperidone can be tried. Valproate also shows promise.
   2. Panic disorder
      a. Antidepressants: First-line therapy. These include the SSRIs (escitalopram, fluoxetine, fluvoxamine, paroxetine, sertraline), venlafaxine, and duloxetine.
      b. Benzodiazepines: High-potency agents; effective; rapid onset
      c. Not effective: Buspirone, β-blockers, antihistamines, antipsychotics, bupropion, trazodone
      d. CBT and other psychotherapies are effective.
      e. Patients with panic disorder tend to have a higher sensitivity to physical symptoms. For this reason, these patients should be initiated on low doses of antidepressants—as low 25 mg of sertraline or 5 mg of paroxetine.
   3. Obsessive-compulsive disorder
      a. Serotonergic agents are effective—SSRIs (escitalopram, fluoxetine, fluvoxamine, paroxetine, and sertraline) and clomipramine
      b. CBT may be effective, but it is secondary to pharmacotherapy.
      c. Alone, SSRIs often fail to control OCD completely. Not many other drugs help. Augmentation with haloperidol or an SGA (olanzapine, quetiapine, or risperidone) may help. In general, high doses need to be used.

4. Posttraumatic stress disorder
   a. SSRIs (fluoxetine, sertraline, and paroxetine) are considered first-line agents.
   b. Augment with other agents to treat specific symptoms (e.g., intermittent explosive behavior with β-blockers or mood stabilizers).
      1. Prazosin is used to treat PTSD-associated nightmares.
      2. Anticonvulsants for aggression, anger, and depression (valproic acid, carbamazepine, lamotrigine, topiramate)
      3. Atypical antipsychotics for psychotic symptoms (olanzapine, quetiapine, risperidone)
   c. Benzodiazepines are not effective.
   d. As with all other anxiety disorders, CBT is integral.
5. Social anxiety disorder
   a. CBT is the most important modality.
   b. Antidepressants: First-line medication for treatment; SSRIs (escitalopram, fluvoxamine, paroxetine, sertraline) and venlafaxine. Response to antidepressants tends to be slow (up to 12 weeks) and has a flat dose-response curve.
   c. Clonazepam may be used as an adjunct.
   d. Gabapentin and pregabalin
6. Specific phobias
   a. Not treated with medication
   b. Systematic desensitization and other behavioral approaches often effective

---

Patient Cases

Questions 16–18 pertain to the following case:

C.D. is a 38-year-old kindergarten teacher who presents to the clinic today with noticeable dark circles under her eyes. She has difficulty with sleep, mainly with staying asleep. It takes her about 20 minutes to fall asleep, but after about 2 hours, she wakes up and cannot fall asleep again for several hours. This pattern has taken a toll on her job, and she feels tired all the time. She once took diphenhydramine for sleep but had to miss work because of extreme drowsiness in the morning. She wonders whether there are any other medications she can take. Her other medical problems include hypothyroidism (levothyroxine 125 mcg at bedtime), hypertension (hydrochlorothiazide 25 mg in the morning), chronic back pain (ibuprofen 800 mg three times daily), and MDD (citalopram 20 mg in the morning).

16. Which agent is most likely contributing to C.D.'s insomnia?
    A. Citalopram.
    B. Hydrochlorothiazide.
    C. Ibuprofen.
    D. Levothyroxine.

17. Which medication used for insomnia is most appropriate to recommend for C.D.?
    A. Eszopiclone.
    B. Trazodone.
    C. Temazepam.
    D. Zaleplon.

Patient Cases *(continued)*

18. Which is the best example of an adverse effect that should concern C.D. when using zolpidem?

A. Orthostasis.

B. Disorientation.

C. Abnormal behaviors while asleep.

D. Seizures with high doses of the drug.

V. INSOMNIA

A. Normal Sleep Patterns and Neurochemistry/Physiology of Sleep
   1. We spend about one-third of our lives asleep. The amount of sleep required varies from individual to individual and changes with age.
   2. Sleep difficulties are common, with up to 35% of the population affected. Of interest, 4%–5% of the population may experience hypersomnia.
   3. People with sleep problems usually experience one or more of the following: insomnia, daytime sleepiness, or abnormal sleep behaviors.
   4. The sleep-wake cycle in humans usually lasts 25 hours, which means that with the 24-hour day-night cycle of the earth's rotation, there must be some internal clock resetting. This resetting is accomplished by cues such as clocks and daylight, which tell the time of day.
   5. The neural networks regulating sleep-wake cycles are located in the brainstem, basal forebrain, and hypothalamus, with projections to the cortex and thalamus.
   6. The reticular activating system maintains wakefulness, and when activity here declines, sleep occurs.
   7. Several neurotransmitters are involved in the sleep-wake cycle. Norepinephrine, acetylcholine, histamine, and neuropeptides operate in the hypothalamus during wakefulness. Neuronal systems in the raphe nuclei, solitary tract, ventricular thalamus, anterior hypothalamus, and basal forebrain promote sleep. As the reticular activating system slows down, serotonin neurotransmission in the raphe nuclei reduces sensory input and inhibits motor activity. Norepinephrine is involved in dreaming, whereas serotonin is active during non-dreaming sleep.
   8. A lot of brain activity occurs during sleep; simultaneous electroencephalograms, electro-oculograms, and electromyograms characterize sleep stages. These are used to measure sleep latency (time to sleep onset), number of awakenings, number of stage shifts during the night, and latency to rapid eye movement (REM). These recordings are termed polysomnography. Stages are as follows:

Table 12. Sleep Stages

State	Characteristics
Wakefulness	Low-voltage EEG, random eye movements, high muscle tone
Non-REM sleep	Low muscle tone, few eye movements
Stage 1	Transition between wakefulness and sleep, low-voltage desynchronized EEG, lasts 0.5–7.0 minute
Stage 2	Low-voltage EEG with sleep spindles and K-complexes
Stages 3 and 4	High-amplitude, slow-wave EEG, "delta sleep"
REM sleep	Low-voltage, mixed-frequency EEG, low muscle tone, REMs, autonomic fluctuations in heart rate and perspiration, and dreaming reported in 80%–90% of subjects

EEG = electroencephalogram; REM = rapid eye movement.

9. Sleep architecture is cyclic. Passing from wakefulness to stage 4 non-REM sleep takes about 45 minutes in young adults. Rapid eye movement usually occurs within 90 minutes of falling asleep; at first, REM lasts 5–7 minutes, but it gets progressively longer through the night. The sleep cycle (non-REM stages 1–4 and REM), which lasts about 70–120 minutes, is repeated four to six times a night. The typical young adult spends about 75% of his or her time in non-REM.

10. Sleep patterns change with age. Elderly patients experience less delta sleep, REM sleep, and total sleep time. They have more nocturnal awakenings and total time awake at night. The incidence of sleep pathology may be as high as 40%.

B. Sleep Disorders

1. The *DSM-5* recognizes several sleep-wake disturbances: insomnia disorder, hypersomnia disorder, narcolepsy, obstructive sleep apnea, hypopnea, central sleep apnea, sleep-related hypoventilation, circadian rhythm sleep-wake disorders, non-REM sleep arousal disorders, nightmare disorder, REM sleep behavior disorder, restless legs syndrome, substance/medication-induced sleep disorder, and several other or unspecified sleep-wake disorders.

2. Insomnia

   a. Insomnia is defined as an inability to initiate or maintain sleep, and it can be associated with problems during the daytime. About one-third of the U.S. population experiences insomnia, with half of those saying it is serious.

   b. More than 40% of those suffering from insomnia self-medicate with over-the-counter medications (discussed below) or with other substances (e.g., alcohol).

   c. Insomnia can be classified according to symptom duration as follows.

Table 13. Types of Insomnia

Type	Duration (weeks)	Likely Causes
Transient	< 1	Acute situational or environmental stressors
Short term	< 4	Continued personal stress
Chronic	> 4	Psychiatric illness, substance abuse Behavioral causes (poor sleep hygiene) Medical causes, primary sleep disorder (e.g., sleep apnea, restless legs syndrome; these are no longer recognized by the *DSM-V* as insomnia)

   d. Transient insomnia is most often associated with acute stressors. It resolves once the acute stressors are removed. Pharmacotherapy may be used for a few days until the situation resolves.

   e. Short-term insomnia is also most often associated with an acute stressor, but it is ongoing. Here, it is important to initiate good sleep hygiene (as below) and avoid stimulants such as caffeine. Pharmacotherapy may be indicated, especially if on an intermittent basis (e.g., skip it after 2 or 3 good nights of sleep). Therapy for 7–10 days is usually sufficient.

   f. Chronic insomnia should be carefully evaluated for an underlying medical or psychiatric cause. If a cause is not present, a common type of chronic insomnia is chronic psychophysiologic insomnia, which is a behavioral problem. The person has usually developed poor sleep hygiene, and the bedroom is associated with an alerting response. Behavioral therapy is important, but pharmacotherapy can be useful in short courses and intermittently. The development of chronic insomnia is a complex process and can be difficult to treat. Pharmacotherapy can be part of the overall treatment approach, but there is no consensus about how effective it is when used long term. Ramelteon, eszopiclone, and zolpidem controlled release all contain language in the package labels suggesting they can be used chronically.

g. The evaluation of insomnia should include an assessment of medical and psychiatric status. Medical causes are many and include thyroid disease and therapy with medications that can interfere with sleep. Several psychiatric conditions can interfere with sleep, including affective and anxiety disorders.

h. For all types of insomnia, patients can be instructed about good sleep hygiene. These principles are listed below:

    i. Maintain regular bedtimes and awakenings.

    ii. Do not go to bed unless you are sleepy.

    iii. Sleep long enough to avoid feeling tired, but no more.

    iv. Optimize the bedroom conditions (e.g., light, temperature, noise).

    v. Develop a bedtime ritual that allows you to unwind.

    vi. If you cannot go to sleep, or if you awaken and cannot go back to sleep, do not stay in bed more than 15–20 minutes; get up and do something else until you are sleepy.

    vii. Do not go to bed hungry, but do not stuff yourself before bed; try a small snack.

    viii. Avoid activities in the bedroom except for sleeping and sex.

    ix. Do not lie there and watch the clock; get one without a luminous dial.

    x. Avoid naps during the day.

    xi. Avoid stimulants such as caffeine and nicotine throughout the day.

    xii. Avoid alcohol because it can lead to "fragmented" sleep.

    xiii. Exercise regularly during the day, but not close to bedtime.

C. Pharmacotherapy of Insomnia

1. Pharmacotherapy is indicated for all forms of insomnia as long as it is part of an overall plan to deal with the causes and is used for well-defined periods. It should be considered adjunctive therapy only for short-term or chronic insomnia.

2. Agents that can depress respiration should be avoided in patients with respiratory disorders, a history of substance abuse, or obstructive sleep apnea. Ramelteon should be avoided in patients with severe sleep apnea.

3. There are several classes of sedative-hypnotics: barbiturates, which are no longer indicated; nonbarbiturates (e.g., chloral hydrate), which have only limited indications; benzodiazepines; and the non-benzodiazepines zolpidem, zaleplon, and eszopiclone, which are often used in clinical practice. Ramelteon is a melatonin receptor 1 and melatonin receptor 2 agonist. Suvorexant is an orexin receptor antagonist.

4. Benzodiazepines: In general, they are safe, effective, and well tolerated by most patients, but they are not considered first line. Although all members of this class can be used as sedatives, only five are FDA approved and marketed as such. These five are primarily used as sedative-hypnotics because they are rapidly absorbed and produce central nervous system actions more quickly than most anxiety agents. The sedative-hypnotic benzodiazepines are listed in Table 15. They are primarily differentiated by their onset of action and half-life in the body. According to their half-life, they are classified as short acting (half-life less than 6 hours), intermediate acting (half-life 6–24 hours), and long acting (half-life more than 24 hours). These are important parameters when selecting therapy. For instance, someone with problems initiating sleep would most likely benefit from an agent with a quick onset but short duration of action. Someone with problems maintaining sleep in the middle of the night might respond better to a drug with a longer half-life. The following table compares the benzodiazepines available in the United States.

Table 14. Benzodiazepines for Insomnia

Drug (Trade)	Usual Dose (mg)	Half-life (hours)	Duration
Triazolam (Halcion)	0.125–0.25	2–6	Short
Temazepam (Restoril)	15–30	8–20	Intermediate
Estazolam (ProSom)	1–2	8–24	Intermediate
Flurazepam (Dalmane)	15–30	48–120	Long
Quazepam (Doral)	7.5–15	48–120	Long

5. These drugs are usually well tolerated. However, several problems still exist.

    a. Tolerance: Tolerance can develop, particularly when the drugs are used consistently for long periods. These drugs are not indicated for chronic use; however, newer evidence is emerging that they may be effective for longer periods than originally thought. Most are effective for 2–4 weeks and, in some cases, longer. An intermittent pattern of use can reduce the development of tolerance. In addition, most people without substance abuse histories do not escalate their doses.

    b. Residual daytime sedation: This is a common complaint of patients using these drugs. It is especially likely with agents having a long half-life. Dose is also an important factor; always use the lowest effective dose.

    c. Rebound insomnia: This can occur when the drug is discontinued abruptly. Insomnia is usually worse than baseline and usually lasts for 1–2 days; tapering the drug may minimize its effect. It is most common after the use of short- and intermediate-acting agents.

    d. Anterograde amnesia: All benzodiazepines appear to impair the acquisition and encoding of new information. They may also impair memory storage and recall. Dosage may be important.

    e. Be careful when using benzodiazepines in elderly patients because they can cause memory problems, increase the risk of falls, and accumulate (agents with a long half-life). Try to avoid use in this population. Idiosyncratic reactions can occur in elderly and pediatric populations with benzodiazepine use.

    f. Withdrawal: Physical dependence will occur if these agents are used long enough. Symptoms of withdrawal include worsening insomnia, anxiety, muscle twitches, photophobia, tinnitus, auditory and visual hypersensitivity, and seizures. Minimize by gradually tapering the drug at discontinuation.

Table 15. Nonbenzodiazepines for Insomnia

Drug	$t_{1/2}$ (hours)	Administration (minutes before sleep)	Indications			CDS Scheduling
			Sleep Onset	Sleep Maintenance	Chronic Therapy	
Doxepin (Silenor)	Doxepin: 15.3 Nordoxepin: 31	30		X		Not controlled
Eszopiclone (Lunesta)	6	Immediately	X	X	X	C-IV
Ramelteon (Rozerem)	1-2.6	30	X		X	Not controlled
Suvorexant (Belsomra)	12	30	X	X		C-IV

Table 15. Nonbenzodiazepines for Insomnia *(continued)*

Drug	t$_{1/2}$ (hours)	Administration (minutes before sleep)	Indications			CDS Scheduling
			Sleep Onset	Sleep Maintenance	Chronic Therapy	
Zaleplon (Sonata)	1	Immediately	X			C-IV
Zolpidem (Ambien)	1.4-6.5 (see below)	Immediately	X	X (CR only)		C-IV

6. Doxepin (Silenor) is a tricyclic antidepressant indicated for the treatment of impaired sleep maintenance. The doses used are lower than those used to treat depression. Chances for morning effects are high due to the long half-life of both doxepin and its active metabolite, nordoxepin..

7. Eszopiclone (Lunesta): This non-benzodiazepine is a GABA$_A$ agonist. Its half-life is 6 hours, so morning effects could result if it is taken late in the night. This drug can be used for chronic insomnia. On May 1, 2014, the FDA reduced the starting dose to 1 mg in order to minimize the amount of next-day impairment. Patients should be counseled to use caution when driving or performing activities that require alertness, particularly with the 2-3 mg doses. It should be taken imeediately before bed, and when the patient will be In bed for at least 7-8 hours.

8. Ramelteon (Rozerem): Melatonin agonist (no activity at the GABA or benzodiazepine receptor). Duration is 2–5 hours. To date, there is no evidence that this melatonin agonist is associated with dependence or tolerance, and it may be used long term. This drug can be used long term for chronic insomnia. It is primarily metabolized by CYP 1A2, but inducers and inhibitors of 2C9 and 3A4 can also affect it.

9. Suvorexant (Belsomra) is a newly approved (August 2014) orexin receptor antagonist. It will be available in 2015. The neuropeptide orexin promotes wakefulness. By blocking the OX1R and OX2R receptors, suvorexant both decreases sleep latency and promotes sleep maintenance. It should be taken within 30 minutes of bedtime, and with at least 7 hours of sleep time. It is metabolized by CYP 3A4, and the dose must be decreased in patient taking concomitant 3A4 inhibitors. C-IV

10. Zaleplon: This is a non-benzodiazepine with a similar pharmacology to zolpidem (see below) and a very short half-life. For patients with sleep maintenance problems, it might not last as long. However, it has a shorter half-life (about 1 hour) and may cause fewer problems in the morning, especially if given late. It shortens onset to sleep, but does not prolong sleep time or number of awakenings. It is indicated only for short-term treatment of insomnia. It has been used in trials for up to 5 weeks. C-IV

11. Zolpidem: This non-benzodiazepine sedative-hypnotic modulates the GABA$_A$ receptor complex. C-IV
    a. Compared with benzodiazepines, zolpidem lacks anticonvulsant action, muscle-relaxant properties, and respiratory depressant effect; it also has a lower risk of tolerance and withdrawal. It should still be avoided in obstructive sleep apnea. It is a good choice for patients in whom benzodiazepines should be avoided.
    b. Zolpidem is available as an immediate release tablet (IR), controlled release tablet (CR), sublingual tablet (Edluar, Intermezzo), and sublingual spray (Zolpimist). The pharmacokinetics and indications vary based upon the dosing form. The sublingual spray has a shorter onset of action, but that of the sublingual tablet is comparable to both the IR and CR tablets.
    c. Indications vary by dosage form. All are indicated to decrease sleep latency. The CR tablets are indicated to improve sleep maintenance and can be used for longer term therapy. Intermezzo Is indicated as a "prn" treatment for patient who have difficulty falling back to sleep, so long as ≥ 4 hours remain.

    d.   The FDA has reduced the dosing recommendations to limit next day impairment. The dosing differs based upon the gender and degree of debility. For women, the nightly dose is 5 mg (IR) or 6.25 mg (CR) For men, it is 5-10 mg (IR) or 6.25-12.5 mg (CR).Debilitated patients should receive 5 mg (IR) or 6.25 mg (CR). Patients should be maintained on the lowest dose needed to benefit.

12. Patients should be warned about the potential risk of engaging in abnormal activities while asleep when taking sedative-hypnotics. Such behaviors may include driving, eating, having sex, or talking on the phone while asleep (with amnesia for the event). Other cautions include anaphylaxis and decreased respiratory drive.

13. Taking any of the agents listed in Table with food can delay onset of effects, thus prolonging the time to onset of sleep and increasing the risk for hangover effects in longer acting agents. Doxepin should be separated from meals by 3 hours.

14. Over-the-counter medications: These are most often antihistamines (doxylamine or diphenhydramine) that are both sedating and anticholinergic. They are possibly effective, but not as effective as benzodiazepines. Their regular use is not recommended. In fact, some data suggest that they do not maintain efficacy beyond a few days. They are associated with a higher incidence of daytime sedation than short- or intermediate-acting benzodiazepines. Diphenhydramine has been a popular agent when benzodiazepines were contraindicated. However, caution should be used in elderly patients because an anticholinergic action can worsen dementia or other medical conditions. In addition, it should not be administered with the cholinesterase inhibitors used for Alzheimer disease.

15. Other non-benzodiazepines: In some situations, antidepressants such as trazodone may be used as sedative-hypnotics. These can be effective, and often, the dose required is lower than that used for depression. However, efficacy has not been fully established through clinical trials. Trazodone has been popular for managing insomnia caused by SSRI antidepressants (see discussion in Depression section). It is also popular by itself as a sleep agent because the potential for dependence is low. However, it is associated with considerable adverse effects, and the data for long-term use are scant.

Patient Cases

Questions 19–22 pertain to the following case:

L.M. is a 50-year-old patient with a 25-year history of alcohol dependence who was found unconscious after his last drinking binge. He was first admitted to the medical unit for alcohol withdrawal symptoms before being transferred to the substance dependence unit. His last drink was 6 hours ago, and fluids have been started. He has had three alcohol withdrawal seizures in the past and an episode of delirium tremens. He also has significant hepatitis, and liver function tests show aspartate aminotransferase (AST) of 220 IU/L and alanine aminotransferase (ALT) of 200 IU/L.

19. Which symptom are you most likely to observe in the medical unit?

    A.   Alcohol craving.

    B.   Delirium tremens.

    C.   Increased heart rate.

    D.   Seizures.

20. Which agent is best for alcohol withdrawal symptoms in L.M. for intramuscular administration?

    A.   Chlordiazepoxide.

    B.   Clonazepam.

    C.   Diazepam.

    D.   Lorazepam.

Patient Cases *(continued)*

21. Before administering fluids with glucose, which agent is most important to administer?

    A. Folate.

    B. Multivitamin supplement.

    C. B_{12}.

    D. Thiamine.

22. Which medication is best to use in L.M. for alcohol dependence?

    A. Acamprosate.

    B. Diazepam.

    C. Disulfiram.

    D. Naltrexone.

VI. SUBSTANCE ABUSE

A. Alcohol
1. Acute Withdrawal
   a. Characteristic symptoms occur after alcohol discontinuation. The symptoms that develop, how quickly they develop, and the degree of severity depend on the level of alcohol abuse and a person's characteristics. Not all patients develop delirium tremens, nor do all develop seizures. However, it is difficult to predict, so detoxification should always be supervised. A history of alcohol withdrawal problems suggests that inpatient detoxification is indicated.
   b. Table 16 lists the stages of acute alcohol withdrawal.

Table 16. Stages of Acute Alcohol Withdrawal

Stage	Onset	Symptoms
1	0–8 hours	Mild tremors, nervousness, tachycardia, nausea
2	12–24 hours	Marked tremors, hyperactivity, hyper-alertness, increased startle response, pronounced tachycardia, insomnia, nightmares, illusions, hallucinations, alcohol cravings
3	12–48 hours	More severe symptoms than observed during stage 2; seizures may occur
4	3–5 days	Delirium tremens: Confusion, agitation, tremor, insomnia, tachycardia, sweating, hyperpyrexia

   c. Delirium tremens, which can be life threatening, should be considered a potential medical emergency and treated promptly.
   d. The seizures that occur are often difficult to control. Status epilepticus can develop; thus, it is important to ensure that these patients have intravenous access. Benzodiazepines are first line for seizure prevention in alcohol withdrawal compared with other anticonvulsants.
2. Treatment of Acute Alcohol Withdrawal
   a. The degree of symptoms and the resulting level of treatment should be individualized, and an accurate history regarding amount, duration, and past withdrawal symptoms including seizures and delirium tremens should guide treatment. If it is believed that complications may arise, treatment should take place in an inpatient setting.

---

b. In determining the level of intervention required, the severity of symptoms is usually assessed. The more severe the symptoms are, the more aggressive the intervention(s).

c. The principle of cross-tolerance is used to advantage in the prevention and treatment of withdrawal symptoms. Benzodiazepines can eliminate many manifestations of withdrawal and are much easier to control with respect to dosing.

    i. Intermittent dosing: Using this regimen, patients are assessed for the severity of withdrawal symptoms; then, the benzodiazepine dose is adjusted to that level. This is probably the most prevalent way of treating these patients.

    ii. Scheduled dosing: Another strategy is to begin a scheduled dose of benzodiazepine on admission, give it regularly, and then taper it down for 3–4 days until symptoms have abated.

    iii. Loading-dose (front loaded) protocol: A new approach during recent years uses a loading-dose strategy for diazepam. Diazepam is given in a dose of 10–20 mg every 1–2 hours until the symptoms of withdrawal are alleviated. Most patients will need two or three doses, especially those with a history of seizures during withdrawal, in which case three doses should be used. The half-life of diazepam is long, and most patients will not need subsequent doses in this protocol once symptoms are relieved. Of course, patients should be monitored closely.

    iv. Table 17 lists the benzodiazepines that may be used. Chlordiazepoxide has the status of the "classic" drug, possibly the oldest, and it can be given either orally or parenterally. However, it has no proven advantages over the other agents; in fact, its long half-life may cause unnecessary sedation. However, for patients with a high risk of withdrawal seizures or delirium tremens, a long-acting benzodiazepine may be preferable. If a shorter-acting agent is used, a round-the-clock schedule would be ideal for high-risk patients. Lorazepam is also safe to administer in patients with liver disease.

Table 17. Benzodiazepines in the Treatment of Acute Alcohol Withdrawal

Drug	Dose	Comments
Lorazepam (Ativan)	1–2 mg PO/IV/IM	Good for general use; less of a problem with liver disease; IM/IV available
Diazepam (Valium)	5–20 mg PO/IV/IM[a]	Use lower dose if liver disease is present; may administer by slow IV; can use a loading-dose strategy
Chlordiazepoxide (Librium)	25–100 mg PO/IV	Long acting; be careful if liver disease is present

[a]IM administration of diazepam is unreliable.

IM = intramuscular(ly); IV = intravenous(ly); PO = orally.

d. Nutritional considerations

    i. Thiamine: This should be given to all patients to prevent Wernicke-Korsakoff syndrome— 100 mg intramuscularly on admission and then orally for 3 days; always give the first dose before glucose because it is a cofactor for the metabolism of glucose.

    ii. Magnesium: Assess by serum chemistry; if low, give intravenous supplement.

    iii. Electrolytes: Assess by serum chemistry and add to intravenous solutions as indicated (e.g., potassium).

    iv. Vitamins: These patients are usually undernourished; a good multivitamin may be indicated (folate and vitamin B_{12} should be monitored).

e. Fluid therapy: The patient may initially be overhydrated, but usually, fluid deficit will follow; replace fluids, usually with intravenous 5% dextrose solution with half-normal saline plus other electrolytes (e.g., potassium, phosphate).

f. Hallucinations: Benzodiazepine will usually manage hallucinations effectively; if not, give haloperidol; however, be cautious because haloperidol can lower the seizure threshold.

g. Seizures: Benzodiazepine will usually prevent seizures. Higher doses (and/or increased frequency) of benzodiazepines can be used if the patient has a history of seizures. If a seizure occurs during withdrawal, increasing the benzodiazepine dose and slowing the taper are options. Other antiepileptics may be used to treat status epilepticus, but their efficacy varies.

h. Other agents
    i. β-Blockers: These agents help with vital signs and blood pressure.
    ii. α-Agonists (e.g., clonidine): These agents may help with some of the withdrawal symptoms.

3. Chronic Therapy
    a. Disulfiram: This drug blocks acetaldehyde dehydrogenase, and if alcohol is used with it, the person will develop symptoms that include nausea/vomiting, flushing, and headache, among others. Adherence is critical, and disulfiram is usually reserved for patients with considerable motivation for adherence. Caution should be exercised in patients with liver disease, particularly if is severe or the patient has cirrhosis. Disulfiram has been associated with hepatotoxicity, although it is not known whether patients with existing liver disease are at an increased risk.
    b. Naltrexone: This drug can also be used chronically and has been shown to reduce cravings. If used, it should be combined with CBT. Liver toxicity is associated with this drug. The extended-release injectable suspension (Vivitrol) is available in an intramuscular formulation and is approved for **the treatment of alcohol dependence in patients who are able to abstain from alcohol in an outpatient setting before treatment initiation.**
    c. Acamprosate (Campral): This drug is a structural analog of GABA. It, too, reduces cravings. It is not metabolized by the liver; however, it must be taken three times daily.

B. Opioid Dependence
    1. In 2013, 1.5 million people used prescription pain relievers for nonmedical reasons. The majority (53%) get their drugs free from friends or relatives. The number of people who received treatment for nonmedical use of prescription pain relievers was 746,000, up from 360,000 in 2002. In 2012, 16,007 deaths due to overdose with opioid analgesics occurred, totally 72% of all deaths due to overdoses with pharmaceuticals.
    2. The potential for abuse led the DEA to reclassify products containing hydrocodone and acteminophen from C-III to C-II, effective October 6, 2014.
    3. Opioid withdrawal is not life-threatening in absence of concomitant medical conditions. Early symptoms may resemble flu and include agitation, anxiety, muscle aches, yawning, sweating, rhinorrhea, and lacrimation. Later symptoms include abdominal cramping, diarrhea, piloerection, dilated pupils, nausea, and vomiting.
       – Pharmacologic therapies for opioid addiction include maintenance therapy with methadone, an opioid agonist; antagonist therapy with naltrexone; detoxification with medications given in rapid taper (e.g., methadone, buprenorphine, or clonidine) to prepare the patient for antagonist or counseling therapy; and partial agonist therapy with buprenorphine or buprenorphine/naloxone.
    4. The use of buprenorphine came about as a result of the Drug Abuse Treatment Act of 2000 (DATA), which allows qualifying physicians to apply for a waiver to treat opioid addiction outside an opioid treatment program using schedule III, IV, and V medications that are FDA approved for this indication.
       a. Only two formulations that qualify under DATA 2000 are FDA approved for opioid dependence: buprenorphine (available as sublingual tablets [Subutex]) and buprenorphine/naloxone (available in 4:1 ratio dosing increments as sublingual tablets [Zubsolv], sublingual film [Suboxone], and buccal film [Bunavail]).

b.   Buprenorphine is a partial agonist at the opioid mu receptor and an antagonist of the kappa receptor. The mu receptor binding affinity is higher than that of full opioid agonists with a lower intrinsic activity. Thus, it will displace morphine, methadone, and other opioid drugs but only gives a fraction of effect that levels out with increasing doses—a ceiling effect. This allows patients enough effect to "feel normal" but minimizes functional impairment. It also makes the drug safer in overdose situations. At high enough doses, the kappa antagonist properties could precipitate withdrawal.

c.   The addition of naloxone reduces abuse potential because naloxone is less potent when given sublingually than by injection. Thus, if the medication is used as intended (sublingually), the likelihood of withdrawal symptoms is low as opposed to dissolving and injecting it.

5.   Treatment with buprenorphine involves three phases: induction, stabilization, and maintenance. Buprenorphine/naloxone is the preferred agent for most patients, including those taking short-acting opioids (hydromorphone, oxycodone, heroin). Patients taking long-acting opioids (methadone, long-acting morphine, long-acting oxycodone) should be tapered to methadone 30 mg/day or less or the equivalent, and transitioned to buprenorphine first. It is recommended that these patients be switched to the combination after no more than 2 days on buprenorphine monotherapy.

a.   Patients should not be intoxicated or feeling effects from their last dose of opioid (~12–24 hours since the last dose of short-acting opioid). They must also be screened for other substance abuse and for appropriateness of buprenorphine therapy. Patients may feel like they are going through early stages of withdrawal. In these cases, the opioid receptors are not fully occupied, and the buprenorphine is less likely to induce withdrawal.

b.   Patients need to receive concomitant counseling and nonpharmacologic treatment support during treatment. Part of the DATA 2000 waiver requires that physicians be able to refer the patient to appropriate supportive services. Counseling should take all psychosocial factors into account.

c.   Induction phase: Find the minimum dose of buprenorphine that minimizes cravings for opioids but prevents withdrawal symptoms. The first dose should be given in the office and the patient observed for 2 hours. The patient is given the 4/1 dose of buprenorphine/naloxone. If withdrawal symptoms are not relieved or return before the 2-hour period, a second dose of 4/1 is given, and the daily dose is established at 8/2. The dose established during the induction phase depends on the presence of withdrawal symptoms on subsequent days, to a maximum of 32/8.

d.   Stabilization phase: Reached when the patient is without withdrawal symptoms, is not experiencing side effects of buprenorphine/naloxone, and no longer has uncontrollable symptoms of craving. Toxicology screens can be used to verify that the patient is not using opioids. Patients should be seen weekly until stable. Doses can be adjusted in 2/0.5 to 4/1 increments. Most patients are maintained on 16/4–24/6.

e.   Maintenance: Once the minimum dose needed to maintain abstinence is reached, the buprenorphine/naloxone therapy can be maintained indefinitely. Nonpharmacologic modalities should continue during this time.

f.   Discontinuation: This should be considered only if the patient is psychologically and medically stable, is able to maintain a drug-free lifestyle, and no longer feels the drug is necessary to remain abstinent. The medication should be tapered slowly to avoid withdrawal symptoms.

6.   Buprenorphine is metabolized by CYP3A4. Use caution with other medications that either induce or inhibit 3A4.

C.   Tobacco Dependence

1.   Tobacco use is the top cause of preventable morbidity and mortality.

2.   It increases the risk of cardiovascular disease (including stroke), chronic obstructive pulmonary disease, and cancer (both lung and nonlung).

3. According to the 2012–2013 National Annual Tobacco Survey, 21.3% of Americans use a tobacco product every day or on most days, and 19.2% used some form of combustible tobacco product. Cigarettes are the most commonly used product. Rates have greatly declined over the past decade. There are more former smokers than current smokers.

4. Smoking cessation counseling is not consistently offered and tends to be directed to patients with tobacco-related conditions. Interventions lasting as little as 3 minutes make a difference. Patient counseling can help prime patients who are not willing to quit to consider it and act on it in the future.

5. As of January 2015, the Joint Commission will require inpatient psychiatric services to screen for tobacco use (TOB-1), offer or provide treatment for tobacco dependence (TOB-2), and provide or offer treatment for tobacco dependence at discharge (TOB-3).

6. It takes an average of seven attempts for a patient to quit successfully.

7. Willingness to quit should be assessed via the five A's: *ask* about tobacco use, *advise* to quit, *assess* willingness to attempt to quit, *assist* in quit attempt, and *arrange* for follow-up.

8. Motivational interviewing is a successful technique that can help identify barriers to change and help the patient overcome them.

9. The five R's can be used to increase motivation to quit: *relevance, risks, rewards, roadblocks,* and *repetition.*

10. Quit lines such as 1-800-QUIT-NOW can facilitate attempts.

11. Seven pharmacologic agents (five nicotine and two nonnicotine) are available to help. They should be used with nonpharmacologic modalities to increase the success of quitting.

12. A usual pack contains 20 cigarettes.

13. Nicotine replacement therapy (NRT): All forms are equally efficacious. Patients should be advised to stop smoking completely before initiating. It comes in the following forms:

    a. Patch: For patients who smoke more than 10 cigarettes/day, start with 21 mg/day for 2 weeks, then 14 mg/day for 2 weeks, then 7 mg/day for 2 weeks. Those who smoke 10 cigarettes/day or less, start with 14 mg/day for 6 weeks, then 7 mg/day for 2 weeks. Patches may be used for longer periods of time if needed to improve success. It is recommended to change the patch upon awakening every day. Rotate sites.

    b. Gum: The gum should be chewed until a "peppery" or flavored taste develops, then "park" the gum between the cheek and gum to facilitate buccal absorption. The gum should be chewed and parked for 30 minutes or until the flavor is gone. The maximum number of pieces of gum is 24 pieces in 24 hours. At least 9 pieces of gum should be used daily to increase the chances of quitting. Patients who smoke 25 cigarettes/day or more should use the 4-mg dose. Those who smoke fewer than 25 cigarettes should use the 2 mg dose. One piece of gum should be used every 1–2 hours for the first 6 weeks of therapy, followed by 1 piece every 2–4 hours for weeks 7–9, then 1 piece every 4–6 hours for weeks 10–12. Acidic beverages (e.g., coffee, juices, and soft drinks) interfere with buccal absorption and should be avoided at least 15 minutes before using the gum. Side effects include soreness, dyspepsia, hiccups, and jaw ache. They are usually mild and can be corrected with changes in chewing technique.

    c. Lozenge: Patients who smoke their first cigarette within 30 minutes of waking should use the 4-mg strength. Otherwise, the 2-mg dose is used. The lozenge should be dissolved in the mouth rather than being chewed or swallowed. The frequency of use and downward titration are the same as for the gum. Side effects are also similar. At least 9 lozenges should be used at the beginning to increase chances of quitting. Only 1 lozenge should be used at one time. No more than 5 lozenges within 6 hours, maximum 20 lozenges/24 hours.

d. Inhaler: Available by prescription only. Each puff delivers 4 mg. Each cartridge delivers 80 inhalations. The recommended dosing is 6–16 cartridges/day. The best results are obtained if the contents of the cartridges are continuously puffed over approximately 20 minutes. Recommended treatment length is 3 months, with reduction in frequency over the last 6–12 weeks. As with the gum and lozenges, patients should not drink acidic beverages or eat within 15 minutes of using the inhaler. Delivery decreases at less than 40°F, so the inhaler should be kept in an inner pocket in cold weather. The most common side effects are sore throat, coughing, and rhinitis. Inhalers should be avoided in patients with reactive airway diseases.

e. Nasal spray: Available by prescription only. The dose is 0.5 mg delivered to each nostril. One to two doses should be used hourly, up to 5 doses. The 24-hour maximum is 40 doses. At least 8 doses should be used at the start of therapy. Each bottle contains 100 doses. Recommended length of therapy is 3–6 months, with downward titration. Risk of dependency is higher than with other forms of nicotine replacement. Inhaling, sniffing, and swallowing can increase the risk of nasal irritation and so should be avoided when taking the spray. Nasal irritation can occur in up to 94% of patients. Although it can resolve, a significant number of patients may have it as much as 8 weeks into therapy. It is not recommended for use in patients with reactive airway diseases or nasal conditions.

f. Nicotine patches can be used with the as-needed dosage forms to increase the chances of quitting.

g. Patients with a history of cardiovascular disease can use nicotine replacement therapies.

h. The treatment of choice in pregnant women is nonpharmacologic. Nicotine has a pregnancy category D rating. NRT has not been shown to be effective in pregnant women.

14. Bupropion sustained release (SR): Bupropion SR should be initiated 7 days before the quit date. Treatment should last for at least 8 weeks but can be continued for up to 6 months to increase chances of quitting. It can also be combined with the nicotine patch if needed.

15. Varenicline: It is a nicotine receptor partial agonist. It blocks the effects of nicotine from smoking. It should be started 1 week before the quit day, although patients can choose to quit smoking up to 35 days after initiating varenicline. It should be continued for a total of 12 weeks. If the patient is successful at smoking cessation, it can be continued for another 12 weeks. Varenicline carries a black box warning for neuropsychiatric symptoms, including depression, suicidal ideation, suicide, psychosis, mood disturbance, and hostility. This can occur in patients with or without preexisting psychiatric conditions. It is associated with an increase in cardiovascular events, particularly in patients with preexisting cardiovascular disease. It must be used with caution in patients with creatinine clearance less than 30 mL/min. Combining it with NRT increases side effects. It can be combined with bupropion.

16. Other agents used include clonidine and nortriptyline.

17. Patients who were unsuccessful in quitting on one form of pharmacologic therapy should be tried on a different method.

REFERENCES

Depression

1. American Psychiatric Association (APA). Practice Guideline for the Treatment of Patients with Major Depressive Disorder, 3rd ed. Washington, DC: APA, 2010. Available at http://psychiatryonline.org/guidelines.aspx. Accessed October 11, 2014. This is the current guideline of the American Psychiatric Association.

2. American Psychiatric Association (APA). Diagnostic and Statistical Manual of Mental Disorders, 5th ed. (DSM-5). Washington, DC: APA, 2013.

3. Teter CJ, Kando JC, Wells BG. Major depressive disorder. In: DiPiro JT, Talbert RL, Hayes PE, et al. Pharmacotherapy: A Pathophysiologic Approach, 9th ed. New York: McGraw-Hill, 2014:chap 51.

Bipolar Disorder

1. American Psychiatric Association (APA). Diagnostic and Statistical Manual of Mental Disorders, 5th ed. (DSM-5). Washington, DC: APA, 2013.

2. Drayton SJ, Pelic CM. Bipolar disorder. In: DiPiro JT, Talbert RL, Hayes PE, et al. Pharmacotherapy: A Pathophysiologic Approach, 9th ed. New York: McGraw-Hill, 2014:chap 52.

3. Pacchiarotti I, Bond DJ, Baldessarini RJ, et al. The International Society for Bipolar Disorders (ISBD) Task Force Report on Antidepressant Use in Bipolar Disorders. 2013;170(11):1249-62.

4. Yatham LN, Kennedy SH, Parikh SV, et al. Canadian Network for Mood and Anxiety Treatments (CANMAT) and International Society for Bipolar Disorders (ISBD) collaborative update of CANMAT guidelines for the management of patients with bipolar disorder: update 2013. Bipolar Disorders 2013;15:1-44.

Schizophrenia

1. Buchanan RW, Kreyenbuhl JM, Kelly DL, et al. The 2009 schizophrenia PORT psychopharmacological treatment. Recommendations and summary statements. Schizophrenia Bull 2010;36:71-93.

2. Crismon ML, Argo TR, Buckley PF. Schizophrenia. In: DiPiro JT, Talbert RL, Hayes PE, et al. Pharmacotherapy: A Pathophysiologic Approach, 9th ed. New York: McGraw-Hill, 2014:chap 50.

Anxiety Disorders

1. Bandelow B, Zohar J, Hollander E, et al. World Federation of Societies of Biological Psychiatry (WFSBP) guidelines for the pharmacological treatment of anxiety, obsessive-compulsive and post-traumatic stress disorders, first revision. World J Biol Psychiatry 2008;9:248-312.

2. Melton ST, Kirkwood CK. Anxiety disorders I: generalized anxiety, panic, and social anxiety disorders. In: DiPiro JT, Talbert RL, Hayes PE, et al. Pharmacotherapy: A Pathophysiologic Approach, 9th ed. New York: McGraw-Hill, 2014:chap 53.

3. Kirkwood CK, Melton ST, Wells BG. Anxiety disorders II: posttraumatic stress disorder and obsessive-compulsive disorder. In: DiPiro JT, Talbert RL, Hayes PE, et al. Pharmacotherapy: A Pathophysiologic Approach, 9th ed. New York: McGraw-Hill, 2014:chap 54.

Insomnia

1. Dopp JM, Philips BG. Sleep disorders. In: DiPiro JT, Talbert RL, Hayes PE, et al. Pharmacotherapy: A Pathophysiologic Approach, 9th ed. New York: McGraw-Hill, 2014:chap 55.

2. Sateia M, Nowell P. Insomnia. Lancet 2004;364:1959-73. This is a good review of the pathophysiology and treatment of insomnia. It also includes a discussion of nondrug interventions.

3. Schutte-Rodin S, Broch L, Buysse D, et al. Clinical guideline for the evaluation and management of chronic insomnia in adults. J Clin Sleep Med 2008;4:487-504.

Substance Abuse

1. Miller NS. Detoxification and Substance Abuse Treatment. TIP 45. Rockville, MD: U.S. Department of Health and Human Services, 2013.

2. Doering P, Li RM. Substance-related disorders I: overview, depressants, stimulant and hallucinogens. In: DiPiro JT, Talbert RL, Hayes PE, et al. Pharmacotherapy: A Pathophysiologic Approach, 9th ed. New York: McGraw-Hill, 2014:chap 48.

3. Doering P, Li RM. Substance-related disorders II: alcohol, nicotine, and caffeine. In: DiPiro JT, Talbert RL, Hayes PE, et al. Pharmacotherapy: A Pathophysiologic Approach, 9th ed. New York: McGraw-Hill, 2014:chap 49.

4. Kosten T, O'Connor P. Management of drug and alcohol withdrawal. N Engl J Med 2003;348:1786-95. A good general review of the management of the most common syndromes.

5. Fiore MC, Jaén CR, Baker TB, et al. Treating tobacco use and dependence: 2008 update—A clinical practice guideline. Rockville, MD: U.S. Department of Health and Human Services; 2008 May.

6. McNicholas L. Clinical Guidelines for the Use of Buprenorphine in the Treatment of Opioid Addiction TIP 40. Rockville, MD: U.S. Department of Health and Human Services, 2004.

ANSWERS AND EXPLANATIONS TO PATIENT CASES

1. Answer: C

Paroxetine has the most interaction with this patient's current medications because of its interaction with hydrocodone by inhibition of the CYP2D6 isoenzyme. This will result in a lack of analgesic effects from the opiate. Fluvoxamine is a CYP1A2 inhibitor that has no interaction with thiazides, metformin, or opiates. Citalopram has no appreciable effects on any of this patient's medications. The effect of sertraline, although it may compete with that of hydromorphone (metabolite of hydrocodone) through CYP3A4, is less than that of paroxetine.

2. Answer: C

Mirtazapine is appropriate because it can improve this patient's insomnia and poor appetite. In addition, mirtazapine does not have a drug-drug interaction with the patient's current medications. Fluoxetine, bupropion, and venlafaxine would worsen her insomnia. Venlafaxine would worsen hypertension, and bupropion would worsen decreased appetite.

3. Answer: B

The citalopram dose should be increased to 40 mg/day because this patient has had some initial response to the drug (improvement in insomnia and appetite) but may not have reached the maximal tolerated dose. The patient has been taking citalopram for only 4 weeks, possibly at a subtherapeutic dose. Bupropion can be added later, after the patient has reached a maximal tolerated dose of citalopram for 6–8 weeks (which is a therapeutic trial). Switching SSRIs may also be an option after the maximal tolerated dose of citalopram is reached.

4. Answer: B

The patient still needs an antidepressant, and discontinuing citalopram without an alternative agent at 6 months is inappropriate. Bupropion can be added to treat the anorgasmia and may even provide augmentation effects. Switching to a different SSRI may also produce the same adverse effect because the anorgasmia appears to be caused by serotonergic activity. Switching to mirtazapine is not appropriate because the patient has had a therapeutic response and has been doing well for 6 months.

5. Answer: C

Lithium should be initiated to treat the current manic phase and prevent future episodes. Carbamazepine is effective for maintenance treatment but considered second or third line for acute mania. Divalproex is also good for maintenance treatment, but given this patient's history of hepatitis C, it is not a good choice. Lamotrigine is also effective for maintenance but not effective for treating the patient's current manic phase.

6. Answer: B

Coarse tremor may indicate lithium toxicity and would require an immediate evaluation of the patient's lithium level. Lithium can cause hyperthyroidism, severe acne, and weight gain, but these can generally be managed with lifestyle modifications or medications.

7. Answer: C

This patient appears to be showing symptoms of lithium toxicity, and a lithium level should be ordered immediately. Certainly, medications that may worsen the condition (e.g., lisinopril, ibuprofen, zolpidem) may be discontinued later.

8. Answer: A

Benztropine or another anticholinergic should be given to reverse the symptoms of EPS (neck stiffness, extreme restlessness). Giving more antipsychotics only worsens the symptoms of EPS.

9. Answer: B

Risperidone has less risk of EPS than haloperidol/FGAs, but it has the greatest risk among SGAs. Risperidone is effective for negative symptoms, like other SGAs, and can be dosed once daily after reaching the target dose. However, for this patient with a significant history of nonadherence, the most likely reason for initiating risperidone is to eventually convert him to the long-acting injection formulation (Risperdal Consta), given twice a month.

10. Answer: C

Risperidone is more likely to cause EPS than other SGAs. Risperidone may cause some sedation but not appreciably so. Anticholinergic effects are minimal with risperidone. Although all antipsychotics can potentially cause QTc prolongation, they rarely cause problems in patients without risk factors.

11. Answer: D

Quetiapine is most appropriate given the patient's history of dystonia and akathisia with haloperidol. Quetiapine has a lower risk of causing EPS than FGAs such as fluphenazine. Clozapine and olanzapine have low risks of EPS as well, but clozapine is reserved for treatment-resistant cases. Olanzapine is not preferred because of the significant metabolic risks in this young patient.

12. Answer: A

Paroxetine should be continued at this time because the patient is being successfully treated for depression, and paroxetine is considered a first-line agent for PTSD. Sertraline also treats PTSD, but there is no reason to discontinue paroxetine. Adding adjunctive agents such as lorazepam and buspirone is not indicated because it has been only 3 weeks since paroxetine was initiated.

13. Answer: C

Anticonvulsants such as divalproex sodium are often used to treat symptoms of irritability and aggression in patients with PTSD. Buspirone is generally ineffective for these symptoms of PTSD and is used for GAD. Clonazepam can be used for short periods for anxiety; however, it is generally not used to target these symptoms of aggression. Lithium may be able to control the mood lability, but it requires close monitoring.

14. Answer: D

Buspirone is not a benzodiazepine and does not have much dependence potential. Buspirone does not work in relieving nightmares, and it is dosed three times daily. It also takes about 2 weeks for the onset of effect.

15. Answer: A

Clomipramine is the most serotonergic drug of the choices provided and is highly effective for OCD.

16. Answer: D

The patient is taking levothyroxine at nighttime, which is most likely to be contributing to the insomnia. Hydrochlorothiazide and ibuprofen are not significantly associated with causing insomnia. Citalopram may contribute to insomnia in certain patients, but this patient is taking it in the morning, which decreases the risk.

17. Answer: A

The patient does not want a drug with significant daytime sedation, but she needs a drug that will help her stay asleep throughout the night. Eszopiclone is the best option. Trazodone has a long half-life that will help her stay asleep but has fewer efficacy data for insomnia. Temazepam causes daytime sedation. Zaleplon does not cause daytime sedation, but the short half-life of the drug will not help her stay asleep.

18. Answer: C

Zolpidem and other sedative-hypnotics have been associated with causing abnormal behaviors such as eating, driving, having sex, and talking on the telephone while asleep. Zolpidem may cause orthostasis and disorientation, but when taken appropriately, it does not cause significant problems. Zolpidem at high doses has been associated with seizures, but this patient does not have a history of drug abuse or of using high doses of medications.

19. Answer: C

The initial symptoms of alcohol withdrawal include hemodynamic instability such as elevated heart rate and blood pressure. Alcohol craving, delirium tremens, and seizures generally occur after 12 hours of being abstinent.

20. Answer: D

Lorazepam can be given intramuscularly and is appropriate because of the patient's liver abnormalities. Lorazepam undergoes glucuronidation and does not rely on oxidative pathways for metabolism. Chlordiazepoxide and diazepam are not available in intramuscular formulations and should be avoided in patients with liver disease. Clonazepam is generally not used for alcohol withdrawal and not given intramuscularly.

21. Answer: D

Thiamine should be administered before fluids containing glucose to prevent Wernicke-Korsakoff syndrome. Folate, a multivitamin supplement, and B_{12} are also helpful but can be given after fluids.

22. Answer: A

Given the patient's liver disease, acamprosate is most appropriate because it does not rely on hepatic metabolism. Disulfiram and naltrexone are not generally recommended in patients with liver disease. Diazepam is not used for alcohol dependence but is used during alcohol withdrawal.

ANSWERS AND EXPLANATIONS TO SELF-ASSESSMENT QUESTIONS

1. Answer: B

Fluoxetine has a side effect profile that most closely counteracts the patient's symptoms. She additionally has anxiety, so the fluoxetine may concomitantly relieve her symptoms of anxiety and allow her to stop her benzodiazepine. Paroxetine can increase appetite and cause somnolence, as can mirtazapine. Although her suicidal ideation is intermittent and passive, desipramine could be fatal in an overdose situation.

2. Answer: B

Duloxetine is the best choice because it is also indicated for diabetic neuropathy. Although nortriptyline is also used to treat neuropathy, it is not a good choice in a patient with cardiovascular disease. It could also cause weight gain. Although bupropion is either weight neutral or can lead to some weight loss, the data are not strong for use in neuropathy. Sertraline is safe in this patient and could be used as an alternative to citalopram but has no utility in the treatment of neuropathy.

3. Answer: D

L.J. is experiencing serotonin syndrome (myoclonus, agitation, diaphoresis). The symptoms are probably caused by adding dextromethorphan to paroxetine. In addition to the serotonergic activity of both agents, paroxetine inhibits CYP2D6, which is responsible for metabolizing dextromethorphan. This further increases the serotonergic activity. None of the other choices represents a combination of serotonergic agents, nor do they interact in a fashion that would cause a rise in serotonergic activity.

4. Answer: C

H.G. is experiencing an acute depressive episode despite therapeutic lithium concentrations. He has been taking lithium long enough to derive any antidepressant effects. Quetiapine is FDA indicated for depression associated with bipolar disorder. Its onset of action is more rapid than that of lamotrigine, which requires a slow titration to reach therapeutic doses. Unlike for unipolar depression, data for aripiprazole suggest it is not effective for bipolar depression. The efficacy of antidepressants in treating bipolar disorder type I is questionable, and treatment with an SNRI could lead to a switch to mania.

5. Answer: A

H.K. is experiencing hypothyroidism, as indicated by her elevated thyroid-stimulating hormone (TSH). This is probably induced by her lithium. Although olanzapine can cause a metabolic syndrome with glucose intolerance and obesity, it would not cause an elevation in her TSH. Lithium-induced hypothyroidism is not dose-dependent, and the patient's lithium level is on the lower side of the 0.6–1.0 mEq/L maintenance range. Yasmin (ethinyl estradiol/drospirenone) is not associated with elevations in TSH.

6. Answer: B

This patient has acute pancreatitis. Although the incidence is rare, divalproex can cause pancreatitis. Patients who develop pancreatitis on divalproex and resolve off it should not be rechallenged. Neither aripiprazole nor lamotrigine is associated with pancreatitis (although I.T.'s lamotrigine dose should have been lowered to prevent Stevens-Johnson syndrome). Despite the temporal relationship with prednisone, it is not likely to be contributing to the current clinical picture.

7. Answer: D

The symptoms most closely resemble akathisia. The treatment of choice is a lipophilic β-blocker such as propranolol. Benztropine is an anticholinergic agent that can be used for other movement disorders, such as dystonias or Parkinsonian symptoms, but it is not effective for akathisia. Benzodiazepines might relieve some of the anxiety but will not treat the underlying problems. Dantrolene is used for neuroleptic malignant syndrome.

8. Answer: B

This patient is experiencing severe tardive dyskinesia. The symptoms involve the orofacial muscles and came on slowly after antipsychotics had been started. The symptoms improved with antipsychotic dose reduction. The antipsychotic of choice in patients with severe tardive dyskinesia is clozapine. Chlorpromazine is also a first-generation antipsychotic associated with tardive dyskinesia. Although risperidone is associated with less EPS, it can cause tardive dyskinesia. Quetiapine has a low incidence of tardive dyskinesia but would not be the agent of choice with severe tardive dyskinesia.

9. Answer: D

U.M. has diabetes, dyslipidemia, and obesity, all factors that contribute to metabolic syndrome. With her family history of early coronary artery disease, she would best be served by an antipsychotic with a low incidence of metabolic syndrome. Of the antipsychotics listed, ziprasidone is the best choice. Olanzapine is associated with one of the highest incidences of metabolic syndrome. Quetiapine has a lower incidence but can still cause metabolic abnormalities. Paliperidone, which is structurally related to risperidone, is also associated with an elevated incidence of galactorrhea.

10. Answer: A

N.Y. has panic disorder. Benzodiazepines treat the acute physical symptoms and fear that occur with panic disorder. SSRIs such as paroxetine are first-line treatment for preventing panic attacks but do not play a role in acute treatment. Buspirone is not effective for panic attacks. Hydroxyzine may offer some sedation but is ineffective to treat the underlying anxiety.

11. Answer: D

An antidepressant is the first-line treatment for generalized anxiety disorder (GAD). Venlafaxine is the agent of choice for several reasons. It ha demonstrated efficacy against GAD. In addition, it may offer some relief against T.R.'s vasomotor symptoms. Fluoxetine is an effective choice for GAD but is a strong inhibitor of CYP2D6. This would decrease the efficacy of her tamoxifen. Bupropion is also an inhibitor of CYP2D6 and is not effective against most anxiety disorders. Pregabalin is sometimes used to treat GAD, but only as a second- or 3rd third-line agent.

12. Answer: B

O.P. primarily has difficulty with sleep onset and would benefit from an agent that would decrease sleep latency and not prolong sleep. Ramelteon is the only one of the listed agents that does this. Older adults can have difficulty with circadian rhythm, and a melatonin analog may help regulate this. It is also indicated for treatment of chronic insomnia if needed for a prolonged period. Although eszopiclone decreases time to sleep, it is also designed to improve sleep maintenance and may result in hangover effects. Suvorexant also treats sleep maintenance and could cause a hangover effect. Zolpidem received recent labeling changes for reduced doses and has reduced metabolism in older adults.

13. Answer: D

To avoid withdrawal symptoms, patients who are on long-acting opioids should be tapered to the equivalent of methadone 30 mg/day or less before being switched to a buprenorphine regimen. Starting a patient on buprenorphine at higher doses of methadone may precipitate withdrawal because of the higher binding affinity of buprenorphine for the mu receptor with less activity and the added antagonism at the kappa receptor. Patients on long-acting opioids such as methadone should be switched to buprenorphine monotherapy before being advanced to buprenorphine/naloxone. Naltrexone monotherapy is not appropriate because it can precipitate withdrawal.

14. Answer: D

C.H. has alcoholic hepatitis, as indicated by his AST and ALT values. Liver function is intact, as evidenced by his albumin, prothrombin time, and platelet values. Presumably this would improve with abstinence. Naltrexone can be given to patients with hepatic dysfunction. Hepatic function would need to be monitored. Disulfiram should be used with caution in patients with active liver disease. It also requires a strong commitment on the part of the patient to abstain from drinking. This patient has a history of several failed attempts. Acamprosate would need to be adjusted downward for the patient's renal function. Chlordiazepoxide is used during acute alcohol detoxification but has no role in maintenance therapy.

15. Answer: A

J.Z.'s previous quit attempt with nicotine gum was probably unsuccessful because the gum strength (2 mg) and frequency of use (less than 9 pieces/day) were too low to support a successful attempt. Thus, his previous use of nicotine gum is not a true treatment failure. Nevertheless, he has concomitant depression, so bupropion is a reasonable choice. His MI is not a contraindication to using nicotine products and could be added to bupropion if monotherapy fails. Coronary artery disease is not a contraindication to varenicline therapy, but because bupropion has not been previously used, it should be tried first.